T0211095

Folate in Health and Disease

Second Edition

Folate in Health and Disease

Second Edition

Edited by
Lynn B. Bailey

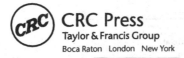

CRC Press
Taylor & Francis Group
Boca Raton London New York

CRC Press is an imprint of the
Taylor & Francis Group, an **informa** business

CRC Press
Taylor & Francis Group
6000 Broken Sound Parkway NW, Suite 300
Boca Raton, FL 33487-2742

First issued in paperback 2017

© 2010 by Taylor and Francis Group, LLC
CRC Press is an imprint of Taylor & Francis Group, an Informa business

No claim to original U.S. Government works

ISBN 13: 978-1-138-11188-2 (pbk)
ISBN 13: 978-1-4200-7124-5 (hbk)

Library of Congress Cataloging-in-Publication Data

Folate in health and disease / edited by Lynn B. Bailey. -- 2nd ed.
    p. ; cm.
Includes bibliographical references and index.
ISBN 978-1-4200-7124-5 (alk. paper)
    1. Folic acid in human nutrition. 2. Folic acid deficiency. 3. Folic acid--Therapeutic use. 4. Folic acid--Metabolism. I. Bailey, Lynn B., 1948-
    [DNLM: 1. Folic Acid--metabolism. 2. Folic Acid--therapeutic use. 3. Diet Therapy. 4. Folic Acid Deficiency--metabolism. 5. Nutritional Requirements. QU 188 F6633 2010]

QP772.F6F623 2010
613.2'86--dc22   2009024346

**Visit the Taylor & Francis Web site at
http://www.taylorandfrancis.com**

**and the CRC Press Web site at
http://www.crcpress.com**

Contents

Preface

More than a decade has passed since the first edition of *Folate in Health and Disease* was published. During this time there have been thousands of new research studies related to folate and its link to disease and birth defect risk, thus providing the impetus for an updated interpretation of this large body of scientific evidence. The public health implications of these new findings are enormous; therefore, the second edition of *Folate in Health and Disease* bridges basic science with clinical medicine and public health.

The first several chapters in the new edition are organized to provide the reader with background knowledge related to folate chemistry, metabolism, bioavailability, and the influence of genetic polymorphisms. Folate's role in reproduction and birth defect prevention is then reviewed, followed by a separate chapter in which epidemiological evidence linking specific birth defects and folate status is evaluated. Intriguing research findings related to basic mechanisms provide insight regarding potential etiologies of folate-responsive birth defects. Folic acid fortification, which was implemented after the first edition of this book was published, is described from a global perspective as it relates to neural tube defect risk reduction.

Chronic disease is covered in a similar manner to that of birth defects; epidemiological data are first critiqued in separate chapters related to cancer, vascular, and neurological diseases, coupled with subsequent chapters in which proposed mechanisms are presented. The potential for folic acid to affect mortality and morbidity associated with the recurrence of vascular disease and cancer has been the focus of ongoing controlled intervention trials. This new edition of *Folate in Health and Disease* is timely in that the findings from these studies can now be described and interpreted to benefit investigators in both the clinical/public health and basic science arenas.

The interrelationships between folate and other nutrients required for normal one-carbon metabolism are covered in several chapters, and the biochemical and clinical ramifications of alterations in status are highlighted. The interaction between folate and vitamin B12 is addressed from a biochemical and public health perspective. The complexities of diagnosis and treatment of a clinical folate deficiency are discussed, followed by a related chapter on the effect of alcohol on folate and methionine metabolism. Choline is covered in a separate chapter that presents evidence related to the metabolic interaction between folate and choline and the implications for health maintenance.

Dietary intake recommendations for select countries worldwide are compared with an overview of the approaches used by the Institute of Medicine's committee to estimate the Dietary Reference Intakes. Changes in folate status over time within the US population are a focus of this chapter with attention given to the influence of folic acid fortification and supplement use on folate status. Estimated dietary folate intakes for the US population and specific population subgroups are presented.

A critique of experimental approaches and an evaluation of studies of one-carbon metabolism provide a new understanding of the knowledge regarding the rates of folate utilization and how to best investigate factors that may influence these rates. Established and new methods for the measurement of folate/folic acid in food and physiological fluids are critiqued in the final chapter as a means to evaluate and compare results from studies in which different methodologies were used. In addition to providing insight into the interpretation of published data, this chapter provides research scientists with guidelines regarding the most appropriate method for future research studies.

In summary, the second edition of *Folate in Health and Disease* integrates and provides an interpretation of basic and applied knowledge related to folate and its role in health maintenance and disease prevention. The interdisciplinary approach taken in this new book results in a valuable resource for both basic and applied research scientists and nutritionists in academics, clinical medicine, and public health.

Editor

Lynn B. Bailey, PhD, is a professor in the Food Science and Human Nutrition Department, University of Florida, Gainesville, Florida. Before joining the faculty at the University of Florida, she received a PhD from Purdue University, an MS from Clemson University, and a BS from Winthrop University. The focus of Dr. Bailey's research program is the estimation of folate requirements involving metabolic studies conducted with human subjects of all ages. Evaluation of the impact of genetic variants on folate requirements and biomarkers for disease and birth defect risk is a key research emphasis.

Dr. Bailey has served as a member of the Institute of Medicine's Dietary Reference Intake committee for folate, vitamin 12, and other B vitamins, and she was a member of the Food and Drug Administration's Folic Acid Advisory Committee. She has served as a scientific advisor for the Centers for Disease Control and Birth Defect Prevention, as well as for other organizations, including the March of Dimes and the Pan American Health Organization, on projects focused on neural tube defect prevention in the United States and developing countries. Dr. Bailey has received numerous awards, including the USDA Superior Achievement Award; the March of Dimes' Agnes Higgins Award, Maternal-Fetal Nutrition; the American Society for Nutrition's Centrum Science Award for influence on current scientific knowledge of folate status and requirements of humans; and the University of Florida's Teacher Scholar of the Year award.

Contributors

Lynn B. Bailey, PhD
Professor, Department of Food Science and Human Nutrition, University of Florida, Gainesville, Florida

Johnathan L. Ballard, PhD
Assistant Research Scientist, Center for Environmental and Genetic Medicine, Institute of Biosciences and Technology, Texas A&M Health Science Center, Houston, Texas

Robert J. Berry, MD, MPHTM
Medical Epidemiologist, Birth Defects Epidemiology Team Leader, National Center on Birth Defects and Developmental Disabilities, Centers for Disease Control and Prevention, Atlanta, Georgia

Teodoro Bottiglieri, PhD
Director of Neuropharmacology Laboratory, Adjunct Professor of Biomedical Studies, Baylor University Medical Center, Institute of Metabolic Disease, Dallas, Texas

Marie A. Caudill, PhD, RD
Associate Professor, Division of Nutritional Sciences, Cornell University, Ithaca, New York

Jia Chen, ScD
Associate Professor, Departments of Community and Preventive Medicine, Pediatrics and Oncological Science, Mount Sinai School of Medicine, New York, New York

Karen E. Christensen, PhD
Postdoctoral Fellow, Departments of Human Genetics and Pediatrics, McGill University, Montreal, Quebec, Canada

Eric Ciappio, MS, RD
Doctoral Student, Friedman School of Nutrition Science Policy, Tufts University; Vitamins & Carcinogenesis Laboratory, Jean Mayer USDA Human Nutrition Research Center on Aging at Tufts University, Boston, Massachusetts

Vanessa R. da Silva, BS
Doctoral Student, Department of Food Science and Human Nutrition, University of Florida, Gainesville, Florida

Megan L. Diaz, MS, RD, LD
Graduate Assistant, University of Florida, Gainesville, Florida

Farah Esfandiari, PhD
Research Faculty, Department of Internal Medicine, University of California Davis, Davis, California

Zia Fazili, MPhil, PhD
Research Chemist, Nutritional Biomarkers Branch, Division of Laboratory Sciences, Centers for Disease Control and Prevention, Atlanta, Georgia

Richard H. Finnell, PhD
Regents Professor, Center for Environmental and Genetic Medicine, Institute of Biosciences and Technology, Texas A&M Health Science Center, Houston, Texas

Alla V. Glushchenko, MD, PhD
Postdoctoral Fellow, Department of Cell Biology, Lerner Research Institute, Cleveland Clinic, Cleveland, Ohio

Jesse F. Gregory III, PhD
Professor, Department of Food Science and Human Nutrition, University of Florida, Gainesville, Florida

Charles H. Halsted, MD
Professor, Departments of Internal Medicine and Nutrition, University of California Davis, Davis, California

Heather C. Hamner, MS, MPH
Nutrition Epidemiologist, Division of Birth Defects and Developmental Disabilities, National Center on Birth Defects and Developmental Disabilities, Centers for Disease Control and Prevention, Atlanta, Georgia

Luciana Hannibal, BSc
Doctoral Student, Department of Cell Biology, Lerner Research Institute, Cleveland Clinic, Cleveland, Ohio; and School of Biomedical Sciences, Kent State University, Kent, Ohio

Charlotte A. Hobbs, MD, PhD
Professor, Department of Pediatrics, College of Medicine, University of Arkansas for Medical Sciences, Little Rock, Arkansas

Donald W. Jacobsen, PhD, FAHA
Staff, Department of Cell Biology, Lerner Research Institute, and Department of Cardiovascular Medicine, Heart and Vascular Institute, Cleveland Clinic, Cleveland, Ohio; Professor of Molecular Medicine, Department of Molecular Medicine,

Cleveland Clinic Lerner College of Medicine, Case Western Reserve University, Cleveland, Ohio

Paul F. Jacques, ScD
Senior Scientist and Director, Nutritional Epidemiology, Jean Myer USDA Human Nutrition Research Center on Aging, and Professor, Friedman School of Nutrition Science and Policy, Tufts University, Boston, Massachusetts

Sari R. Kalin, MS, RD, LDN
Program Coordinator, Department of Nutrition, Harvard School of Public Health, Boston, Massachusetts

Gail P. A. Kauwell, PhD, RD, LDN
Professor, Food Science and Human Nutrition Department, University of Florida, Gainesville, Florida

Yvonne Lamers, PhD
Postdoctoral Associate, Department of Food Science and Human Nutrition, University of Florida, Gainesville, Florida

Edward J. Lammer, MD
Associate Scientist, Children's Hospital Oakland Research Institute, Oakland, California

Amy Liu, MPH
Doctoral Student, Department of Epidemiology, University of Washington, Seattle, Washington

Joel B. Mason, MD
Associate Professor, Schools of Medicine and Nutritional Science & Policy, Tufts University; Director, Vitamins & Carcinogenesis Laboratory, Jean Mayer USDA Human Nutrition Research Center on Aging at Tufts University, Boston, Massachusetts

Michelle Kay McGuire, PhD
Associate Professor, School of Molecular Biosciences, Washington State University, Pullman, Washington

Helene McNulty, PhD, RD
Professor, Northern Ireland Centre for Food and Health, School of Biomedical Sciences, University of Ulster, Coleraine, Northern Ireland

Valentina Medici, MD
Assistant Professor, Department of Internal Medicine, Division of Gastroenterology and Hepatology, University of California Davis Medical Center, Sacramento, California

Anne Molloy, PhD
Research Senior Lecturer, Department of Clinical Medicine, School of Medicine, Trinity College, Dublin, Ireland

Martha Savaria Morris, PhD
Epidemiologist, Nutritional Epidemiology Program, Jean Mayer USDA Human Nutrition Research Center on Aging at Tufts University, Boston, Massachusetts

Bridget S. Mosley, MPH
Epidemiologist, Department of Pediatrics, College of Medicine, University of Arkansas for Medical Sciences, Little Rock, Arkansas

Joseph Mulinare, MD, MSPH
Chief, Prevention Research & Health Communications Team, National Center on Birth Defects and Developmental Disabilities, Centers for Disease Control and Prevention, Atlanta, Georgia

Kristina Pentieva, MD, PhD
Senior Lecturer, Northern Ireland Centre for Food and Health, School of Biomedical Sciences, University of Ulster, Coleraine, Northern Ireland

Christine M. Pfeiffer, PhD
Chief of Nutritional Biomarkers Branch, Division of Laboratory Sciences, Centers for Disease Control and Prevention, Atlanta, Georgia

Mary Frances Picciano, PhD
Senior Nutrition Research Scientist, Office of Dietary Supplements, National Institutes of Health, Bethesda, Maryland

Edward Reynolds, MD, FRCP, FRCPsych
Honorary Senior Lecturer, Department of Neurology, King's College, University of London, London, England

Eric B. Rimm, ScD
Associate Professor of Medicine, Harvard Medical School, Channing Laboratory, Brigham and Women's Hospital; Associate Professor of Epidemiology and Nutrition, Director, Program in Cardiovascular Epidemiology, Harvard School of Public Health, Boston, Massachusetts

Rima Rozen, PhD, FCCMG
James McGill Professor, Departments of Human Genetics and Pediatrics, McGill University, Montreal, Quebec, Canada

Barry Shane, PhD
Professor, Department of Nutritional Sciences and Toxicology, University of California, Berkeley, California

Gary M. Shaw, DrPH
Professor, Department of Pediatrics, Stanford University, Palo Alto, California

Sally P. Stabler, MD
Co-Division Head of Hematology, Professor of Medicine, Department of Medicine, University of Colorado at Denver, Aurora, Colorado

Patrick J. Stover, PhD
Professor of Nutritional Biochemistry, Division of Nutritional Sciences, Cornell University, Ithaca, New York

Tsunenobu Tamura, MD
Professor, Department of Nutrition Sciences, University of Alabama at Birmingham, Birmingham, Alabama

Cornelia M. Ulrich, PhD
Full Member, Cancer Prevention Program, Fred Hutchinson Cancer Research Center, Seattle, Washington; Head, Division of Preventive Oncology, German Cancer Research Center, and Co-Director, National Center for Tumor Diseases, Heidelberg, Germany

Deeann Wallis, PhD
Research Scientist, Texas A&M Institute for Genomic Medicine, Texas A&M Health Science Center, Houston, Texas

Martha M. Werler, ScD
Professor, Epidemiology, Slone Epidemiology Center at Boston University, Boston, Massachusetts

Xinran Xu, PhD
Research Fellow, Department of Community and Preventive Medicine, Mount Sinai School of Medicine, New York, New York

Quanhe Yang, PhD
Epidemiologist, Office of Public Health Genomics, Centers for Disease Control and Prevention, Atlanta, Georgia

Ming Zhang, MD
Research Microbiologist, Nutritional Biomarkers Branch, Division of Laboratory Sciences, Centers for Disease Control and Prevention, Atlanta, Georgia

1 Folate Chemistry and Metabolism

Barry Shane

CONTENTS

I. INTRODUCTION

The vitamin folic acid was initially investigated as a dietary antianemia factor, and early studies on folic acid [1] and the establishment of its role as a cofactor in one-carbon metabolism [2] have been reviewed. Because of the role of folate coenzymes in the synthesis of DNA precursors, folate antagonists have found widespread clinical use as antiproliferative and antimicrobial agents. It has been known for many years that the pernicious anemia that results from defects in vitamin B12 availability is caused by induction of a secondary functional folate deficiency [3] with a concomitant defect in DNA synthesis in erythroid cells. More recently, the demonstration [4] that periconceptional supplementation with folic acid dramatically reduces the incidence of neural tube defects has generated considerable clinical and public health interest and has led to fortification with folic acid of the food supply in the United States and some other countries. The metabolic basis for this reduction in birth defects is not understood, and some concerns have been raised about possible adverse effects of increased folic acid intake [5].

Regimens for the treatment of folate-related disorders and the use of folate antagonists, as well as the advantages and potential disadvantages of folate fortification, require an understanding of normal folate metabolism and the metabolic consequences of derangements in folate metabolism. This chapter presents an overview of current knowledge on the mechanisms by which folate is handled in the body and how tissue folate concentration levels and homeostasis are established and regulated. The role of folates as coenzymes in one-carbon metabolism and the clinical consequences of derangements in folate metabolism are discussed in greater detail in subsequent chapters.

II. CHEMISTRY

Folic acid (pteroylmonoglutamate, PteGlu) consists of a 2-amino-4-hydroxy-pteridine (pterin) moiety linked via a methylene group at the C-6 position to a p-aminobenzoyl-glutamate moiety. Folate metabolism involves the reduction of the pyrazine ring of the pterin moiety to the coenzymatically active tetrahydro form (Figure 1.1), the elongation of the glutamate chain by the addition of glutamate residues in γ-peptide linkage, and the acquisition and oxidation or reduction of one-carbon units at the N-5 and/or N-10 positions (Figure 1.2). Folate coenzymes function as acceptors and donors of one-carbon moieties in reactions involving nucleotide and amino acid metabolism. These reactions, known as one-carbon metabolism, are discussed in Chapter 3. The active coenzymatic species used in these reactions are folylpolyglutamates [6,7]. Folylpolyglutamates are much more effective substrates and inhibitors than pteroylmonoglutamates of almost all folate-dependent enzymes, the exception being dihydrofolate (DHF) reductase, and usually exhibit greatly increased affinity and lower K_m values for these enzymes. Some of the enzymes involved in folate metabolism are multifunctional, with multiple catalytic sites on a single protein, or are part of multiprotein complexes. For some of these complexes, the longer polyglutamate derivatives allow channeling of substrates between active sites without release of intermediate products from the complex. The polyglutamate tail is thought

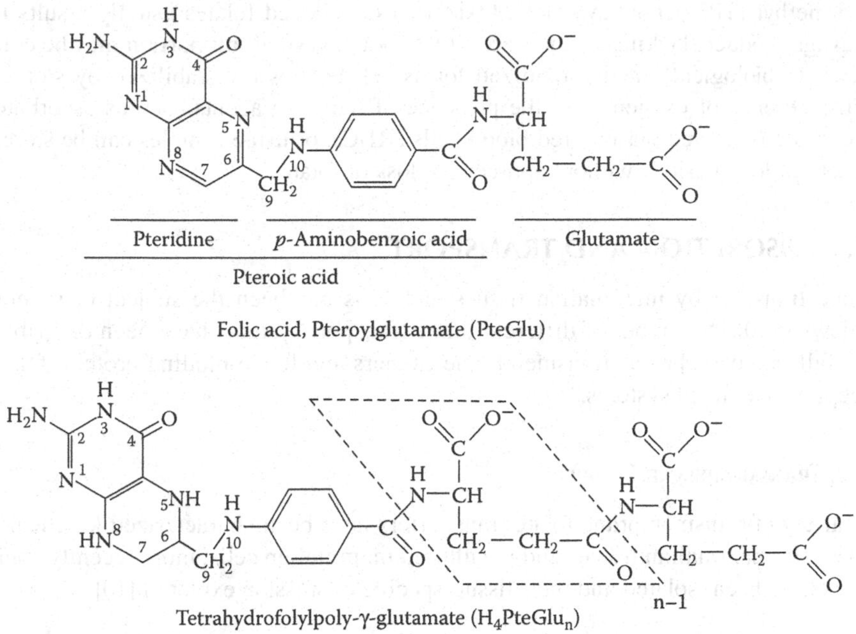

FIGURE 1.1 Structure of folates.

One carbon substituent		Position	Oxidation state
Methyl	$-CH_3$	N-5	Methanol
Methylene	$-CH_2-$	N-5, N-10	Formaldehyde
Methenyl	$-CH=$	N-5, N-10	Formate
Formyl	$-CHO$	N-5 or N-10	Formate
Formimino	$HN=CH-$	N-5	Formate

FIGURE 1.2 One-carbon folate derivatives.

to be anchored to a site on the complex, and channeling of substrates between active sites prevents the accumulation of intermediate products in bulk cell water and increases the efficiency of metabolic pathways. Folylpolyglutamates are also preferentially retained by tissues, whereas the monoglutamates are the transport forms.

Mammals lack the ability to synthesize folates de novo and require preformed folates in the diet. Folates are synthesized in microorganisms and plants as the DHF derivative. All naturally occurring folates are reduced derivatives, and consequently the fully oxidized folic acid form found in supplements is only found in the diet when foodstuffs are fortified with folic acid or when dietary folates are oxidized. Reduced folates are generally less stable than folic acid, and their stability varies depending on the one-carbon substitution. Folinic acid (5-formyl-tetrahydrofolate [THF]) is a stable reduced folate, and a stabilized salt of other reduced folates such as 5-methyl-THF is now available. Oxidation of reduced folates usually results in cleavage products lacking vitamin activity, although a small proportion may be converted to biologically active oxidized forms [8]. Folates are stabilized by storage in the absence of oxygen or in the presence of reducing agents such as ascorbate. Ascorbate-protected plasma, red blood cells (RBC), or urine samples can be stored frozen for long periods without appreciable loss of folate.

III. ABSORPTION AND TRANSPORT

Folate transport by mammalian tissues and cells has been the subject of several reviews [9,10]. A number of different folate transport systems have been described that fall into two classes: transmembrane carriers and folate-binding protein (folate receptor)–mediated systems.

A. TRANSMEMBRANE CARRIERS

A variety of transmembrane folate transporters have been characterized kinetically in various mammalian tissues and in cultured mammalian cells; more recently, their genes have been isolated and their tissue-specific expression explored [10].

1. Reduced Folate Carrier

The reduced folate carrier (RFC1) gene encodes a transmembrane anionic exchanger that functions optimally at physiological pH and is essentially inactive below pH 6.5. It is a facilitative carrier, and folate transport into cells is stimulated by high levels of intracellular organic anions (e.g., adenine nucleotides), whereas extracellular organic anions are inhibitory [11,12]. The relatively high concentration of intracellular anions makes folate transport essentially unidirectional. The other two members of the RFC1 gene family are facilitative thiamin transporters and do not transport folate. Whereas thiamin is not transported by RFC1, thiamin pyrophosphate is, and high intracellular levels of thiamin pyrophosphate stimulate folate transport into cells [13]. RFC1 has been the most extensively studied of the folate transporters. It is expressed in tissue culture cells, is found in some tumor cells and fetal tissues, and is ubiquitously expressed in normal adult tissues, although it may not be responsible for the bulk of folate transport in all tissues (see below). The transporter is saturable and has a fairly low affinity for folate with K_t values in the low micromolar range (approximately 3 µM) for reduced folates and a similar affinity for the antifolate methotrexate [11,14]. The carrier has a greatly reduced affinity for folic acid (K_t approximately 200 µM), which explains why most cultured cells require much higher levels of folic acid compared with reduced folates for growth.

2. Proton Coupled Folate Transporter

The proton coupled folate transporter (PCFT) is a recently identified transmembrane folate carrier that functions at acidic pH and has reduced or negligible activity at pH 7.4 [15], depending on the folate form. It was originally identified as a putative heme transporter. Unlike RFC1, this carrier has similar affinity for reduced folates and folic acid (K_t values 0.5–0.8 μM at pH 5.5). At pH 6.5, 5-methyl-THF is transported more effectively than folic acid. PCFT is highly expressed in the small intestine, particularly in the jejunum and duodenum, kidney, liver, placenta, and brain, and is also expressed in other tissues. Proton coupling allows the concentrative transport of folates at acidic pH [10,15].

3. ATP Binding Cassette Exporters and Other Exporters

A family of low-affinity membrane carriers (multidrug resistance-associated protein [MRP] 1–4) can serve as folate exporters from tissues. These proteins were originally identified as being responsible for multidrug resistance of cells to chemotherapeutic agents [16,17]. The affinity of folates for these carriers is very low (K_t values 0.2–2 mM), but they have a high capacity for folate transport. A number of other organic anion transporters, such as the solute carriers SLC21 and SLC22, may potentially play a role in folate transport or efflux [10].

4. Mitochondrial Folate Transporter

The transmembrane transporter responsible for folate uptake by the mitochondrion is distinct from the other folate transporters [18]. It is specific for reduced folates, and folic acid and methotrexate are not transported [19,20]. Mammalian cells with a defect in this transporter (Chinese hamster ovary [CHO] *gly*B) are glycine auxotrophs and are defective in both mitochondrial and cytosolic one-carbon metabolism [21].

5. Lysosomal Folate Transporter

A transporter that is responsible for methotrexate polyglutamate uptake by lysosomes has been reported [22] but has received little further attention. The role, if any, of this transporter in folate transport or turnover is not known.

B. FOLATE RECEPTORS

A family of three high-affinity closely related folate receptors (FRs) (α, β, and γ), also known as folate-binding proteins, are expressed in some epithelial cells [23]. In normal tissues, the distribution of FR-α is usually limited to the apical membrane where it would not be in contact with the general circulation [10]. High concentrations are found in the choroid plexus (basolateral membrane). The protein is also found in kidney proximal tubules, erythropoietic cells, vas deferens, ovaries, fallopian tubes, uterine epididymis, trophoblastic cells of the placenta, lung alveolar, acinar cells of the breast, submandibular salivary and bronchial cells, and retinal pigment epithelial cells (basolateral membrane) [24]. Low levels are found in the thyroid gland, and very low levels may be present in gut mucosal cells. FR-α is expressed in fetal and adult tissues and in some tumors. FR-β is primarily found in the placenta, spleen, and thymus, and in some monocytes. It is expressed during normal myelopoiesis, and high levels are found in some acute myelogenous leukemia blasts. FR-β is also expressed in fetal tissue.

Transport via the FR is a relatively slow process compared with transport via the transmembrane transporters, and, apart from its well-established role in kidney folate reabsorption [25, see below], the extent to which this receptor is involved in folate transport is not well established. It clearly plays an important role in development as deletion of the mouse gene equivalent to *FR-α* results in embryonic lethality and embryos develop neural tube defects, whereas deletion of *FR-β* has no obvious phenotype [26].

FRs were originally identified as a high-affinity soluble plasma folate-binding protein, also found in milk [27]. Normally, FRs are attached to the plasma membrane of cells via a glycosylphosphatidylinositol anchor and can be released from the membrane by a specific phospholipase C [28]. The binding proteins show high affinity for a variety of folates with K_ds in the nanomolar range. Folic acid shows the highest affinity (K_d 1–10 nM). The affinity of 5-methyl-THF for FR-α is slightly lower, and its affinity is reduced about 50-fold further for FR-β. Methotrexate has relatively poor affinity for these proteins [10].

Although most tissue culture cells express RFC1, some cells of epithelial origin also express folate-binding protein, and the protein can be induced by culturing cells in medium containing very low levels of folic acid [29]. The level of the binding protein may also be regulated by cell differentiation [30]. Antisera to the binding protein inhibits folate uptake and reduces intracellular folate accumulation in erythroid progenitor cells [31].

Folate transport via the folate-binding protein occurs via a receptor-mediated process, but the mechanism is not fully understood. In studies with some tissues and cells, the binding protein–folate complex has been shown to internalize via a non–clathrin-mediated classical endocytotic pathway not involving lysosomes [32]. Folate is released from the vesicle into the cytosol, and the binding protein rapidly recycles back to the plasma membrane. The mechanism by which folate is transported out of these vesicles has not been definitively established. It has been suggested that acidification of the vesicles effects release of folate from the binding protein and that the vesicles may also contain the low-pH PCFT carrier [10]. As folate would be concentrated in the vesicles, this would allow efficient transport of folate via the PCFT carrier. This plausible mechanism would allow cells and tissues to accumulate folate at exogenous folate concentrations that would be inefficiently transported if the cell was dependent solely on the lower-affinity transmembrane carriers. However, if PCFT is involved in the endocytotic transport of folate, it is not clear why infants with hereditary folate malabsorption (HFM) disease resulting from a defect in *PCFT* [33, see below] do not display the fetal abnormalities associated with deletion of the *FR-α* gene.

C. Intestinal Absorption and Transport

Most dietary folates are polyglutamate derivatives and are hydrolyzed to monoglutamate forms in the gut before absorption across the intestinal mucosa. The bioavailability of food folate and folic acid in fortified foods is discussed in Chapter 2. The hydrolysis of dietary folylpolyglutamates, which is catalyzed by a brush-border membrane γ-glutamyl hydrolase (γ-GH, glutamate carboxypeptidase II [*GCPII*]) in humans and pigs, and the intestinal absorption of pteroylmonoglutamates are also described in Chapter 2. The *GCPII* gene encodes a protein identical to prostate-specific membrane (PSM) antigen, a marker for prostate cancer, and

N-acetylated α-linked acidic dipeptidase (NAALADase), a brain enzyme that regulates glutamate neurotransmission [34]. As far as is known, the functions of PSM and NAALADase are unrelated to folate metabolism. In other species, such as the rat, the hydrolase activity is secreted in the bile. This latter activity is similar to a γ-GH activity found in the lysosomes of all tissues.

The mechanism by which folate crosses the mucosal cell and is released across the basolateral membrane into the portal circulation is not totally understood, although some features have been clarified recently. Extensive metabolism of folic acid and reduced folates to 5-methyl-THF can occur during this process, but metabolism is not required for transport. The degree of metabolism in the intestinal mucosa is dependent on the folate dose given. When pharmacological doses of various folates are given, most of the transported vitamin appears unchanged in the portal circulation [35]. Some of this can be metabolized to 5-methyl-THF in liver, but some can appear unchanged in the peripheral circulation.

Both PCFT and RFC1 are expressed on the apical membranes of the intestinal mucosa, and their mRNAs are up-regulated under conditions of folate depletion [10]. However, transport into the mucosal cell appears to occur primarily via the PCFT carrier. The mucosal cell is bathed by an acid microclimate. Intestinal folate transport has a pH optimum of about 5.5, and folic acid is transported as effectively as reduced folate monoglutamates. All of these are consistent with transport by the PCFT carrier. RFC1 would not be an effective transporter under these conditions. HFM disease is a rare autosomal recessive disorder in which there is impaired folate absorption leading to a severe systemic folate deficiency and impaired folate transport into the brain with very low folate levels in the cerebrospinal fluid (CSF) [33]. CSF folate concentrations are normally higher than in plasma. It has recently been shown that the molecular basis for this disease is loss-of-function mutations in the *PCFT* gene [36]. Symptoms develop several months after birth and include anemia, developmental defects, and seizures. Infants can be treated with low-dose parenteral folate or with high-dose oral methyl-THF, suggesting that some intestinal transport can occur via the RFC1 carrier, but also indicating that PCFT is normally responsible for the bulk of folate transport in the intestine. Normalization of CSF folate levels in subjects with HFM disease requires very high plasma folate concentrations.

RFC1 and PCFT are not expressed on the basolateral membrane of the intestinal mucosal cell, and folate efflux into the portal circulation is believed to be mediated by MRP3, one of the low-affinity, high-capacity transporters [37].

D. TRANSPORT INTO TISSUES

Pteroylmonoglutamates, primarily 5-methyl-THF, are the circulating forms of folate in plasma, and mammalian cells are not believed to transport polyglutamates of chain length three and above. After folate absorption into the portal circulation, much of this folate can be taken up by the liver, where it is either metabolized to polyglutamate derivatives and retained, or it is released into blood or bile. An enterohepatic circulation of folate has been described involving release of hepatic 5-methyl-THF into bile via MRP2 [38] with reabsorption in the small intestine [10]. The predominance of 5-methyl-THF in plasma probably reflects that this is the major cytosolic folate in mammalian tissues and consequently is the major form that would be released (Section IV.E.3, Folate Status and Effects of High Folate Intake). The extent, if any, of release of short-chain folylpolyglutamates from tissues is unknown. Plasma contains γ-GH activity, and any polyglutamate released into plasma would be hydrolyzed to the monoglutamate.

A variable proportion of plasma folate is bound to low-affinity protein binders, primarily albumin, which accounts for about 50% of bound folate. This proportion is increased in folate deficiency [39]. Plasma also contains low concentrations of a soluble form of the FR. The levels of this high-affinity binder are increased in pregnancy and are very high in some leukemia patients [39]. Increased concentrations of the high-affinity binder may reflect tissue damage or incidental release from tissues, and the effect of plasma protein binding on folate availability for tissues remains an open question.

RBCs contain much higher levels of folate than plasma, and practically all RBC folates are normally 5-methyl-THF polyglutamates. 10-Formyl-THF polyglutamates have been detected in RBCs of some subjects homozygous for the T variant of the 677C→T polymorphism in methylene-THF reductase [40]. Mature RBCs have a negligible capacity to transport and accumulate folate, and their folate stores accumulate during erythropoiesis and appear to be retained, probably as a result of hemoglobin binding, through the life span of the cell. Because of this, RBC folate concentrations are often used as a measure of long-term folate status. Fasting plasma folate levels are also a good indicator of status, but plasma concentrations can also be influenced by recent dietary intake.

Mammalian tissues appear to possess a diverse range of folate transporters with differing affinities for various folate derivatives. Folate transport in hepatocytes is energy dependent and complex with saturable and nonsaturable components [41]. Basolateral (sinusoidal) membranes from rat and human liver, which transport folate from the portal circulation, express high levels of PCFT [10] and possess an electroneutral folate-H⁺ cotransporter for reduced and oxidized folates and methotrexate [42]. Transport is minimal at pH 7.4, and it appears that PCFT is responsible for folate uptake by hepatocytes. How the proton gradient required for transport is set up remains an open question.

Transport into peripheral tissues primarily uses RFC1 [10]. As both the RFC1 and PCFT transporters have affinities for reduced folates in the micromolar range, and plasma folate concentrations are in the nanomolar range, these transporters would not be saturated by folate under any physiological conditions. This would be the case even when folate intake is very high, and folate influx into tissues should be responsive to any elevation in plasma folate levels found after folate supplementation. However, tissues dependent on RFC1 for folate transport would be ineffective in removing any circulating folic acid from plasma.

The choroid plexus, which supplies folate to the CSF, expresses high levels of FR-α and PCFT on the basolateral membrane and RFC1 on the apical membrane [10], and infants with HFM disease have low levels of CSF folate [33]. Clearly, PCFT plays a role in folate transport into the CSF. Whether this role involves direct transport from plasma or a coupled transport with FR-α is not clear. In either case, this would allow transport of any free folic acid in plasma into the choroid plexus. Transport from the choroid plexus into the CSF could be mediated by RFC1. PCFT and RFC1 are also expressed in the vascular blood-brain barrier, which supplies folate to the brain parenchyma. FR-α was thought to mediate folate uptake into the brain, but FR-α is not found in the blood-brain barrier or in the brain [43]. It is not known whether PCFT or RFC1 is responsible for folate uptake into the brain. Uptake is inhibited by low levels of 5-methyl-THF or folic acid, which suggests involvement of PCFT. However, the neutral pH at the interface would be more consistent with RFC1-mediated transport.

Normally folate is effectively reabsorbed in the kidney proximal tubules, and little or no folate is lost in the urine at normal folate intakes. This reabsorption is mediated by FR-α [25], and clearance rates for folates are inversely proportional to their affinities for FR-α [44]. Because of the high affinity of the receptor for folic acid, this form of the vitamin can accumulate to high levels in the kidney.

IV. TISSUE ACCUMULATION

Endogenous folates in mammalian tissues are almost entirely folylpolyglutamate derivatives, whereas pteroylmonoglutamates are the only forms in plasma and urine [7]. Although pentaglutamates are the predominant derivatives in rat liver, longer-chain derivatives are found in most other mammalian tissues, including human cells. Intracellular metabolism to polyglutamates is required for the retention and concentration of transported folate. Plasma folate concentrations in humans are usually in the 10 to 30 nM range, whereas hepatic levels, practically all polyglutamates, are reported to range from about 10 to 30 μM [45]. Although metabolism to polyglutamate derivatives might be considered a mechanism for folate storage, folylpolyglutamates are the active coenzyme species, and metabolism to polyglutamates is required for normal one-carbon metabolism, and there is no real store for excess folate. Total body stores of folate in humans have been estimated to range from 10 to 100 mg, with 3 to 16 mg in liver [45–47].

Tissue folate accumulation, which is summarized in Figure 1.3, requires folate metabolism to polyglutamate derivatives in the cytosol and mitochondria of cells.

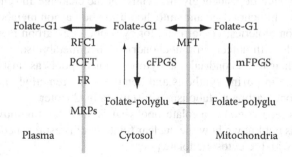

FIGURE 1.3 Overview of folate homeostasis. Folate-G1, folate monoglutamate; Folate-polyglu, folypolyglutamate; FPGS, folypolyglutamate synthetase (mitochondrial and cytosolic isozymes); FR, folate receptor (folate-binding protein); MFT, mitochondrial folate transporter; MRP, multidrug resistance protein; PCFT, proton coupled folate transporter; RFC1, reduced folate carrier.

The mitochondrial folate transporter competes with the cytosolic folylpolygluta-mate synthetase for the entering folate monoglutamate [21]. After transport into tis-sues, monoglutamate derivatives are interconverted to other monoglutamates via the enzymes of one-carbon metabolism (Chapter 3). Some folates are metabolized to polyglutamate derivatives and retained. Any not metabolized to longer-chain poly-glutamate species are lost from the cell. Folate monoglutamates compete very poorly with cellular folylpolyglutamates for the enzymes of one-carbon metabolism; thus, the extent of metabolism of monoglutamates will depend on the folylpolyglutamate pools in the cell. Similarly, the ability to metabolize folates to retainable polygluta-mate derivatives will be inhibited by competition with cellular folate pools. Tissues contain folate-binding proteins, primarily the enzymes of one-carbon metabolism, and it has been estimated that the folate-binding capacity of these proteins normally exceeds the folate concentration in tissues. Binding of cellular folylpolyglutamates to these proteins will reduce their competition with monoglutamate derivatives and allow more extensive metabolism of monoglutamates and their conversion to retainable polyglutamate derivatives. The ability of tissues to accumulate high levels of the vitamin, that is, levels in excess of that required for normal metabolism, is limited ([48], Section IV.E.3, Folate Status and Effects of High Folate Intake). Under conditions of very high folate intake, the protein binding capacity is probably exceeded; polyglutamylation is impaired; and there is increased turnover of folate pools.

A. FOLATE DISTRIBUTION

A significant proportion of cellular folate, up to 50% depending on the tissue or cell type, is associated with the mitochondria [49,50]. The mitochondrial folate pool is distinct from the cytosolic pool and displays a distinct one-carbon distribution. Practically all the cellular 5-methyl-THF polyglutamate is in the cytosol, whereas most of the cellular 10-formyl-THF polyglutamate is in the mitochondria [49]. Mitochondria contain folylpolyglutamates that are of longer glutamate chain length than cytosolic folates [50]. Although 5-methyl-THF is transported into the mitochon-dria, it is not metabolized to retainable polyglutamates and does not accumulate in this organelle. Folate-dependent glycine synthesis and cleavage and choline degrada-tion occur in the mitochondria, and mitochondrial one-carbon metabolism also pro-vides one-carbon moieties, via formate, for cytosolic one-carbon metabolism ([51], Chapter 3). Cells with defects in mitochondrial folate metabolism contain a higher proportion of their mitochondrial and cytosolic folate pools as unsubstituted THF and are defective in purine synthesis and homocysteine remethylation. The role of mitochondrial one-carbon metabolism is discussed in Chapter 3.

The nucleus also contains a folate pool that is used for thymidylate synthesis (Chapter 3). It is not known how the nuclear folate pool is established, but it may be in equilibrium with the cytosolic folate pool.

B. FOLYLPOLY-γ-GLUTAMATE SYNTHETASE

The synthesis of folylpolyglutamates, as well as factors that regulate this synthesis, plays a major role in the regulation of folate homeostasis and in the regulation of cellular folate pools. Mammalian cells possess two enzyme activities that can potentially directly regulate this process: folylpolyglutamate synthetase, which catalyzes the synthesis of folylpoly-γ-glutamates, and γ-GH, a lysosomal peptidase that can hydrolyze the folate polypeptide chain. The general properties of both these activities have been the subject of reviews [6,7]. The potential role of γ-GH is discussed in Section IV.D, Role of γ-Glutamyl Hydrolase.

Mammalian CHO cell mutants that lack folylpolyglutamate synthetase activity have greatly reduced folate pools because of an inability to retain folates and are auxotrophic for methionine, glycine, purines, and thymidine [52]. This auxotrophy is not relieved by elevating intracellular pteroylmonoglutamate to folate concentrations typically found in wild-type CHO cells [48], indicating that the auxotrophy is not caused solely by low folate levels but is also the result of an inability to synthesize folylpolyglutamates. Although wild-type CHO cells normally contain hexa- and heptaglutamates, metabolism of folate to the triglutamate is sufficient for normal cellular folate retention [52], and triglutamates function almost as effectively as the longer-chain derivatives in the metabolic cycles of purine, thymidine, and glycine synthesis [48]. However, longer polyglutamate derivatives are required for methionine synthesis (homocysteine remethylation). Folylpolyglutamate synthetase activity is highest in liver, and appreciable levels are found in most mammalian tissues, although it appears to be absent or present in negligible amounts in muscle tissue and mature blood cells [53].

Folylpolyglutamate synthetase is located in the cytosol and mitochondria of mammalian tissues and cells, and the mitochondrial isozyme is required for the accumulation of normal mitochondrial folate pools [50]. Although folylpolyglutamates cannot be transported into the mitochondria, folylpolyglutamates synthesized in the mitochondria are slowly released into the cytosol. Model cells expressing folylpolyglutamate synthetase solely in the mitochondria have normal cytosolic and mitochondrial folate pools [21]. Folylpolyglutamate synthetase is encoded by a single human gene, and cytosolic and mitochondrial isozymes are generated by alternate transcription start sites for the gene [54,55] and by alternate translational start sites for its mRNA [58].

Mammalian folylpolyglutamate synthetases are very low abundance proteins. The most effective pteroylmonoglutamate substrates for the mammalian enzymes are THF and DHF. 10-Formyl-THF has a reduced k_{cat}, whereas 5-substituted folates, such as 5-methyl- and 5-formyl-THF, and folic acid are very poor substrates [54,57]. Increasing the glutamate chain length of the folate molecule causes a decrease in catalytic rate. The k_{cat} values for polyglutamates of THF, DHF, and folic acid decrease with increasing glutamate chain length, although long-chain folylpolyglutamates still retain affinity for the protein. The substrate specificity of the enzyme for pteroylmonoglutamate derivatives is not necessarily a good indicator of which compounds are the most effective polyglutamate substrates. Activity decreases faster with elongation of the polyglutamate chain of DHF and 10-formyl-THF than with THF. THF polyglutamates are the only effective long-chain substrates for the enzyme [54,58]. 5-Methyl-THF is a relatively poor substrate, and its diglutamate derivative is essentially inactive. Folic acid is a relatively poor substrate for the human enzyme. Although its diglutamate derivative is a poor substrate, it does possess some activity;

thus, folic acid can be metabolized directly to retainable polyglutamate derivatives, whereas the ability to metabolize 5-methyl-THF to a retainable form is practically nonexistent.

4-Aminofolates, such as aminopterin and methotrexate, are more effective substrates of folylpolyglutamate synthetase than their parent 4-oxo-pteroylmono-glutamate derivatives (folic acid and 10-methyl–folic acid) [54,59–61]. However, the 4-amino substitution significantly impairs catalysis with polyglutamate derivatives, and the diglutamate derivatives of all the 4-amino-folates tested have proven to be poor substrates for the enzyme. The human enzyme is more effective in handling diglutamate substrates than other mammalian enzymes. As metabolism of folate derivatives to the triglutamate is required for cellular retention, this explains why human cells are more sensitive than rodent cells to antifolates such as methotrexate.

C. INTRACELLULAR FOLATE-BINDING PROTEINS

Binding of folylpolyglutamates to cellular proteins, primarily enzymes of one-carbon metabolism, would be expected to reduce the availability of some of these compounds for other enzymes of one-carbon metabolism and would assist in folate retention by tissues. Liver contains five major folate-binding proteins [27]. A large proportion of hepatic mitochondrial THF polyglutamate is associated with sarcosine and dimethylglycine dehydrogenases [62]. The major cytoplasmic folate-binding protein, glycine N-methyltransferase, is present in high concentrations and contains bound 5-methyl-THF polyglutamate, which is an inhibitor of the enzyme [63,64]. Liver contains additional cytosolic folate-binding proteins, including 10-formyl-THF dehydrogenase [65]. This enzyme binds THF polyglutamate, which is a product, and consequently an inhibitor, of the enzyme. Serine hydroxymethyltransferase is also a high abundance protein in liver cytosol and mitochondria [66] but has not been identified as a folate-binding protein despite the high affinity of folylpolyglutamates for the enzyme. 5-Methyl-THF polyglutamate is a tight-binding potent inhibitor of this enzyme. Dilution of proteins and cellular metabolites occurs under the conditions used to isolate and identify binding proteins. Under normal cellular conditions, a significant proportion of hepatic folates could potentially be associated with this enzyme and other enzymes of one-carbon metabolism. Based on the affinities reported for folylpolyglutamates for enzymes involved in one-carbon metabolism, it is probable that a large proportion, if not most, of the intracellular folate is associated with proteins under physiological conditions; this proportion is likely to be increased when tissue folate levels are low. For example, most of the hepatic 5-methyl-THF polyglutamate is associated with glycine methyltransferase in folate-depleted rats [67].

Many of the enzymes of one-carbon metabolism are present at much higher levels in liver than in other tissues. This probably reflects their role in hepatic gluconeogenesis. Peripheral tissues have lower levels of both folate-binding proteins and cellular folate. Because protein binding limits the availability of folate substrates for various enzymes of one-carbon metabolism, it is not always intuitive how changes in folate availability influence folate and one-carbon metabolism. Some recent modeling studies have attempted to address this and suggest that protein binding may partially buffer one-carbon metabolism over a wide range of physiological tissue folate concentrations [68,69], making one-carbon metabolism less responsive to changes in folate concentration.

D. Role of γ-Glutamyl Hydrolase

Mammalian tissues contain γ-GH (conjugases) that can hydrolyze the polygluta-mate chain of folates. The properties of these enzymes, which are distinct from the GCPII hydrolase involved in intestinal absorption of folate in humans, have been previously reviewed [6]. The hydrolases lack specificity for the pterin moiety and will hydrolyze p-aminobenzoylpolyglutamates with equal efficacy. Longer-chain folylpolyglutamates are usually better substrates than the shorter glutamate chain length derivatives. γ-GHs in most tissues are located in the lysosome, have an acid pH optimum, and appear to be primarily endopeptidases [6]. Some plasma γ-GHs function at physiological pH. There is no evidence for the existence of cytoplasmic hydrolases that function at physiological pH, although this has not been rigorously addressed.

The role of lysosomal γ-GH in folate homeostasis has not been well established but presumably is involved, at a minimum, in catabolism of folate cleavage products (see Section V, Turnover and Excretion). Addition of putative γ-GH inhibitors or lysosomal function inhibitors to CHO cells does not influence folate or antifolate accumulation or metabolism [20,48], and it is unlikely that the hydrolase plays a role in modulating the glutamate chain of folates to effect regulation of metabolic cycles of one-carbon metabolism in this cell line. However, methotrexate metabolism in some tumor cell lines is influenced by γ-GH inhibitors [70], and increased hydrolase activity has been reported as a mechanism for resistance to antifolate agents [71]. Differences between cell lines may reflect that most tissue culture cells secrete γ-GH into the medium and are depleted in the lysosomal enzyme [72], and this enzyme could play a role in folate turnover in tissues. As described above, a lysosomal uptake system for methotrexate polyglutamates has been characterized [22], which is pre-sumed to be involved in methotrexate polyglutamate turnover in the cell. It is pos-sible that this transporter could transport folylpolyglutamates into the lysosome for conversion to monoglutamate derivatives. If so, the monoglutamates could then be released into the cytosol via the PCFT transporter.

E. Physiological and Pharmacological Factors Affecting Tissue Folate Accumulation

The ability of tissues to accumulate folate depends on the level and specificity of the folate transporter in the tissue and on the level of folylpolyglutamate synthetase activity. Both of these processes will be influenced by folate intake and status and by the level of intracellular folate-binding proteins. Under some conditions, transport would be limiting; under others, metabolism to retainable polyglutamates becomes limiting.

1. Folate Transporter Levels and Specificity

The rate of entry of folate into tissues depends on the level and specificity of the folate transporter expressed in the tissue. Because the major tissue transporters, RFC1 and PCFT, are not saturated by reduced folate monoglutamates under physiological conditions, even when very high doses of folate are provided, influx of folate into tissues that use these transporters will be proportional to the plasma folate level and the expressed level of the transporter. Because folic acid has very poor affinity for RFC1 [11,14], tissues dependent on RFC1 for transport would not be expected to be effective in taking up any folic acid that might be in the circulation. Folic acid would be removed primarily by tissues such as liver that use PCFT [15] and by tissues that use the FR for transport.

The FR has affinities for reduced folates in the physiological plasma folate concentration range [10]. Transport via this receptor would be somewhat responsive to increased plasma folate levels but would saturate when high doses of folate are given. Folic acid has very high affinity for this receptor, and folic acid transport would be saturated even at low levels of folic acid in plasma.

2. Folylpolyglutamate Synthetase Activity

The effect of folylpolyglutamate synthetase activity on folate accumulation has been investigated using model CHO transfectants expressing various levels of human folylpolyglutamate synthetase activity [48,52]. Under conditions in which medium folate mimics physiological conditions, there is little effect of folylpolyglutamate synthetase activity on folate accumulation, and accumulation is limited primarily by influx via the RFC1. Essentially all transported folate is metabolized to retained polyglutamate derivatives. Folate accumulation only becomes limited by folylpolyglutamate synthetase activity when activity levels are low [48].

Because folylpolyglutamate synthetase catalyzes the stepwise addition of glutamate moieties to the folate molecule, the product of the reaction has to compete with the substrate for further glutamate chain elongation. Metabolism of a diglutamate product to a retainable triglutamate (or longer) product would be in competition with entering monoglutamate and with the endogenous folylpolyglutamate pool. Competition with the endogenous folate pool would be relieved to some extent by binding of these derivatives to intracellular binding proteins. However, competition and inhibition of conversion of entering monoglutamate to retainable forms would be expected to be most pronounced when tissues are exposed to high levels of folate and contain high intracellular folate pools. This effect is observed when cells are exposed to high levels of folate. Under these conditions, competition between entering folate and diglutamate in the cell limits the extent of metabolism to retainable polyglutamates (triglutamates and longer), and only a small proportion of the folate that is transported is retained by the cell [48]. This competition limits the ability of the cell to accumulate high levels of folate despite high folate concentrations in the medium. Folate accumulation under these conditions is directly proportional to the level of folylpolyglutamate synthetase activity.

As the level of folylpolyglutamate synthetase activity found in many tissues is lower than that typically found in cultured cells, accumulation of folate would be expected to be limited by the level of folylpolyglutamate synthetase activity and, in some tissues, by the activity of the tissue's folate transporter(s). Although developing blood cells accumulate folate, mature human blood cells possess negligible folylpo- lyglutamate synthetase activity and do not accumulate exogenous folate. Mitogen- stimulated human lymphocytes regain the ability to accumulate folate, and the time course of mitogen activation of folate accumulation correlates with an induction of folylpolyglutamate synthetase mRNA [73]. Polyglutamate formation is more rapid in dividing cell cultures [74], probably reflecting that folylpolyglutamate synthetase levels appear to be growth related and are higher in growing cells and decrease when cells are induced to differentiate [75].

Elevated expression of folylpolyglutamate synthetase should increase the accumulation of pharmacological levels of folate and the accumulation and metab- olism of poor substrates of the enzyme, such as 4-amino-folates. Methotrexate uptake and metabolism in tissue culture cells, as well as the cytotoxic efficacy of methotrexate, are directly correlated with enzyme activity levels [20]. Decreased polyglutamylation of methotrexate in cells from patients resistant to this drug has been described, and several tumor cell lines have been described in which resis- tance to methotrexate is caused by decreased folylpolyglutamate synthetase levels [76–78].

3. Folate Status and Effects of High Folate Intake

Endogenous folate levels are reduced in the livers of folate-depleted animals [79], but the chain lengths of endogenous folylpolyglutamates are increased. This phe- nomenon reflects that the synthesis of very long-chain folylpolyglutamates occurs at a slow rate and is limited by competition with entering pteroylmonoglutamate and shorter-chain folylpolyglutamates, which are preferred substrates for folylpolygluta- mate synthetase. Under folate-restricted conditions, this competition is decreased.

A major factor that limits polyglutamylation and consequently folate retention by tissues is the very poor substrate activity of 5-methyl-THF, and in particular its diglutamate derivative, for folylpolyglutamate synthetase. Under most dietary condi- tions, much of the absorbed folate is metabolized to 5-methyl-THF in the intestine and/or liver, and this is the major form of the vitamin available for peripheral tis- sues. Although some metabolism to the diglutamate of 5-methyl-THF can occur, its retention by cells requires its metabolism via the methionine synthase reaction to THF, the most effective substrate for folylpolyglutamate synthetase. 5-Methyl-THF polyglutamate, the major intracellular form of folate in the cytosol of cells, has much higher affinity for methionine synthase than the mono- and diglutamate forms and potently inhibits the use of the mono- and diglutamates by methionine synthase [80]. The inability to "demethylate" 5-methyl-THF results in its efflux from tissues. This inhibition occurs under conditions of normal folate status and is exacerbated when tissue folate levels increase; it also serves as a homeostatic mechanism to control tissue folate levels.

Plasma folate concentrations increase as folate intake increases, whereas tissue folate levels saturate (or near saturate) at high folate intakes [81]. Although folate absorption and tissue influx are not limited, a decreased ability to convert the enter- ing folate in tissues to retainable polyglutamate forms leads to release of much of the transported folate back to the plasma. Hepatic folate levels in rats receiving 100 times the recommended daily allowance (RDA) in the diet increase only 50% compared with animals on the RDA diet, while plasma concentrations are maintained at a very high level (S. Yoo and B. Shane, unpublished data). When very large pharmacological doses are administered to tumor-bearing experimental animals, tissue folate concentrations are increased to only a limited extent (1.5- to 4-fold). In humans, large doses of folinate (50 or 100 mg) are given as an adjunct to fluorouracil treatment. These doses elevate plasma folate to very high concentrations, but tumor folate levels increase only 50%–100%. Again, plasma folate levels increase to very high levels in the first 4 hours after the dose and then decrease. Clearance of folate from plasma is rapid. When high doses are given, much of the initial loss is the result of exceeding the renal capacity for reabsorption. Pharmacological doses of 5-formyl-THF are more effective than 5-methyl-THF or folic acid at elevating tissue folate levels [82].

These homeostatic mechanisms allow polyglutamylation to proceed effectively when tissue concentrations of folate are low but limit the accumulation of folate when tissue levels are adequate. Folate supplements will increase tissue folate levels, but the increase will be modest in those subjects receiving a good dietary folate intake. Although modest, these increases can have a metabolic effect and increase the one-carbon metabolic flux through some of the pathways of one-carbon metabolism, such as the methionine cycle (Chapter 3).

4. Differences in the Handling of Folic Acid versus Reduced Folates

Most of the folic acid from supplements or fortified foods is metabolized to reduced folates, primarily 5-methyl-THF, during its passage across the intestinal mucosa and/or first pass in the liver, and would behave identically to natural reduced folates. However, low levels of free folic acid are found in fasted plasma when the diet contains folic acid, and higher levels are present in nonfasted samples [83]. When pharmacological amounts of folic acid are taken, plasma levels of folic acid are initially very high [82]. As described above, the fate of plasma folic acid differs from 5-methyl-THF and other reduced folates because of differences in specificity for folate transmembrane transporters and the FR. Folic acid itself can be metabolized to short-chain retainable polyglutamates in mammalian tissues, but these derivatives would then be metabolized to reduced folates. Although concerns have been raised about the presence of this unnatural form of the vitamin in the circulation, there is no evidence currently available to suggest that it has any harmful effects unique to folic acid itself as opposed to high levels of other forms of the vitamin. It is possible that the extremely tight binding of folic acid to the FR could interfere with the transport of other folates that use the FR for entry into tissues.

Folic acid has to be reduced to DHF to enter the naturally occurring folate pool. This reduction, as well as its further reduction to THF, is catalyzed by DHF reductase [84]. DHF reductase evolved to reduce DHF to THF, and folic acid is a very poor substrate for this enzyme; thus, the initial reduction of folic acid to DHF is very slow compared with its further reduction to THF. Some bacterial DHF reductases will not reduce folic acid. Because of the poor substrate activity of folic acid, it would be predicted that folic acid use would be very sensitive to changes in the level of DHF reductase and to gene variants that influence DHF reductase activity. Recently, a fairly common 19-base pair deletion in the *DHFR* gene was shown to be associated with increased free folic acid in plasma and reduced RBC folate levels [83].

5. Vitamin B12 Deficiency

Tissue folate retention is also regulated by physiological and nutritional factors that affect the types of folate one-carbon derivatives that accumulate in tissues. In humans and experimental animals, vitamin B12 deficiency induces a secondary folate deficiency, and tissue levels of folate are reduced up to 60%. The interaction between the vitamins is best explained by the methyl trap hypothesis [3]. Vitamin B12 deficiency reduces the activity of methionine synthase, and a functional folate deficiency results because of accumulation of 5-methyl-THF polyglutamate, a substrate for methionine synthase, at the expense of other folate one-carbon forms, including THF polyglutamate [3,85]. The megaloblastic anemia that occurs in humans can be explained by a lack of folate coenzymes for DNA precursor synthesis in blood cells. The reduction in tissue levels of folate is caused by an impaired ability to retain folate rather than impaired tissue uptake of the vitamin [3]. The impaired retention of folate can be explained by the decreased level of THF under these conditions and the poor substrate activity of 5-methyl-THF for folylpolyglutamate synthetase, as well as the almost complete lack of substrate activity with polyglutamate forms of this compound.

High levels of methionine ameliorate some of the effects of vitamin B12 deficiency in experimental animals and correct abnormal hepatic folate metabolism in the rat. Methionine acts via *S*-adenosylmethionine, which inhibits methylene-THF reductase, the enzyme responsible for the synthesis of 5-methyl-THF [86]. *S*-Adenosylmethionine inhibition of this enzyme would slow the formation of 5-methyl-THF and its consequent "trapping" when methionine synthase activity is inhibited, thus slowing the synthesis of a very poor substrate for folylpolyglutamate synthetase.

In animals exposed to nitrous oxide, which inactivates methionine synthase, cytosolic folates are almost completely trapped as 5-methyl-THF polyglutamate [85]. Hepatic folate accumulation is reduced by up to 85% in the nitrous oxide–treated rat regardless of the type of folate administered, and all folates are trapped as 5-methyl-THF polyglutamate (S. Yoo and B. Shane, unpublished data).

V. TURNOVER AND EXCRETION

A. MECHANISM OF TURNOVER

Folylpolyglutamates turn over in mammalian cells and tissues, but the mechanism of turnover has not been well characterized. Hepatic folate stores turn over rapidly in rats fed a very high folate diet (half-life 1.5 days), whereas turnover is very slow in folate-depleted animals (S. Yoo and B. Shane, unpublished data), which may reflect an increased proportion of tissue folate bound to folate-binding proteins. Mitochondrial folate pools turn over at the same rate as cytosolic pools. The half-life of labeled folates, primarily folylpolyglutamates, in cultured cells is similar to the generation time of the cells when cells accumulate levels of folate that support normal rates of growth, whereas the half-life is reduced, indicative of folate efflux, when cells contain high levels of folate [52].

The major route of whole-body folate turnover appears to be via catabolism to cleavage products [87–89], and this occurs at a much slower rate than tissue turnover in humans with a half-life of 100 to 200 days, depending on folate intake [46,47]. This suggests that much of tissue turnover involves folate hydrolysis to monoglutamates with release of intact folates into the circulation followed by reuptake by tissues. Plasma clearance of folate in humans is rapid [47], reflecting uptake and reuptake into tissues rather than elimination from the body. After administration of a labeled folate dose to animals, a small amount of the dose is recovered as intact folate derivatives in urine in the first 24 to 48 hours. The bulk of the dose is recovered as pterin derivatives and N-acetamidobenzoyl-glutamate with a smaller amount of p-aminobenzoyl-glutamate [90]. These cleavage products account for the bulk of whole-body folate turnover in humans and experimental animals. It was thought that the initial step in folate catabolism involves the oxidative cleavage of intracellular folylpolyglutamates at the C9–N10 bond, presumably as a result of oxidative damage, and the resulting p-aminobenzoylpolyglutamates are hydrolyzed to the monoglutamate by lysosomal γ-GH, and the monoglutamate is N-acetylated in liver before excretion. Although this catabolic pathway was thought to be initiated by nonenzymatic cleavage of labile folate derivatives, recent studies have suggested that several enzyme-mediated systems may be involved in this process and that formyl derivatives of folate may be the immediate substrates for the cleavage reactions [91]. Metabolic conditions or manipulations that cause an accumulation of 5- or 10-formyl-THF polyglutamates result in increased folate catabolism. In addition, heavy chain ferritin has been demonstrated to cleave folates to pterin derivatives [92]. Metabolic conditions that influence the folate one-carbon distribution in tissues or ferritin levels may influence folate catabolism, and hence requirements.

B.   FOLATE EXCRETION

Folate is freely filtered at the glomerulus and is reabsorbed in the proximal renal tubule [93,94]. The net effect is that most of the secreted folate is reabsorbed. The renal clearance of folate derivatives is inversely proportional to their affinities for the folate-binding protein in the kidney proximal tubes [44]. Increased excretion of folate has been reported in alcoholic subjects, although it is unclear whether this reflects increased secretion or impaired reabsorption or whether this significantly depletes body stores of the vitamin [95]. As described above, although urine does contain some folate derivatives, the bulk of the excretion products in humans are folate cleavage products [87].

Biliary excretion of folate has been estimated at up to 100 μg/day in humans [35,93]. Much of this would be reabsorbed in the small intestine, but loss of folate via this route could be significant in malabsorption syndromes. Fecal folate excretion is variable and is not a measure of folate availability as a result of folate biosynthesis by the intestinal flora. The ability of this endogenously synthesized folate to contribute to folate stores in humans is not known. In experimental animals, sulfa drug treatment is required to produce a complete folate deficiency, and it has been demonstrated that bacterially synthesized folates contribute to hepatic folate stores, although the extent of this contribution has not be quantitated [96,97].

VI. SUMMARY

This chapter has summarized our current understanding of the mechanisms by which folate stores in tissues and in the body are regulated. During the past few years, considerable progress has been made in our understanding of the properties of the folate transporters responsible for folate influx into tissues, as well as on the mechanisms by which folate is metabolized and retained in tissues. Our understanding of potential defects in these processes under pathological conditions is more limited. The mechanisms governing folate turnover and excretion are still poorly understood.

ACKNOWLEDGMENTS

Some of the described studies were supported by National Institutes of Health Grant DK42033.

REFERENCES

1. Wills L. Treatment of "pernicious anemia of pregnancy" and "tropical anemia" with special reference to yeast extract as a curative agent. *BMJ* 1931; 1:1059–64.
2. Stokstad ELR. Historical perspective on key advances in the biochemistry and physiology of folates. In: Picciano MF, Stokstad ELR, Gregory JF, eds., *Contemporary Issues in Clinical Nutrition, vol. 13, Folic Acid Metabolism in Health and Disease.* New York: Wiley-Liss, 1990:1–21.
3. Shane B, Stokstad ELR. Vitamin B12-folate interrelationships. *Ann Rev Nutr* 1985; 5:115–41.
4. MRC Vitamin Study Research Group. Prevention of neural tube defects: Results of the Medical Research Council Vitamin Study. *Lancet* 1991; 338:131–37.
5. Mason JB, Dickstein A, Jacques PF, Haggarty P, Selhub J, Dallal G, Rosenberg IH. A temporal association between folic acid fortification and an increase in colorectal cancer rates may be illuminating important biological principles: A hypothesis. *Cancer Epidemiol Biomarkers Prev* 2007; 16:1325–29.
6. McGuire JJ, Coward JK. Pteroylpolyglutamates: Biosynthesis, degradation, and function. In: Blakley RL, Benkovic SJ, eds., *Folates and Pterins, vol. 1, Chemistry and Biochemistry of Folates.* New York: John Wiley & Sons, 1984:135–90.
7. Shane B. Folylpolyglutamate synthesis and role in the regulation of one carbon metabolism. *Vitam Horm* 1989; 45:263–335.
8. Gregory JF. Chemical and nutritional aspects of folate research: Analytical procedures, methods of folate synthesis, stability, and bioavailability of dietary folates. *Adv Food Nutr Res* 1989; 33:1–101.
9. Sirotnak FM, Tolner B. Carrier-mediated membrane transport of folates in mammalian cells. *Annu Rev Nutr* 1999; 19:91–122.
10. Zhao R, Matherly LH, Goldman ID. Membrane transporters and folate homeostasis: Intestinal absorption and transport into systemic compartments and tissues. *Expert Rev Mol Med* 2009; 11:e4, DOI: 10.1017/S1462399409000969.
11. Matherly LH, Goldman DI. Membrane transport of folates. *Vitam Horm* 2003; 66:403–56.

12. Matherly LH, Hou Z, Deng Y. Human reduced folate carrier: Translation of basic biology to cancer etiology and therapy. *Cancer Metastasis Rev* 2007; 26:111–28.

13. Sirotnak FM, Tolner B. Carrier-mediated membrane transport of folates in mammalian cells. *Annu Rev Nutr* 1999; 19:91–122.

14. Zhao R, Gao F, Goldman ID. Reduced folate carrier transports thiamine monophosphate: An alternative route for thiamine delivery into mammalian cells. *Am J Physiol Cell Physiol* 2002; 282:C1512–17.

15. Qiu A, Jansen M, Sakaris A, Min SH, Chattopadhyay S, Tsai E, Sandoval C, Zhao R, Akabas MH, Goldman ID. Identification of an intestinal folate transporter and the molecular basis for hereditary folate malabsorption. *Cell* 2006; 127:917–28.

16. Kruh GD, Belinsky MG. The MRP family of drug efflux pumps. *Oncogene* 2003; 22:7537–52.

17. Assaraf YG. The role of multidrug resistance efflux transporters in antifolate resistance and folate homeostasis. *Drug Resist Update* 2006; 9:227–46.

18. Titus SA, Moran RG. Retrovirally mediated complementation of the *glyB* phenotype. Cloning of a human gene encoding the carrier for entry of folates into mitochondria. *J Biol Chem* 2000; 47:36811–17.

19. Horne DW, Holloway RS, Said HM. Uptake of 5-formyltetrahydrofolate in isolated rat liver mitochondria is carrier-mediated. *J Nutr* 1992; 122:2204–09.

20. Kim J-S, Lowe KE, Shane B. Regulation of folate and one carbon metabolism in mammalian cells. 4. Role of folylpolyglutamate synthetase in antifolate metabolism and cytotoxicity. *J Biol Chem* 1993; 268:21680–85.

21. Lin BF, Shane B. Expression of *Escherichia coli* folylpolyglutamate synthetase in the Chinese hamster ovary cell mitochondrion. *J Biol Chem* 1994; 269:9705–13.

22. Barrueco JR, O'Leary DF, Sirotnak FM. Metabolic turnover of methotrexate polyglutamates in lysosomes derived from S180 cells. *J Biol Chem* 1992; 267:19986–91.

23. Kamen BA, Smith AK. A review of folate receptor alpha cycling and 5-methyltetrahydrofolate accumulation with an emphasis on cell models in vitro. *Adv Drug Deliv Rev* 2004; 56:1085–97.

24. Chancy CD, Kekuda R, Huang W, Prasad PD, Kuhnel JM, Sirotnak FM, Roon P, Ganapathy V, Smith SB. Expression and differential polarization of the reduced-folate transporter-1 and the folate receptor alpha in mammalian retinal pigment epithelium. *J Biol Chem* 2000; 275:20676–84.

25. Birn H, Selhub J, Christensen EI. Internalization and intracellular transport of folate-binding protein in rat kidney proximal tubule. *Am J Physiol* 1993; 264:C302–10.

26. Finnell RH. Embryonic development of folate binding protein-1 (Folbp1) knockout mice: Effects of the chemical form, dose, and timing of maternal folate supplementation. *Dev Dyn* 2004; 231:221–31.

27. Wagner C. Proteins binding pterins and folates. In: Blakley RL, Whitehead VM, eds., *Folates and Pterins, vol. 3, Nutritional, Pharmacological, and Physiological Aspects.* New York: John Wiley & Sons, 1986:251–96.

28. Lee H-C, Shoda R, Krall JA, Foster JD, Selhub J, Rosenberry TL. Folate binding protein from kidney brush border membranes contains components of a glycoinositol phospholipid anchor. *Biochemistry* 1992; 31:3236–43.

29. Weitman SD, Weinberg AG, Coney LR, Zarawski VR, Jennings DS, Kamen BA. Cellular localization of the folate receptor: Potential role in drug toxicity and folate homeostasis. *Cancer Res* 1992; 52:6708–11.

30. Sirotnak FM, Jacobsen DM, Yang C-H. Alteration of folate analogue transport following induced maturation of HL-60 leukemia cells. Early decline in mediated influx, relationship to commitment, and functional dissociation of entry and exit routes. *J Biol Chem* 1986; 261:11150–55.

31. Antony AC, Bruno E, Briddell RA, Brandt JE, Verma RS, Hoffman R. Effect of perturbation of specific folate receptors during in vitro erythropoiesis. *J Clin Invest* 1987; 80:1618–23.
32. Rothberg KG, Ying Y, Kolhouse JF, Kamen BA, Anderson RGW. The glycophospholipid-linked folate receptor internalizes folate without entering the clathrin-coated pit endocytic pathway. *J Cell Biol* 1990; 110:637–49.
33. Geller J, Kronn D, Jayabose S, Sandoval C. Hereditary folate malabsorption: Family report and review of the literature. *Medicine (Baltimore)* 2002; 81:51–68.
34. Devlin AM, Ling EH, Peerson JM, Fernando S, Clarke R, Smith AD, Halsted CH. Glutamate carboxypeptidase II: A polymorphism associated with lower levels of serum folate and hyperhomocysteinemia. *Hum Mol Genet* 2000; 9:2837–44.
35. Herbert V, Das KC. Folic acid and vitamin B12. In: Shils ME, Olson JA, Shike M, eds., *Modern Nutrition in Health and Disease*, 8th ed. Philadelphia: Lea and Febiger, 1994:402–25.
36. Zhao R, Min SH, Qiu A, Sakaris A, Goldberg GL, Sandoval C, Malatack JJ, Rosenblatt DS, Goldman ID. The spectrum of mutations in the PCFT gene, coding for an intestinal folate transporter, that are the basis for hereditary folate malabsorption. *Blood* 2007; 110:1147–52.
37. Rost D, Mahner S, Sugiyama Y, Stremmel W. Expression and localization of the multidrug resistance-associated protein 3 in rat small and large intestine. *Am J Physiol Gastrointest Liver Physiol* 2002; 282:G720–26.
38. Masuda M, I'izuka Y, Yamazaki M, Nishigaki R, Kato Y, Ni'inuma K, Suzuki H, Sugiyama Y. Methotrexate is excreted into the bile by canalicular multispecific organic anion transporter in rats. *Cancer Res* 1997; 57:3506–10.
39. Ratnam M, Freisheim JH. Proteins involved in the transport of folates and antifolates by normal and neoplastic cells. In: Picciano MF, Stokstad ELR, Gregory JF, eds., *Contemporary Issues in Clinical Nutrition, vol. 13, Folic Acid Metabolism in Health and Disease*. New York: Wiley-Liss, 1990:91–120.
40. Quinlivan EP, Davis SR, Shelnutt KP, Henderson GN, Ghandour H, Shane B, Selhub J, Bailey LB, Stacpoole PW, Gregory JF III. Methylene-tetrahydrofolate reductase 677C->T polymorphism and folate status affect one-carbon incorporation into human DNA deoxynucleosides. *J Nutr* 2005; 135:389–96.
41. Horne DW, Briggs WT, Wagner C. Transport of 5-methyltetrahydrofolic acid and folic acid in freshly isolated hepatocytes. *J Biol Chem* 1978; 253:3529–35.
42. Horne DW, Reed KA, Hoefs J, Said HM. 5-Methyltetrahydrofolic acid transport in basolateral membrane vesicles from human liver. *Am J Clin Nutr* 1993; 58:80–84.
43. Weitman SD, Frazier KM, Kamen BA. The folate receptor in central nervous system malignancies of childhood. *J Neurooncol* 1994; 21:107–12.
44. Selhub J, Emmanouel D, Stavropoulos T, Arnold R. Renal folate absorption and the kidney folate binding protein. *Am J Physiol* 1987; 252:F750–56.
45. Hoppner K, Lampi B. Folate levels in human liver from autopsies in Canada. *Am J Clin Nutr* 1980; 33:862–64.
46. von der Porten AE, Gregory JF, Toth JP, Cerda JJ, Curry SH, Bailey LB. In vivo folate kinetics during chronic supplementation of human subjects with deuterium-labeled folic acid. *J Nutr* 1992; 122:1293–99.
47. Lin Y, Dueker SR, Follett JR, Fadel JG, Arjomand A, Schneider PD, Miller JW, et al. Quantitation of in vivo folate metabolism. *Am J Clin Nutr* 2004; 80:690–91.
48. Lowe KE, Osborne CB, Lin B-F, Kim J-S, Hsu J-C, Shane B. Regulation of folate and one carbon metabolism in mammalian cells. 2. Effect of folylpolyglutamate synthetase substrate specificity and level on folate metabolism and folylpolyglutamate specificity of metabolic cycles of one carbon metabolism. *J Biol Chem* 1993; 268:21665–73.

49. Horne DW, Patterson D, Cook RJ. Effect of nitrous oxide inactivation of vitamin B12-dependent methionine synthetase on the subcellular distribution of folate coenzymes in rat liver. *Arch Biochem Biophys* 1989; 270:729–33.

50. Lin B-F, Huang R-FS, Shane B. Regulation of folate and one carbon metabolism in mammalian cells. 3. Role of mitochondrial folylpolyglutamate synthetase. *J Biol Chem* 1993; 268:21674–79.

51. Appling DR. Compartmentation of folate-mediated one-carbon metabolism in eukaryotes. *FASEB J* 1991; 5:2645–51.

52. Osborne CB, Lowe KE, Shane B. Regulation of folate and one carbon metabolism in mammalian cells. 1. Folate metabolism in Chinese hamster ovary cells expressing *Escherichia coli* or human folylpoly-g-glutamate synthetase activity. *J Biol Chem* 1993; 268:21657–64.

53. Moran RG, Colman PD. Measurement of folylpolyglutamate synthetase in mammalian tissues. *Anal Biochem* 1984; 140:326–42.

54. Chen L, Qi H, Korenberg J, Garrow TA, Choi YJ, Shane B. Purification and properties of human cytosolic folylpoly-γ-glutamate synthetase and organization, localization, and differential splicing of its gene. *J Biol Chem* 1996; 271:13077–87.

55. Freemantle SJ, Taylor SM, Krystal G, Moran RG. Upstream organization of and multiple transcripts from the human folylpoly-γ-glutamate synthetase gene. *J Biol Chem* 1995; 270:9579–84.

56. Qi H, Atkinson I, Xiao S, Choi Y-J, Tobimatsu T, Shane B. Folylpoly-γ-glutamate synthetase: Generation of isozymes and role in one carbon metabolism and antifolate cytotoxicity. *Adv Enz Reg* 1999; 39:263–73.

57. Cichowicz DJ, Shane B. Mammalian folylpoly-γ-glutamate synthetase. 2. Substrate specificity and kinetic properties. *Biochemistry* 1987; 26:513–21.

58. Cook JD, Cichowicz DJ, George S, Lawler A, Shane B. Mammalian folylpoly-γ-glutamate synthetase. 4. In vitro and in vivo metabolism of folates and analogues and regulation of folate homeostasis. *Biochemistry* 1987; 26:530–39.

59. McGuire JJ, Hsieh P, Coward JK, Bertino JR. Enzymatic synthesis of folylpoly-glutamates. Characterization of the reaction and its products. *J Biol Chem* 1980; 255:5776–88.

60. Moran RG, Colman PD. Mammalian folylpolyglutamate synthetase: Partial purification and properties of the mouse liver enzyme. *Biochemistry* 1984; 23:4580–89.

61. George S, Cichowicz DJ, Shane B. Mammalian folylpoly-γ-glutamate synthetase. 3. Specificity for folate analogues. *Biochemistry* 1987; 26:522–29.

62. Wittwer AJ, Wagner C. Identification of the folate-binding proteins of rat liver mitochondria as dimethylglycine dehydrogenase and sarcosine dehydrogenase. Purification and folate-binding characteristics. *J Biol Chem* 1981; 256:4102–08.

63. Cook RJ, Wagner C. Glycine-*N*-methyltransferase is a folate binding protein of rat liver cytosol. *Proc Natl Acad Sci USA* 1984; 81:3631–34.

64. Wagner C, Briggs WT, Cook RJ. Inhibition of glycine N-methyltransferase activity by folate derivatives: Implications for regulation of methyl group metabolism. *Biochem Biophys Res Commun* 1985; 127:746–52.

65. Min H, Shane B, Stokstad ELR. Identification of 10-formyl-tetrahydrofolate dehydrogenase-hydrolase as a major folate binding protein in liver cytosol. *Biochim Biophys Acta* 1988; 967:348–53.

66. Schirch L. Folates in serine and glycine metabolism. In: Blakley RL, Benkovic SJ, eds., *Folates and Pterins, vol. 1, Chemistry and Biochemistry of Folates*. New York: John Wiley & Sons, 1984:399–432.

67. Zamierowski MM, Wagner C. Effect of folacin deficiency on folacin-binding proteins in the rat. *J Nutr* 1977; 107:1937–45.

68. Nijhout HF, Reed MC, Ulrich CM. Mathematical models of folate-mediated one-carbon metabolism. *Vitam Horm* 2008; 79:45–82.

69. Reed MC, Nijhout HF, Neuhouser, ML, Gregory JF III, Shane B, James SJ, Boynton A, Ulrich CM. A mathematical model gives insights into nutritional and genetic aspects of folate-mediated one-carbon metabolism. *J Nutr* 2006; 136:2653–61.
70. Whitehead VM, Kalman TI, Vuchich M-J. Inhibition of gamma-glutamyl hydrolases in human cells by 2-mercaptomethylglutaric acid. *Biochem Biophys Res Commun* 1987; 144:292–97.
71. Rhee MS, Wang Y, Nair MG, Galivan J. Acquisition of resistance to antifolates caused by enhanced g-glutamyl hydrolase activity. *Cancer Res* 1993; 53:1–3.
72. O'Conner BM, Rotundo RF, Nimec Z, McGuire JM, Galivan J. Secretion of g-glutamyl hydrolase in vitro. *Cancer Res* 1991; 51:3874–81.
73. Fort DW, Lark RH, Smith AK, Marling-Cason M, Weitman SD, Shane B, Kamen BA. Accumulation of 5-methyltetrahydrofolic acid and folylpolyglutamate synthetase expression by mitogen stimulated human lymphocytes. *Br J Haematol* 1993; 84:595–601.
74. Galivan J, Nimec Z, Balinska M. Regulation of methotrexate polyglutamate accumulation in vitro: Effects of cellular folate content. *Biochem Pharm* 1983; 32:3244–47.
75. Egan MG, Sirlin S, Rumberger BG, Shane B, Sirotnak FM. Decreasing levels of folylpolyglutamate synthetase gene expression during induction of differentiation of HL-60 cells. *Proc Am Assoc Cancer Res* 1993; 34:275.
76. Pizzorno GP, Mini E, Coronella M, McGuire JJ, Moroson BA, Cashmore AR, Dreyer RN, et al. Impaired polyglutamylation of methotrexate as a cause of resistance in CCRF-CEM cells after short-term, high-dose treatment with this drug. *Cancer Res* 1988; 48:2149–55.
77. McCloskey DE, McGuire JJ, Russell CA, Rowan BG, Bertino JR, Pizzorno G, Mini E. Decreased folylpolyglutamate synthetase activity as a mechanism of methotrexate resistance in CCRF-CEM human leukemia sublines. *J Biol Chem* 1991; 266:6181–87.
78. Pizzorno G, Chang Y-M, McGuire JJ, Bertino JR. Inherent resistance of human squamous carcinoma cell lines to methotrexate as a result of decreased polyglutamylation of this drug. *Cancer Res* 1989; 49:5275–80.
79. Cassady IA, Budge MM, Healy MJ, Nixon PF. An inverse relationship of rat liver folate polyglutamate chain length to nutritional folate sufficiency. *Biochim Biophys Acta* 1980; 633:258–68.
80. Matthews RG. Methionine biosynthesis. In: Blakley RL, Benkovic SJ, eds., *Folates and Pterins, vol. 1, Chemistry and Biochemistry of Folates*. New York: John Wiley & Sons, 1984:497–554.
81. Clifford AJ, Heid MK, Muller HG, Bills ND. Tissue distribution and prediction of total body folate of rats. *J Nutr* 1990; 120:1633–39.
82. Houghton JA, Williams LG, de Graaf SS, Cheshire PJ, Rodman JH, Maneval DC, Wainer IW, Jadaud P, Houghton PJ. Relationship between dose rate of [6RS]Leucovorin administration, plasma concentrations of reduced folates, and pools of 5,10-methylenetetrahydrofolates and tetrahydrofolates in human colon adenocarcinoma xenografts. *Cancer Res* 1990; 50:3493–502.
83. Kalmbach RD, Choumenkovitch SF, Troen AP, Jacques PF, D'Agostino R, Selhub J. A 19-base pair deletion polymorphism in dihydrofolate reductase is associated with increased unmetabolized folic acid in plasma and decreased red blood cell folate. *J Nutr* 2008; 138:2323–27.
84. Blakley RL. Dihydrofolate reductase. In: Blakley RL, Benkovic SJ, eds., *Folates and Pterins, vol. 1, Chemistry and Biochemistry of Folates*. New York: Wiley, 1984: 191–244.
85. Wilson SD, Horne DW. Effect of nitrous oxide inactivation of vitamin B12 on the levels of folate coenzymes in rat bone marrow, kidney, brain, and liver. *Arch Biochem Biophys* 1986; 244:248–53.

86. Kutzbach C, Stokstad ELR. Mammalian methylenetetrahydrofolate reductase. Partial purification, properties, and inhibition by S-adenosylmethionine. *Biochem Biophys Acta* 1971; 250:459–77.
87. Scott JM. Catabolism of folates. In: Blakley RL, Benkovic SJ, eds., *Folates and Pterins, vol. 1, Chemistry and Biochemistry of Folates.* New York: John Wiley & Sons, 1984:307–27.
88. McNulty H, McPartlin JM, Weir DG, Scott JM. Folate catabolism is increased during pregnancy in rats. *J Nutr* 1993; 123:1089–93.
89. Suh JR, Herbig AK, Stover PJ. New perspectives on folate catabolism. *Annu Rev Nutr* 2001; 21:255–82.
90. Murphy M, Keating M, Boyle P, Weir DG, Scott JM. The elucidation of the mechanism of folate catabolism in the rat. *Biochem Biophys Res Commun* 1976; 71:1017–24.
91. Anguera MC, Field MS, Perry C, Ghandour H, Chiang E-P, Selhub J, Shane B, Stover PJ. Regulation of folate-mediated one-carbon metabolism by 10-formyltetrahydrofolate dehydrogenase. *J Biol Chem* 2006; 281:18335–42.
92. Suh JR, Oppenheim EW, Girgis S, Stover PJ. Purification and properties of a folate-catabolizing enzyme. *J Biol Chem* 2000; 275:35646–55.
93. Whitehead VM. Pharmacokinetics and physiological disposition of folate and its derivatives. In: Blakley RL, Whitehead VM, eds., *Folates and Pterins, vol. 3, Nutritional, Pharmacological, and Physiological Aspects.* New York: John Wiley & Sons, 1986:177–205.
94. Williams WM, Huang KC. Renal tubular transport of folic acid and methotrexate in the monkey. *Am J Physiol* 1982; 242:F484–90.
95. Eisenga BH, Collins TD, McMartin KE. Effect of acute ethanol on urinary excretion of 5-methyltetrahydrofolic acid and folate derivatives in the rat. *J Nutr* 1989; 119:1498–505.
96. Camilo E, Zimmerman J, Mason JB, Golner B, Russell R, Selhub J, Rosenberg IH. Folate synthesized by bacteria in the human upper small intestine is assimilated by the host. *Gastroenterology* 1996; 110:991–98.
97. Rong N, Selhub J, Goldin BR, Rosenberg IH. Bacterially synthesized folate in rat large intestine is incorporated into host tissue folyl polyglutamates. *J Nutr* 1991; 121:1955–59.

2 Folate Bioavailability

Helene McNulty and Kristina Pentieva

CONTENTS

I. INTRODUCTION

Bioavailability can be defined as the proportion of an ingested nutrient that is absorbed and becomes available for metabolic processes or storage. Natural food folates are a mixture of reduced forms of the vitamin, typically involving one-carbon substitution of the pteridine ring (most predominantly 5-methyltetrahydrofolate [5-methyl-THF]) and usually in the polyglutamylated form containing a variable number of glutamate residues. The synthetic form, folic acid, is a monoglutamate found in the human diet only in fortified foods and supplements. Whereas natural food folates are labile and prone to oxidative cleavage at the C9-N10 bond [1], folic acid is a fully oxidized molecule and as such is stable and relatively resistant to destruction [2]. These structural differences have a major impact on folate bioavailability, and there is widespread agreement that the bioavailability of folates from natural food sources is incomplete when compared with folic acid. However, published estimates from controlled long-term feeding trials of the extent of lower bioavailability of food folates compared with folic acid (relative bioavailability) vary greatly, ranging between 30% and 98% [3–7]. Thus, there remains uncertainty regarding folate bioavailability [8] and controversy regarding the extent to which the bioavailability of folate from natural food sources is reduced relative to folic acid.

Folate bioavailability is a concern for policy makers. Incomplete bioavailability of food folates can hinder the achievement of optimal folate status, a current priority for public health, and particularly so in populations with limited or no access to fortified foods. The bioavailability of food folates is also a consideration for those with the task of revising dietary folate recommendations, specifically with reference to expressing recommended intakes in terms of dietary folate equivalents (DFEs) [9]. In countries taking this approach, the DFE is defined as the quantity of natural food folate plus 1.7 times the quantity of folic acid in the diet. Meaningful estimates of relative bioavailability of food folate are necessary to confirm the robustness of the DFE value.

This chapter considers the many factors that potentially contribute to the bioavailability of different folate forms. The various experimental approaches for investigating folate bioavailability, their main findings, and study limitations are reviewed. The priorities and challenges for future bioavailability studies are also considered.

II. FACTORS INFLUENCING THE BIOAVAILABILITY OF FOOD FOLATES

The bioavailability of folates from various foods is considered to be dependent on a number of potential factors, including intestinal hydrolysis of polyglutamyl folates, the extent of conjugation of food folate sources, folate absorption in the small and large intestine, the food matrix, the instability of certain labile folates during digestion (or before ingestion), and the presence of certain dietary constituents that may enhance folate stability during digestion (Table 2.1).

A. INTESTINAL HYDROLYSIS OF POLYGLUTAMYL FOLATES

Dietary folates exist predominantly in the polyglutamyl form containing up to seven glutamate residues. Approximately two-thirds of total folate intake from a mixed unfortified diet is estimated to be in the polyglutamyl form, derived mainly from vegetables [10,11]. The intestinal absorption of dietary folates is a two-step process that involves the hydrolysis of folate polyglutamates to the corresponding monoglutamyl derivatives followed by their transport through the intestinal membranes into the enterocyte (Figure 2.1).

Hydrolysis of the polyglutamyl chain is an obligatory step in folate absorption because only monoglutamyl forms are able to cross cell membranes. The hydrolysis of polyglutamyl folates occurs in the proximal part of the jejunum with the

TABLE 2.1

Factors Considered to Influence the Bioavailability of Food Folates

1. Intestinal Factors

Hydrolysis of Polyglutamyl Folates

- pH of jejunum
- Organic acids
- Nucleic acids
- Heat-activated inhibitors (pulses)
- Drugs (diphenylhydantoin, salicylazosulfapyridine)
- Alcohol
- Disease (atrophic gastritis, celiac sprue)
- GCPII polymorphism

Folate Absorption in the Small Intestine

- pH of jejunum
- Disease (atrophic gastritis)
- Age
- Dietary intake of folate
- Food components (tea catechins)
- Mutations in the transporter protein genes

2. Food Matrix
- Mechanical processing of foods
- Dietary fiber
- Ingestion with other foods

3. Chemical Instability of Folates
- Losses during cooking
- Losses during intestinal digestion
- Stabilizing food ingredients (ascorbic acid, folate-binding protein)

4. Other Factors
- Gender
- Ethnicity
- Polymorphisms in genes involved in folate metabolism

involvement of the brush-border enzyme glutamate carboxypeptidase II (GCPII; EC 3.4.17.21), previously also known as folate hydrolase, folylpolyglutamate hydrolase, pteroylpolyglutamate hydrolase, or pteroylpoly-γ-glutamate carboxypeptidase. The enzyme is a transmembrane glycoprotein expressed in pig and human small intestine (predominantly in the proximal jejunum). It acts as an exopeptidase, cleaving terminal γ-linked glutamate residues from polyglutamyl folates in a progressive stepwise way to release folates with different glutamate chain lengths [12,13]. GCPII has an optimal pH of 6.5 [12], and studies have shown that the maintenance of this optimal

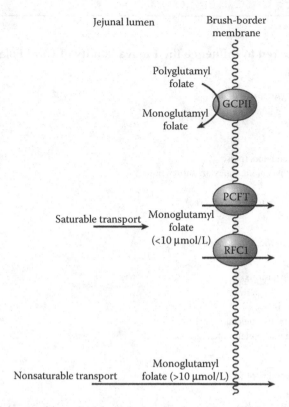

FIGURE 2.1 Scheme of intestinal hydrolysis and absorption of folate. GCPII, glutamate carboxypeptidase II; PCFT, proton coupled folate transporter; RFC1, reduced folate carrier. (Adapted from Alemdaroglu NC, et al., *Biopharm Drug Dispos* 2008; 29:335–48.)

pH is critical for the complete deconjugation of polyglutamyl folates in the jejunum [12,14].

Tamura et al. [14] found a marked reduction in the bioavailability of heptaglutamyl folate compared with monoglutamyl folate ingested simultaneously with orange juice at a pH of 3.7, whereas the bioavailability was found to be similar for the two folate forms when the pH of the mixture was increased to 6.8. Thus, gastrointestinal diseases that alter the pH of the intestinal lumen, such as atrophic gastritis, have the potential to impair the hydrolysis of polyglutamyl folates. However, jejunal perfusion studies with labeled mono- and polyglutamyl folates have not shown any differences in the disappearance from the intestinal lumen of the two folate forms and no detectable difference in the activity of GCPII between younger and older subjects [15], although atrophic gastritis is much more common in older adults. It is possible, therefore, that GCPII activity is influenced only under extreme circumstances, such as the ingestion of unusually high portion sizes of acidic/alkaline foods or pathological conditions that provoke a change in the jejunal pH milieu.

Some food components and certain drugs have been reported to act as inhibitors of GCPII activity. Studies with stable isotopes in humans [16] and in vitro experiments with porcine jejunal brush-border membrane [17] indicate that organic acid ions (citrate, malate, ascorbate, and phytate) present in orange juice have a combined inhibitory effect on the activity of GCPII. Nucleic acids in yeast ingested in large doses were also reported to decrease the activity of GCPII [18]. A naturally occurring heat-activated GCPII inhibitor in the skin of various pulses was also reported [19]; however, later bioavailability studies in humans did not detect any effect of beans on the use of heptaglutamates [20]. There is also evidence that some drugs (e.g., salicylazosulfapyridine) [21] and ethanol [22] competitively inhibit GCPII, whereas the effect on GCPII activity of other drugs reported to impair folate status, such as anticonvulsants, is unclear [23].

Recently a polymorphism (1561C→T) in the gene encoding GCPII has been identified, and in vitro studies found that COS-7 cells expressing the mutant variant had 53% lower GCPII enzyme activity than cells with the wild genotype [24]. However, the frequency of the homozygous mutant genotype for this polymorphism in the general population is very low (0.6%), and its in vivo effects on dietary folate digestion and folate status remain unclear because various human studies have shown contradictory results [24–29]. Another polymorphism in the *GCPII* gene, the 484A→G mutation, is much more common (47.6% of the general population are carriers for the G allele) and has been associated with only a slight increase in plasma homocysteine concentrations and no significant effect on blood folate concentrations [29]. Thus, there is no convincing evidence that polymorphisms in the *GCPII* gene influence folate bioavailability in humans to any significant degree.

Marked differences have been reported in the activity of intestinal GCPII among different animal species. A high GCPII activity was found in humans and pigs, whereas very low or no enzyme activity was detected in rats and monkeys [30]. There is evidence that in species without intestinal GCPII activity (i.e., rats), the main route for hydrolysis of dietary folates is through pancreatic γ-glutamyl hydrolase (γ-GH; EC 3.4.19.9) [31,32], another enzyme present in the small intestine. Like GCPII, γ-GH is capable of hydrolyzing polyglutamyl folates, but the two enzymes have very different characteristics [33–35]. However, the role of γ-GH in the intestinal digestion of dietary folates in humans is unknown [33].

B. THE EXTENT OF CONJUGATION OF FOOD FOLATES

The question of whether polyglutamyl folates are less bioavailable than monoglutamyl folates (i.e., in the absence of specific inhibitors of GCPII) is a controversial aspect of folate bioavailability [36]. This specific issue has been explored in different studies using various approaches with inconsistent results. Earlier acute studies [20,37,38], together with two recent chronic studies [39,40], all using synthetic folate forms, indicated that the bioavailability of polyglutamyl folate was 50% to 80% lower than that of monoglutamyl folate. In contrast, no difference in the bioavailability of monoglutamyl and polyglutamyl folates was reported by researchers in acute studies using unlabeled [41] and labeled [16,42,43] synthetic folates. Such findings, suggesting that folate polyglutamates are not inherently less bioavailable than monoglutamates, are supported by the results of studies that have compared monoglutamyl and polyglutamyl folates in their natural forms. In an acute study of ileostomy subjects, Konings et al. [44] reported similar bioavailability for spinach containing 60% polyglutamate and spinach pretreated before ingestion to convert all folates to the monoglutamate form. Likewise, results from a randomized cross-over trial in our laboratory, using an area-under-the-curve (AUC) protocol to measure intestinal absorption, showed no difference in the bioavailability of folate from three representative food folate sources (egg yolk, spinach, and yeast) with a measured polyglutamyl folate content of 0%, 50%, and 100% [45]. An earlier 30-day controlled feeding trial from our laboratory with two natural food folate sources, spinach (50% polyglutamate) and yeast (100% polyglutamate), had also failed to provide any evidence to support the view that the extent of glutamylation per se is a factor that limits the bioavailability of folates from natural food sources [46]. In fact, evidence reported much earlier by Reisenauer and Halsted [47] indicated that the activity of human intestinal GCPII exceeded the demands for hydrolysis of polyglutamyl folates within the range of dietary intake and, therefore, was not rate limiting in the absorption process under normal circumstances (e.g., absence of specific inhibitors of GCPII or any food matrix effect). The disagreement in the findings of the various studies in this area is most likely related to differences in the protocols used and to problems with accurate measurement of the folate treatment dose [36]. The relevant question in relation to the mixed diet is whether naturally occurring monoglutamyl folates are inherently more bioavailable than naturally occurring polyglutamyl folates. In our view, the balance of evidence would appear to suggest that they are not.

C.   FOLATE ABSORPTION IN THE SMALL INTESTINE

Folate monoglutamates are absorbed in the intestine through saturable and nonsaturable transport mechanisms. The saturable transport operates at the dietary range of folate intake (concentrations <10 μmol/L) mainly in the duodenum and upper jejunum [48]. It is a carrier-mediated process with a pH optimum within the mildly acidic range (pH 6.0) [49]. In addition, evidence shows that oxidized and reduced folates are transported with similar affinity [50], with several studies (both acute and chronic) specifically addressing the comparative bioavailability in humans of folic acid and reduced folate forms as discussed below. Reduced folate carrier (RFC1) and the recently identified proton coupled folate transporter (PCFT) reported by Qui et al. [51] are considered to be the transmembrane proteins involved in this process. The exact mechanism of folate transport through the intestine is not known, but evidence suggests that PCFT plays a primary role because it is functionally expressed in the apical brush border of duodenum and jejunum (the principal sites of folate absorption) and has characteristics consistent with the requirements for folate transport (acidic pH optimum, high and similar affinity for folic acid and reduced folates) [52]. In addition, mutations in the gene encoding the PCFT are reported to be associated with the rare autosomal recessive disorder characterized by severe folate deficiency, hereditary folate malabsorption [53].

Information on the factors that potentially influence folate absorption is limited. In vitro and in vivo perfusion studies have shown that slight deviations from the mildly acidic pH in the jejunum result in decreased folate transport [54]. Low intestinal absorption of folate was also reported in people suffering from atrophic gastritis with hypochlorhydria [55] and in users of antacid drugs [56]. Conversely, an increased rate of folate absorption was reported in patients with pancreatic insufficiency compared with healthy controls, which was related to the maintenance of an acidic environment in the duodenum and jejunum resulting from impaired production of alkaline pancreatic juice [57]. Changes in the pH of the jejunum probably impact the carrier protein PCFT, which operates within a mildly acidic pH, but as yet there is no direct evidence for this assumption.

There are conflicting data regarding the effect of age on monoglutamyl folate absorption. One investigation found no difference in the luminal disappearance of labeled folic acid between younger and older adults [15]. In contrast, a more recent study reported a 20% lower folate absorption (calculated by kinetic modeling based on plasma folate concentrations recorded for 6 hours) in subjects aged ≥50 years compared with younger adults [58].

Some evidence indicates that fluctuations in dietary folate intake influence the rate of folate absorption. Studies with rats and in vitro experiments with human intestinal cell lines have shown that folate deficiency results in significant and specific up-regulation of transepithelial transport of folate because of an induction of carrier-mediated folate uptake [59,60]. Furthermore, human-derived intestinal cells maintained for five generations in a high folic acid growth medium (100 μmol/L) showed down-regulation in intestinal folate uptake together with a reduction in expressions of the carrier proteins RFC1 and PCFT compared with cells grown under folate-sufficient conditions [61]. The adaptive regulation of intestinal uptake according to the provision of a nutrient is known to exist for some other micronutrients such as iron [62]; however, in vivo human studies are needed to confirm the relevance of such a mechanism in relation to folate absorption.

There are also reports that certain foods can influence folate absorption. For example, green and black tea extract coadministered with an oral folic acid dose of 400 μg have been found to reduce, by 26.6% and 17.9%, respectively, the AUC of serum folate response monitored for 8 hours [63]. Likewise, an in vitro study provided evidence of reduced folate uptake in intestinal cell lines incubated with tea catechins and crude tea extracts [64]. The authors speculated that their observations might be the result of suppression of the active folate transport system in the intestine by tea extract; however, it is also possible that an interaction between folate and some component of tea makes folate less available for absorption.

A nonsaturable transport of folate functions at concentrations of folate within the supraphysiological and pharmacological range of intake (>10 μmol/L), occurring in the ileum without the involvement of any specific transporter [65]. There are no data showing that nonsaturable transport is affected by any dietary or physiological factors; thus, it is considered an important route for folate absorption in patients with impaired saturable transport (e.g., hereditary folate malabsorption, celiac disease).

D. Folate Absorption in the Large Intestine

Another potential source of folate is that produced by microorganisms in the large intestine. A considerable folate pool is reported to exist in the colon of different species, including rats [66], piglets [67], and human infants. The predominant derivative in the folate pool in piglets and infants was shown to be 5-methyl-THF, of which 30% to 50% is in the monoglutamate form [67]. Studies using [^{3}H]*para*-aminobenzoic acid (a precursor for folate synthesis by colonic microorganisms) injected into the cecum of rats and piglets found that 6.9% and 12.6%, respectively, of bacterially synthesized folate was absorbed in the large intestine and incorporated into animal tissues [66,68]. Direct evidence for the absorption of folate across the large intestine in humans was provided for the first time by a recent study in subjects infused with a physiological dose of stable folate isotope during colonoscopy [69]. Based on the appearance of the labeled derivative 5-methyl-THF in plasma, the authors estimated that the amount of folate absorbed in the colon accounted for 5% of the average folate requirement for healthy adults [69]. This new evidence is generally consistent with the results from an earlier epidemiological study showing a positive relationship between serum folate concentrations in young women and the level of consumption of soluble fiber (a dietary component that increases the amount of fermentable substrate and microbial growth in the colon) [70]. It is reasonable to assume that folate absorbed through the colon has the potential to influence folate status in humans.

E. THE FOOD MATRIX AND RELATED FACTORS

Because folates are covalently bound to macromolecules in foods, the food matrix as a whole and its components can also influence folate bioavailability through entrapment of folate in the matrix, thereby hindering diffusion to the absorptive surface during digestion. Thus, incomplete release from plant cellular structure may be a factor influencing folate bioavailability from plant foods. Two independent studies demonstrated that folate bioavailability from minced, chopped, or enzymatically liquefied spinach was higher than that from whole spinach leaves when equal amounts of spinach folates were provided to human volunteers [71,72]. The effects of wheat bran and dietary fiber on folate bioavailability were explored in various acute and chronic studies in humans, but the results are inconsistent [20,42,72]. In vitro studies with intestinal brush-border membrane vesicles indicated that dietary fiber did not affect the activity of GCPII [71].

Apart from any food matrix effect, the presence of other foods in the intestinal milieu may inhibit folate absorption. For example, Pfeiffer et al. [74] reported a small reduction (15%) in the absorption of [^{13}C5]folic acid when administered after a light breakfast meal compared with the absorption rate when administered without food.

F. CHEMICAL STABILITY OF FOOD FOLATES

Unlike folic acid, which is a fully oxidized molecule, natural folates are a mixture of reduced forms that are structurally labile and prone to oxidative cleavage at the C9-N10 bond [1]. One consequence is that extensive losses of folate can occur during cooking and preparation of foods, considerably reducing the folate content of a food before it is even ingested. Folate losses in the range of 50% to 80% were reported in green vegetables after boiling [75–78] and in processed legumes [79]. In addition to such losses, in vitro studies mimicking the intestinal digestion of folates from various foods [80] suggest that the instability of certain labile food folates after they are ingested may be considerable. Thus, the instability of labile folate species in vivo may be an important factor contributing to the incomplete bioavailability of natural food folates.

Conversely, the presence of some dietary constituents such as ascorbic acid and components of milk may enhance folate bioavailability by increasing the stability of food folates during food processing and during digestion in the gastrointestinal tract [81,82]. Consistent with the findings that folate-binding protein stabilizes tetrahydrofolates in vitro [83], one recent study provided evidence that the inclusion of cow's milk in the diet of healthy women for 8 weeks enhanced the bioavailability of food folate as assessed by red blood cell (RBC) folate and plasma homocysteine responses [84].

G. OTHER POTENTIAL FACTORS AFFECTING FOLATE BIOAVAILABILITY

Long-term interventions with doses of folic acid in the range of 50 µg to 800 µg indicated that the RBC folate response was 5% to 10% less in men than in women [85]. These findings are in general agreement with the results of a meta-analysis of homocysteine lowering in response to intervention with folic acid, where the homocysteine response was significantly greater in women than in men [86]. The mechanism for such gender differences is unclear, but it may relate to differences in body size [85].

Factors such as ethnicity and race are reported to be important determinants of folate status. A recent chronic intervention study showed that under strictly controlled folate intake of 400 and 800 µg DFE/day, blood folate concentrations and urinary folate excretion were consistently lower in African American women than in white and Mexican American women [87]. The mechanism for this ethnic/racial effect is unknown but probably relates to differences in the frequencies of polymorphisms in genes involved in regulating folate absorption or metabolism. For example, the common 677C→T variant in the methylenetetrahydrofolate reductase (*MTHFR*) gene is known to impair folate metabolism in vivo. Homozygous individuals (TT genotype, the frequency of which varies from 3% to 32% in populations worldwide) [88] have reduced MTHFR activity, resulting in elevated homocysteine concentrations [89]. They also have lower RBC folate concentrations, suggesting that the dietary folate requirement may be somewhat higher in individuals with this genetic predisposition [90].

III. EXPERIMENTAL APPROACHES TO FOLATE BIOAVAILABILITY AND THEIR FINDINGS

Acute and chronic protocols have been used to study folate bioavailability. They involve the administration of reduced folates either in the form of foods or commercial preparations corresponding to the major food folate forms (usually 5-methyl-THF). Typically the bioavailability of natural folates is compared with that of folic acid because the latter is assumed to be highly bioavailable.

A. ACUTE STUDIES

The protocol used in acute folate bioavailability studies is similar to that used in studies testing the pharmacokinetics of drugs. In most cases, in a crossover or parallel design, a single reference dose of natural folates or folic acid is administered to humans, and the changes in blood and/or urinary folate concentrations are monitored at various time points. The responses between the different treatments can then be compared by calculating AUC for plasma/serum folate and urinary folate responses, the maximal plasma/serum folate concentration (C_{max}), and the time required to achieve C_{max}. Acute studies may be divided into those that have used labeled or unlabeled folates.

1. Acute Studies with Unlabeled Folates

Findings from early nonisotopic acute studies using folate compounds in the physiological range of intake are varied. Perry and Chanarin [91] and Brown et al. [92] demonstrated higher serum responses to reduced folates compared with folic acid, whereas Tamura and Stokstad [41] did not report significant differences between natural folate forms and folic acid based on 24-hour urinary folate excretion. However, the validity of these results may be questioned given the lack of placebo treatment and the fact that the period of monitoring (2–3 hours) was insufficient to quantify the full plasma folate response [91,92]. In a later acute study using a very extended period of blood folate monitoring (3 days) and a much higher folate dose (1,000 μg), the bioavailability of 5-formyl-THF and folic acid was found to be similar based on AUC for plasma folate response to treatment [93]. Likewise, findings from a more recent study from our laboratory indicated equivalent bioavailability for 5-methyl-THF and folic acid based on the plasma folate response measured for a 10-hour period and using a lower folate dose of 500 μg [94].

The bioavailability of folate from different foods has also been explored using acute protocols. In early studies by Tamura and Stokstad [41], estimates of folate bioavailability varied considerably based on urinary folate excretion measured up to 24 hours after the consumption of 12 different food items. Of the food items studied, bananas and lima beans were reported to contain highly bioavailable folates (82%–96% relative to folic acid), whereas the bioavailability of folates from other foods such as romaine lettuce, orange juice, cabbage, soybean meal, and wheat germ was much lower (25%–47%). In more recent studies based on serum folate responses (AUC), the bioavailability of folate from wheat aleurone flour [95] and from spinach [44] was found to be similar to that of folic acid provided as a tablet. The reported differences in folate bioavailability between studies are probably the result of differences in the protocols used, together with any inherent differences between the foods administered, including the food matrices and other potential factors influencing folate bioavailability (e.g., GCPII inhibitors, pH).

When reviewing or designing nonisotopic acute studies, a number of important methodological considerations that have been described comprehensively by others [8,96,97] should be considered. They include the administration of a folate dose that is sufficiently high to elicit measurable folate responses in blood or urine (but not so high as to exceed the physiologically relevant range); the use of a folate presaturation protocol (otherwise, the ingested dose may be preferentially directed toward depleted folate pools); sufficient monitoring (in terms of both frequency and duration, usually over 8 hours) of the folate response after ingestion of the test dose to ensure that the peak response is not missed, as well as to allow sufficient time for folate concentrations to return to baseline values; a sufficient sample size for statistical power given the variability in the folate response; avoidance of fasting, which may provoke an increase in plasma folate concentrations by interrupting the enterohepatic folate circulation; strict control of dietary folate intake during the treatment period; and the inclusion of a placebo group to control for any changes in folate measurements as a result of the study conditions.

2. Acute Studies with Labeled Folates

Isotopic studies, which became particularly attractive after the introduction of stable isotope folate forms (which are considered safe for human use), offer the advantage of high specificity because the only source of labeled folate detected in the blood/ urine is the ingested folate isotope [8]. However, most stable isotope folate forms are not commercially available and need to be synthesized and purified by the investigators [98,99]. The methodological requirements for stable isotope folate studies have been reviewed elsewhere [100,101].

In general, the results of these studies suggest differential bioavailability of folic acid compared with reduced derivatives. However, recent isotopic studies by Wright et al. [102,103] raise questions regarding the validity of comparing responses to orally administered reduced folates with a reference dose of folic acid in acute bioavailability protocols. These authors examined the rate and extent of appearance of labeled and unlabeled folates in plasma following oral doses of folic acid, 5-formyl-THF, or intrinsically labeled spinach folates and showed a marked difference in the absorption of folic acid versus the natural folates. However, all forms caused an increase in unlabeled plasma folate, and the extent of this phenomenon differed between folic acid and the natural folates, leading the authors to conclude that there was a different hepatic first-pass effect between folic acid and the reduced folate forms. In addition, the investigators indicated that this was a potential limitation in interpreting the results of acute studies that have used folic acid as the reference treatment [102,103]. Newer methodology based on accelerator mass spectrometry (AMS) may potentially overcome this experimental problem. In contrast to traditional nonlabeled and stable isotope protocols requiring the use of folic acid doses greater than 200 μg, AMS is extremely sensitive, allowing the use of a very small dose of labeled folic acid (i.e., 35 μg) [104]. Such a small dose is well below the threshold level recently reported in humans at which unmetabolized folic acid starts to appear in the circulation when the metabolic capacity of intestinal cells to reduce folic acid is exceeded [105], thereby ensuring that only reduced folates will reach the liver and overcoming the problem of a differential first-pass effect associated with the more traditional acute protocols using folic acid as the reference. However, although AMS has been used successfully as a technique for investigating folate kinetics and metabolism [106,107], its applicability in bioavailability studies needs to be confirmed.

B. Chronic Studies

Chronic bioavailability studies involve interventions over extended periods of 4 weeks or more to examine the effects of comparable doses of folic acid and reduced folates on biomarkers of folate status (usually one or more of serum folate, RBC folate, and plasma homocysteine concentrations). Treatments can involve specific food folates, mixed diets, or commercial preparations corresponding to the major food folate forms. Chronic studies involving interventions with specific food folate sources or mixed diets are probably the most meaningful but present major challenges. Similar bioavailability has been reported in response to chronic supplementation for commercial folate preparations of folic acid and 5-methyl-THF at doses in the range of 100 to 400 µg/day [108–111].

1. Chronic Studies: Feeding Trials Involving the Provision of Folate-Rich Foods to Free-Living Participants

The interpretation of studies involving the provision of folate-rich foods to free-living subjects (i.e., not designed to examine folate bioavailability per se) may be particularly problematic as a result of a number of confounding effects. These include the poor stability of food folates during cooking [78], potentially resulting in considerable folate losses before ingestion and large inter- and intrasubject variation in ingested folate over the intervention period. In contrast, folic acid supplements (against which responses to food folates are typically compared) provide a very stable and consistent source of the vitamin. In addition, poor compliance of subjects with demanding intervention protocols in chronic studies or dietary displacement of usual food folate sources with intervention foods may result in considerably less food folate being consumed than the intended amount [112,113]. However, compliance with folic acid treatment is often found to be excellent because it is far less demanding than manipulations of dietary folate intakes [112]. These issues are most problematic in the case of those studies designed to evaluate the effectiveness of different options for achieving optimal folate status in practice rather than to assess the relative bioavailability of different food sources of folate [112–114]. Once published, such studies have often been interpreted by others to generate estimates of folate bioavailability. This is inappropriate because the amount of folate ingested by the various treatment groups was not controlled, a necessity when estimating the relative bioavailability of food folates.

2. Chronic Studies: Controlled Feeding Trials with Food Folates

Even controlled chronic feeding trials designed to examine folate bioavailability result in great variation in estimates of the bioavailability of food folates compared with folic acid (relative bioavailability) (30%–98%) [3–7]. Estimates of food folate bioavailability from controlled chronic feeding trials are summarized in Table 2.2. Data from one landmark study in which the bioavailability of natural folates from a mixed diet was compared with that of folic acid in nonpregnant women in a metabolic unit for 92 days indicate that food folate is no more than 50% that of folic acid [3]. Although based on a sample size of just 10 subjects (divided into three parallel groups), the intense nature of the study, the highly controlled environment in which

TABLE 2.2
Estimates of Food Folate Bioavailability from Controlled Chronic
Feeding Trials

Study Reference	Participants	Intervention and Control	Estimated Food Folate Bioavailability
Sauberlich et al. [3]	*Country*: United States *Participants*: Nonpregnant women aged 21–40 years, maintained in a metabolic unit for 92 days *No. included*: 10 divided into three treatment groups	*Intervention*: Depletion (very low folate diet: 9.5 μg/day) followed by phased, controlled repletion (over 64 days) with increasing levels of folic acid or food folate (from a mixed diet) to a total intake of 300 μg/day *Duration of intervention*: 92 days (28 days depletion followed by 64 days repletion)	<50% that of folic acid *Comment*: Relative bioavailability based on plasma folate responses
Brouwer et al. [4]	*Country*: The Netherlands *Participants*: Healthy men and women aged 18–45 years *No. included*: 66 divided into three treatment groups	*Intervention*: Three treatment groups: (1) dietary folate group (560 μg/day); (2) folic acid group (500 μg/day folic acid on alternate days) plus low folate diet, 210 μg/day); (3) placebo (placebo tablet plus low folate diet) *Duration of intervention*: 4 weeks	60%–98% that of folic acid *Comment*: Relative bioavailability varied according to the response biomarker used: homocysteine (60%); plasma folate (78%); and erythrocyte folate (98%)
Hannon-Fletcher et al. [5]	*Country*: Northern Ireland *Participants*: Men aged 18–45 years recruited from university staff and students and local community *No. included*: 73 divided into four treatment groups	*Intervention*: Four treatment groups: (1) placebo tablet; (2) 200 μg/day folic acid as a tablet; (3) 200 μg/day food folate as spinach; or (iv) as yeast; the two food sources were chosen to represent the extent to which folates are conjugated in a mixed diet (spinach and yeast; 50% and 100% polyglutamyl folate) respectively) *Duration of intervention*: 30 days	45% that of folic acid *Comment*: Relative bioavailability based on serum folate or plasma homocysteine gave similar responses but varied according to the food folate source: spinach (30%) and yeast (59%)

continued

TABLE 2.2 (continued)
Estimates of Food Folate Bioavailability from Controlled Chronic Feeding Trials

Study Reference	Participants	Intervention and Control	Estimated Food Folate Bioavailability
Yang et al. [6]	*Country*: United States *Participants*: Women aged 18–45 years recruited from university staff and students and local community *No. included*: 42 divided into six treatment groups	*Intervention*: Depletion (low folate diet: 135 μg/day) followed by randomization to six treatment groups where participants received either 400 or 800 μg DFE/day from food folate or folic acid in various combinations *Duration of intervention*: 14 weeks (2 weeks depletion followed by 12 weeks repletion)	52% that of folic acid 60% that of added folic acid* *Comment*: Estimates were similar whether based on serum folate or erythrocyte folate responses
Winkels et al. [7]	*Country*: The Netherlands *Participants*: Men and women recruited from university staff and students and local community *No. included*: 72 divided into four treatment groups	*Intervention*: Four treatment groups: (1) high folate diet, 369 μg/day, plus placebo capsule; (2–4) low folate diet, 73 μg/day, plus folic acid at doses of 92, 191, and 289 μg/day, respectively; in addition, all treatment groups were administered a daily capsule with 58 μg [$^{13}C_{11}$] labeled folic acid *Duration of intervention*: 4 weeks	78%–85% that of folic acid *Comment*: Relative bioavailability was 85% based on serum folate response and 78% based on percentage of labeled folate in total plasma folate pool

* Relative bioavailability calculated as DFE, which assumes that folic acid added to food is 85%, and food folate 50%, as bioavailable as free folic acid; thus, the 1.7 multiplier was used to convert folic acid to DFE.

it was conducted, and the absence of a more reliable estimate of relative food folate bioavailability at the time resulted in this study providing the basis for units derived by the Institute of Medicine to express dietary folate intake recommendations, now expressed in terms of DFE values [9]. The concept of DFE recognizes the differences in bioavailability between natural food folates and folic acid added to foods during fortification. Results from a controlled (but not metabolic) 30-day intervention study from our laboratory [5] based on administering two representative food folate sources (spinach and yeast; 50% and 100% polyglutamyl folate, respectively) estimated the bioavailability of food folate to be approximately 45% relative to that of folic acid, generally consistent with the estimate of "<50%" used to generate the DFE value [3]. A subsequent controlled feeding study by Yang et al. [6], which provided various combinations of food folate and folic acid for a 12-week intervention, also supports the validity of the DFE value. Importantly, the consistency in estimates of food folate bioavailability when measured at two different doses (400 or 800 μg DFE/day) increases the robustness of the conclusions of the latter study [6]. However, the results of two other controlled studies [4,7] do not support the estimate of relative food folate bioavailability used to generate the DFE value; both estimated the bioavailability of food folates to be approximately 80%, far higher than found in the other studies [3,5,6]. It is possible that the disagreement in estimates of food folate bioavailability among studies relates to differences in the methods used for folate analysis of foods. However, the administration in one of these studies [4] of the folic acid treatment on alternate days at a dose of 500 μg/day (for an assumed intake of 250 μg/day folic acid) is likely to have confounded the interpretation of the results by underestimating the biomarker response to folic acid, thereby overestimating the relative bioavailability of food folates.

IV. FUTURE BIOAVAILABILITY STUDIES: PRIORITIES AND CHALLENGES

Folate bioavailability is a concern for policy makers for two reasons. First, incomplete bioavailability of food folate can hinder the achievement of optimal folate status in populations. The achievement of optimal folate status in turn is a current priority for public health, not only because of its well-established role in the prevention of neural tube defects (NTDs) [115,116] but also because of its other potential protective roles in cardiovascular disease and stroke in particular [117], certain cancers [118], bone disease [119], and cognitive decline [120]. However, typical folate intakes are suboptimal, in that although adequate in preventing clinical folate deficiency (i.e., megaloblastic anemia) in most people, they are generally insufficient to achieve a folate status associated with the lowest risk of NTDs. This is especially true for those populations without access to fortified food who are therefore reliant on natural food folates as a means to optimize status.

The incomplete bioavailability of food folates is also a consideration for those involved in revising dietary folate recommendations. The DFE is defined as the quantity of natural food folate plus 1.7 times the quantity of folic acid in the diet, a definition based on the assumption that the bioavailability of folic acid added to food is greater than that of natural food folate by a factor of 1.7 [9]. There are sound reasons for basing emerging recommendations on DFEs to adjust for the differences in bioavailability between natural food folates and folic acid added to food. In a recent observational study of 440 healthy adults in Northern Ireland, for example, folic acid was found to be a much more important determinant than natural food folate of RBC folate concentrations, and only participants with higher folic acid intakes from fortified foods were able to achieve an average RBC folate concentration that would be considered optimal in terms of preventing NTDs [121]. However, only controlled bioavailability studies can provide meaningful estimates of the relative bioavailability of food folate to confirm the robustness of the DFE value for emerging folate recommendations.

Thus, assessment of folate bioavailability in mixed diets should be a priority for future research; however, there are major challenges involved. Perhaps the greatest of these is ensuring that food folates and folic acid are delivered at equivalent doses throughout the intervention period. Studies conducted in a metabolic unit offer the best means of achieving this, but they require specialist facilities and are extremely costly and labor intensive. Whether or not a study is conducted in a metabolic unit, all food consumed during the intervention period should ideally be prepared and analyzed *before* consumption. The alternative, verifying the folate content of the intervention diet after it is administered (e.g., by duplicate meal analysis), has proven to be problematic even in highly controlled bioavailability studies [4] because analysis of administered meals often reveals folate intakes that differ from the target dose. The major reason why the amount of folate in a meal has been found on analysis to differ from that targeted is primarily because of the well-documented underestimation of the folate content of foods in current food tables used for dietary analysis. Using more up-to-date food folate methodology based on trienzyme (protease, amylase, and conjugase) treatment [122], our research group reported much higher values for folates in various plant and animal foods and in composite meals [45] compared with published folate values generated using traditional folate methodology. Such findings may have major implications for the calculation of dietary folate intake (and therefore folate recommendations) and require further investigation.

V. SUMMARY

It is widely recognized that the bioavailability of folate from natural food sources is incomplete when compared with folic acid. A number of factors have been reported as potentially contributing to the incomplete bioavailability of various food folates, but their relevance in influencing the bioavailability of folate from a mixed diet is poorly understood. Apart from their lower bioavailability when compared with folic acid, the poor stability of natural folates under typical cooking conditions may also contribute to the limited ability of unfortified foods to enhance folate status, a factor often overlooked in published studies. These are important issues given the established and emerging roles for folate in disease prevention on one hand, and the widespread underprovision of folate in typical diets in most European countries on the other.

A number of methodological approaches have been used to address folate bioavailability, but depending on the experimental approach used, there may be important limitations that can confound the interpretation of many published studies. Long-term studies in humans aimed at determining the relative bioavailability of food folates are notoriously difficult to conduct but are likely to give the most meaningful results in future research, as long as they are based on robust analytical methods and highly controlled protocols to ensure that the target intakes of food folate and folic acid are maintained throughout the intervention period. In addition, the accurate assessment of dietary folate intake in the general population remains an issue because food tables in most countries (used for dietary analysis purposes) are based on folate determinations carried out before the introduction of newer food folate methodology based on trienzyme treatment, leading to an underestimation of folate intakes in dietary surveys. These challenges are considerable but need to be addressed if folate bioavailability in whole diets is to be accurately assessed to provide quantifiable data on which to base emerging dietary recommendations for folate.

ACKNOWLEDGMENTS

We thank the UK Food Standards Agency for supporting our folate bioavailability research (project number NO503).

REFERENCES

1. Murphy M, Keating M, Boyle P, Weir DG, Scott JM. The elucidation of the mechanism of folate catabolism in the rat. *Biochem Biophys Res Commun* 1976; 71:1017–24.
2. Colman N, Green R, Metz J. Prevention of folate deficiency by food fortification. II. Absorption of folic acid from fortified staple foods. *Am J Clin Nutr* 1975; 28:459–64.
3. Sauberlich HE, Kretsh MJ, Skala JH, Johnson HL, Taylor PC. Folate required and metabolism in nonpregnant women. *Am J Clin Nutr* 1987; 46:1016–28.
4. Brouwer IA, van Dusseldorp M, West CE, Meyboom S, Thomas CM, Duran M, van het Hof KH, Eskes TK, Hautvast JG, Steegers-Theunissen RP. Dietary folate from vegetables and citrus fruit decreases plasma homocysteine concentrations in humans in a dietary controlled trial. *J Nutr* 1999; 129:1135–39.
5. Hannon-Fletcher MP, Armstrong NC, Scott JM, Pentieva K, Bradbury I, Ward M, Strain JJ, et al. Determining bioavailability of food folates in a controlled intervention study. *Am J Clin Nutr* 2004; 80:911–18.
6. Yang TL, Hung J, Caudill MA, Urrutia TF, Alamilla A, Perry CA, Li R, Hata H, Cogger EA. A long-term controlled feeding study in young women supports the validity of the 1.7 multiplier in the dietary folate equivalency equation. *J Nutr* 2005; 135:1139–45.
7. Winkels RM, Brouwer IA, Siebelink E, Katan MB, Verhoef P. Bioavailability of food folates is 80% of that of folic acid. *Am J Clin Nutr* 2007; 85:465–73.
8. Gregory JF. Case study: Folate bioavailability. *J Nutr* 2001; 131:1376S–1382S.
9. Institute of Medicine, Panel on Folate, Other B Vitamins, and Choline. *Dietary Reference Intake: Thiamine, Riboflavin, Niacin, Vitamin B6, Folate, Vitamin B12, Pantothenic Acid, Biotin, and Choline.* Washington, DC: National Academy Press, 1998.
10. Melse-Boonstra A, de Bree A, Verhoef P, Bjorke-Monsen AL, Verschuren WMM. Dietary monoglutamate and polyglutamate folate are both associated with plasma folate concentrations in Dutch men and women aged 20-65 y. *J Nutr* 2002; 132:1307–12.
11. Stockstad ELR, Shin YS, Tamura T. Distribution of folate forms in food and folate availability. In: *Food and Nutrition Board, National Research Council. Folic Acid: Biochemistry and Physiology in Relation to the Human Nutrition Requirement.* Washington, DC: National Academy of Sciences, 1977:56–68.
12. Chandler CJ, Wang TT, Halsted CH. Pteroylpolyglutamate hydrolase from human jejunal brush borders. Purification and characterization. *J Biol Chem* 1986; 261:928–33.
13. Gregory JF, Ink SL, Cerda JJ. Comparison of pteroylpolyglutamate hydrolase (folate conjugase) from porcine and human brush border membrane. *Comp Biochem Physiol* 1987; 88B:1135–41.
14. Tamura T, Shin YS, Buehring KU, Stokstad ELR. The availability of folate in man: Effect of orange juice supplement on intestinal conjugase. *Br J Haematol* 1976; 32:123–33.
15. Bailey LB, Cerda JJ, Bloch BS, Busby MJ, Vargas L, Chandler CJ, Halsted CH. Effect of age on poly- and monoglutamyl folacin absorption in human subjects. *J Nutr* 1984; 114: 1770–76.

16. Wei MM, Bailey LB, Toth JP, Gregory JF. Bioavailability for humans of deuterium-labeled monoglutamyl and polyglutamyl folates is affected by selected foods. *J Nutr* 1996; 126:3100–08.

17. Wei MM, Gregory JF. Organic acids in selected foods inhibit intestinal brush border pteroylpolyglutamate hydrolase in vitro: Potential mechanism affecting the bioavailability of dietary polyglutamyl folate. *J Agr Food Chem* 1998; 46:211–19.

18. Rosenberg IH, Godwin HA. Inhibition of intestinal γ-glutamyl carboxypeptidase by yeast nucleic acid: An explanation of variability in utilisation of dietary polyglutamyl folate. *J Clin Invest* 1971; 50:78a.

19. Butterworth CE, Newman AJ, Krumdieck CL. Tropical sprue: A consideration of possible etiologic mechanisms with emphasis on pteroylpolyglutamate metabolism. *Transam Clin Climatol Assoc* 1974; 86:11–22.

20. Keagy PM, Shane B, Oace SM. Folate bioavailability in humans: Effect of wheat bran and beans. *Am J Clin Nutr* 1988; 47:80–88.

21. Reisenauer AM, Halsted CH. Human brush border folate conjugase: Characteristics and inhibition by salicylazosulfapyridine. *Biochem Biophys Acta* 1981; 659:62–69.

22. Halsted CH, Villanueva JA, Devlin AM, Carol J, Chandler CJ. Metabolic interactions of alcohol and folate. *J Nutr* 2002; 132:2367S–72S.

23. Halsted CH. Intestinal absorption of dietary folates. In: Picciano MF, Stockstad ELR, Gregory JF, eds. *Folic Acid Metabolism in Health and Disease.* New York: Wiley-Liss, 1990:23–45.

24. Devlin AM, Ling E, Peerson JM, Fernando S, Clarke R, Smith AD, Halsted CH. Glutamate carboxypeptidase II: A polymorphism associated with lower levels of serum folate and hyperhomocysteinemia. *Hum Mol Gen* 2000; 9:2837–44.

25. Lievers KJA, Kluijtmans LAJ, Boers GHJ, Verhoef P, den Heijer M, Trijbels FJM, Blom HJ. Influence of glutamate carboxypeptidase II (GCPII) polymorphism (1561C→T) on plasma homocysteine, folate and vitamin B_{12} levels and its relationship to cardiovascular disease risk. *Atherosclerosis* 2002; 164:269–73.

26. Vargas-Martinez C, Ordovas JM, Wilson PW, Selhub J. The glutamate carboxypeptidase gene II (C>T) polymorphism does not affect folate status in the Framingham offspring cohort. *J Nutr* 2002; 132:1176–79.

27. Afman LA, Frans JM, Trijbels, Blom HJ. The H475Y polymorphism in the glutamate carboxypeptidase II gene increases plasma folate without affecting the risk for neural tube defects in humans. *J Nutr* 2003; 133:75–77.

28. Fodinger M, Dierkes J, Skoupy S, Rohrer C, Hagen W, Puttinger H, Hauser AC, Vychytil A, Sunder-Plassmann G. Effect of glutamate carboxypeptidase II and reduced folate carrier polymorphisms on folate and total homocysteine concentrations in dialysis patients. *J Am Soc Nephrol* 2003; 14:1314–19.

29. Halsted CH, Wong DH, Peerson JM, Warden CH, Refsum H, Smith DA, Nygard OK, Ueland PM, Vollset SE, Tell GS. Relations of glutamate carboxypeptidase II (GCPII) polymorphisms to folate and homocysteine concentrations and to scores of cognition, anxiety, and depression in a homogeneous Norwegian population: The Hordaland homocysteine study. *Am J Clin Nutr* 2007; 86:514–21.

30. Wang TT, Reisenauer AM, Halsted CH. Comparison of folate conjugase activities in human, pig, rat and monkey intestine. *J Nutr* 1985; 115:814–19.

31. Kesavan V, Noronha JM. Folate malabsorption in aged rats related to low levels of pancreatic folyl conjugase. *Am J Clin Nutr* 1983; 37:262–67.

32. Shafizadeh TB, Halsted CH. γ-Glutamyl hydrolase, not glutamate carboxypeptidase II, hydrolyzes dietary folate in the small intestine. *J Nutr* 2007; 137:1149–53.

33. Elsenhans B, Ahmad O, Rosenberg IH. Isolation and characterisation of pteroylpolyglutamate hydrolase from rat intestinal mucosa. *J Biol Chem* 1984; 259:6364–68.

34. Wang TT, Chandler CJ, Halsted CH. Intracellular pteroylpolyglutamate hydrolase from human jejunal mucosa. Isolation and characterization. *J Biol Chem* 1986; 261:13551–55.

35. Halsted CH, Ling E, Carter RL, Vilanueva JA, Gardner JM, Coyle JT. Folylpoly-γ-glutamate carboxypeptidase from pig jejunum molecular characterisation and relation to glutamate carboxypeptidase II. *J Biol Chem* 1998; 273:20417–24.

36. Gregory JF III, Quinlivan EP, Davis SR. Integrating the issue of folate bioavailability, intake and metabolism in the era of fortification. *Trends Food Sci Technol* 2005; 16:229–40.

37. Godwin HA, Rosenberg IH. Comparative studies of the intestinal absorption of [³H] pteroylmonoglutamate and [³H]pteroylheptaglutamate in man. *Gastroenterology* 1975; 69:364–73.

38. Gregory JF, Bhandari SD, Bailey LB, Toth JP, Baumgartner TG, Cerda JJ. Relative bioavailability of deuterium-labeled monoglutamyl and hexaglutamyl folates in human subjects. *Am J Clin Nutr* 1991; 53:736–40.

39. Melse-Boonstra A, West CE, Katan MB, Kok FJ, Verhoef P. Bioavailability of hepta-glutamyl relative to monoglutamyl folic acid in healthy adults. *Am J Clin Nutr* 2004; 79:424–29.

40. Melse-Boonstra A, Verhoef P, West CE, van Rhijn JA, van Breemen RB, Lasaroms JJP, Garbis SD, Katan MB, Kok FJ. A dual-isotope-labeling method of studying the bioavailability of hexaglutamyl folic acid relative to that of monoglutamyl folic acid in humans by using multiple orally administered low doses. *Am J Clin Nutr* 2006; 84:1128–33.

41. Tamura T, Stokstad ELR. The availability of food folate in man. *Br J Haematol* 1973; 25:513–32.

42. Bailey LB, Barton LE, Hillier SE, Cerda JJ. Bioavailability of mono and polyglutamyl folate in human subjects. *Nutr Rep Intern* 1988; 38:509–18.

43. Boodie AM, Dedlow ER, Nackashi JA, Opalko FJ, Kauwel GP, Gregory JF 3rd, Bailey LB. Folate absorption in women with a history of neural tube defect-affected pregnancy. *Am J Clin Nutr* 2000; 72:154–58.

44. Konings EJM, Troost FJ, Castenmiller JJM, Roomans HHS, van den Brandt PA, Saris WHM. Intestinal absorption of different types of folate in healthy subjects with an ileostomy. *Br J Nutr* 2002; 88:235–42.

45. McKillop DJ, McNulty H, Scott JM, McPartlin JM, Strain JJ, Bradbury I, Girvan J, et al. The rate of intestinal absorption of natural food folates is not related to the extent of folate conjugation. *Am J Clin Nutr* 2006; 84:167–73.

46. Hannon-Fletcher MPA, Armstrong NC, Scott JM, Ward'M, Strain JJ, Pentieva K, Dunn AA, Molloy AM, Scullion M, McNulty H. A controlled intervention study to determine the bioavailability of food folates. *J Inher Metab Dis* 2003; 26(Suppl 1):11.

47. Reisenauer AM, Halsted CH. Issues and opinions in nutrition: Human folate requirements. *J Nutr* 1987; 117:600–02.

48. Rosenberg IH, Zimmerman J, Selhub J. Folate transport. *Chemioterapia* 1985; 4: 354–58.

49. Smith ME, Matty AJ, Blair JA. The transport of pteroylglutamic acid across the small intestine of the rat. *Biochem Biophys Acta* 1970; 219:124–29.

50. Bhandari SD, Gregory JF. Folic acid, 5-methyltetrahydrofolate and 5-formyltetrahydrofolate exhibit equivalent intestinal absorption, metabolism and in vivo kinetics in rats. *J Nutr* 1992; 122:1847–54.

51. Qui A, Jansen M, Sakaris A, Min SH, Chattopadhyay S, Tsai E, Sandoval C, Zhao R, Akabas MH, Goldman ID. Identification of an intestinal folate transporter and the molecular basis for hereditary folate malabsorption. *Cell* 2006; 127:917–28.

52. Subramanian VS, Marchant JS, Said HM. Apical membrane targeting and trafficking of the human proton-coupled transporter in polarized epithelia. *Am J Physiol Cell Physiol* 2008; 294:C233–40.

53. Zhao R, Min SH, Qiu A, Sakaris A, Goldberg GL, Sandoval C, Malatack JJ, Rosenblatt DS, Goldman ID. The spectrum of mutations in the PCFT gene, coding for an intestinal

folate transporter, that are the basis for hereditary folate malabsorption. *Blood* 2007; 110:1147–52.

54. Said HM, Hollander D, Katz D. Absorption of 5-methyltetrahydrofolatein rat jejunum with intact blood and lymphatic vessels. *Biochem Biophys Acta* 1984; 775:402–08.

55. Russell RM, Kransinski SD, Samloff IM, Jacob RA, Hartz SC, Brovender SR. Folic acid malabsorption in atrophic gastritis. Possible compensation by bacterial folate synthesis. *Gastroenterology* 1986; 91:1476–82.

56. Russell RM, Golner BB, Kransinski SD, Sadowski JA, Suter PM, Braun CL. Effect of antacid and H2 receptor antagonists on the intestinal absorption of folic acid. *J Lab Clin Med* 1988; 112:458–63.

57. Russell RM, Dhar GJ, Dutta SK, Rosenberg IH. Influence of intraluminal pH on folate absorption: Studies in control subjects and in patients with pancreatic insufficiency. *J Lab Clin Med* 1979; 93:428–36.

58. de Meer K, Smulders YM, Dainty JR, Smith DEC, Kok RM, Stehouwer CDA, Finglas PM, Jakobs C. [6S]5-Methyltetrahyrofolate or folic acid supplementation and absorption and initial elimination of folate in young and middle-aged adults. *Eur J Clin Nutr* 2005; 59:1409–16.

59. Said HM, Chatterjee N, Hag RU, Subramanian VS, Ortiz A, Matherly LH, Sirotnak FM, Halsted C, Rubin SA. Adaptive regulation of intestinal folate uptake: Effect of dietary folate deficiency. *Am J Physiol Cell Physiol* 2000; 279:C1889–95.

60. Subramanian VS, Chatterjee N, Said HM. Folate uptake in the human intestine: Promoter activity and effect of folate deficiency. *J Cell Physiol* 2003; 196:403–08.

61. Ashokkumar B, Mohammed ZM, Vaziri ND, Said HM. Effect of folate oversupplementation on folate uptake by human intestinal and renal epithelial cells. *Am J Clin Nutr* 2007; 86:159–66.

62. Fleming RE. Advances in understanding the molecular basis for the regulation of dietary iron absorption. *Curr Opin Gastroenterol* 2005; 21:201–06.

63. Alemdaroglu NC, Dietz U, Wolffram S, Spahn-Langguth H, Langguth P. Influence of green and black tea on folic acid pharmacokinetics in healthy volunteers: Potential risk of diminished folic acid bioavailability. *Biopharm Drug Dispos* 2008; 29:335–48.

64. Alemdaroglu NC, Wolffram S, Boissel JP, Closs E, Spahn-Langguth H, Langguth P. Inhibition of folic acid uptake by catechins and tea extracts in Caco-2 cells. *Planta Med* 2007; 73:27–32.

65. Mason JB, Rosenberg IH. Intestinal absorption of folate. In: Johnson LR, ed. *Physiology of the Gastrointestinal Tract*, 3d ed. New York: Raven Press, 1994:1979–96.

66. Rong N, Selhub J, Goldin BR, Rosenberg IH. Bacterially synthesized folate in rat large intestine is incorporated into host tissue folyl polyglutamates. *J Nutr* 1991; 121:1955–59.

67. Kim TH, Yang J, Darling PB, O'Connor DL. A large pool of available folate exists in the large intestine of human infants and piglets. *J Nutr* 2004; 134:1389–94.

68. Asrar FM, O'Connor DL. Bacterially synthesized folate and supplemental folic acid are absorbed across the large intestine in piglets. *J Nutr Biochem* 2005; 16:587–93.

69. Aufreiter S, Gregory JF, Pfeiffer CM, Fazili Z, Kim YI, Marcon N, Kamalaporn P, Pencharz PB, O'Connor DL. Folate is absorbed across the large intestine in adults: Evidence from cecal infusion of 13C-labeled [6S]-5-formyltetrahydrofolate. *Am J Clin Nutr* 2009; 90:116–23.

70. Houghton LA, Green TJ, Donovan UM, Gibson RS, Stephen AM, O'Connor DL. Association between dietary fiber intake and the folate status of a group of female adolescents. *Am J Clin Nutr* 1997; 66:1414–21.

71. van het Hof KH, Tijburg LBM, Pietrzik K, Weststrate JA. Influence of feeding different vegetables on plasma levels of carotenoids, folate and vitamin C. Effect of disruption of the vegetable matrix. *Br J Nutr* 1999; 82:203–12.

72. Castenmiller JJM, van de Poll CJ, West CE, Brouwer IA, Thomas CMG, van Dusseldorp M. Bioavailability of folate from processed spinach in humans. *Ann Nutr Metab* 2000; 44:163–69.
73. Bhandari SD, Gregory JF. Inhibition by selected food components of human and porcine intestinal pteroylpolyglutamate hydrolase activity. *Am J Clin Nutr* 1990; 51:87–94.
74. Pfeiffer CM, Rogers LM, Bailey LB, Gregory JF. Absorption of folate from fortified cereal-grain products and of supplemental folate consumed with or without food determined by using a dual-label stable-isotope protocol. *Am J Clin Nutr* 1997; 66:1388–97.
75. Hurdle ADF, Barton D, Searles IH. A method for measuring folate in foods and its application to a hospital diet. *Am J Clin Nutr* 1968; 21:1202–07.
76. Leichter J, Switzer VP, Landymore AF. Effect of cooking on folate content of vegetables. *Nutr Rep Intern* 1978; 8:475–79.
77. De Souza SC, Eitenmiller RR. Effects of processing and storage on the folate content of spinach and broccoli. *J Food Sci* 1986; 51:626–28.
78. McKillop D, Pentieva K, Daly D, McPartlin JM, Hughes J, Strain JJ, Scott JM, McNulty H. The effect of different cooking methods on folate retention in various foods which are amongst the major contributors to folate intake in the UK diet. *Br J Nutr* 88:681–88.
79. Dang J, Arcot J, Shrestha A. Folate retention in selected processed legumes. *Food Chem* 2000; 68:295–98.
80. Seyom E, Selhub J. Properties of food folates determined by stability and susceptibility to intestinal pteroylpolyglutamate hydrolase action. *J Nutr* 1998; 128:1956–60.
81. Andersson A, Oste R. Loss of ascorbic acid, folate and vitamin B12, and changes in oxygen content of UHT-milk. II. Results and discussion. *Milchwissenschaft* 1992; 47: 299–302.
82. Verwei M, Arkbage K, Mocking H, Havenaar R, Groten J. The FBP binding characteristics during gastric passage are different for folic acid and 5-methyltetrahydrofolate as studied in a dynamic in vitro gastrointestinal model. *J Nutr* 2004; 134:31–37.
83. Jones ML, Nixon PF. Tetrahydrofolates are greatly stabilized by binding to bovine milk folate-binding protein. *J Nutr* 2002; 132:2690–94.
84. Picciano MF, West SG, Ruch AL, Kris-Etherton PM, Zhao G, Johnston KE, Maddox DH, Fishell VK, Dirienzo DB, Tamura T. Effect of cow milk on food folate bioavailability in young women. *Am J Clin Nutr* 2004; 80:1565–69.
85. Winkels RM, Brouwer IA, Verhoef P, van Oort FVA, Durga J, Katan MB. Gender and body size affect the response of erythrocyte folate to folic acid treatment. *J Nutr* 2008; 138:1456–61.
86. Homocysteine Lowering Trialists' Collaboration. Dose-dependent effects of folic acid on blood concentrations of homocysteine: A meta-analysis of the randomized trials. *Am J Clin Nutr* 2005; 82:806–12.
87. Perry CA, Renna SA, Khitun E, Ortiz M, Moriarty DJ, Caudill MA. Ethnicity and race influence the folate status response to controlled folate intakes in young women. *J Nutr* 2004; 134:1786–92.
88. Wilcken B, Bamforth F, Li Z, Zhu H, Ritvanen A, Redlund M, Stoll C, et al. Geographical and ethnic variation of the 677C→T allele of 5, 10 methylenetetrahydrofolate reductase (MTHFR): Findings from over 7000 newborns from 16 areas world wide. *J Med Genet* 2003; 40:619–25.
89. Frosst P, Blom HJ, Milos R, Goyette P, Sheppard CA, Matthews RG, Boers GJH, et al. A candidate genetic risk factor for vascular disease: A common mutation in methylenetetrahydrofolate reductase. *Nat Genet* 1995; 10:111–13.
90. Molloy AM, Daly S, Mills JL, Kirke PN, Whitehead AS, Ramsbottom D, Conley MR, Weir DG, Scott JM. Thermolabile variant of 5,10-methylenetetrahydrofolate reductase associated with low red-cell folates: Implications for folate intake recommendations. *Lancet* 1997; 349:1591–93.

91. Perry J, Chanarin I. Intestinal absorption of reduced folate compounds in man. *Br J Haematol* 1970; 18:329–39.
92. Brown JP, Scott JM, Foster FG, Weir DG. Ingestion and absorption of naturally occurring pteroylmonoglutamates (folates) in man. *Gastroenterology* 1973; 64:223–32.
93. Pietrzik K, Remer T. Zur Bioverfugbarkeitsprufung von Mikronahrstoffen (Bioavailability study of micronutrients). *Z Ernahrungswiss* 1989; 28:130–41.
94. Pentieva K, McNulty H, Reichert R, Ward M, Strain JJ, McKillop D, McPartlin JM, Connolly E, Molloy A, Krämer K, Scott JM. The short-term bioavailabilities of [6S]-5-methyltetrahydrofolate and folic acid are equivalent in men. *J Nutr* 2004; 134: 580–85.
95. Fenech M, Noakes M, Clifton P, Topping D. Aleurone flour is a rich source of bioavailable folate in humans. *J Nutr* 1999; 129:1114–19.
96. Gregory JF. The bioavailability of folate. In: Bailey LB, ed. *Folate in Health and Disease*. New York: Marcel Dekker, 1995:195–235.
97. Pietrzik K, Hages M, Remer T. Methodological aspects in vitamin bioavailability testing. *J Micronutr Anal* 1990; 7:207–22.
98. Gregory JF. Improved synthesis of [3′, 5′-2H2] folic acid: Extent and specificity of deuterium labelling. *J Agr Food Chem* 1990; 38:1073–76.
99. Maunder P, Finglas PM, Mallet AI, Mellon FA, Razzaque MA, Ridge B, Vahteristo L, Witthoft C. The synthesis of folic acid, multiply labelled with stable isotopes, for bioavailability studies in human nutrition. *J Chem Soc Perkin Transact* 1999; 1:1311–23.
100. Gregory JF, Toth JP. Stable-isotopic methods for in vivo investigation of folate absorption and metabolism. In: Picciano MF, Stokstad ELR, Gregory JF, eds. *Folic Acid Metabolism in Health and Disease*. New York: Wiley-Liss Inc, 1990:151–69.
101. Gregory JF, Quinlivan EP. In vivo kinetics of folate metabolism. *Ann Rev Nutr* 2002; 22:199–220.
102. Wright AJA, Finglas PM, Dainty JR, Hart DJ, Wolfe CA, Southon S, Gregory JF. Single oral doses of 13C forms of pteroylmonoglutamic acid and 5-formyltetrahydrofolic acid elicit differences in short-term kinetics of labelled and unlabelled folates in plasma: Potential problems in interpretation of folate bioavailability studies. *Br J Nutr* 2003; 90:363–71.
103. Wright AJ, Finglas PM, Dainty JR, Wolfe CA, Hart DJ, Wright DM, Gregory JF. Differential kinetic behaviour and distribution for pteroylglutamic acid and reduced folates: A revised hypothesis of the primary site of PteGlu metabolism in humans. *J Nutr* 2005; 135:619–23.
104. Dueker SR, Lame M, Lin Y, Clifford AJ, Buchholz BA, Vogel JS. Traditional and accelerator mass spectrometry for quantitation of human folate pools. *Trends Food Sci Technol* 2005; 16:267–70.
105. Sweeney MR, McPartlin J, Scott J. Folic acid fortification and public health: Report on threshold doses above which unmetabolized folic acid appear in serum. *BMC Public Health* 2007; 7:41–47.
106. Buchholz BA, Arjomand A, Dueker SR, Schneider PD, Clifford AJ, Vogel JS. Intrinsic erythrocyte labelling and attomole pharmacokinetic tracing of 14C-labeled folic acid with accelerator mass spectrometry. *Anal Biochem* 1999; 269:348–52.
107. Lin Y, Dueker SR, Follett JR, Fadel JG, Arjomand A, Schneider PD, Miller JW, et al. Quantitation of in vivo human folate metabolism. *Am J Clin Nutr* 2004; 80:680–91.
108. Venn BJ, Green TJ, Moser R, McKenzie JE, Skeaff CM, Mann J. Increases in blood folate indices are similar in women of childbearing age supplemented with [6S]-5-methyltetrahydrofolate and folic acid. *J Nutr* 2002; 132:3353–55.
109. Venn BJ, Green TJ, Moser R, Mann JI. Comparison of the effect of low-dose supplementation with L-5-methyltetrahydrofolate or folic acid on plasma homocysteine: A randomized placebo-controlled study. *Am J Clin Nutr* 2003; 77:658–62.

110. Lamers Y, Prinz-Langenohl R, Moser R, Pietrzik K. Supplementation with [6S]-5-methyltetrahydrofolate or folic acid equally reduces plasma total homocysteine concentrations in healthy women. *Am J Clin Nutr* 2004; 79:473–78.

111. Houghton LA, Sherwood KL, Pawlosky R, Ito S, O'Connor DL. [6S]-5-Methyltetra-hydrofolate is at least as effective as folic acid in preventing a decline in food folate concentrations during lactation. *Am J Clin Nutr* 2006; 83: 842–50.

112. Cuskelly GJ, McNulty H, Scott JM. Effect of increasing dietary folate on red-cell folate: Implications for prevention of neural tube defects. *Lancet* 1996; 347:657–59.

113. Ashfield-Watt PAL, Whiting JM, Clark ZE, Moat SJ, Newcombe RG, Burr ML, McDowell IFW. A comparison of the effect of advice to eat either '5-a-day' fruit and vegetables or folic acid-fortified foods on plasma folate and homocysteine. *Eur J Clin Nutr* 2003; 57:316–23.

114. Riddell LJ, Chisholm A, Williams S, Mann JI. Dietary strategies for lowering homo-cysteine concentrations. *Am J Clin Nutr* 2000; 71:1448–54.

115. Medical Research Council Vitamin Study Research Group. Prevention of neural tube defects: Results of the Medical Research Council Vitamin Study. *Lancet* 1991; 338:131–37.

116. Czeizel AE, Dudas I. Prevention of first occurrence of neural tube defects by pericon-ceptional vitamin supplementation. *N Engl J Med* 1992; 327:1832–35.

117. Wang X, Qin X, Demirtas H, Li J, Mao G, Huo Y, Sun N, Liu L, Xu X. Efficacy of folic acid supplementation in stroke prevention: A meta-analysis. *Lancet* 2007; 369:1876–82.

118. Ericson U, Sonestedt E, Gullberg B, Olsson H, Wirfalt E. High folate intake is associ-ated with lower breast cancer incidence in postmenopausal women in the Malmo Diet and Cancer cohort. *Am J Clin Nutr* 2007; 86:434–43.

119. Sato Y, Honda Y, Iwamoto J, Kanoko T, Satoh K. Effect of folate and mecobalamin on hip fractures in patients with stroke: A randomized controlled trial. *JAMA* 2005; 293:1082–88.

120. Durga J, van Boxtel MPJ, Schouten EG, Kok FJ, Jolles J, Katan MB, Verhoef P. Effect of 3-year folic acid supplementation on cognitive function in older adults in the FACIT trial: A randomised, double blind, controlled trial. *Lancet* 2007; 369:208–16.

121. Hoey L, McNulty H, Askin N, Dunne A, Ward M, Pentieva K, Strain JJ, Molloy AM, Flynn CA, Scott JM. Impact of a voluntary food fortification policy on folate, related B-vitamin status and homocysteine in healthy adults. *Am J Clin Nutr* 2007; 86:1405–13.

122. Tamura T, Mizuno Y, Johnston KE, Jacob RA. Food folate assay with protease, α-amylase and folate conjugase treatments. *J Agr Food Chem* 1997; 45:135–39.

3 Folate Biochemical Pathways and Their Regulation

Patrick J. Stover

CONTENTS

I. INTRODUCTION

Tetrahydrofolate (THF) polyglutamates function in cells as a family of coenzymes that activate and carry single carbons on the N-5 and/or N-10 position. THF-activated one-carbons are carried at three different oxidation states for one-carbon transfer reactions. THF carries activated formate as 10-formyl-THF, 5-formyl-THF, or 5,10-methenyl-THF. In addition, THF transports activated formaldehyde as 5,10-methylene-THF and activated methanol as 5-methyl-THF. Once transported into the cell, folate monoglutamate molecules are modified with a covalently bound glutamate polypeptide that consists of three to eight glutamate residues that are polymerized through unusual γ-linked peptide bonds. The addition of the glutamate polypeptide is necessary to generate functional coenzymes; the polyglutamate peptide is essential for high-affinity binding to many folate-dependent enzymes and binding proteins, as well as for cellular and intracellular compartment retention of folate coenzymes [1].

THF polyglutamates accept and transfer one-carbons in a network of biosynthetic and catabolic reactions known as folate-mediated one-carbon metabolism. Folate coenzymes and one-carbon pathways function in three cellular compartments: the cytoplasm (Figures 3.1 and 3.2), mitochondria (Figure 3.3), and nucleus (Figure 3.1). Folate coenzymes do not readily exchange among the cellular compartments, and each compartment carries out specialized metabolic functions. Mitochondrial one-carbon metabolism generates one-carbons in the form of formate through the catabolism of serine, glycine, and choline. Cytoplasmic one-carbon metabolism uses mitochondrially derived formate for nucleotide biosynthesis and for the remethylation of homocysteine to methionine. Nuclear folate metabolism generates thymidylate during DNA replication and repair. Despite their specialized functions, all the folate-dependent pathways and intracellular compartments are interdependent [2–5]. This interdependence results from the shuttling of common metabolic intermediates among compartments, including serine, glycine, and formate, and the competition among compartments and folate-dependent biosynthetic pathways for a limiting pool of folate coenzymes. Even under folate-replete conditions, the concentration of cellular folate-binding proteins exceeds that of folate coenzymes, indicating that the concentration of free folate is negligible [6,7]. Proteins that bind THF cofactors function in folate-dependent one-carbon metabolism and have one or more of the following functions: (1) generate THF-activated one-carbons; (2) interconvert one-carbon–activated THF cofactors; (3) catalyze one-carbon transfer reactions; and (4) bind and/or sequester THF cofactors without metabolizing them (Figures 3.1 and 3.2).

II. ONE-CARBON METABOLISM IN THE CYTOPLASM

Folate-mediated one-carbon metabolism in the cytoplasm includes three interdependent biosynthetic pathways that catalyze the de novo synthesis of purines, thymidylate, and the remethylation of homocysteine to methionine (Figure 3.1). Methionine is a precursor for the synthesis of S-adenosylmethionine (AdoMet or SAM), a cofactor and methyl group donor for numerous methylation reactions, including the methylation of DNA, RNA, neurotransmitters and other small molecules, phospholipids, and proteins including histones. Many AdoMet-dependent methylation reactions serve

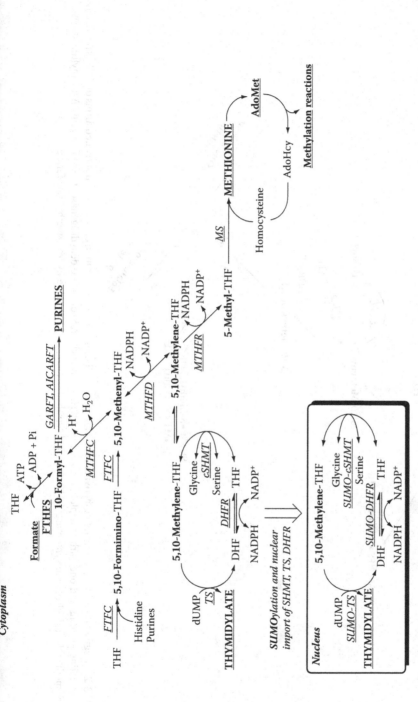

FIGURE 3.1 Compartmentation of folate-mediated one-carbon metabolism in the cytoplasm and nucleus. One-carbon metabolism in the cytoplasm is required for the de novo synthesis of purines and thymidylate, and for the remethylation of homocysteine to methionine. One-carbon metabolism in the nucleus synthesizes dTMP from dUMP and serine. AdoHcy, S-adenosylhomocysteine; AdoMet, S-adenosylmethionine; AICARFT, phosphoribosylamin- oimidazolecarboxamide formyltransferase; cSHMT, cytoplasmic serine hydroxymethyltransferase; DHFR, dihydrofolate reductase; dTMP, deoxythymidine monophosphate; dUMP, deoxyuridine monophosphate; FTCT, glycine forminotransferase/formiminoyltetrahydrofolate cyclodeaminase and glutamate formiminotransferase/formiminoyltetrahydrofolate cyclodeaminase; FTHFS, 10-formyltetrahydrofolate synthetase; GARFT, phosphoribosylglycinamide formyltransferase; MS, methionine synthase; MTHFC, methenyltetrahydrofolate cyclohydrolase; MTHFD, methylenetetrahydrofolate dehydrogenase; MTHFR, methylenetetrahydrofolate reductase; SUMO, small ubiquitin-like modifier; THF, 5-formyl-tetrahydrofolate; TS, thymidylate synthase.

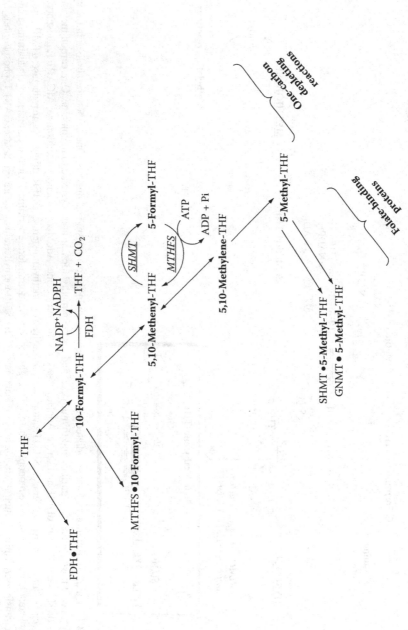

FIGURE 3.2 Regulation of cytoplasmic folate-activated one-carbon pools. The relative concentration of one-carbon activated forms of THF is regulated by folate-binding proteins and one-carbon depleting reactions. FDH, 10-formyltetrahydrofolate dehydrogenase; GNMT, glycine N-methyltransferase; MTHFS, methenyltetrahydrofolate synthetase; THF, 5-formyl-tetrahydrofolate; SHMT, serine hydroxymethyltransferase.

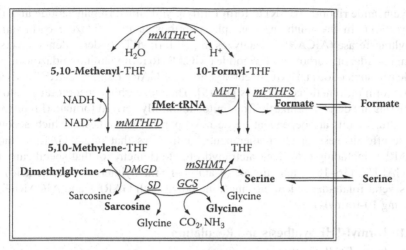

FIGURE 3.3 Compartmentation of folate-mediated one-carbon metabolism in mitochondria. One-carbon metabolism in mitochondria is required to generate formate for one-carbon metabolism in the cytoplasm, to generate the amino acid glycine, and to synthesize formylmethionyl-tRNA for protein synthesis in mitochondria. DMGD, dimethylglycine dehydrogenase; GSC, glycine cleavage system; mFTHFS, mitochondrial formyltetrahydrofolate synthetase; mMTHFC, mitochondrial methenyltetrahydrofolate cyclohydrolase; mMTHFD, mitochondrial methylenetetrahydrofolate dehydrogenase; mSHMT, mitochondrial serine hydroxymethyltransferase; M-tRNA-FT, methionyl-tRNA formyltransferase; SD, sarcosine dehydrogenase.

regulatory functions by affecting gene transcription and genome stability [8], protein localization [9], and the degradation of small molecules [10]. Although mitochondria are a primary source of one-carbons for these biosynthetic pathways, one-carbons can be generated directly in the cytoplasm from histidine, purine, and serine catabolism.

A. 10-FORMYL-THF AND PURINE BIOSYNTHESIS

1. Purine Biosynthesis

Purine nucleotides are precursors for DNA and RNA synthesis and serve as coenzymes and regulatory factors. There are two purine nucleotide synthesis pathways: (1) the salvage pathway, which may be the major source of purines in differentiated mammalian cells [11]; and (2) the de novo pathway, which provides most of the adenine and guanine nucleotides during human embryonic development [12]. The formyl group of 10-formyl-THF is incorporated into the C-2 and C-8 positions of the purine ring during de novo purine biosynthesis. The enzymes involved in this 10-step pathway exist in a "purinosome" complex that converts 5-phosphoribosylpyrophosphate to inosine monophosphate, which is the precursor of adenine and guanine nucleotides [13]. In the third reaction, phosphoribosylglycinamide formyltransferase (GARFT) catalyzes the 10-formyl-THF–dependent conversion of glycinamide ribotide (GAR) to form formylglycinamide ribonucleotide and THF (Figure 3.1). In the ninth reaction, phosphoribosylaminoimidazole carboxamide formyltransferase (AICARFT) catalyzes the 10-formyl-THF–dependent conversion of aminoimidazole carboxomide ribotide (AICAR) to formylaminoimidazolecarbox-omide ribonucleotide and THF. In eukaryotic cells, GARFT and AICARFT activities are part of multifunctional enzymes [14,15]. The one-carbons incorporated into the purine ring are derived primarily from mitochondrially derived formate (Figure 3.1). Transformed cells are dependent on de novo purine biosynthesis, which accounts for the effectiveness of chemotherapeutic antifolates that target GARFT and/or AICARFT, including 6-R-dideazatetrahydrofolate (lometrexol that specifically targets GARFT) [16–18]. Methotrexate (4-amino-10-methylpteroylglutamic acid) targets several folate-dependent enzymes, including both GARFT and AICARFT, by depleting 10-formyl-THF.

2. 10-Formyl-THF Synthesis and Regulation

a. 10-Formyl-THF Synthetase

Cytoplasmic 10-formyl-THF synthetase (FTHFS) activity is the primary entry point of one-carbons for cytoplasmic folate-dependent biosynthetic reactions [5]. The enzyme catalyzes the adenosine 5′-triphosphate (ATP)–dependent conversion of THF and formate to 10-formyl-THF, adenosine 5′-diphosphate (ADP), and inorganic phosphate (Figure 3.1). 10-Formyl-THF synthetase activity resides on the C-terminal domain of a trifunctional enzyme, C_1-THF synthase, which also contains 5,10-methenyl-THF cyclohydrolase (MTHFC) and 5,10-methylene-THF dehydrogenase (MTHFD) activities on the N-terminal domain of the protein [19]. C_1-THF synthase is encoded by the *Mthfd1* gene, which is expressed ubiquitously and is transcriptionally up-regulated in response to conditions that require DNA synthesis [20]. 10-Formyl-THF is a required cofactor for de novo purine biosynthesis [21], or the one-carbon can be dehydrated and reduced for use in the biosynthesis of thymidylate and methionine (Figure 3.1). FTHFS is an essential activity; mice lacking FTHFS exhibit an early embryonic lethal phenotype (P. J. Stover and B. Shane, unpublished results).

A common variant of *Mthfd1*, G1958A, contains the coding substitution R653Q, which is present in the FTHFS domain of C_1-THF synthase. The effect of this substitution on the physical and/or catalytic properties is not known. The polymorphism does not affect homocysteine concentrations, plasma folate, or red blood cell folate concentrations [22] but does confer increased maternal risk for having a neural tube defect (NTD)–affected pregnancy [22–24], severe placental abruption, and unexplained second trimester loss [25,26].

b. Glutamate Formiminotransferase Cyclodeaminase and Glycine Formiminotransferase Cyclodeaminase

The catabolism of histine and purines generates one-carbon units that enter the cytoplasmic folate-activated one-carbon pool as 5,10-methenyl-THF, which exists in chemical equilibrium with 10-formyl-THF (Figure 3.1). During their catabolism, the imidazole ring of histidine, adenine, and guanine is converted to a formimino group, which is transferred to THF, forming 5-formimino-THF, which is subsequently converted to 5,10-methenyl-THF by the cyclodeaminase activity of the protein. The quantitative contribution of purine and histidine catabolism to the cytoplasmic folate-activated one-carbon pool is not known, although severe inborn errors of metabolism are associated with impairments in histidine and purine catabolism. Histidinemia and glutamate formiminotransferase deficiency are autosomal recessive disorders resulting from mutations in the histidase and formiminotransferase/cyclodeaminase genes, respectively. Both are characterized by mental retardation, speech impairment, and developmental delay; severe glutamate formiminotransferase deficiency is also associated with elevated serum folate concentrations [27].

c.   10-Formyl-TFH Dehydrogenase

10-Formyl-THF dehydrogenase (FDH) catalyzes the irreversible and nicotinamide-adenine dinucleotide phosphate, oxidized form (NADP+)-dependent oxidation of 10-formyl-THF to THF and CO_2. FDH contains two active sites. FDH catalyzes the hydrolysis of 10-formyl-THF to THF and formate through the hydrolase catalytic site located on the N-terminal domain, and the NADP+-dependent dehydrogenase reaction that oxidizes formate to CO^2 is catalyzed on the C-terminal domain [28,29]. The two active sites function in concert through a 4'-phosphopantetheine swinging arm that is bound through a phosphoester bond to Ser354. The swinging arm transfers formate between the two active sites [28]. FDH is one of the most abundant folate enzymes and is expressed in the liver, kidney, and central nervous system [30]. Once generated, the product of the reaction, THF, remains tightly bound to FDH (Figure 3.2) but can be channeled efficiently to serine hydroxymethyltransferase (SHMT) 1 or FTHFS to regenerate an activated one-carbon (Figure 3.1) [31].

FDH has been proposed to have several metabolic roles. These include (1) recycling THF cofactors by removing excess 10-formyl-THF; (2) protecting the cell from formate toxicity through its conversion to CO_2; (3) regulating of de novo purine biosynthesis by depleting 10-formyl-THF pools; (4) removing of excess one-carbon units from folate metabolism in the form of CO_2; and (5) sequestering and storing cellular folate in the form of THF. These proposed physiological functions have been investigated in cultured cells. FDH has been demonstrated to regulate cellular concentrations of 10-formyl-THF and the homocysteine remethylation cycle, presumably by regulating the supply of folate-activated one-carbon units; FDH appears to regulate de novo purine biosynthesis in some but not all cell types [32–34]. FDH is not an essential gene in mice [35].

d.   5,10-Methenyl-THF Synthetase

5,10-Methenyl-THF synthetase (MTHFS) catalyzes the ATP-dependent and irreversible conversion of 5-formyl-THF to 5,10-methenyl-THF. It is the only enzyme known to use 5-formyl-THF as a substrate and is expressed ubiquitously [36]. 5-Formyl-THF is not a coenzyme for one-carbon transfer reactions but may be a stable storage form of excess formyl folates [37,38]. The MTHFS reaction and the SHMT-catalyzed synthesis of 5-formyl-THF from 5,10-methenyl-THF constitute a futile cycle that serves to regulate intracellular 5-formyl-THF concentrations [39] (Figure 3.2). MTHFS also binds 10-formyl-THF tightly and thereby inhibits its catalytic activity [38]. MTHFS enhances de novo purine biosynthesis through two distinct mechanisms. First, MTHFS activity reduces cellular concentrations of 5-formyl-THF, an inhibitor of AICARFT [40]. Second, MTHFS enhances purine biosynthesis by enriching cellular 10-formyl-THF pools and/or by channeling 10-formyl-THF to AICARFT and/or GARFT [38]. *MTHFS* is an essential gene in mice; mice lacking MTHFS activity exhibit an early embryonic lethal phenotype (P. J. Stover, unpublished results).

B.   5,10-METHYLENE-THF AND THYMIDYLATE BIOSYNTHESIS

1.   Thymidylate Biosynthesis

The one-carbon carried by 5,10-methylene-THF is transferred to deoxyuridine monophosphate (dUMP) to form deoxythymidine 5'-triphosphate monophosphate (dTMP) and dihydrofolate (DHF) in a reaction catalyzed by thymidylate synthase (TS) [41] (Figure 3.1). This is the only folate-dependent reaction for which the folate coenzyme also serves as a source of reducing equivalents. DHF is reduced back to THF through the activity of DHF reductase (DHFR) (Figure 3.1). 5,10-Methylene-THF pools are derived from the reduction of 10-formyl-THF catalyzed by methenyl-THF dehydrogense/methenyl-THF cyclohydrolase in equilibrium with 5,10-methylene-THF derived from the THF-dependent conversion of serine to glycine catalyzed by SHMT, and both pools contribute to de novo thymidylate biosynthesis (Figure 3.1) [42].

TS protein concentrations increase from the G_1 to the S phase of the cell cycle for the provision of deoxythymidine 5'-triphosphate (dTTP) during DNS synthesis [43–45]. In G_0 and G_1, the transcription factor E2F interacts with the retinoblastoma tumor suppressor, histone deacetylase, and SWItch/Sucrose NonFermentable (SWI/SNF) chromatin remodeling proteins, forming a repressor complex that inhibits transcription [46]. In mice, the LSF element is required for the S phase expression in growth-stimulated cells [47]. TS expression is also regulated through mRNA stability and translational repression. An antisense RNA (rTSα) transcribed from the *rTS* gene that overlaps with the 3' end of the *TS* gene down-regulates TS expression by inducing the site-specific cleavage of TS RNA [48]. TS also autoregulates its own translation by binding to its mRNA and repressing its translation [49]. Several chemotherapeutic agents that target TS have been developed, including the fluoropyrimidines 5-fluorouracil and 5-fluoro-2-deoxyuridine, as well as the antifolates raltitrexed, pemetrexed, and methotrexate. These agents have proven effective in the treatment of head, neck, breast, stomach, and colon cancers [50]. These agents decrease TS catalytic function while also increasing cellular TS concentrations [51,52] by preventing TS from binding to its mRNA and/or by decreasing the rate of ubiquitin-independent enzyme degradation [53,54].

Loss of TS enzymatic activity, resulting from gene polymorphisms or chemotherapeutic agents, results in decreased rates of DNA synthesis, increased rates of uracil misincorporation into DNA, chromosome damage, fragile site induction, and apoptotic cell death [55,56]. A common 28-nucleotide G/C-rich tandem repeat polymorphism within the sequence that encodes the 5' untranslated region in the *TS* gene affects its transcription and response to TS-based chemotherapy. The most common TS variants contain two (2R) or three (3R) copies of the repeat sequences. The repeats contain USF-1 transcription factor-binding sites, which stimulate TS transcription and translation [57]. The 2R/2R genotype is associated with lower TS protein concentrations than the 3R/3R genotype [58,59] and better response to fluoropyrimidine and methotrexate therapy [60,61]. The second repeat of the 3R allele and the first repeat of the 2R allele contain a G→C polymorphism that disrupts USF-1 binding and lowers *TS* expression [57,62,63]. The *TS* gene also contains a 6-base pair insertion/deletion polymorphism that is present in the 3' untranslated region of the transcript [64] that affects mRNA stability and translation [48] and decreases *TS* expression [65]. The homozygous insertion genotype increases risk for NTDs, especially when present in combination with the 2R/2R genotype [66].

2. 5,10-Methylene-THF Synthesis and Regulation

a. 5,10-Methenyl-THF Cyclohydrolase and 5,10-Methylene-THF Dehydrogenase

C1-THF synthase is the primary source of cytoplasmic 5,10-methylene-THF, which is generated from 10-formyl-THF through its MTHFC and MTHFD activities (Figure 3.1) encoded by *Mthfd1* [67]. MTHFC catalyzes the reversible interconversion of 10-formyl-THF and 5,10-methenyl-THF, whereas MTHFD catalyzes the nicotinamide-adenine dinucleotide phosphate, reduced form (NADPH)-dependent and reversible interconversion of 5,10-methenyl-THF and 5,10-methylene-THF. The dehydrogenase reaction is driven in the reductive direction in vivo by the cytoplasmic NADPH/NADP+ ratio (Figure 3.1). MTHFC and MTHFD are essential for the provision of folate-activated one-carbons for thymidylate biosynthesis and homocysteine remethylation from 10-formyl-THF.

b. Serine Hydroxymethyltransferase

SHMT catalyzes the reversible and pyridoxal-phosphate–dependent interconversion of serine and THF to glycine and methylene-THF (Figure 3.1). Mammals express cytoplasmic serine hydroxy methyltransferase (cSHMT, encoded by *SHMT1*) and mitochondrial serine hydroxy methyltransferase (mSHMT, encoded by *SHMT2*) isozymes that share 63% amino acid sequence identity [68]. *SHMT1* expression is limited to liver, kidney, intestine, and skeletal muscle, whereas *SHMT2* is expressed ubiquitously [69]. Recently, the *SHMT2* gene was shown to express ubiquitously a cytoplasmic protein through an alternate promoter located in intron 1. Transcription from the alternate promoter produces transcript that lacks exon 1, which encodes the mitochondrial leader sequence (D. D. Andersen and P. J. Stover, unpublished results). This finding indicates that all cells contain cSHMT activity that can be derived from *SHMT1* or *SHMT2*.

cSHMT-derived 5,10-methylene-THF supports thymidylate biosynthesis and homocysteine remethylation when converted to 5-methyl-THF by methylene-THF reductase (MTHFR) (Figure 3.1). cSHMT-derived one-carbons do not make significant contributions to purine biosynthesis because the reductive environment (NADPH/NADP+ ratio) in the cytoplasm does not support the conversion of 5,10-methylene-THF to 10-formyl-THF [20]. Stable isotope tracer studies using cultured cells indicate that 5,10-methylene-THF derived from SHMT in the cytoplasm is preferentially directed to thymidylate biosynthesis relative to homocysteine remethylation [42,70]. This preferential partitioning of cSHMT-derived one-carbons to thymidylate synthesis may be achieved through the localization of the thymidylate synthesis pathway in the nucleus [71] (Figure 3.1) (see Section II.B.2.d, Nuclear Folate-Dependent

Thymidylate Biosynthesis). cSHMT can also deplete 5,10-methylene-THF pools when catalyzing serine synthesis, which impairs AdoMet synthesis and regenerates unsubstituted THF for purine biosynthesis [42,72]. The SHMT-catalyzed conversion of glycine to serine supports gluconeogenesis; glycine is a glucogenic amino acid through its conversion to serine [73]. SHMT activity is suppressed by the tight-binding inhibitors 5-formyl-THF and 5-methyl-THF (Figure 3.2).

SHMT1 expression and cSHMT activity are regulated by several nutrients and metabolic factors, including pyridoxal phosphate (vitamin B6), retinoic acid, zinc, and ferritin. Vitamin B6 deficiency was shown to decrease cSHMT activity in rat liver [74] and protein concentrations in cultured cells [75]. Retinoic acid, which inhibits proliferation and induces differentiation during vertebrate development, reduces cSHMT mRNA concentrations [76]. In contrast, zinc induces *SHMT1* transcription by acting through a metal regulatory element present within the promoter [77]. The heavy chain subunit of the iron-storage protein ferritin was also shown to increase cSHMT protein concentrations [70] by stimulating the cap-independent translation of the transcript through a ferritin-responsive internal ribosome entry site (IRES) [78]. More recent studies have demonstrated that the cSHMT IRES is induced by exposure to ultraviolet radiation and that cSHMT is essential for efficient DNA repair (P. J. Stover and J. T. Fox, unpublished results).

c. Dihydrofolate Reductase

DHFR catalyzes the NADPH-dependent conversion of DHF to THF and completes the thymidylate synthesis cycle (Figure 3.1). This reaction is essential to regenerate the functional THF coenzymes and is highly efficient in cells, as DHF is not known to accumulate except following exposure to antifolate chemotherapeutic agents that target DHFR, including methotrexate [79]. Although there is no evidence that DHFR activity is rate limiting in the thymidylate synthesis cycle, it has been an effective target for the development of antimicrobial and anticancer agents [80]. DHFR has been shown to autoregulate its translation by binding to its mRNA in a manner similar to that described for TS translational autoregulation [81,82]. The *DHFR* gene contains a 19-bp deletion polymorphism in intron 1 [83]. This polymorphism is associated with a 1.6-fold increase in DHFR expression in lymphoblast cell lines in one study [84] with no effect on expression in another study [85]. Polymorphisms in the DHFR promoter are associated with worse outcomes following methotrexate therapy in childhood acute lymphoblastic leukemia (ALL), likely resulting from higher DHFR expression [80].

d. Nuclear Folate-Dependent Thymidylate Biosynthesis

De novo thymidylate biosynthesis occurs in both the nucleus and cytoplasm (Figure 3.1). Approximately 10% of cellular folate resides in the nucleus, and TS and cSHMT have been localized to the nucleus in several mammalian cell types in S phase [71,86–90]. The enzymes that constitute the TS cycle (cSHMT, TS, and DHFR) are substrates for UBC9-mediated modification with the small ubiquitin-like modifier (SUMO), which targets proteins for nuclear localization during S phase [4,71]. Nuclear TS was shown to form part of a putative "replitase complex" along with DNA polymerase α, ribonucleotide reductase, thymidylate kinase, nucleoside diphosphate kinase, and the folate-dependent enzyme DHFR [87,91,92]. Nuclear de novo thymidylate synthesis may occur directly at the replication fork during S phase and lower uracil misincorporation into DNA. A common *SHMT1* variant, C1420T, has been shown to be protective against adult ALL [93] and malignant lymphoma [94]. This single-nucleotide polymorphism (SNP) results in an amino acid substitution, L474F, which prevents cSHMT SUMOylation [4]. When present in combination with the *MTHFR* C677T polymorphism (see below), *SHMT1* C1420T is a risk factor for cardiovascular disease [95].

C. 5-METHYL-THF AND HOMOCYSTEINE REMETHYLATION

1. Methionine Synthesis

5-Methyl-THF is a required cofactor for the Zn^{+2}- and cobalamin (vitamin B12)-dependent remethylation of homocysteine to methionine catalyzed by methionine synthase (MS) [96–99].

Although MS metabolic function is partially redundant with betaine homocysteine methyltransferase (BHMT), which remethylates homocysteine to form methionine in a folate-independent reaction, the expression of BHMT is limited primarily to the liver and kidney, whereas MS displays ubiquitous expression [100]. MS serves several important functions, including (1) regeneration of the THF cofactor and prevention of 5-methyl-THF accumulation; (2) synthesis of the essential amino acid methionine; and (3) removal of cellular homocysteine, which is a risk factor for cardiovascular disease [101], NTDs [102], and Alzheimer's disease [103]. Mice lacking MS expression exhibit embryonic lethality, indicating that MS is an essential enzyme for mammals [104].

Relatively little is known about the regulation of MS expression. Vitamin B12 elevates MS protein concentrations by stabilizing MS protein and by stimulating MS translation through an IRES located within the 5′-untranslated region (UTR) of the transcript [105]. The 5′ leader sequence of human MS mRNA also contains two upstream open reading frames that recruit the 40S ribosomal subunit and cause it to stall and inhibit the MS translation [106].

Loss of MS activity, resulting from vitamin B12 deficiency or destruction of the cobalamin cofactor by radicals including nitrous oxide exposure, inhibits nucleotide biosynthesis because of the accumulation of cytoplasmic folate cofactors such as 5-methyl-THF. This effect is referred to as a "5-methyl-THF trap" [107,108] and occurs because the MTHFR reaction is irreversible in vivo, and MS is the only 5-methyl-THF-using enzyme (Figure 3.1).

Rare gene mutations that result in low MS activity are associated with an autosomal recessive disease that presents with homocysteinemia, homocystinuria, hypomethioninemia, megaloblastic anemia, neural dysfunction, and mental retardation [109]. The common polymorphic variant, A2756G, which affects the domain involved in methylation and reactivation of the vitamin B12 cofactor [110], results in decreased plasma homocysteine concentrations [111] and is a risk factor for systemic lupus erythematosus [112], bipolar disorder, schizophrenia [113], and for having a child with spina bifida [114], orofacial clefts [115], and Down syndrome [116].

2.   5-Methyl-THF Synthesis and Regulation

a.   5,10-Methylene-THF Reductase

5-Methyl-THF is generated through the NADPH-dependent reduction of 5,10-methylene-THF catalyzed by the flavoenzyme MTHFR. The N-terminal domain catalyzes the NADPH-dependent reduction of 5,10-methylene-THF to 5-methyl-THF for the remethylation of homocysteine to methionine. The C-terminal domain of the protein contains the binding site for AdoMet, which serves as an allosteric inhibitor of its catalytic activity, which ensures 5,10-methylene-THF is spared for thymidylate biosynthesis when AdoMet concentrations are adequate. The MTHFR reaction is virtually irreversible in vivo and therefore commits one-carbon units to methionine biosynthesis [5,117]. Mice lacking MTHFR survive gestation to birth, have elevated serum homocysteine, are smaller, and exhibit developmental retardation with cerebellar pathology but do not exhibit NTDs [118].

MTHFR regulation is complex and occurs at multiple levels. At the enzyme level, feedback inhibition of MTHFR by AdoMet protects against "trapping" of cellular folate as 5-methyl-THF by inhibiting MTHFR and thereby preventing the depletion of 5,10-methylene-THF pools required for thymidylate biosynthesis. The feedback inhibition of AdoMet also ensures that, during times when methionine is abundant, one-carbon units are spared for the synthesis of DNA precursors [119]. AdoMet binds MTHFR in the inactive T state and thereby increases the T/R ratio in the cell [120]. Phosphorylation of the MTHFR N-terminal domain at Thr34 reduces the inhibition of enzymatic activity by AdoMet by inducing conformational changes in the protein that favor the active R state conformation of the enzyme [121].

The MTHFR undergoes extensive alternative splicing, generating transcripts that vary in the length of their 5′-UTR [122], which influences translational efficiency [123]. MTHFR contains two distinct promoters that generate two isoforms of the MTHFR protein that differ in their molecular mass [122]. MTHFR transcription from the downstream promoter is regulated by nuclear factor κB in a tissue-specific manner [124].

Mild MTHFR deficiency, as characterized by an enzyme with 35% to 45% residual activity, is the most common inborn error of folate metabolism, affecting 5% to 20% of North Americans and Europeans [125]. The primary cause is a common C to T substitution at nucleotide 677, which results in the amino acid change A222V in the catalytic domain of the protein [126]. The 677C→T SNP enhances the loss of the flavin adenine dinucleotide (FAD) cofactor [125,127,128], creating a thermolabile protein [129]. Mild MTHFR deficiency is associated with mild hyperhomocysteinemia, especially in those with low folate concentrations [130], and decreased plasma and red cell folate concentrations [131,132]. Clinically, 677C→T has been shown, in some cases, to be associated with an increased risk for cardiovascular disease [133–135], neural tube defects [136–138], cleft lip and palate [102,139], thrombosis [140–142], and schizophrenia [143–146]. It has also been shown to be protective against several types of cancers, including ALL [147], childhood acute leukemia [148], and colorectal cancer [149,150]. Another common *MTHFR* SNP, 1298A→C (E429A), exists in strong linkage disequilibrium with 677C→T [151]. The 1298 A→C SNP affects the regulatory (C-terminal) domain of the protein [128].

3. Glycine *N*-Methyltransferase and Serine Hydroxymethyltransferase

Both SHMT and glycine *N*-methyltransferase (GNMT) bind tightly but do not metabolize 5-methyl-THF. GNMT is an abundant protein that catalyzes the AdoMet-dependent methylation of glycine to sarcosine and thereby governs transmethylation reactions by regulating and buffering the AdoMet/*S*-adenosylhomocysteine (AdoHcy) ratio, which is referred to as the cellular "methylation potential." GNMT is allosterically regulated by 5-methyl-THF. Under conditions of adequate AdoMet concentrations, AdoMet inhibits MTHFR and limits 5-methyl-THF synthesis to decrease rates of methionine synthesis. GNMT remains active under these conditions and metabolizes excess AdoMet. In contrast, when AdoMet concentrations are low, the production of 5-methyl-THF by MTHFR inhibits GNMT activity and conserves the limited amount of methionine for essential methylation reactions [3]. 5-Methyl-THF is sequestered by SHMT and may compete with MS for this coenzyme [152]. Increased *SHMT1* expression elevates cellular concentrations of 5-methyl-THF at the expense of other one-carbon forms of folate while depleting AdoMet concentrations [42]. This observation is consistent with cSHMT serving as a 5-methyl-THF-binding protein in the cytoplasm and thereby limiting the availability of 5-methyl-THF for homocysteine remethylation (Figure 3.1) [42].

III. ONE-CARBON METABOLISM IN MITOCHONDRIA

Our knowledge of one-carbon metabolism in mitochondria, as well as its regulation, is limited compared with that of the cytoplasmic compartment. Many of the enzyme activities associated with cytoplasmic one-carbon metabolism have mitochondrial isozymes that arose through gene duplications. However, unlike the cytoplasm, the interconversion of one-carbon-substituted folates in mitochondria is driven in the oxidative direction toward formate production and differs with respect to the source of reducing equivalents [5,20]. Approximately 40% of total cellular folates are found in mitochondria [153,154]. The primary functions of mitochondrial one-carbon metabolism are (1) to generate one-carbon units in the form of formate for one-carbon metabolism in the cytoplasm; (2) to generate the amino acid glycine; and (3) to synthesize formylmethionyl-tRNA for protein synthesis in mitochondria (Figure 3.3).

The role of mitochondria in the folate-dependent conversion of serine to glycine and formate was established by demonstrating that isolated mitochondria convert serine to glycine and formate [155,156]. The essentiality of mitochondria for glycine synthesis was demonstrated by the generation of mutant Chinese hamster ovary (CHO) cell complementation groups that were glycine auxotrophs. Characterization of these cell lines identified mitochondrial folate-dependent proteins *SHMT2* (*glyA*) [157] and the mitochondrial folate transporter (*glyB*) [158] as essential for glycine synthesis. However, the definitive pathway for the generation of formate from serine in mitochondria has yet to be established [20], and not all the enzymes and their associated genes required for this pathway have been identified.

A.   5,10-METHYLENE-THF SYNTHESIS IN MITOCHONDRIA

1.   Mitochondrial Serine Hydroxymethyltransferase

The C3 of serine is a primary source of folate-activated one-carbon units [159]. The cleavage of serine to formate and glycine in mitochondria is initiated by the pyridoxal-phosphate–dependent mSHMT, which is encoded by *SHMT2*. Loss of the mSHMT isozyme creates a glycine auxotrophy in CHO cells [160], indicating that cSHMT is not a primary source of glycine and that cSHMT cannot compensate for mSHMT function [42,157]. mSHMT may also function in the conversion of glycine to serine during gluconeogenesis [20,73]. *SHMT2* is ubiquitously expressed in human tissues [161]. Its activity is sensitive to pyridoxal-phosphate concentrations [32,74], and its transcription is *myc* responsive, consistent with its role in generating one-carbons for cytoplasmic metabolism. Expression of the *SHMT2* cDNA in c-myc-null cells partially complements the growth inhibition associated with loss of myc expression [162].

2.   Glycine Cleavage System, Aminomethyltransferase

The glycine cleavage system (GCS) is a multienzyme complex that generates folate-activated one-carbons by catalyzing the reversible oxidation of glycine to CO_2, ammonia, and 5,10-methylene-THF [163]. GCS comprises four proteins: (1) the P-protein, which catalyzes the pyridoxal-phosphate–dependent decarboxylation of glycine; (2) the H-protein, a lipoic acid–dependent hydrogen carrier; (3) the T-protein, which exhibits THF-dependent aminomethyltransferase (AMT) activity; and (4) the L-protein, a lipoamide dehydrogenase. The complex localizes to the inner mitochondrial membrane in the liver, kidney, glia-astrocyte lineage of the brain, and neuroepithelium during development [164]. In humans, GCS accounts for nearly 40% of overall glycine flux, and the one-carbon produced makes major contributions to cytoplasmic THF-dependent purine and thymidylate biosynthesis [165]. GCS is essential for normal embryonic development; loss of GCS activity is associated with nonketotic hyperglycinemia, an inborn error of metabolism. This autosomal recessive disorder presents with severe mental retardation, seizures, apnea, and hypotonia resulting from the accumulation of glycine in all tissues, including the central nervous system [166].

3.   Dimethylglycine Dehydrogenase and Sarcosine Dehydrogenase

Oxidative choline catabolism occurs through the sequential conversion of choline → betaine → dimethylglycine → sarcosine → glycine. Both dimethylglycine and sarcosine catabolism are sources of one-carbons for folate metabolism, which occurs in the liver mitochondria matrix through the activity of dimethylglycine dehydrogenase (DMGD) and sarcosine dehydrogenase (SD), respectively. These enzymes contain a covalently bound FAD and are folate-binding proteins [167]. The quantitative contribution of choline degradation to the cytoplasmic folate-activated one-carbon pool is not known. DMGD and SD deficiency are associated with inborn errors of metabolism. DMGD deficiency results in muscle fatigue and body odor, whereas sarcosinemia is a rare autosomal disorder with a broad and variable spectrum of symptoms, including mental retardation and growth failure [168].

B. 10-FORMYL-THF SYNTHESIS FROM 5,10-METHYLENE-THF IN MITOCHONDRIA

1. Mitochondrial Methenyl-THF Cyclohydrolase and Methylene-THF Dehydrogenase

The generation of 10-formyl-THF from 5,10-methylene-THF requires MTHFD and MTHFC activities. *Mthfd2*, which arose through gene duplication and mutation of *Mthfd1*, encodes the mitochondrial isozymes of MTHFD and MTHFC [169,170]. *Mthfd2* differs from *Mthfd1* in that it does not encode FTHFS activity, and the mitochondrial methylene-THF dehydrogenase (mMTHFD) activity is NAD-dependent, which serves to drive the reaction in the oxidative direction to generate 10-formyl-THF [20]. *Mthfd2* is an essential gene during mouse development, but its expression appears to be limited to embryonic and transformed cells [171]. Deletion in murine embryonic fibroblasts creates a glycine auxotrophy, consistent with its role in generating formate from serine. The gene encoding mMTHFD and mitochondrial methenyl-THF cyclohydrolase (mMTHFC) activities in adult tissues remains to be identified.

C. FORMATE SYNTHESIS FROM 10-FORMYL-THF IN MITOCHONDRIA

1. Mitochondrial 10-Formyl-THF Synthetase

The final step in the conversion of 5,10-methylene-THF to formate in mitochondria requires the hydrolysis of formate from 10-formyl-THF [5]. The reverse reaction of FTHFS generates formate, which is driven by a favorable ADP/ATP ratio in mitochondria [5]. The mitochondrial 10-formyl-THF synthetase (mFTHFS) isozyme is encoded by *Mthfd1L*, which encodes a monofunctional enzyme that is expressed ubiquitously in mammalian cells [172]. Functional studies of this recently identified FTHFS enzyme will be required to determine whether its primary function is to generate formate from 10-formyl-THF.

D. METHIONYL-tRNA$_F$^{MET} FORMYLTRANSFERASE

The initiation of protein synthesis in mitochondria requires formyl-methionyl-tRNA (fMet-tRNA), which is formed by the 10-formyl-THF–dependent formylation of Met-tRNA–catalyzed methionyl-tRNA$_f$^{Met} formyltransferase [173,174]. The formylation of Met-tRNA increases its affinity for initiation factor 2 by 25-fold, and mitochondrial ribosomes bind fMet-tRNA 50-fold tighter than Met-tRNA in the presence of initiation factor 2 [175].

IV. SUMMARY

Impaired folate metabolism is associated with several pathologies and developmental anomalies, including NTDs [176,177], cardiovascular disease [178–180], and cancer [56,181–184]. One-carbon metabolism can be disrupted by folate and other B-vitamin deficiencies and/or common, penetrant genetic mutations and polymorphisms [176,185–187]. However, the biochemical mechanisms and causal metabolic pathways responsible for the initiation and/or progression of folate-associated pathologies have yet to be established, although they likely involve gene–nutrient interactions. There are still knowledge gaps in our fundamental understanding of one-carbon metabolism and its regulation. Little is known about the interactions among mitochondrial, cytoplasmic, and nuclear one-carbon metabolism and their role in gene expression and genome stability. Furthermore, the entire metabolic pathway for the folate-dependent conversion of serine to formate and glycine has yet to be established. Future studies in genetically engineered mice will be required to model and elucidate the gene–nutrient interactions and associated mechanisms that underlie folate-related pathologies.

ACKNOWLEDGMENTS

This work was supported by Public Health Service DK58144.

REFERENCES

1. Schirch V, Strong WB. Interaction of folylpolyglutamates with enzymes in one-carbon metabolism. *Arch Biochem Biophys* 1989; 269:371–80.
2. Shane B. Folylpolyglutamate synthesis and role in the regulation of one-carbon metabolism. *Vitam Horm* 1989; 45:263–335.
3. Porter DH, Cook RJ, Wagner C. Enzymatic properties of dimethylglycine dehydrogenase and sarcosine dehydrogenase from rat liver. *Arch Biochem Biophys* 1985; 243:396–407.
4. Woeller CF, Anderson DD, Szebenyi DM, Stover PJ. Evidence for small ubiquitin-like modifier-dependent nuclear import of the thymidylate biosynthesis pathway. *J Biol Chem* 2007; 282:17623–31.
5. Appling DR. Compartmentation of folate-mediated one-carbon metabolism in eukaryotes. *FASEB J* 1991; 5:2645–51.
6. Scott JM, Dinn JJ, Wilson P, Weir DG. Pathogenesis of subacute combined degeneration: A result of methyl group deficiency. *Lancet* 1981; 2:334–37.
7. Suh JR, Herbig AK, Stover PJ. New perspectives on folate catabolism. *Annu Rev Nutr* 2001; 21:255–82.
8. Miranda TB, Jones PA. DNA methylation: The nuts and bolts of repression. *J Cell Physiol* 2007; 213:384–90.
9. Winter-Vann AM, Kamen BA, Bergo MO, Young SG, Melnyk S, James SJ, Casey PJ. Targeting Ras signaling through inhibition of carboxyl methylation: An unexpected property of methotrexate. *Proc Natl Acad Sci USA* 2003; 100:6529–34.
10. Stead LM, Jacobs RL, Brosnan ME, Brosnan JT. Methylation demand and homocysteine metabolism. *Adv Enzyme Regul* 2004; 44:321–33.
11. Meredith M, Rabaglia M, Metz S. Cytosolic biosynthesis of GTP and ATP in normal rat pancreatic islets. *Biochim Biophys Acta* 1995; 1266:16–22.
12. Brodsky G, Barnes T, Bleskan J, Becker L, Cox M, Patterson D. The human GARS-AIRS-GART gene encodes two proteins which are differentially expressed during human brain development and temporally overexpressed in cerebellum of individuals with Down syndrome. *Hum Mol Genet* 1997; 6:2043–50.
13. An S, Kumar R, Sheets ED, Benkovic SJ. Reversible compartmentalization of de novo purine biosynthetic complexes in living cells. *Science* 2008; 320:103–06.
14. Aimi J, Qiu H, Williams J, Zalkin H, Dixon JE. De novo purine nucleotide biosynthesis: Cloning of human and avian cDNAs encoding the trifunctional glycinamide ribonucleotide synthetase-aminoimidazole ribonucleotide synthetase-glycinamide ribonucleotide

transformylase by functional complementation in *E. coli. Nucleic Acids Res* 1990; 18:6665–72.

15. Schild D, Brake AJ, Kiefer MC, Young D, Barr PJ. Cloning of three human multifunctional de novo purine biosynthetic genes by functional complementation of yeast mutations. *Proc Natl Acad Sci USA* 1990; 87:2916–20.

16. Beardsley GP, Moroson BA, Taylor EC, Moran RG. A new folate antimetabolite, 5,10-dideaza-5,6,7,8-tetrahydrofolate is a potent inhibitor of de novo purine synthesis. *J Biol Chem*1989; 264:328–33.

17. Erba E, Sen S, Sessa C, Vikhanskaya FL, D'Incalci M. Mechanism of cytotoxicity of 5,10-dideazatetrahydrofolic acid in human ovarian carcinoma cells in vitro and modulation of the drug activity by folic or folinic acid. *Br J Cancer* 1994; 69:205–11.

18. Zhao R, Goldman ID. Resistance to antifolates. *Oncogene* 2003; 22:7431–57.

19. Howard KM, Muga SJ, Zhang L, Thigpen AE, Appling DR. Characterization of the rat cytoplasmic C1-tetrahydrofolate synthase gene and analysis of its expression in liver regeneration and fetal development. *Gene* 2003; 319:85–97.

20. Christensen KE, MacKenzie RE. Mitochondrial one-carbon metabolism is adapted to the specific needs of yeast, plants and mammals. *Bioessays* 2006; 28:595–605.

21. Smith GK, Mueller WT, Benkovic PA, Benkovic SJ. On the cofactor specificity of glycinamide ribonucleotide and 5-aminoimidazole-4-carboxamide ribonucleotide transformylase from chicken liver. *Biochemistry* 1981; 20:1241–45.

22. Brody LC, Conley M, Cox C, Kirke PN, McKeever MP, Mills JL, Molloy AM, et al. A polymorphism, R653Q, in the trifunctional enzyme methylenetetrahydrofolate dehydrogenase/methenyltetrahydrofolate cyclohydrolase/formyltetrahydrofolate synthetase is a maternal genetic risk factor for neural tube defects: Report of the Birth Defects Research Group. *Am J Hum Genet* 2002; 71:1207–15.

23. De Marco P, Merello E, Calevo MG, Mascelli S, Raso A, Cama A, Capra V. Evaluation of a methylenetetrahydrofolate-dehydrogenase 1958G>A polymorphism for neural tube defect risk. *J Hum Genet* 2006; 51:98–103.

24. Parle-McDermott A, Kirke PN, Mills JL, Molloy AM, Cox C, O'Leary VB, Pangilinan F, et al. Confirmation of the R653Q polymorphism of the trifunctional C1-synthase enzyme as a maternal risk for neural tube defects in the Irish population. *Eur J Hum Genet* 2006; 14:768–72.

25. Parle-McDermott A, Mills JL, Kirke PN, Cox C, Signore CC, Kirke S, Molloy AM, et al. MTHFD1 R653Q polymorphism is a maternal genetic risk factor for severe abruptio placentae. *Am J Med Genet A* 2005; 132:365–68.

26. Parle-McDermott A, Pangilinan F, Mills JL, Signore CC, Molloy AM, Cotter A, Conley M, et al. A polymorphism in the MTHFD1 gene increases a mother's risk of having an unexplained second trimester pregnancy loss. *Mol Hum Reprod* 2005; 11:477–80.

27. Hilton JF, Christensen KE, Watkins D, Raby BA, Renaud Y, de la Luna S, Estivill X, MacKenzie RE, Hudson TJ, Rosenblatt DS. The molecular basis of glutamate formiminotransferase deficiency. *Hum Mutat* 2003; 22:67–73.

28. Donato H, Krupenko NI, Tsybovsky Y, Krupenko SA. 10-Formyltetrahydrofolate dehydrogenase requires a 4'-phosphopantetheine prosthetic group for catalysis. *J Biol Chem* 2007; 282:34159–66.

29. Cook RJ, Lloyd RS, Wagner C. Isolation and characterization of cDNA clones for rat liver 10-formyltetrahydrofolate dehydrogenase. *J Biol Chem* 1991; 266:4965–73.

30. Mackenzie RE. Biogenesis and interconversion of substituted tetrahydrofolates. In: Blakley RL, Benkovic SJ, eds., *Folates and Pterins, vol. 1, Chemistry and Biochemistry of Folates*. New York: Wiley-Interscience, 1984:255–306.

31. Kim DW, Huang T, Schirch D, Schirch V. Properties of tetrahydropteroylpentaglutamate bound to 10-formyltetrahydrofolate dehydrogenase. *Biochemistry* 1996; 35:15772–83.

32. Anguera MC, Field MS, Perry C, Ghandour H, Chiang EP, Selhub J, Shane B, Stover PJ. Regulation of folate-mediated one-carbon metabolism by 10-formyltetrahydrofolate dehydrogenase. *J Biol Chem* 2006; 281:18335–42.

33. Krupenko SA, Oleinik NV. 10-Formyltetrahydrofolate dehydrogenase, one of the major folate enzymes, is down-regulated in tumor tissues and possesses suppressor effects on cancer cells. *Cell Growth Differ* 2002; 13:227–36.

34. Oleinik NV, Krupenko SA. Ectopic expression of 10-formyltetrahydrofolate dehydrogenase in A549 cells induces G1 cell cycle arrest and apoptosis. *Mol Cancer Res* 2003; 1:577–88.

35. Champion KM, Cook RJ, Tollaksen SL, Giometti CS. Identification of a heritable deficiency of the folate-dependent enzyme 10-formyltetrahydrofolate dehydrogenase in mice. *Proc Natl Acad Sci USA* 1994; 91:11338–42.

36. Anguera MC, Liu X, Stover PJ. Cloning, expression, and purification of 5,10-methenyltetrahydrofolate synthetase from *Mus musculus. Protein Expr Purif* 2004; 35:276–83.

37. Field MS, Szebenyi DM, Perry CA, Stover PJ. Inhibition of 5,10-methenyltetrahydrofolate synthetase. *Arch Biochem Biophys* 2007; 458:194–201.

38. Field MS, Szebenyi DM, Stover PJ. Regulation of de novo purine biosynthesis by methenyltetrahydrofolate synthetase in neuroblastoma. *J Biol Chem* 2006; 281:4215–21.

39. Stover P, Kruschwitz H, Schirch V. Evidence that 5-formyltetrahydropteroylglutamate has a metabolic role in one-carbon metabolism. *Adv Exp Med Biol* 1993; 338:679–85.

40. Bertrand R, Jolivet J. Methenyltetrahydrofolate synthetase prevents the inhibition of phosphoribosyl 5-aminoimidazole 4-carboxamide ribonucleotide formyltransferase by 5-formyltetrahydrofolate polyglutamates. *J Biol Chem* 1989; 264:8843–46.

41. Carreras CW, Santi DV. The catalytic mechanism and structure of thymidylate synthase. *Annu Rev Biochem* 1995; 64:721–62.

42. Herbig K, Chiang EP, Lee LR, Hills J, Shane B, Stover PJ. Cytoplasmic serine hydroxymethyltransferase mediates competition between folate-dependent deoxyribonucleotide and *S*-adenosylmethionine biosyntheses. *J Biol Chem* 2002; 277:38381–89.

43. Ash J, Liao WC, Ke Y, Johnson LF. Regulation of mouse thymidylate synthase gene expression in growth-stimulated cells: Upstream S phase control elements are indistinguishable from the essential promoter elements. *Nucleic Acids Res* 1995; 23:4649–56.

44. Jenh CH, Geyer PK, Johnson LF. Control of thymidylate synthase mRNA content and gene transcription in an overproducing mouse cell line. *Mol Cell Biol* 1985; 5:2527–32.

45. Navalgund LG, Rossana C, Muench AJ, Johnson LF. Cell cycle regulation of thymidylate synthetase gene expression in cultured mouse fibroblasts. *J Biol Chem* 1980; 255:7386–90.

46. Angus SP, Wheeler LJ, Ranmal SA, Zhang X, Markey MP, Mathews CK, Knudsen ES. Retinoblastoma tumor suppressor targets dNTP metabolism to regulate DNA replication. *J Biol Chem* 2002; 277:44376–84.

47. Powell CM, Rudge TL, Zhu Q, Johnson LF, Hansen U. Inhibition of the mammalian transcription factor LSF induces S-phase-dependent apoptosis by downregulating thymidylate synthase expression. *EMBO J* 2000; 19:4665–75.

48. Chu J, Dolnick BJ. Natural antisense (rTSalpha) RNA induces site-specific cleavage of thymidylate synthase mRNA. *Biochim Biophys Acta* 2002; 1587:183–93.

49. Chu E, Koeller DM, Casey JL, Drake JC, Chabner BA, Elwood PC, Zinn S, Allegra CJ. Autoregulation of human thymidylate synthase messenger RNA translation by thymidylate synthase. *Proc Natl Acad Sci USA* 1991; 88:8977–81.

50. Takemura Y, Jackman AL. Folate-based thymidylate synthase inhibitors in cancer chemotherapy. *Anticancer Drugs* 1997; 8:3–16.

51. Gorlick R, Metzger R, Danenberg KD, Salonga D, Miles JS, Longo GS, Fu J, et al. Higher concentrations of thymidylate synthase gene expression are observed in pulmonary as

compared with hepatic metastases of colorectal adenocarcinoma. *J Clin Oncol* 1998; 16:1465–69.

52. Van der Wilt CL, Pinedo HM, Smid K, Peters GJ. Elevation of thymidylate synthase following 5-fluorouracil treatment is prevented by the addition of leucovorin in murine colon tumors. *Cancer Res* 1992; 52:4922–28.

53. Forsthoefel AM, Pena MM, Xing YY, Rafique Z, Berger FG. Structural determinants for the intracellular degradation of human thymidylate synthase. *Biochemistry* 2004; 43:1972–79.

54. Kitchens ME, Forsthoefel AM, Rafique Z, Spencer HT, Berger FG. Ligand-mediated induction of thymidylate synthase occurs by enzyme stabilization. Implications for autoregulation of translation. *J Biol Chem* 1999; 274:12544–47.

55. Hori T, Ayusawa D, Shimizu K, Koyama H, Seno T. Chromosome breakage induced by thymidylate stress in thymidylate synthase-negative mutants of mouse FM3A cells. *Cancer Res* 1984; 44:703–09.

56. Blount BC, Mack MM, Wehr CM, MacGregor JT, Hiatt RA, Wang G, Wickramasinghe SN, Everson RB, Ames BN. Folate deficiency causes uracil misincorporation into human DNA and chromosome breakage: Implications for cancer and neuronal damage. *Proc Natl Acad Sci USA* 1997; 94:3290–95.

57. Mandola MV, Stoehlmacher J, Muller-Weeks S, Cesarone G, Yu MC, Lenz HJ, Ladner RD. A novel single nucleotide polymorphism within the 5′ tandem repeat polymorphism of the thymidylate synthase gene abolishes USF-1 binding and alters transcriptional activity. *Cancer Res* 2003; 63:2898–904.

58. Horie N, Aiba H, Oguro K, Hojo H, Takeishi K. Functional analysis and DNA polymorphism of the tandemly repeated sequences in the 5′-terminal regulatory region of the human gene for thymidylate synthase. *Cell Struct Funct* 1995; 20:191–97.

59. Kawakami K, Watanabe G. Identification and functional analysis of single nucleotide polymorphism in the tandem repeat sequence of thymidylate synthase gene. *Cancer Res* 2003; 63:6004–07.

60. Krajinovic M, Costea I, Chiasson S. Polymorphism of the thymidylate synthase gene and outcome of acute lymphoblastic leukaemia. *Lancet* 2002; 359:1033–34.

61. Pullarkat ST, Stoehlmacher J, Ghaderi V, Xiong YP, Ingles SA, Sherrod A, Warren R, Tsao-Wei D, Groshen S, Lenz HJ. Thymidylate synthase gene polymorphism determines response and toxicity of 5-FU chemotherapy. *Pharmacogenomics J* 2001; 1:65–70.

62. Kawakami K, Omura K, Kanehira E, Watanabe Y. Polymorphic tandem repeats in the thymidylate synthase gene is associated with its protein expression in human gastrointestinal cancers. *Anticancer Res* 1999; 19:3249–52.

63. Lincz LF, Scorgie FE, Garg MB, Ackland SP. Identification of a novel single nucleotide polymorphism in the first tandem repeat sequence of the thymidylate synthase 2R allele. *Int J Cancer* 2007; 120:1930–34.

64. Ulrich CM, Bigler J, Velicer CM, Greene EA, Farin FM, Potter JD. Searching expressed sequence tag databases: Discovery and confirmation of a common polymorphism in the thymidylate synthase gene. *Cancer Epidemiol Biomarkers Prev* 2000; 9:1381–85.

65. Mandola MV, Stoehlmacher J, Zhang W, Groshen S, Yu MC, Iqbal S, Lenz HJ, Ladner RD. A 6 bp polymorphism in the thymidylate synthase gene causes message instability and is associated with decreased intratumoral TS mRNA levels. *Pharmacogenetics* 2004; 14:319–27.

66. Volcik KA, Shaw GM, Zhu H, Lammer EJ, Laurent C, Finnell RH. Associations between polymorphisms within the thymidylate synthase gene and spina bifida. *Birth Defects Res A Clin Mol Teratol* 2003; 67:924–28.

67. Tan LU, Drury EJ, MacKenzie RE. Mcthylenetetrahydrofolate dehydrogenase-methenyltetrahydrofolate cyclohydrolase-formyltetrahydrofolate synthetase. A multifunctional protein from porcine liver. *J Biol Chem* 1977; 252:1117–22.

68. Garrow TA, Brenner AA, Whitehead VM, Chen XN, Duncan RG, Korenberg JR, Shane B. Cloning of human cDNAs encoding mitochondrial and cytosolic serine hydroxymethyltransferases and chromosomal localization. *J Biol Chem* 1993; 268:11910–16.

69. Girgis S, Nasrallah IM, Suh JR, Oppenheim E, Zanetti KA, Mastri MG, Stover PJ. Molecular cloning, characterization and alternative splicing of the human cytoplasmic serine hydroxymethyltransferase gene. *Gene* 1998; 210:315–24.

70. Oppenheim EW, Adelman C, Liu X, Stover PJ. Heavy chain ferritin enhances serine hydroxymethyltransferase expression and de novo thymidine biosynthesis. *J Biol Chem* 2001; 276:19855–61.

71. Anderson DD, Woeller CF, Stover PJ. Small ubiquitin-like modifier-1 (SUMO-1) modification of thymidylate synthase and dihydrofolate reductase. *Clin Chem Lab Med* 2007; 45:1760–63.

72. Strong WB, Schirch V. In vitro conversion of formate to serine: Effect of tetrahydropteroylpolyglutamates and serine hydroxymethyltransferase on the rate of 10-formyltetrahydrofolate synthetase. *Biochemistry* 1989; 28:9430–39.

73. Nijhout HF, Reed MC, Lam SL, Shane B, Gregory JF 3rd, Ulrich CM. In silico experimentation with a model of hepatic mitochondrial folate metabolism. *Theor Biol Med Model* 2006; 3:40.

74. Scheer JB, Mackey AD, Gregory JF 3rd. Activities of hepatic cytosolic and mitochondrial forms of serine hydroxymethyltransferase and hepatic glycine concentration are affected by vitamin B-6 intake in rats. *J Nutr* 2005; 135:233–38.

75. Perry C, Yu S, Chen J, Matharu KS, Stover PJ. Effect of vitamin B6 availability on serine hydroxymethyltransferase in MCF-7 cells. *Arch Biochem Biophys* 2007; 462:21–27.

76. Nakshatri H, Bouillet P, Bhat-Nakshatri P, Chambon P. Isolation of retinoic acid-repressed genes from P19 embryonal carcinoma cells. *Gene* 1996; 174:79–84.

77. Perry C, Sastry R, Nasrallah IM, Stover PJ. Mimosine attenuates serine hydroxymethyltransferase transcription by chelating zinc. Implications for inhibition of DNA replication. *J Biol Chem* 2005; 280:396–400.

78. Woeller CF, Fox JT, Perry C, Stover PJ. A ferritin-responsive internal ribosome entry site regulates folate metabolism. *J Biol Chem* 2007; 282:29927–35.

79. Kompis IM, Islam K, Then RL. DNA and RNA synthesis: Antifolates. *Chem Rev* 2005; 105:593–620.

80. Dulucq S, St-Onge G, Gagne V, Ansari M, Sinnett D, Labuda D, Moghrabi A, Krajinovic M. DNA variants in the dihydrofolate reductase gene and outcome in childhood ALL. *Blood* 2008; 111:3692–700.

81. Tai N, Ding Y, Schmitz JC, Chu E. Identification of critical amino acid residues on human dihydrofolate reductase protein that mediate RNA recognition. *Nucleic Acids Res* 2002; 30:4481–88.

82. Tai N, Schmitz JC, Liu J, Lin X, Bailly M, Chen TM, Chu E. Translational autoregulation of thymidylate synthase and dihydrofolate reductase. *Front Biosci* 2004; 9:2521–26.

83. Johnson WG, Stenroos ES, Spychala JR, Chatkupt S, Ming SX, Buyske S. New 19 bp deletion polymorphism in intron-1 of dihydrofolate reductase (DHFR): A risk factor for spina bifida acting in mothers during pregnancy? *Am J Med Genet A* 2004; 124:339–45.

84. Parle-McDermott A, Pangilinan F, Mills JL, Kirke PN, Gibney ER, Troendle J, O'Leary VB, et al. The 19-bp deletion polymorphism in intron-1 of dihydrofolate reductase (DHFR) may decrease rather than increase risk for spina bifida in the Irish population. *Am J Med Genet A* 2007; 143:1174–80.

85. van der Linden IJ, Nguyen U, Heil SG, Franke B, Vloet S, Gellekink H, Heijer M, Blom HJ. Variation and expression of dihydrofolate reductase (DHFR) in relation to spina bifida. *Mol Genet Metab* 2007; 91:98–103.

86. Brown SS, Neal GE, Williams DC. Subcellular distribution of some folic acid-linked enzymes in rat liver. *Biochem J* 1965; 97:34C–36C.

87. Prem veer Reddy G, Pardee AB. Multienzyme complex for metabolic channeling in mammalian DNA replication. *Proc Natl Acad Sci USA* 1980; 77:3312–16.
88. Samsonoff WA, Reston J, McKee M, O'Connor B, Galivan J, Maley G, Maley F. Intracellular location of thymidylate synthase and its state of phosphorylation. *J Biol Chem* 1997; 272:13281–85.
89. Wong NA, Brett L, Stewart M, Leitch A, Longley DB, Dunlop MG, Johnston PG, Lessells AM, Jodrell DI. Nuclear thymidylate synthase expression, p53 expression and 5FU response in colorectal carcinoma. *Br J Cancer* 2001; 85:1937–43.
90. Bissoon-Haqqani S, Moyana T, Jonker D, Maroun JA, Birnboim HC. Nuclear expression of thymidylate synthase in colorectal cancer cell lines and clinical samples. *J Histochem Cytochem* 2006; 54:19–29.
91. Boorstein RJ, Pardee AB. Coordinate inhibition of DNA synthesis and thymidylate synthase activity following DNA damage and repair. *Biochem Biophys Res Commun* 1983; 117:30–36.
92. Noguchi H, Prem veer Reddy G, Pardee AB. Rapid incorporation of label from ribonucleoside disphosphates into DNA by a cell-free high molecular weight fraction of animal cell nuclei. *Cell* 1983; 32:443–51.
93. Skibola CF, Smith MT, Hubbard A, Shane B, Roberts AC, Law GR, Rollinson S, Roman E, Cartwright RA, Morgan GJ. Polymorphisms in the thymidylate synthase and serine hydroxymethyltransferase genes and risk of adult acute lymphocytic leukemia. *Blood* 2002; 99:3786–91.
94. Hishida A, Matsuo K, Hamajima N, Ito H, Ogura M, Kagami Y, Taji H, Morishima Y, Emi N, Tajima K. Associations between polymorphisms in the thymidylate synthase and serine hydroxymethyltransferase genes and susceptibility to malignant lymphoma. *Haematologica* 2003; 88:159–66.
95. Lim U, Peng K, Shane B, Stover PJ, Litonjua AA, Weiss ST, Gaziano JM, et al. Polymorphisms in cytoplasmic serine hydroxymethyltransferase and methylenetetrahydrofolate reductase affect the risk of cardiovascular disease in men. *J Nutr* 2005; 135:1989–94.
96. Drennan CL, Huang S, Drummond JT, Matthews RG, Lidwig ML. How a protein binds B12: A 3.0 A x-ray structure of B12-binding domains of methionine synthase. *Science* 1994; 266:1669–74.
97. Goulding CW, Postigo D, Matthews RG. Cobalamin-dependent methionine synthase is a modular protein with distinct regions for binding homocysteine, methyltetrahydrofolate, cobalamin, and adenosylmethionine. *Biochemistry* 1997; 36: 8082–91.
98. Peariso K, Huang S, Matthews RG, Penner-Hahn JE. Characterization of the zinc binding site in methionine synthase enzymes of *Escherichia coli*: The role of zinc in the methylation of homocysteine. *J Am Chem Soc* 1998; 120:8410–16.
99. Ludwig ML, Matthews RG. Structure-based perspectives on B12-dependent enzymes. *Annu Rev Biochem* 1997; 66:269–313.
100. Chen LH, Liu ML, Hwang HY, Chen LS, Korenberg J, Shane B. Human methionine synthase. cDNA cloning, gene localization, and expression. *J Biol Chem* 1997; 272:3628–34.
101. Refsum H, Ueland PM, Nygard O, Vollset SE. Homocysteine and cardiovascular disease. *Annu Rev Med* 1998; 49:31–62.
102. Mills JL, McPartlin JM, Kirke PN, Lee YJ, Conley MR, Weir DG, Scott JM. Homocysteine metabolism in pregnancies complicated by neural-tube defects. *Lancet* 1995; 345:149–51.
103. Clarke R, Smith AD, Jobst KA, Refsum H, Sutton L, Ueland PM. Folate, vitamin B12, and serum total homocysteine concentrations in confirmed Alzheimer disease. *Arch Neurol* 1998; 55:1449–55.

104. Swanson DA, Liu ML, Baker PJ, Garrett L, Stitzel M, Wu J, Harris M, Banerjee R, Shane B, Brody LC. Targeted disruption of the methionine synthase gene in mice. *Mol Cell Biol* 2001; 21:1058–65.

105. Oltean S, Banerjee R. A B12-responsive internal ribosome entry site (IRES) element in human methionine synthase. *J Biol Chem* 2005; 280:32662–68.

106. Col B, Oltean S, Banerjee R. Translational regulation of human methionine synthase by upstream open reading frames. *Biochim Biophys Acta* 2007; 1769:532–40.

107. Lassen HC, Henriksen E, Neukirch F, Kristensen HS. Treatment of tetanus: Severe bone-marrow depression after prolonged nitrous-oxide anaesthesia. *Lancet* 1956; 270:527–30.

108. Shane B, Stokstad EL. Vitamin B12-folate interrelationships. *Annu Rev Nutr* 1985; 5:115–41.

109. Gulati S, Brody LC, Banerjee R. Posttranscriptional regulation of mammalian methionine synthase by B12. *Biochem Biophys Res Commun* 1999; 259:436–42.

110. Leclerc D, Campeau E, Goyette P, Adjalla CE, Christensen B, Ross M, Eydoux P, Rosenblatt DS, Rozen R, Gravel RA. Human methionine synthase: cDNA cloning and identification of mutations in patients of the cblG complementation group of folate/cobalamin disorders. *Hum Mol Genet* 1996; 5:1867–74.

111. Harmon DL, Shields DC, Woodside JV, McMaster D, Yarnell JW, Young IS, Peng K, Shane B, Evans AE, Whitehead AS. Methionine synthase D919G polymorphism is a significant but modest determinant of circulating homocysteine concentrations. *Genet Epidemiol* 1999; 17:298–309.

112. Burzynski M, Duriagin S, Mostowska M, Wudarski M, Chwalinska-Sadowska H, Jagodzinski PP. MTR 2756 A > G polymorphism is associated with the risk of systemic lupus erythematosus in the Polish population. *Lupus* 2007; 16:450–54.

113. Kempisty B, Sikora J, Lianeri M, Szczepankiewicz A, Czerski P, Hauser J, Jagodzinski PP. MTHFD 1958G>A and MTR 2756A>G polymorphisms are associated with bipolar disorder and schizophrenia. *Psychiatr Genet* 2007; 17:177–81.

114. Doolin MT, Barbaux S, McDonnell M, Hoess K, Whitehead AS, Mitchell LE. Maternal genetic effects, exerted by genes involved in homocysteine remethylation, influence the risk of spina bifida. *Am J Hum Genet* 2002; 71:1222–26.

115. Mostowska A, Hozyasz KK, Jagodzinski PP. Maternal MTR genotype contributes to the risk of non-syndromic cleft lip and palate in the Polish population. *Clin Genet* 2006; 69:512–17.

116. Bosco P, Gueant-Rodriguez RM, Anello G, Barone C, Namour F, Caraci F, Romano A, Romano C, Gueant JL. Methionine synthase (MTR) 2756 (A --> G) polymorphism, double heterozygosity methionine synthase 2756 AG/methionine synthase reductase (MTRR) 66 AG, and elevated homocysteinemia are three risk factors for having a child with Down syndrome. *Am J Med Genet A* 2003; 121:219–24.

117. Wagner C. Biochemical role of folate in cellular metabolism. In: Bailey LB, ed., *Folate in Health and Disease*. New York: Marcel Dekker, Inc, 1995:23–42.

118. Chen Z, Karaplis AC, Ackerman SL, Pogribny IP, Melnyk S, Lussier-Cacan S, Chen MF, et al. Mice deficient in methylenetetrahydrofolate reductase exhibit hyperhomocysteinemia and decreased methylation capacity, with neuropathology and aortic lipid deposition. *Hum Mol Genet* 2001; 10:433–43.

119. Kutzbach C, Stokstad EL. Mammalian methylenetetrahydrofolate reductase. Partial purification, properties, and inhibition by S-adenosylmethionine. *Biochim Biophys Acta* 1971; 250:459–77.

120. Jencks DA, Mathews RG. Allosteric inhibition of methylenetetrahydrofolate reductase by adenosylmethionine. Effects of adenosylmethionine and NADPH on the equilibrium between active and inactive forms of the enzyme and on the kinetics of approach to equilibrium. *J Biol Chem* 1987; 262:2485–93.

121. Yamada K, Strahler JR, Andrews PC, Matthews RG. Regulation of human methyl-enetetrahydrofolate reductase by phosphorylation. *Proc Natl Acad Sci USA* 2005; 102:10454–59.
122. Tran P, Leclerc D, Chan M, Pai A, Hiou-Tim F, Wu Q, Goyette P, Artigas C, Milos R, Rozen R. Multiple transcription start sites and alternative splicing in the methyl-enetetrahydrofolate reductase gene result in two enzyme isoforms. *Mamm Genome* 2002; 13:483–92.
123. van der Velden AW, Thomas AA. The role of the 5' untranslated region of an mRNA in translation regulation during development. *Int J Biochem Cell Biol* 1999; 31:87–106.
124. Pickell L, Tran P, Leclerc D, Hiscott J, Rozen R. Regulatory studies of murine methyl-enetetrahydrofolate reductase reveal two major promoters and NF-kappaB sensitivity. *Biochim Biophys Acta* 2005; 1731:104–14.
125. Pejchal R, Campbell E, Guenther BD, Lennon BW, Matthews RG, Ludwig ML. Structural perturbations in the Ala --> Val polymorphism of methylenetetrahydrofolate reductase: How binding of folates may protect against inactivation. *Biochemistry* 2006; 45:4808–18.
126. Shivapurkar N, Tang Z, Frost A, Alabaster O. Inhibition of progression of aberrant crypt foci and colon tumor development by vitamin E and beta-carotene in rats on a high-risk diet. *Cancer Lett* 1995; 91:125–32.
127. Guenther BD, Sheppard CA, Tran P, Rozen R, Matthews RG, Ludwig ML. The structure and properties of methylenetetrahydrofolate reductase from *Escherichia coli* suggest how folate ameliorates human hyperhomocysteinemia. *Nat Struct Biol* 1999; 6:359–65.
128. Yamada K, Chen Z, Rozen R, Matthews RG. Effects of common polymorphisms on the properties of recombinant human methylenetetrahydrofolate reductase. *Proc Natl Acad Sci USA* 2001; 98:14853–58.
129. Kang SS, Wong PW, Zhou JM, Sora J, Lessick M, Ruggie N, Grcevich G. Thermolabile methylenetetrahydrofolate reductase in patients with coronary artery disease. *Metabolism* 1988; 37:611–13.
130. Jacques PF, Bostom AG, Williams RR, Ellison RC, Eckfeldt JH, Rosenberg IH, Selhub J, Rozen R. Relation between folate status, a common mutation in methylenetetrahydro-folate reductase, and plasma homocysteine concentrations. *Circulation* 1996; 93:7–9.
131. Molloy AM, Daly S, Mills JL, Kirke PN, Whitehead AS, Ramsbottom D, Conley MR, Weir DG, Scott JM. Thermolabile variant of 5,10-methylenetetrahydrofolate reductase associated with low red-cell folates: Implications for folate intake recommendations. *Lancet* 1997; 349:1591–93.
132. Parle-McDermott A, Mills JL, Molloy AM, Carroll N, Kirke PN, Cox C, Conley MR, Pangilinan FJ, Brody LC, Scott JM. The MTHFR 1298CC and 677TT genotypes have opposite associations with red cell folate levels. *Mol Genet Metab* 2006; 88:290–94.
133. Klerk M, Verhoef P, Clarke R, Blom HJ, Kok FJ, Schouten EG. MTHFR 677C-->T polymorphism and risk of coronary heart disease: A meta-analysis. *JAMA* 2002; 288:2023–31.
134. Kluijtmans LA, van den Heuvel LP, Boers GH, Frosst P, Stevens EM, van Oost BA, den Heijer M, Trijbels FJ, Rozen R, Blom HJ. Molecular genetic analysis in mild hyperho-mocysteinemia: A common mutation in the methylenetetrahydrofolate reductase gene is a genetic risk factor for cardiovascular disease. *Am J Hum Genet* 1996; 58:35–41.
135. Morita H, Taguchi J, Kurihara H, Kitaoka M, Kaneda H, Kurihara Y, Maemura K, et al. Genetic polymorphism of 5,10-methylenetetrahydrofolate reductase (MTHFR) as a risk factor for coronary artery disease. *Circulation* 1997; 95:2032–36.
136. Christensen B, Arbour L, Tran P, Leclerc D, Sabbaghian N, Platt R, Gilfix BM, et al. Genetic polymorphisms in methylenetetrahydrofolate reductase and methionine syn-thase, folate concentrations in red blood cells, and risk of neural tube defects. *Am J Med Genet* 1999; 84:151–57.

137. Ou CY, Stevenson RE, Brown VK, Schwartz CE, Allen WP, Khoury MJ, Rozen R, Oakley GP Jr, Adams MJ Jr. 5,10 Methylenetetrahydrofolate reductase genetic polymorphism as a risk factor for neural tube defects. *Am J Med Genet* 1996; 63:610–14.

138. van der Put NM, Steegers-Theunissen RP, Frosst P, Trijbels FJ, Eskes TK, van den Heuvel LP, Mariman EC, den Heyer M, Rozen R, Blom HJ. Mutated methylenetetrahydrofolate reductase as a risk factor for spina bifida. *Lancet* 1995; 346:1070–71.

139. Zhu J, Ren A, Hao L, Pei L, Liu J, Zhu H, Li S, Finnell RH, Li Z. Variable contribution of the MTHFR C677T polymorphism to non-syndromic cleft lip and palate risk in China. *Am J Med Genet A* 2006; 140:551–57.

140. Keijzer MB, den Heijer M, Blom HJ, Bos GM, Willems HP, Gerrits WB, Rosendaal FR. Interaction between hyperhomocysteinemia, mutated methylenetetrahydrofolatereductase (MTHFR) and inherited thrombophilic factors in recurrent venous thrombosis. *Thromb Haemost* 2002; 88:723–28.

141. Quere I, Perneger TV, Zittoun J, Bellet H, Gris JC, Daures JP, Schved JF, et al. Red blood cell methylfolate and plasma homocysteine as risk factors for venous thromboembolism: A matched case-control study. *Lancet* 2002; 359:747–52.

142. Zalavras ChG, Giotopoulou S, Dokou E, Mitsis M, Ioannou HV, Tzolou A, Kolaitis N, Vartholomatos G. Lack of association between the C677T mutation in the 5,10-methylenetetrahydrofolate reductase gene and venous thromboembolism in Northwestern Greece. *Int Angiol* 2002; 21:268–71.

143. Lewis SJ, Zammit S, Gunnell D, Smith GD. A meta-analysis of the MTHFR C677T polymorphism and schizophrenia risk. *Am J Med Genet B Neuropsychiatr Genet* 2005; 135:2–4.

144. Muntjewerff JW, Hoogendoorn ML, Kahn RS, Sinke RJ, Den Heijer M, Kluijtmans LA, Blom HJ. Hyperhomocysteinemia, methylenetetrahydrofolate reductase 677TT genotype, and the risk for schizophrenia: A Dutch population based case-control study. *Am J Med Genet B Neuropsychiatr Genet* 2005; 135:69–72.

145. Muntjewerff JW, Kahn RS, Blom HJ, den Heijer M. Homocysteine, methylenetetrahydrofolate reductase and risk of schizophrenia: A meta-analysis. *Mol Psychiatry* 2006; 11:143–49.

146. Scher AI, Terwindt GM, Verschuren WM, Kruit MC, Blom HJ, Kowa H, Frants RR, et al. Migraine and MTHFR C677T genotype in a population-based sample. *Ann Neurol* 2006; 59:372–75.

147. Skibola CF, Smith MT, Kane E, Roman E, Rollinson S, Cartwright RA, Morgan G. Polymorphisms in the methylenetetrahydrofolate reductase gene are associated with susceptibility to acute leukemia in adults. *Proc Natl Acad Sci USA* 1999; 96:12810–15.

148. Wiemels JL, Smith RN, Taylor GM, Eden OB, Alexander FE, Greaves MF. Methylenetetrahydrofolate reductase (MTHFR) polymorphisms and risk of molecularly defined subtypes of childhood acute leukemia. *Proc Natl Acad Sci USA* 2001; 98:4004–09.

149. Chen J, Giovannucci E, Kelsey K, Rimm EB, Stampfer MJ, Colditz GA, Spiegelman D, Willett WC, Hunter DJ. A methylenetetrahydrofolate reductase polymorphism and the risk of colorectal cancer. *Cancer Res* 1996; 56:4862–64.

150. Ma J, Stampfer MJ, Giovannucci E, Artigas C, Hunter DJ, Fuchs C, Willett WC, Selhub J, Hennekens CH, Rozen R. Methylenetetrahydrofolate reductase polymorphism, dietary interactions, and risk of colorectal cancer. *Cancer Res* 1997; 57:1098–102.

151. Stegmann K, Ziegler A, Ngo ET, Kohlschmidt N, Schroter B, Ermert A, Koch MC. Linkage disequilibrium of MTHFR genotypes 677C/T-1298A/C in the German population and association studies in probands with neural tube defects (NTD). *Am J Med Genet* 1999; 87:23–29.

152. Stover P, Schirch V. 5-Formyltetrahydrofolate polyglutamates are slow tight binding inhibitors of serine hydroxymethyltransferase. *J Biol Chem* 1991; 266:1543–50.

153. Horne DW, Patterson D, Cook RJ. Effect of nitrous oxide inactivation of vitamin B12-dependent methionine synthetase on the subcellular distribution of folate coenzymes in rat liver. *Arch Biochem Biophys* 1989; 270:729–33.
154. Lin BF, Huang RF, Shane B. Regulation of folate and one-carbon metabolism in mammalian cells. III. Role of mitochondrial folylpoly-gamma-glutamate synthetase. *J Biol Chem* 1993; 268:21674–79.
155. Barlowe CK, Appling DR. Nitrous oxide exposure reduces hepatic C1-tetrahydrofolate synthase expression in rats. *Biochem Biophys Res Commun* 1988; 157:245–49.
156. Garcia-Martinez LF, Appling DR. Characterization of the folate-dependent mitochondrial oxidation of carbon 3 of serine. *Biochemistry* 1993; 32:4671–76.
157. Pfendner W, Pizer LI. The metabolism of serine and glycine in mutant lines of Chinese hamster ovary cells. *Arch Biochem Biophys* 1980; 200:503–12.
158. Titus SA, Moran RG. Retrovirally mediated complementation of the glyB phenotype. Cloning of a human gene encoding the carrier for entry of folates into mitochondria. *J Biol Chem* 2000; 275:36811–17.
159. Davis SR, Stacpoole PW, Williamson J, Kick LS, Quinlivan EP, Coats BS, Shane B, Bailey LB, Gregory JF 3rd. Tracer-derived total and folate-dependent homocysteine remethylation and synthesis rates in humans indicate that serine is the main one-carbon donor. *Am J Physiol Endocrinol Metab* 2004; 286:E272–79.
160. Chasin LA, Feldman A, Konstam M, Urlaub G. Reversion of a Chinese hamster cell auxotrophic mutant. *Proc Natl Acad Sci USA* 1974; 71:718–22.
161. Girgis S, Suh JR, Jolivet J, Stover PJ. 5-Formyltetrahydrofolate regulates homocysteine remethylation in human neuroblastoma. *J Biol Chem* 1997; 272:4729–34.
162. Nikiforov MA, Chandriani S, O'Connell B, Petrenko O, Kotenko I, Beavis A, Sedivy JM, Cole MD. A functional screen for Myc-responsive genes reveals serine hydroxymethyltransferase, a major source of the one-carbon unit for cell metabolism. *Mol Cell Biol* 2002; 22:5793–800.
163. Okamura-Ikeda K, Hosaka H, Yoshimura M, Yamashita E, Toma S, Nakagawa A, Fujiwara K, Motokawa Y, Taniguchi H. Crystal structure of human T-protein of glycine cleavage system at 2.0 A resolution and its implication for understanding non-ketotic hyperglycinemia. *J Mol Biol* 2005; 351:1146–59.
164. Ichinohe A, Kure S, Mikawa S, Ueki T, Kojima K, Fujiwara K, Iinuma K, Matsubara Y, Sato K. Glycine cleavage system in neurogenic regions. *Eur J Neurosci* 2004; 19:2365–70.
165. Lamers Y, Williamson J, Gilbert LR, Stacpoole PW, Gregory JF 3rd. Glycine turnover and decarboxylation rate quantified in healthy men and women using primed, constant infusions of [1,2-(13)C2]glycine and [(2)H3]leucine. *J Nutr* 2007; 137: 2647–52.
166. Dinopoulos A, Matsubara Y, Kure S. Atypical variants of nonketotic hyperglycinemia. *Mol Genet Metab* 2005; 86:61–69.
167. Wittwer AJ, Wagner C. Identification of folate binding protein of mitochondria as dimethylglycine dehydrogenase. *Proc Natl Acad Sci USA* 1980; 77:4484–88.
168. Binzak BA, Wevers RA, Moolenaar SH, Lee YM, Hwu WL, Poggi-Bach J, Engelke UF, Hoard HM, Vockley JG, Vockley J. Cloning of dimethylglycine dehydrogenase and a new human inborn error of metabolism, dimethylglycine dehydrogenase deficiency. *Am J Hum Genet* 2001; 68:839–47.
169. Di Pietro E, Wang XL, MacKenzie RE. The expression of mitochondrial methylenetetrahydrofolate dehydrogenase-cyclohydrolase supports a role in rapid cell growth. *Biochim Biophys Acta* 2004; 1674:78–84.
170. Di Pietro E, Sirois J, Tremblay ML, MacKenzie RE. Mitochondrial NAD-dependent methylenetetrahydrofolate dehydrogenase-methenyltetrahydrofolate cyclohydrolase is essential for embryonic development. *Mol Cell Biol* 2002; 22:4158–66.

171. Peri KG, MacKenzie RE. NAD(+)-dependent methylenetetrahydrofolate dehydroge-nase-cyclohydrolase: Detection of the mRNA in normal murine tissues and transcriptional regulation of the gene in cell lines. *Biochim Biophys Acta* 1993; 1171:281–87.

172. Christensen KE, Patel H, Kuzmanov U, Mejia NR, MacKenzie RE. Disruption of the mthfd1 gene reveals a monofunctional 10-formyltetrahydrofolate synthetase in mammalian mitochondria. *J Biol Chem* 2005; 280:7597–602.

173. Bianchetti R, Lucchini G, Crosti P, Tortora P. Dependence of mitochondrial protein synthesis initiation on formylation of the initiator methionyl-tRNAf. *J Biol Chem* 1977; 252:2519–23.

174. Takeuchi N, Kawakami M, Omori A, Ueda T, Spremulli LL, Watanabe K. Mammalian mitochondrial methionyl-tRNA transformylase from bovine liver. Purification, charac-terization, and gene structure. *J Biol Chem* 1998; 273:15085–90.

175. Spencer AC, Spremulli LL. Interaction of mitochondrial initiation factor 2 with mitochondrial fMet-tRNA. *Nucleic Acids Res* 2004; 32:5464–70.

176. van der Put NM, Blom HJ. Neural tube defects and a disturbed folate dependent homo-cysteine metabolism. *Eur J Obstet Gynecol Reprod Biol* 2000; 92:57–61.

177. Scott JM. Evidence of folic acid and folate in the prevention of neural tube defects. *Bibl Nutr Dieta* 2001:192–95.

178. Ueland PM, Refsum H, Beresford SA, Vollset SE. The controversy over homocysteine and cardiovascular risk. *Am J Clin Nutr* 2000; 72:324–32.

179. Gerhard GT, Duell PB. Homocysteine and atherosclerosis. *Curr Opin Lipidol* 1999; 10:417–28.

180. Lindenbaum J, Allen RH. Clinical spectrum and diagnosis of folate deficiency. In: Bailey LB, ed., *Folate in Health and Disease*. New York: Marcel Dekker, Inc., 1995:43–73.

181. Ames BN. DNA damage from micronutrient deficiencies is likely to be a major cause of cancer. *Mutat Res* 2001; 475:7–20.

182. Choi SW, Mason JB. Folate and carcinogenesis: An integrated scheme. *J Nutr* 2000; 130:129–32.

183. Pogribny IP, Basnakian AG, Miller BJ, Lopatina NG, Poirier LA, James SJ. Breaks in genomic DNA and within the p53 gene are associated with hypomethylation in livers of folate/methyl-deficient rats. *Cancer Res* 1995; 55:1894–901.

184. Kim YI. Folate and cancer prevention: A new medical application of folate beyond hyperhomocysteinemia and neural tube defects. *Nutr Rev* 1999; 57:314–21.

185. Bailey LB. Folate requirements and dietary recommendations. In: Bailey LB, ed., *Folate in Health and Disease*. New York: Marcel Dekker, Inc, 1995:123–151.

186. McNulty H. Folate requirements for health in different population groups. *Br J Biomed Sci* 1995; 52:110–19.

187. Scott JM. How does folic acid prevent neural tube defects? *Nat Med* 1998; 4:895–96.

4 Genetic Variation

Effect on Folate Metabolism and Health

Karen E. Christensen and Rima Rozen

CONTENTS

I.   INTRODUCTION

Folate (tetrahydrofolate, THF) has long been known to play an important role in human health. Its role in the prevention of megaloblastic anemia has been recognized since the 1930s, and it was first suggested to prevent neural tube defects (NTDs) in the 1960s [1]. Severe deficiencies of enzymes in folate metabolism are known to cause classic hereditary disorders such as homocystinuria. These severe deficiencies are extremely rare and for the most part are linked to deletions, nonsense mutations, and nonsynonymous mutations that result in major or complete loss of enzyme activity [2]. The importance of dietary folate and the deleterious effects of inborn errors have stimulated a great deal of research on folate metabolism and on the impact of genetic variation in folate-dependent proteins on human health and disease.

Folate metabolism includes enzymes involved in the uptake and retention of folates, the conversion of one-carbon substituted folates between oxidation states, and the transfer of one-carbon units in synthetic reactions (Figure 4.1; for review, see reference [3]). Folates are involved in a wide variety of metabolic processes, including amino acid and nucleotide synthesis, and in the methylation cycle. The generation of methionine through the remethylation of homocysteine (Hcy) is particularly important; not only does this process detoxify Hcy but it also serves to synthesize S-adenosylmethionine (SAM), the ubiquitous methyl donor used in hundreds of cellular reactions, including the methylation of DNA, and the synthesis of neurotransmitters, membrane phospholipids, and creatine [4].

In the past 15 years, genetic polymorphisms (variants present in greater than 1% of alleles in a population) in folate metabolism have been identified. Although these variants have much more subtle phenotypes than the rare mutations causing inborn errors of folate metabolism, they may have a greater impact on population health because they have been linked to a wide variety of common multifactorial disorders. The 677C→T polymorphism in methylenetetrahydrofolate reductase (*MTHFR*) was first identified in 1995 [5] as a potential risk factor for vascular disease and was shortly thereafter reported to increase the risk of NTD [6]. Since then, gene variants in folate metabolism have been the subject of intense investigation as risk factors for many disorders; approximately 300 articles on *MTHFR* variants are still published every year (Figure 4.2). Although the majority of publications on folate variants concern *MTHFR*, interest in other genetic variants has increased in recent years.

The most investigated genes in folate metabolism are highlighted in Figure 4.1. The pathways can be divided into two segments: one primarily concerned with the methylation cycle and the other with nucleotide synthesis. These segments are bridged by MTHFR, which catalyzes the reduction of methylene-THF to methyl-THF. Methyl-THF is used by methionine synthase (MTR) to methylate Hcy, forming methionine; the proper function of MTR is maintained by methionine synthase reductase (MTRR). Most tissues depend on folate-dependent enzymes for Hcy remethylation; alternatively, in some tissues, betaine can be used as a carbon donor for Hcy remethylation by betaine-homocysteine methyltransferase (BHMT) [7]. Hcy can also be metabolized by the transsulfuration pathway, the first committed step of which is catalyzed by cystathionine-β-synthase (CBS) [8].

The MTHFR substrate methylene-THF is generated in the cytoplasm by 5,10-methylene-THF dehydrogenase 1 (MTHFD1; a trifunctional enzyme encoding dehydrogenase, cyclohydrolase, and synthetase activities) or by serine hydroxymethyltransferase 1 (SHMT1). The SHMT1 reaction is reversible; therefore, methylene-THF can also be used to make serine from glycine as required.

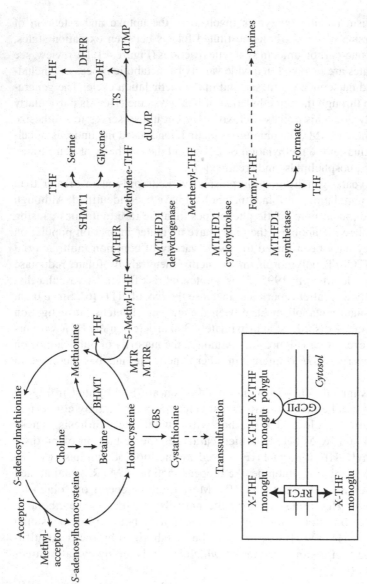

FIGURE 4.1 Folate metabolism. The methylation cycle is shown on the left of the figure, and the nucleotide synthesis pathways is shown on the right. Proteins involved in folate transport are shown in the inset. The reactions catalyzed by proteins with gene variants attracting the most recent interest (10 or more journal articles since 2001) are labeled and discussed in this chapter. BHMT, betaine-homocysteine methyltransferase; CBS, cystathionine-β-synthase; DHFR, dihydrofolate reductase; dUMP, deoxyuridine monophosphate; dTMP, deoxythymidine monophosphate; GCPII, glutamate carboxy-peptidase II; MTHFD1, methylene-THF dehydrogenase–methenyl-THF cyclohydrolase–formyl-THF synthetase; MTHFR, methylenetetrahydrofolate reductase; MTR, methionine synthase; MTRR, methionine synthase reductase; RFC1, reduced folate carrier; SHMT1, serine hydroxymethyltrans-ferase; TS, thymidylate synthase.

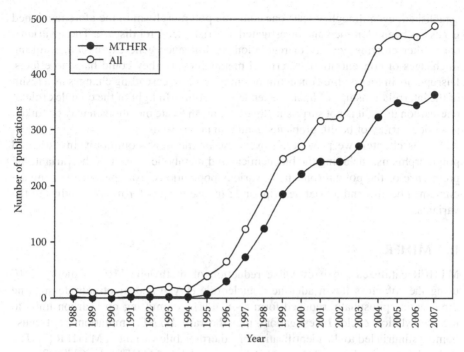

FIGURE 4.2 Publications on variants of genes in folate metabolism from 1988 to 2007. Publications were identified by literature searches of articles in the MEDLINE database by using the search terms (folate or folic acid or MTHFR or methylenetetrahydrofolate reductase or 5-methyltetrahydrofolate-homocysteine S-methyltransferase or methionine synthase or TS or thymidylate synthase or MTRR or methionine synthase reductase or cystathionine beta synthase or methylenetetrahydrofolate dehydrogenase or formyltetrahydrofolate synthetase or serine hydroxymethyltransferase or reduced folate carrier or SLC19A1 or betaine homocysteine methyltransferase or GCPII or FolH1 or folate hydrolase or glutamate carboxypeptidase II) and (polymorphism* or variant or mutation or genotype or thermolabile) for "All" or (MTHFR or methylenetetrahydrofolate reductase) and (polymorphism* or variant or mutation or genotype or thermolabile) for "MTHFR," and limiting the search to publications on humans.

Methylene-THF can also be used as a one-carbon donor by thymidylate synthase (TS) to synthesize deoxythymidine monophosphate (dTMP) from deoxyuridine monophosphate (dUMP), or it can be oxidized to formyl-THF by MTHFD1 for de novo purine synthesis [3]. During the TS reaction, THF is oxidized to DHF, which requires reduction by dihydrofolate reductase (DHFR) for use as an enzyme cofactor. The reduced folate carrier 1 (RFC1) and glutamate carboxypeptidase II (GCPII) are involved in the uptake and transport of naturally occurring folates from the diet.

Hundreds of single nucleotide polymorphisms (SNPs) have been identified in these genes; more than 30 have been found in the coding region of *MTHFR* alone (dbSNP build 129) [9]. The biochemical impact of the majority of these variants has yet to be established, even though at least one common polymorphism in the aforementioned genes has been identified and investigated as a risk factor for disease. These variants could alter enzyme activity or regulation, or influence gene expression, resulting in changes of concentrations of critical metabolites, or they could have no effects. Disruptions in metabolite concentrations may result in cascading changes as a result of the interrelationships of folate-dependent reactions. In light of the complex role of one-carbon units, it is not surprising that variants in folate metabolism may be linked to a wide variety of health problems in human populations.

In this chapter, we provide an overview of the most commonly investigated polymorphisms, including the biochemical and metabolic impact of the variant, the prevalence of the polymorphisms in various populations, examples of their impact on human health, and a brief description of mouse models for in vivo studies of the variants.

II. MTHFR

MTHFR catalyzes the irreversible reduction of methylene-THF to methyl-THF using the cofactors flavin adenine dinucleotide (FAD) and nicotinamide-adenine dinucleotide phosphate, reduced form (NADPH), committing one-carbon units to the methylation cycle. Investigations into the rare *MTHFR* mutations that cause homocystinuria led to the identification of a thermolabile variant of MTHFR [2]. The molecular genetic change that encoded the thermolabile MTHFR, the 677C→T variant, was also shown to be associated with an elevation in plasma Hcy and therefore first suggested as a risk factor for cardiovascular disease [5]. Since that first report, the *MTHFR* 677C→T polymorphism has become the most extensively investigated variant in folate metabolism.

A.   *MTHFR* 677C→T

1.   Identification and Prevalence of the *MTHFR* 677C→T Variant

The *MTHFR* 677C→T variant (dbSNP ID: rs1801133) is a nonsynonymous mutation in exon 4 resulting in an alanine to valine substitution (A222V) in the catalytic domain [5]. Using the standard notation that designates the A of the initiator methionine codon as nucleotide 1, the numbering of this variant would be 665C→T (reference sequence NM_005957.3). However, the numbering is based on the sequence of the original cDNA (reference sequence U09806.2) [10], resulting in the 677C→T notation.

The prevalence of the 677TT genotype varies widely between regions and ethnic groups [2,11–16]. The frequency has been reported as 8% to 14% in whites in North America. In European populations, the frequency appears to increase from north to south: 6% to 14% in northern Europe and 15% to 24% in southern Europe. The genotype is particularly common in Mexican and other Hispanic populations at 15% to 35%, whereas less than 2% of African and African American populations are homozygous for the variant. In Asia, the reported frequencies range from 12% to 18%.

2. Biochemical Impact of the *MTHFR* 677C→T Variant

The *MTHFR* 677C→T substitution results in a thermolabile enzyme with reduced enzyme activity in vivo [5,17,18]. The thermolabile MTHFR retains only about 30% of wild-type activity after heating at 46°C [5,17]. In addition, individuals with the 677TT genotype have only about 30% of activity in lymphocyte extracts as compared with 677CC individuals [5,19,20]. The catalytic function of the purified A222V protein does not differ from the wild-type in vitro, but it is more likely to lose its FAD cofactor, which may explain the reduced activity in vivo [17]. The addition of methyl-THF and/or FAD decreases the thermolability of the A222V variant and protects against FAD loss. Inhibition of MTHFR by SAM is unaffected by the variant, although SAM does protect the variant enzyme from FAD loss [17].

The 677C→T variant may have a number of deleterious effects on the methylation cycle because MTHFR is the sole producer of 5-methyl-THF. Reduced MTHFR activity increases Hcy concentrations by decreasing the methyl-THF available for Hcy methylation (Figure 4.1). Elevations in Hcy by as much as 70% in 677TT compared with 677CC individuals have been reported in numerous studies, particularly when folate concentrations are low [5,15,16,18,21–25]. The difference in Hcy concentrations between TT and CC individuals has been shown to increase as folate concentrations decrease and may only be significant when folate concentrations are low. This relationship most likely reflects the stabilization of the variant protein by increased folate concentrations [17].

Low riboflavin, the FAD precursor, in TT individuals may also lead to increased Hcy, particularly when folate concentrations are also low [24,26]. Again, this relationship likely reflects the stabilization of the variant protein by increased cofactor concentrations [17]. Deficiency of vitamin B12, the cofactor of MTR, has also been linked to elevated Hcy in TT individuals when folate concentrations are low [15,24]. Homozygosity for this variant may also reduce plasma betaine [23], likely a result of an increased reliance on BHMT to remethylate Hcy.

Reduced MTHFR activity could alter the distribution of folate derivatives, with a decrease in methyl-THF and an increase in methylene-THF. The methylene-THF can then be used for dTMP synthesis or converted to other folate forms, such as formyl-THF, for de novo purine synthesis and other processes. Increased dTMP synthesis [27] and altered folate distributions in red blood cells (RBCs) have been observed in TT individuals [22,27–29]. In general, the amount of methyl-THF decreases, whereas the concentrations of other folates not normally found in RBCs, such as formyl-THF, increase. As methyl-THF is the major transport form of folate, reduced MTHFR activity is expected to decrease the amount of circulating folate. Therefore, the variant may contribute to low folate concentrations, possibly exacerbating its metabolic impact. Altered distribution of folate forms appears to confound the measurement of total RBC folate by certain assay methods [30], leading to conflicting results on the association between MTHFR variants and RBC folate [31]. However, the measurement of folate in plasma/serum is unaffected by these technical difficulties; the TT genotype is usually associated with a 10% to 35% reduction in circulating folate [15,16,23,31].

Methylation activity may decrease when MTHFR activity is reduced because of decreased SAM and increased S-adenosylhomocysteine (SAH), a known inhibitor of methyltransferases [4]. Although disruption of methylation could have wide-ranging effects, a major focus has been the effect of *MTHFR* variants on the methylation of DNA. Altered DNA methylation has been shown to change gene expression and alter chromatin conformation, and it is commonly observed in neo-plasias [4]. Increased genetic instability [32] and reductions in DNA methylation in TT individuals have been reported [29]. However, neither DNA methylation nor SAM/SAH concentrations were affected by the 677C→T genotype in two studies examining the effects of variable folate intake [22,33]. Other important methyla-tion reactions, such as choline synthesis or protein methylation, have not been examined.

Therefore, the *MTHFR* 677C→T variant may influence disease risk by a number of mechanisms associated with reduced enzyme activity. Increased Hcy, decreased folate, altered folate distributions, abnormal nucleotide synthesis, and decreased capacity for methylation reactions may all contribute to the clinical consequences of the variant.

3. Impact of the *MTHFR* 677C→T Variant on Health

a. NTDs and Other Birth Defects

The variant was first implicated as a risk factor for NTD in 1995 [6]. Since then, multiple meta-analyses have confirmed that the TT and CT genotypes, either in the mother or in the child, increase the risk for NTDs [11,12,34]. Odds ratios associated with the TT genotype range from 1.4 to 1.9 for the child and 1.6 to 2.0 for the mother. However, the link between the variant and NTD is not always observed, possibly because of various modifiers. Ethnicity [11], site or type of NTD [35,36], interactions with other variants in the pathways [12,37], and vitamin use/folate concentrations [35,38,39] have all been found to modify the risk for NTD associated with this variant. The TT genotype in both the mother and the child may also increase NTD risk [18,38].

The 677C→T variant has also been investigated as a risk factor for congenital heart defects (CHDs) with mixed results. Recent meta-analyses have found weak associations between the variant and all types of CHD [40,41]. As the incidence of CHD may be increased by elevated Hcy [40], it is not surprising that folate intake has been observed to modify the risk for CHD [42]. The risk associated with this variant also appears to differ depending on the specific type of CHD [42,43]. Again, the heterogeneity of the type of defect, as well as the folate status of the mother, should be considered when examining the potential impact of gene vari-ants on risk.

Other birth defects thought to be influenced by folate metabolism, such as cleft lip and palate and Down syndrome [34,40], have also been examined for an association with the 677C→T variant with inconclusive results. Folate intake may also modify the impact of this variant on these disorders, making it more difficult to identify links between *MTHFR* 677C→T and birth defects, particularly in populations with folic acid fortification of food.

b. Cardiovascular Disease

The variant has been investigated extensively as a risk factor for a variety of cardio-vascular diseases (CVDs), including coronary artery disease (CAD), stroke, venous thrombosis, and hypertension. The TT genotype has been found by meta-analyses to increase the risk for CAD by 20%, likely a result of the increased Hcy [44–46]. This increase in risk varies between populations; the effect of the TT genotype appears to be greater in Asian populations than European ones and is often not seen in North American populations [45,46]. Some of these discrepancies may be explained by dif-ferences in folate intake, as low folate concentrations together with the TT genotype have been associated with an increased risk for CAD [45,47]. Another factor that is not always considered is matched ethnicity between cases and controls, particularly in populations with considerable admixture. The TT genotype may be a more impor-tant risk factor in early-onset CAD, as would be expected for a genetic determinant [48,49]. Other known CAD risk factors may also obscure the effect of the variant; in general, it has been found to significantly increase CAD risk primarily in the absence of other known risk factors [48,50].

The variant appears to increase risk for stroke by about 30% in a number of meta-analyses [51,52]. Similarly, it increases risk for venous thrombosis 1.2- to 1.5-fold [44,50,53,54]. As with CAD, the effects of the variant may be obscured by other known risk factors for thrombosis [50,53], and it may not be a risk factor in North Americans because of increased folate intake [54].

c. Colorectal and Other Cancers

The relationship between colorectal cancer (CRC) and the *MTHFR* 677C→T vari-ant has been investigated extensively following initial reports of a possible protec-tive effect of the TT genotype [55,56]. In general, it appears that the TT genotype reduces the risk of CRC if folate concentrations are high, but that protection is lost, or the TT genotype may become a risk factor, if folate concentrations are low [14,57]. The protective effect of this variant may be caused by an increase in methylene-THF for conversion of dUMP to dTMP, reducing DNA damage resulting from uracil misincorporation into DNA [55,58]. Alternatively, increased Hcy or its metabolites could increase apoptosis in transformed cells in the intestine (A. K. Lawrance and R. Rozen, unpublished data). Recent meta-analyses have shown that the TT genotype reduces CRC risk by about 20% [57,59]. Several factors have been reported to modify this protective effect, including folate concentrations [56,60], tumor location [61], alcohol intake [55], and ethnicity [59]. The variant may not affect risk for colorectal adenoma, which suggests that it may help prevent adenomas from developing into carcinomas [14,59].

In contrast to CRC, the *MTHFR* 677C→T variant may increase risk for gastric cancer by 40% to 50% [62,63]. Again, the effect of the variant may be altered by folate concentrations [62,63] and by tumor site [63]. Reports are emerging on the impact of the variant on other types of cancers such as breast cancer and leukemia, but additional studies are required before conclusions can be reached. The influence of the 677C→T variant on cancer risk may depend on the mechanisms by which a specific cancer develops.

d.   Other Effects on Health

The variant has been investigated as a risk factor for most folate- or nutrition-related disorders; sufficient studies have been performed to allow for meta-analyses for some of these conditions. The TT genotype may increase the risk for schizophrenia [64,65] and depression [65] by as much as 40%. Similarly, it may increase the risk for pregnancy complications such as recurrent pregnancy loss [66] and severe hypertension or preeclampsia [67]. For many of these disorders, the mechanism is likely through hyperhomocysteinemia [64,66]. The variant may also have pharmacogenetic effects that influence the response to treatment with antifolate chemotherapeutics (methotrexate, 5-fluorouracil), anticonvulsants, and other drugs [68].

B.   MTHFR 1298A→C

1.   Identification and Prevalence of the MTHFR 1298A→C Variant

The *MTHFR* 1298A→C variant (rs1801131) is a nonsynonymous mutation in exon 7 resulting in a glutamate to alanine substitution (E429A) in the regulatory domain of MTHFR [19,20]. As for the 677 variant, the numbering is based on the reference sequence U09806.2; using standard notation this variant would be labeled 1286A→C (reference sequence NM_005957.3).

The prevalence of the 1298CC genotype varies with geography and ethnic group [13,15,16]. In white populations in North America and Europe, the frequency ranges from 6% to 11%. It is somewhat lower in African (2%–4%), Asian (1.4%–3.7%), and US Hispanic and Mexican (2%–4%) populations. The *MTHFR* 677C→T and 1298A→C variants are in linkage disequilibrium; the 677T and 1298C alleles are rarely found in the *cis* configuration, and the compound homozygous genotype is rarely reported [13,69].

2.   Biochemical Impact of the MTHFR 1298A→C Variant

The biochemical effects of the 1298A→C variant are much more subtle than the 677C→T variant. This variant has been reported to modestly reduce the specific activity in lymphocyte extracts; 1298CC individuals have 60%–70% of the MTHFR activity of 1298AA, a much smaller effect than the 30% observed in 677TT individuals [19,20]. Unlike the 677C→T variant, the 1298A→C substitution does not result in a thermolabile enzyme [17,20,70]. The E429A protein has been purified and characterized; catalytic function, inhibition by SAM, and rate of FAD release were unaffected, both for E429A alone and in combination with A222V [17]. In most studies the variant does not affect plasma Hcy or folate [15,19,20]. Increased Hcy has been reported in compound heterozygotes of the 677C→T and 1298A→C variants in some populations [20,70] but not in others [16]. In every case, the 677C→T allele was found to have a much bigger effect on Hcy and folate concentrations than the 1298A→C variant, effectively drowning out the impact of the A→C substitution.

3   Impact of the MTHFR 1298A→C Variant on Health

The *MTHFR* 1298A→C variant has not been as extensively studied as the 677 change. Nonetheless, the majority of studies have concluded that it is not an independent risk factor for NTDs [19,20,37,71,72]. A few studies suggest that compound heterozygosity for the two variants increases NTD risk [12,20,72], although this association has not always been observed [71]. The 1298A→C variant has not been found to be a risk factor for other birth defects such as CHD and cleft lip and palate [40] or for CVD [73,74].

Studies on the 1298A→C variant and CRC risk have yielded mixed results, with no effect or a nonsignificant reduction in risk associated with the CC genotype [14,57]. One recent meta-analysis reported a protective effect of the CC genotype [59]. No associations have been found in meta-analyses for gastric cancer risk [62,63].

C. Mouse Model of MTHFR Deficiency

A mouse model for MTHFR deficiency has been established by disrupting the *Mthfr* gene on the Balb/c background [75]. These mice are good models for both severe and mild MTHFR deficiency; *Mthfr*−/− mice mimic the effects of severe MTHFR deficiency and homocystinuria, whereas *Mthfr*+/− mice have metabolic effects similar to the 677C→T variant [75]. *Mthfr*−/− pups are developmentally delayed and have smaller cerebella and reduced survival [75]; however, *Mthfr*−/− pups recently generated on a C57Bl/6 background appear to have normal survival [76]. *Mthfr*+/− mice express 60% of wild-type enzyme activity and appear normal in terms of growth and development [75]. Plasma Hcy is increased in *Mthfr*+/− mice by about 60% compared with wild-type mice [75,77–79]; in liver, Hcy concentrations increase by about 40% [80]. The increase in Hcy is accompanied by decreased SAM/SAH ratios in liver and brain, which may explain the trend toward DNA hypomethylation in liver [75,80]. *Mthfr*+/− mice are more dependent on the transsulfuration pathway for Hcy degradation [75,80], and reduced choline metabolites in liver suggest an increased reliance on Hcy remethylation through the BHMT pathway [77]. Many of the effects of the *Mthfr*+/− genotype are reduced by supplementation with betaine [77,79,80]. MTHFR deficiency in mice alters the distribution of folate forms. The proportion of methyl-THF is reduced in plasma, liver, and brain [75,81]. In contrast, total folate concentrations remain unchanged in liver and brain and were significantly decreased only in plasma of *Mthfr*−/− mice [75,81]. However, these measurements were obtained from mice fed a folate-replete diet and may not reflect the effects of reduced MTHFR activity on folate-restricted diets.

Mthfr+/− mice have been used as a model to examine the relationship between MTHFR deficiency and birth defects. These experiments suggest that the genotype of the mother has a significant effect on the health of her offspring. Resorptions and developmental delay are increased in embryos of *Mthfr*+/− mothers [78]. Embryos at gestational day 14.5 (E14.5) have an increased incidence of CHD, primarily ventricular septal defects [78], and younger embryos have disrupted neural tube development and laterality defects (L. Pickell and R. Rozen, unpublished data). Significant interactions between maternal diet and the phenotype of *Mthfr*−/− pups have also been observed. The cerebellar morphology, survival rate, and development of *Mthfr*−/− pups are improved if the *Mthfr*+/− mother receives a betaine supplement to support Hcy remethylation by BHMT [80]. Supplementation of mothers with mefolinate (a synthetic form of 5-methyl-THF) results in similar improvements in the

Mthfr−/− phenotype; supplementation with folic acid does not [82]. These findings demonstrate that mothers with reduced MTHFR activity are not capable of generating enough 5-methyl-THF to overcome severe MTHFR deficiency in offspring.

This mouse model has also been used to investigate diseases of aging, such as CVD and CRC. *Mthfr*+/− mice have an increased risk for atherosclerotic disease; abnormal lipid deposition in the aorta [75,79], endothelial dysfunction, and stiffer arteries have been observed [83,84]. The *Mthfr*+/− mouse also has reduced apolipoprotein A-I in plasma and liver [85], resulting in reduced high-density lipoprotein cholesterol and increased inflammation, as well as increased nitrotyrosine in the liver, a marker of oxidative stress [79]. Some of these effects of MTHFR deficiency are alleviated by betaine supplementation [79]. Gene–nutrient interactions were also observed when this model was used to investigate MTHFR deficiency and cancer risk. *Mthfr*+/− mice have an increased risk for the development of intestinal tumors while on a low folate diet; 12.5% of wild-type and 28.1% of *Mthfr*+/− mice on a low folate diet developed tumors [86]. In contrast, in mice predisposed to tumorigenesis, the *Mthfr*+/− genotype may reduce tumor development (A. K. Lawrance and R. Rozen, unpublished data).

Pharmacogenetic studies of *MTHFR* variants have also been facilitated with the mouse model. MTHFR deficiency may modify the effects of simvastatin treatment [87], increase sensitivity to methotrexate [76], and reduce the teratogenicity of valproic acid [88]. These experiments underscore the value of the *Mthfr*-deficient mouse in investigating the effects of *MTHFR* variants on human health.

III. METHIONINE SYNTHASE

MTR catalyzes the remethylation of Hcy using methyl-THF as the one-carbon donor and cobalamin (I) (vitamin B12) as a cofactor. MTR is the primary ubiquitous pathway for the remethylation of Hcy [89], unlike BHMT, which is present in liver and kidney [7]. If MTR activity is reduced, such as in cblG patients with deleterious mutations in MTR, Hcy increases [90], and methyl-THF concentrations may increase because the MTR reaction is the only way to remove the methyl group so that THF can be used for other folate-dependent reactions.

A. *MTR* 2756A→G

1. Identification and Prevalence of the *MTR* 2756A→G Variant

The *MTR* 2756A→G polymorphism (rs1805087, reference sequence NM_000254.2) is a nonsynonymous mutation in exon 26 that results in a glutamate to glycine substitution (D919G) [89,91]. The frequency of the GG genotype is fairly consistent worldwide, ranging from 1% to 5% in Asian, European, North American, and Australian populations [14,23,91,92].

2. Biochemical Impact of the *MTR* 2756A→G Variant

The D919G substitution may alter the structure of the protein, but the effect of the variant on MTR activity has not been evaluated [93]. A number of studies have shown an association between the variant and lower Hcy concentrations [14,23,94], although there was no effect in other studies [91,95–98]. *MTR* 2756A→G does not appear to influence the level of folate or B12 [23,95].

3. Impact of the *MTR* 2756A→G Variant on Health

This variant has been investigated as a risk factor for many of the same disorders as the *MTHFR* variant because of their biochemical relationship. The variant in the mother or the child has not been observed to increase risk for NTDs [91,99]. However, two studies have reported that the G allele may further increase NTD risk associated with the *MTRR* 66A→G variant [99,100]. With respect to CVD, the 2756A→G variant does not appear to be a risk factor [94,96,97,101]. The relationship between the variant and cancer may be complicated by a number of confounders. An overall lack of association with CRC has been observed in a number of studies [60,92,93,95,102]. However, the GG genotype has been reported to protect against CRC at specific sites [98] and in men who consume less than one alcoholic drink per day [95]. No significant relationship has been reported with colorectal adenoma [103]. The 2756AA genotype has been reported to increase risk for Alzheimer's disease by about threefold in Europeans [104,105], and interactions with other genetic risk factors may further increase this risk [104,105].

B. Mouse Model of MTR Deficiency

MTR-deficient mice have been generated [106]. The *Mtr*[-/-] mouse is embryonic lethal, and the embryos cannot be rescued by supplementing the mother's diet. The *Mtr*[+/-] mice appear morphologically normal but have slightly increased plasma Hcy and methionine relative to *Mtr*[+/+], particularly on a low folate diet [106,107]. The *Mtr*[+/-] mice show signs of impaired cerebrovascular function on a folate-replete diet [107].

IV. METHIONINE SYNTHASE REDUCTASE

MTRR reactivates the cobalamin cofactor of MTR when it is oxidized to cobalt (II) [90]. MTRR requires NADPH, FAD, and riboflavin 5′-phosphate and uses SAM as a methyl donor [90]. It may also stabilize the MTR apoenzyme and generate its cobalamin cofactor [108]. If cobalamin (II) is not reduced to cobalamin (I) by MTRR, MTR activity is essentially blocked, which could lead to elevated Hcy as it does in cblE patients with deleterious *MTRR* mutations [90].

A. *MTRR* 66A→G

1. Identification and Prevalence of *MTRR* 66A→G

The *MTRR* 66A→G variant (rs1801394, reference sequence NM_002454.2) is a nonsynonymous mutation in exon 2 that results in an isoleucine to methionine substitution (I22M) [109]. Although the reported frequency of the G allele was high (51%), *MTRR* 22M was designated to be the "mutant" protein because of the conservation of isoleucine at this position in other species [109]. The 66GG frequency is highest in whites (20%–38%) and much lower in Asian (7%–10%), African (6%–8%), and Mexican (6%–7%) populations [14,15,23,92,110].

2. Biochemical Impact of the *MTRR* 66A→G Variant

Purified wild-type and I22M proteins have very similar kinetic characteristics, although four times more I22M protein was required to reach maximal activity [90]. This effect does not appear to arise from differences in the reduction kinetics or the stability of the MTR/MTRR interaction; therefore, its reduced efficiency remains unexplained [111,112].

The *MTRR* 66A→G variant does not appear to affect Hcy when considered independently [15,23,32,100,113–115]. An association between modestly elevated Hcy (~20%) and the wild-type 66AA genotype has been reported that may depend on low vitamin B12 concentrations [97,116]. Recently, the 66GG genotype was found to modulate the effects of the *MTHFR* 677C→T variant on Hcy concentrations. This very large study found that non-Hispanic white TT/GG individuals had significantly lower Hcy concentrations (25.6%) than TT/AA individuals [15]. The variant does not appear to affect serum SAM/SAH ratios [115], folate, vitamin B12, or methylmalonic acid (MMA, a marker of intracellular vitamin B12) [15,23,97,113,115].

3. Impact of the *MTRR* 66A→G Variant on Health

In a recent meta-analysis on the potential association between this variant and NTD risk, the 66GG genotype in the mother was shown to increase risk by 55%; the child's genotype had no impact [100]. However, the effect may be influenced by interactions with other folate-related variants and vitamin concentrations. Maternal GG genotype in combination with low vitamin B12 or high MMA concentrations has been found to increase NTD risk about fivefold [100,109]. In contrast, folate intake did not affect the impact. There are some indications that the combination of the 66A→G and *MTHFR* 677C→T variants may affect NTD risk, but the exact relationship is unclear [37,100,109]. The combination of the *MTR* 2756 A→G allele and the 66 A→G allele has also been observed to increase NTD risk [99,100].

The 66A→G variant has been evaluated as a risk factor for CHD. One study reported no significant interactions between this variant and CHD, alone or in combination with vitamin B12 [117]. Another study found that maternal GG genotype in combination with elevated MMA increased the risk for non-conotruncal CHD more than sixfold [118].

The variant has not been extensively studied in CVD. The results on CAD risk have been mixed [97,113,114]. The impact on cancer risk also requires additional studies. Although the variant has been reported to increase CRC risk, this relationship was not observed in two larger studies [60,92,93]. Vitamin concentrations may play a role as interactions between the variant and folate or vitamin B12 intake have been reported to influence the risk of developing colorectal adenoma and lung cancer [103,119].

B. Mouse Model of MTRR Deficiency

A mouse model for MTRR deficiency has been established using a gene trap approach to greatly reduce, rather than eliminate, MTRR, because the complete lack of MTRR may be embryonic lethal [120]. Although the *Mtrr*^{gt/gt} mice are morphologically similar to their *Mtrr*^{+/gt} and *Mtrr*^{+/+} littermates, *Mtrr*^{gt/gt} mice have increased Hcy and decreased methionine in plasma compared with *Mtrr*^{+/+} mice. The same trend in metabolites is observed for the *Mtrr*^{+/gt} mice, although it does not reach significance. There is also a nonsignificant trend toward increased methyl-THF in some tissues, as expected. The SAM/SAH ratio in heart is decreased in *Mtrr*^{gt/gt} mice, unchanged in kidney and brain, and increased in liver. In the kidney and liver, this could be because of BHMT activity.

The mice have been used to investigate the impact of MTRR deficiency on birth defects and pregnancy complications. Reduced maternal MTRR activity increases pregnancy loss and embryonic delays [121]. There is an increased incidence of CHD (specifically ventricular septal defects) and reduced size in embryos of *Mtrr*^{+/gt} and *Mtrr*^{gt/gt} mothers.

V. METHYLENE-THF DEHYDROGENASE–METHENYL-THF CYCLOHYDROLASE–FORMYL-THF SYNTHETASE

Methylene-THF dehydrogenase–methenyl-THF cyclohydrolase–formyl-THF synthetase (MTHFD1) is a trifunctional enzyme with two independent active domains: the dehydrogenase–cyclohydrolase domain and the synthetase domain [122]. The dehydrogenase uses nicotinamide-adenine dinucleotide phosphate as a cofactor to oxidize methylene-THF to methenyl-THF, which is then converted to formyl-THF by the cyclohydrolase. The synthetase domain catalyzes the production of formyl-THF from formate and THF using MgATP as a cofactor. All MTHFD1 activities are reversible. Because methylene-THF is used for dTMP and methyl-THF synthesis, and formyl-THF is required for purine synthesis, MTHFD1 plays a key role in balancing the supply of these one-carbon folates to meet metabolic demands [3]. Therefore, disruptions of MTHFD1 could alter the distribution of one-carbon folates, reduce nucleotide synthesis, and impair methylation.

A. *MTHFD1* 1958G→A

1. Identification and Prevalence of *MTHFD1* 1958G→A

The *MTHFD1* 1958G→A variant (rs2236225, reference sequence NM_005956.1) is a nonsynonymous mutation in exon 20 that results in an arginine to glutamine substitution (R653Q) in the synthetase domain [123]. The frequency of the 1958AA genotype is usually 15% to 21% for European and American white populations [23,110,123–129]. In the Chinese population, the AA frequency is much lower, at 3.8% to 6.4% [110,130,131].

2. Biochemical Impact of the *MTHFD1* 1958G→A Variant

The *MTHFD1* 1958G→A variant protein has been purified and characterized in vitro and found to be less thermostable than the wild-type protein [132]. The stability difference is abolished by high folate concentrations, suggesting the potential for gene–nutrient interactions. The variant was also found to significantly reduce de novo purine synthesis when expressed in cells, demonstrating a metabolic effect of this mutation.

The variant has not been observed to affect Hcy, RBC, or plasma/serum folate [23,123–125,133]. However, in one report, individuals with the A allele had higher SAH and were found to be seven times more susceptible to choline deficiency unless they were given folic acid supplements [133]. These findings suggest that these individuals are more dependent on choline or its metabolite betaine for Hcy remethylation.

3. Impact of the *MTHFD1* 1958G→A Variant on Health

The 1958AA genotype has been reported to be a maternal risk factor for NTD in the Irish population, with an increase in risk of about 50% [124,134]. In contrast, in the Italian population, the A allele in the child may increase the risk for NTD by 76% [128]. In other populations, there was no increase in NTD risk [123,129]. These observations suggest that some secondary factor, such as other polymorphisms or nutrient intake, may modify the effect of the variant. For example, the combination of *MTHFD1* 1958AA and *RFC1* 80GG genotypes was reported to double the risk of having a child with Down syndrome as compared with the *RFC1* 80GG genotype alone [135].

The AA genotype has recently been shown to increase the risk for CHD twofold in Canadian children [132]. This increase was specific for the type of defect; the risks for tetralogy of Fallot and aortic stenosis were increased more than threefold, whereas the risk for ventricular septal defects was unaffected. The maternal genotype did not have an effect on CHD for any of the subtypes in this cohort, whereas in China, the A allele in the mother has been reported to reduce the risk of atrial septal defects [130]. The 1958G→A variant is also linked to an increased risk for pregnancy complications, such as placental abruption and pregnancy loss, in two Irish studies [126,127].

There have been very few studies examining this variant and cancer risk. The 1958G→A variant did not increase risk for CRC, colorectal adenoma, or breast cancer [103,125,136], although it doubled the risk for gastric cancer in one Chinese study [131]. Other studies point to potential gene–gene interactions, e.g., an interaction with the *MTHFR* 677C→T variant in risk for migraine [137] and an interaction with the *TS* 3R variant in response to methotrexate chemotherapy [138].

VI. SHMT1

Cytoplasmic SHMT1 catalyzes the reversible transfer of one-carbon units from methylene-THF to glycine to form serine and THF. This reaction requires pyridoxal phosphate (PLP), the active form of vitamin B6. During the S phase, SHMT1 translocates to the nucleus with TS and DHFR to generate methylene-THF for dTMP synthesis, with serine as the one-carbon donor [139]. At other times, SHMT1 may compete with MTHFR for methylene-THF to make serine and sequester methyl-THF, inhibiting the methylation cycle [140]. Therefore, disruption of SHMT1 could lead to dUMP accumulation and increased DNA damage or alter the distribution of folates for purine synthesis or methylation.

A. SHMT1 1420C→T

1. Identification and Prevalence of SHMT1 1420C→T

The *SHMT1* 1420C→T variant (rs1979277, reference sequence NM_004169.3) is a nonsynonymous polymorphism in exon 13 that results in a leucine to phenylalanine change (L474F) [141]. *SHMT1* has several splice variants that differ in expression between tissues [142]. In the isoform 2 sequence of *SHMT1* (reference sequence NM_148918.1), this variant is L435F (1303C→T). The frequency of the TT genotype is 7% to 13% in white populations [37,72,125,141,143,144], 6.7% in African Americans [144], and 0.2% to 1.7% in Asians [145,146].

2. Biochemical Impact of the SHMT1 1420C→T Variant

Purified *SHMT1* 1420C→T protein behaves like the wild-type in stability, catalysis, and affinity for monoglutamylated folates, glycine, and serine [147]. However, the affinity for the physiological pentaglutamate substrate and the rate of formation of the active holoenzyme from PLP and the apoenzyme are reduced. These reductions could result in decreased function in vivo and suggest that the effects of the variant may be influenced by vitamin B6. The variant also impairs the modification of SHMT1 with the small ubiquitin-like modifier (SUMO) that is required for import into the nucleus; this interference could affect dTMP synthesis and increase SHMT1 in cytoplasm where it can compete with MTHFR for substrate and sequester methyl-THF, inhibiting methylation [139].

A consistent effect of the variant on Hcy concentrations has not been observed [125,141,148]. This could be a result of the influence of other folate variants because the 1420 TT genotype has been reported to act synergistically with the *MTHFR* 677TT genotype to increase Hcy concentrations [148]. Mixed results have been observed for RBC and plasma folate concentrations [72,125,141].

3. Impact of the SHMT1 1420C→T Variant on Health

There are limited studies of this variant and disease risk. The relationship with NTD risk is unclear [37,72,141]. The maternal 1420T allele has been reported to double the risk of preterm birth of whites in the United States [144]. The same study did not observe an effect for African American women, except in combination with low folate intake. The variant does not appear to influence CVD risk on its own, but in combination with the *MTHFR* 677 variant, the 1420TT genotype increased CVD risk 5 to 10-fold [148].

The variant does not appear to influence risk for CRC or colorectal adenoma [103,125]. The T allele has been reported to protect against other cancers, especially when combined with the *TS* 3R variant [145,146]. These findings are intriguing because they suggest that SHMT1 interacts closely with TS in the prevention of DNA damage, perhaps by limiting dUMP accumulation.

B. MOUSE MODEL OF SHMT1 DEFICIENCY

SHMT1-deficient mice have recently been generated. Unlike several other mouse models of deficiencies in the pathway, the *Shmt1$^{-/-}$* mice are viable and have normal fertility and litter sizes [149]. However, they have a fourfold increase in the SAM/SAH ratio in liver. In addition, uracil misincorporation was increased in livers of *Shmt1$^{+/-}$* mice.

Therefore, reduced SHMT1 activity may provide more methylene-THF for methyl-THF synthesis and methylation reactions at the expense of dTMP synthesis.

VII. TS

TS catalyzes the methylation of dUMP to dTMP using methylene-THF as the carbon donor. If TS activity is reduced, dUMP may accumulate and be misincorporated into DNA, resulting in DNA damage [58]. Variants in *TS* are of particular clinical interest because the enzyme is the target of fluoropyrimidine chemotherapeutics such as 5-fluorouracil (5-FU).

Two major *TS* variants have been described: the 2R/3R 28–basepair (bp) repeat in the 5′-untranslated region (UTR) (reference sequence NM_00107.2, rs45445694) [150] and a 6-bp deletion at c.1494 in the 3′-UTR (reference sequence X02308.1, rs34489327) [151]. The 2R variant is in linkage disequilibrium with the 3′-UTR 6-bp deletion; the 2R and 6-bp deletion alleles are rarely found together [152,153]. In addition, a G→C substitution that modifies the effects of the 2R/3R variation has recently been identified within the 28-bp repeats (rs34743033) [154]. The 3R G allele is also in linkage disequilibrium with the 3′-UTR variant; it is frequently associated with the 6-bp deletion [153]. The 2R/3R variant is the best-studied *TS* polymorphism.

A.   TS 2R/3R Repeat/Insertion

1. Identification and Prevalence of *TS* 2R/3R

The 5′-UTR of *TS* contains a repeated 28-bp sequence, required for efficient gene expression, which is usually found in triplicate 8 bp upstream of the start codon in a region called the TS enhancer region (TSER) [150]. This sequence is referred to as the triple tandem repeat (3R). The double repeat (2R) polymorphism was first described in 1995 [150]; higher numbers of repeats have also been reported. The frequency of the 2R/2R genotype varies by ethnicity; it is less common in Asians (2%–10%) than in African (14%–19%) or white (18%–23%) populations [14,102,145,155].

2. Biochemical Impact of the *TS* 2R/3R Variant

Protein expression from the 2R TSER is three- to fourfold less efficient than the 3R [150,154,156]. TS activity or mRNA concentrations are higher in those with colorectal tumors with the 3R/3R genotype than in those with the 2R allele [156,157]. The relationship between 2R/2R genotype and plasma folate is unclear [158,159]. Hcy concentrations appear to be unaffected by this variant [158,159].

3. Impact of the *TS* 2R/3R Variant on Health

The 2R/2R genotype may reduce risk of CRC by 1.4- to 1.7-fold compared with the 3R/3R genotype, particularly in men or individuals with low folate intake [102,158]. It does not independently influence risk for colorectal adenoma [143,152], although there may be an interaction of genotype with folate intake [152].

Much of the research on *TS* variants has focused on their impact in response to fluoropyrimidines. CRC patients with the 3R/3R genotype may benefit less from 5-FU than those with the 2R allele in terms of survival [160,161], although these results are not consistent [162]. Similar studies with variable conclusions have been reported for gastric cancer [163,164].

B. MOUSE MODEL OF TS OVEREXPRESSION

A transgenic mouse that overexpresses human TS has been generated [165]. High concentrations of enzyme are found in the pancreas, with low concentrations in other tissues. The transgenic mice appear normal and have a normal life span but were found to develop pancreatic tumors after about 1 year. Even though pancreatic cancer in humans has been associated with a low TS-expressing genotype rather than a high TS-expressing genotype [155], this model may be useful for studying cancer treatments as well as gene–gene and gene–nutrient interactions.

VIII. RFC1

RFC1 (gene name *SLC19A1*) is a bidirectional folate transporter that preferentially transports reduced folates such as methyl-THF and formyl-THF across cell membranes [166]. RFC1 has a relatively low affinity for oxidized folates such as folic acid [166]. Decreased activity may reduce the uptake of circulating methyl-THF into cells and disturb folate metabolism by reducing the cellular pool of one-carbon donors.

A. *RFC1* 80A→G

1. Identification and Prevalence of *RFC1* 80A→G

The *RFC1* 80A→G polymorphism (rs1051266, reference sequence NM_194255.1) is a nonsynonymous mutation in exon 2 that results in a histidine to arginine (H27R) substitution in a region that may be important for function [166,167]. The variant is referred to as R27H in some studies. In North America, the frequencies of the GG genotype are 24% to 33% in whites, about 20% in African Americans, and 26% to 32% in Hispanics [102,166,168–170]. In northern Europe, the frequency of the GG genotype is 26% to 41% [23,25,37,72], whereas in Italy it has been reported as 18% [135]. The GG frequency in Asia ranges from 19% to 33% [171,172]. It is unclear whether these large frequency ranges are caused by biological differences or differences in nomenclature of the variant.

2. Biochemical Impact of the *RFC1* 80A→G Variant

The effects of the *RFC1* 80A→G variant on transport have been measured in transfected cells and in white blood cells from individuals with the three genotypes [167,173]. Methotrexate and formyl-THF transport are unaffected by this variant in transfected cells [167]. Similarly, the sensitivity of these cells to antifolates did not differ, even though approximately twofold decreases in affinity for these substrates were observed for the H27 (wild-type) protein. One study has reported a reduction in methotrexate uptake in cultured cells from GG individuals [173].

The variant does not appear to have significant impact on Hcy, SAM/SAH, or RBC and plasma folate concentrations [23,25,72,115,166,168]. However, it may modulate the effects of the *MTHFR* 677C→T polymorphism; increased Hcy concentrations were observed in 677TT individuals homozygous for the G allele as compared with 677TT individuals homozygous for the A allele [25,166]. Other folate transporters may compensate for reduced RFC1 activity; therefore, the variant may affect folate metabolism only under specific circumstances.

3. Impact of the *RFC1* 80A→G Variant on Health

The *RFC1* GG genotype has been linked to a 2.5-fold increase in NTD risk [171,174], although this association has not been routinely observed [72,170,175]. The inconsistency may be because of potential interaction between maternal genotype and folate intake. The combination of low folate intake and maternal GG genotype may increase risk for NTD (from no risk up to as much as 4.6-fold) [168,171,175]. In addition, the effects of the variant may be specific for the type and location of NTD and modified by the presence of other gene variants, such as *CBS* c.844ins68 [37]. Similarly, the variant may not be an independent risk factor for Down syndrome [176], but combined with other variants (*MTHFR* 677C→T or *MTHFD1* 1958G→A) or other risk factors such as maternal age, the GG genotype may increase risk for this disorder [135,176]. The *RFC1* 80A→G variant may also be a folate-responsive risk factor for CHD [169,172].

The effects of the 80A→G variant on cancer risk have not been studied extensively. To date it does not appear to affect the risk for CRC [102,177]. However, it may be significant in chemotherapy treatment outcomes. The A allele has been associated with shorter event-free survival times and increased hepatotoxicity following methotrexate treatment [178,179].

B. MOUSE MODEL OF RFC1 DEFICIENCY

Two RFC1-deficient mouse lines have been established [180,181]. The null mutation is embryonic lethal; in the absence of folic acid supplementation, mice die before E9.5 [180,182]. If the mothers are supplemented with folic acid during gestation, the null mice may survive until E18.5, although they display developmental abnormalities, such as NTD, CHD, and defects in hematopoietic tissues [180,182]. *Rfc1*+/− mice are morphologically normal and do not exhibit significant changes in plasma or tissue folate, although plasma SAM/SAH ratio is reduced [181]. The lack of folate deficiency in these mice confirms that RFC1 is not solely responsible for the uptake of folate from the diet. However, the other effects of RFC1 deficiency make it clear that the other folate transporters cannot completely compensate for an absent RFC1.

Rfc1+/− mice have increased proliferation of cells in the colon relative to *Rfc1*+/+ and develop more precancerous lesions and larger adenocarcinomas in response to carcinogen exposure [181]. In contrast, when these mice are crossed with the Apc−/+ mouse model for colon cancer, Apc^min/+ *Rfc*+/− mice develop fewer adenomas than Apc^min/+ *Rfc1*+/+ mice [183].

IX. VARIANTS IN OTHER GENES OF FOLATE METABOLISM

The following three variants have not been as thoroughly investigated as the aforementioned polymorphisms and are presented briefly. Glutamate carboxypeptidase II

(*GCPII*) 1561 C→T, *BHMT* 742G→A, and the *DHFR* 19-bp deletion have attracted recent interest because of their effects on the protein or on disease risk.

A. *GCPII* 1561C→T

GCPII (also known as folate hydrolase 1, *N*-acetylated α-linked acidic dipeptidase 1 [NAALADase] and prostate-specific membrane antigen) catalyzes the sequential removal of glutamates from its substrates [184]. The protein removes the polyglutamate tail from folates to allow efficient transport of dietary and circulating folates into cells. Reduced GCPII activity could lead to a generalized folate deficiency.

1. Identification and Prevalence of the *GCPII* 1561C→T Variant

The *GCPII* 1561C→T variant is numbered from the first base of the reference sequence AF176574.1 [185]; it would be the 1424C→T variant using standard notation. This nonsynonymous mutation in exon 13 results in a histidine to tyrosine substitution (H475Y) in the putative catalytic region [185]. The variant is not common worldwide; the reported frequency of the TT genotype ranges from less than 0.5% to 2% [25,37,103,110,125,168,177,186,187].

2. Biochemical Impact of the *GCPII* 1561C→T Variant

The activity of the H475Y variant protein has been shown to be about 50% of the wild-type when evaluated in vitro [185], although it does not appear to affect the bioavailability of polyglutamylated folates in CT individuals as compared with CC individuals [187]. Most studies have found that the T allele either increases or has no effect on plasma and RBC folate concentrations [25,125,168,186,187] and that it decreases or has no effect on Hcy concentrations [25,125,168,177,186,187].

3. Impact of the *GCPII* 1561C→T Variant on Health

The variant does not appear to have a major influence on health thus far. An association with NTD risk has not been observed [37,168], and it does not appear to increase risk for CVD [186], CRC [125,177], or colorectal adenoma [103].

4. Mouse Models of GCPII Deficiency

Two GCPII-deficient mouse lines have been established: the first by disrupting exons 1 and 2 [188] and the second by disrupting exons 9 and 10 [184]. The first mouse lacks the folate hydrolase activity of GCPII, but the *GcpII*$^{-/-}$ mice appear normal, likely because a second NAALADase compensates for GCPII in brain [188]. The *GcpII* disruption in the second mouse is embryonic lethal and cannot be rescued by folate supplementation; the difference in phenotype was suggested to result from dominant negative inhibition of the second NAALADase [184].

B. *BHMT* 742G→A

BHMT, primarily found in liver and kidney [7], uses the choline metabolite betaine as a carbon donor to remethylate Hcy, producing dimethylglycine and methionine. BHMT is inhibited by excess SAM [189], sparing choline for other uses. Reduced

BHMT activity could lead to increased dependence on folate for Hcy remethylation or increased use of the transsulfuration pathway for Hcy disposal.

1. Identification and Prevalence of *BHMT* 742G→A

The *BHMT* 742G→A variant (rs3733890, reference sequence NM_001713.1) is a nonsynonymous mutation in exon 6 that results in an arginine to glutamine substitution (R239Q) [190,191]. The numbering for this variant starts at the first nucleotide of the reference sequence; using standard notation, this variant is 716G→A. The frequency of the AA genotype is 9% to 13% in North American and European populations [23,103,190–194].

2. Biochemical Impact of the *BHMT* 742G→A Variant

The R239Q variant expressed in bacteria and examined in crude extracts did not show changes in kinetics or thermostability [191], although it is possible that such effects would be apparent using purified protein. The variant does not appear to affect circulating Hcy, folate, or vitamin B12 concentrations [23,190–192]. However, dimethylglycine has been reported to decrease significantly in GA and AA individuals, suggesting that the variant may reduce BHMT activity in vivo [23].

3. Impact of the *BHMT* 742G→A Variant on Health

The 742AA genotype does not appear to be an independent risk factor for NTD [192,193]. One report has identified an increased risk of placental abruption in AA women [194]. The variant does not appear to modulate the risk for CVD [190]. The A allele has been reported to decrease risk for colorectal adenoma in individuals with a high folate/methyl group diet [103]. The variant does not appear to influence breast cancer risk but may reduce mortality in breast cancer patients [195,196].

4. Mouse Model of BHMT Overexpression

A transgenic mouse that overexpresses human BHMT outside the liver has been established [197]. These mice appear morphologically normal and do not have significant changes in liver betaine or plasma Hcy concentrations. They are protected against alcohol- or high methionine/low folate–induced increases in Hcy.

C.   *DHFR* 19-bp Deletion

DHFR catalyzes the reduction of oxidized folates, such as folic acid and DHF, to THF. Therefore, the benefits of folic acid supplementation are dependent on DHFR activity. DHFR is also required to reduce the DHF produced by TS to regenerate THF.

1. Identification and Prevalence of the *DHFR* 19-bp Deletion Variant

The 19-bp deletion in intron 1 (c.86+60del19 or 19-bp del) was reported in 2004 [198]. The current reference sequence of *DHFR* (NC_000005.8) contains the 19-bp deletion allele. The homozygosity frequency of the 19-bp deletion allele in whites is 17% to 22% [198–201].

2. Biochemical Impact of the *DHFR* 19-bp Deletion Variant

The 19-bp deletion variant removes a putative binding site for the transcription factor Sp1 and therefore may affect DHFR expression [198]. Two studies have observed an increase in DHFR expression as a result of the 19-bp deletion allele, whereas a third reported no effect [200–202]. Research findings related to the effect of the del/del genotype on Hcy and folate concentrations are inconclusive [199,200].

3. Impact of the *DHFR* 19-bp Deletion Variant on Health

Studies on the 19-bp deletion variant and NTD risk have yielded conflicting results [198,200,202]. In a large cohort, the combination of the del/del genotype and multivitamin use was associated with a 50% increase in breast cancer risk [201].

X. CONCLUSIONS

Genetic variation in folate metabolism has become an important area of investigation, largely because of the potential impact on many common conditions, including CVD, birth defects, and cancer. Despite the hundreds of studies that are appearing every year on folate-related variants and disorders, it is often difficult to confirm the impact of a particular variant on disease risk because of confounders in clinical studies. Therefore, it is essential that studies on polymorphisms consider the biological impact of the variant on the gene product and on outcomes in a model system in vivo. With the advent of genome-wide technology worldwide, there will be many more polymorphisms identified in genes of folate metabolism and numerous association studies to evaluate their impact in a variety of populations. In addition to the comprehensive biological approach already suggested, the genetic and nongenetic variation in a population should be carefully considered when evaluating polymorphisms. This is particularly important when studying a variant involved in nutritional health because the impact of a folate-related variant may depend on concentrations of several nutrients in addition to folate (e.g., riboflavin, choline, betaine, and vitamin B12). Gene–gene and gene–nutrient interactions may become more apparent as additional large-scale population studies are performed; many of the studies discussed in this chapter suffer from small cohorts. It is also possible that the impact of a genetic variant is subtle and can only be teased out when the system is under stress, such as during periods of rapid growth, drug treatment, oxidative stress, or inflammation.

Despite the various confounders and inconsistent conclusions, it has become evident that some variants in folate metabolism affect human health. The deleterious effect(s) of these variants raises the question of why they have been maintained in human populations, particularly the variants that are relatively common. As a clearer understanding of the interaction of these variants with their genetic and nongenetic environment emerges, it is possible that subtle beneficial effects may become apparent.

REFERENCES

1. Hoffbrand AV, Weir DG. The history of folic acid. *Br J Haematol* 2001; 113:579–89.
2. Leclerc D, Sibani S, Rozen R. Molecular biology of methylenetetrahydrofolate reductase (MTHFR) and overview of mutation/polymorphisms. In: Ueland PM, Rozen R, eds., *MTHFR Polymorphisms and Disease.* Georgetown, TX: Landes Bioscience, 2005:1–20.
3. Christensen KE, MacKenzie RE. Mitochondrial one-carbon metabolism is adapted to the specific needs of yeast, plants and mammals. *Bioessays* 2006; 28:595–605.
4. James SJ. The molecular dynamics of abnormal folate metabolism and DNA methylation: Implications for disease susceptibility and progression. In: Ueland PM, Rozen R, eds., *MTHFR Polymorphisms and Disease.* Georgetown, TX: Landes Bioscience, 2005:78–99.
5. Frosst P, Blom HJ, Milos R, Goyette P, Sheppard CA, Matthews RG, Boers GJ, et al. A candidate genetic risk factor for vascular disease: A common mutation in methylenetetrahydrofolate reductase. *Nat Genet* 1995; 10:111–13.
6. van der Put NM, Steegers-Theunissen RP, Frosst P, Trijbels FJ, Eskes TK, van den Heuvel LP, Mariman EC, den Heyer M, Rozen R, Blom HJ. Mutated methylenetetrahydrofolate reductase as a risk factor for spina bifida. *Lancet* 1995; 346:1070–71.
7. Sunden SL, Renduchintala MS, Park EI, Miklasz SD, Garrow TA. Betaine-homocysteine methyltransferase expression in porcine and human tissues and chromosomal localization of the human gene. *Arch Biochem Biophys* 1997; 345:171–74.
8. Bao L, Vlcek C, Paces V, Kraus JP. Identification and tissue distribution of human cystathionine beta-synthase mRNA isoforms. *Arch Biochem Biophys* 1998; 350:95–103.
9. Database of Single Nucleotide Polymorphisms (dbSNP). Bethesda, MD: National Center for Biotechnology Information, National Library of Medicine (dbSNP Build ID: 129). Available at http://www.ncbi.nlm.nih.gov/SNP/.
10. Goyette P, Sumner JS, Milos R, Duncan AM, Rosenblatt DS, Matthews RG, Rozen R. Human methylenetetrahydrofolate reductase: Isolation of cDNA, mapping and mutation identification. *Nat Genet* 1994; 7:195–200.
11. Amorim MR, Lima MA, Castilla EE, Orioli IM. Non-Latin European descent could be a requirement for association of NTDs and *MTHFR* variant 677C → T: A meta-analysis. *Am J Med Genet A* 2007; 143A:1726–32.
12. Botto LD, Yang Q. 5,10-Methylenetetrahydrofolate reductase gene variants and congenital anomalies: A HuGE review. *Am J Epidemiol* 2000; 151:862–77.
13. Ogino S, Wilson RB. Genotype and haplotype distributions of *MTHFR* 677C→T and 1298A→C single nucleotide polymorphisms: A meta-analysis. *J Hum Genet* 2003; 48:1–7.
14. Sharp L, Little J. Polymorphisms in genes involved in folate metabolism and colorectal neoplasia: A HuGE review. *Am J Epidemiol* 2004; 159:423–43.
15. Yang QH, Botto LD, Gallagher M, Friedman JM, Sanders CL, Koontz D, Nikolova S, Erickson JD, Steinberg K. Prevalence and effects of gene-gene and gene-nutrient interactions on serum folate and serum total homocysteine concentrations in the United States: Findings from the Third National Health and Nutrition Examination Survey DNA Bank. *Am J Clin Nutr* 2008; 88:232–46.
16. Gueant-Rodriguez RM, Gueant JL, Debard R, Thirion S, Hong LX, Bronowicki JP, Namour F, et al. Prevalence of methylenetetrahydrofolate reductase 677T and 1298C alleles and folate status: A comparative study in Mexican, West African, and European populations. *Am J Clin Nutr* 2006; 83:701–07.
17. Yamada K, Chen Z, Rozen R, Matthews RG. Effects of common polymorphisms on the properties of recombinant human methylenetetrahydrofolate reductase. *Proc Natl Acad Sci USA* 2001; 98:14853–58.

18. van der Put NM, van den Heuvel LP, Steegers-Theunissen RP, Trijbels FJ, Eskes TK, Mariman EC, den Heyer M, Blom HJ. Decreased methylene tetrahydrofolate reductase activity due to the 677C→T mutation in families with spina bifida offspring. *J Mol Med* 1996; 74:691–94.

19. Weisberg I, Tran P, Christensen B, Sibani S, Rozen R. A second genetic polymorphism in methylenetetrahydrofolate reductase (*MTHFR*) associated with decreased enzyme activity. *Mol Genet Metab* 1998; 64:169–72.

20. van der Put NM, Gabreels F, Stevens EM, Smeitink JA, Trijbels FJ, Eskes TK, van den Heuvel LP, Blom HJ. A second common mutation in the methylenetetrahydrofolate reductase gene: An additional risk factor for neural-tube defects? *Am J Hum Genet* 1998; 62:1044–51.

21. Jacques PF, Bostom AG, Williams RR, Ellison RC, Eckfeldt JH, Rosenberg IH, Selhub J, Rozen R. Relation between folate status, a common mutation in methylenetetrahydrofolate reductase, and plasma homocysteine concentrations. *Circulation* 1996; 93:7–9.

22. Davis SR, Quinlivan EP, Shelnutt KP, Maneval DR, Ghandour H, Capdevila A, Coats BS, et al. The methylenetetrahydrofolate reductase 677C→T polymorphism and dietary folate restriction affect plasma one-carbon metabolites and red blood cell folate concentrations and distribution in women. *J Nutr* 2005; 135:1040–44.

23. Fredriksen A, Meyer K, Ueland PM, Vollset SE, Grotmol T, Schneede J. Large-scale population-based metabolic phenotyping of thirteen genetic polymorphisms related to one-carbon metabolism. *Hum Mutat* 2007; 28:856–65.

24. Hustad S, Midttun O, Schneede J, Vollset SE, Grotmol T, Ueland PM. The methylenetetrahydrofolate reductase 677C→T polymorphism as a modulator of a B vitamin network with major effects on homocysteine metabolism. *Am J Hum Genet* 2007; 80:846–55.

25. Devlin AM, Clarke R, Birks J, Evans JG, Halsted CH. Interactions among polymorphisms in folate-metabolizing genes and serum total homocysteine concentrations in a healthy elderly population. *Am J Clin Nutr* 2006; 83:708–13.

26. Jacques PF, Kalmbach R, Bagley PJ, Russo GT, Rogers G, Wilson PW, Rosenberg IH, Selhub J. The relationship between riboflavin and plasma total homocysteine in the Framingham offspring cohort is influenced by folate status and the C677T transition in the methylenetetrahydrofolate reductase gene. *J Nutr* 2002; 132:283–88.

27. Quinlivan EP, Davis SR, Shelnutt KP, Henderson GN, Ghandour H, Shane B, Selhub J, Bailey LB, Stacpoole PW, Gregory JF III. Methylenetetrahydrofolate reductase 677C→T polymorphism and folate status affect one-carbon incorporation into human DNA deoxynucleosides. *J Nutr* 2005; 135:389–96.

28. Bagley PJ, Selhub J. A common mutation in the methylenetetrahydrofolate reductase gene is associated with an accumulation of formylated tetrahydrofolates in red blood cells. *Proc Natl Acad Sci USA* 1998; 95:13217–20.

29. Friso S, Choi SW, Girelli D, Mason JB, Dolnikowski GG, Bagley PJ, Olivieri O, et al. A common mutation in the 5,10-methylenetetrahydrofolate reductase gene affects genomic DNA methylation through an interaction with folate status. *Proc Natl Acad Sci USA* 2002; 99:5606–11.

30. Molloy AM, Mills JL, Kirke PN, Whitehead AS, Weir DG, Scott JM. Whole-blood folate values in subjects with different methylenetetrahydrofolate reductase genotypes: Differences between the radioassay and microbiological assays. *Clin Chem* 1998; 44:186–88.

31. Jacques PF, Choumenkovitch SF. Mild MTHFR deficiency and folate status. In: Ueland PM, Rozen R, eds., *MTHFR Polymorphisms and Disease*. Georgetown, TX: Landes Bioscience, 2005:54–70.

32. Botto N, Andreassi MG, Manfredi S, Masetti S, Cocci F, Colombo MG, Storti S, Rizza A, Biagini A. Genetic polymorphisms in folate and homocysteine metabolism as risk factors for DNA damage. *Eur J Hum Genet* 2003; 11:671–78.

33. Shelnutt KP, Kauwell GP, Gregory JF 3rd, Maneval DR, Quinlivan EP, Theriaque DW, Henderson GN, Bailey LB. Methylenetetrahydrofolate reductase 677C→T polymorphism affects DNA methylation in response to controlled folate intake in young women. *J Nutr Biochem* 2004; 15:554–60.

34. Vollset SE, Botto LD. Neural tube defects, other congenital malformations and single nucleotide polymorphisms in the 5,10 methylenetetrahydrofolate reductase (*MTHFR*) gene: A meta-analysis. In: Ueland PM, Rozen R, eds., *MTHFR Polymorphisms and Disease.* Georgetown, TX: Landes Bioscience, 2005:125–43.

35. Volcik KA, Shaw GM, Lammer EJ, Zhu H, Finnell RH. Evaluation of infant methylenetetrahydrofolate reductase genotype, maternal vitamin use, and risk of high versus low level spina bifida defects. *Birth Defects Res A Clin Mol Teratol* 2003; 67:154–57.

36. Wenstrom KD, Johanning GL, Owen J, Johnston KE, Acton S, Cliver S, Tamura T. Amniotic fluid homocysteine levels, 5,10-methylenetetrahydrafolate reductase genotypes, and neural tube closure sites. *Am J Med Genet* 2000; 90:6–11.

37. Relton CL, Wilding CS, Pearce MS, Laffling AJ, Jonas PA, Lynch SA, Tawn EJ, Burn J. Gene-gene interaction in folate-related genes and risk of neural tube defects in a UK population. *J Med Genet* 2004; 41:256–60.

38. Christensen B, Arbour L, Tran P, Leclerc D, Sabbaghian N, Platt R, Gilfix BM, et al. Genetic polymorphisms in methylenetetrahydrofolate reductase and methionine synthase, folate levels in red blood cells, and risk of neural tube defects. *Am J Med Genet* 1999; 84:151–57.

39. Shaw GM, Rozen R, Finnell RH, Wasserman CR, Lammer EJ. Maternal vitamin use, genetic variation of infant methylenetetrahydrofolate reductase, and risk for spina bifida. *Am J Epidemiol* 1998; 148:30–37.

40. Verkleij-Hagoort A, Bliek J, Sayed-Tabatabaei F, Ursem N, Steegers E, Steegers-Theunissen R. Hyperhomocysteinemia and *MTHFR* polymorphisms in association with orofacial clefts and congenital heart defects: A meta-analysis. *Am J Med Genet A* 2007; 143A:952–60.

41. van Beynum IM, den Heijer M, Blom HJ, Kapusta L. The *MTHFR* 677C→T polymorphism and the risk of congenital heart defects: A literature review and meta-analysis. *QJM* 2007; 100:743–53.

42. van Beynum IM, Kapusta L, den Heijer M, Vermeulen SH, Kouwenberg M, Daniels O, Blom HJ. Maternal *MTHFR* 677C→T is a risk factor for congenital heart defects: Effect modification by periconceptional folate supplementation. *Eur Heart J* 2006; 27:981–87.

43. Junker R, Kotthoff S, Vielhaber H, Halimeh S, Kosch A, Koch HG, Kassenbohmer R, Heineking B, Nowak-Gottl U. Infant methylenetetrahydrofolate reductase 677TT genotype is a risk factor for congenital heart disease. *Cardiovasc Res* 2001; 51:251–54.

44. Wald DS, Law M, Morris JK. Homocysteine and cardiovascular disease: Evidence on causality from a meta-analysis. *BMJ* 2002; 325:1202.

45. Klerk M, Verhoef P, Clarke R, Blom HJ, Kok FJ, Schouten EG. *MTHFR* 677C→T polymorphism and risk of coronary heart disease: A meta-analysis. *JAMA* 2002; 288:2023–31.

46. Lewis SJ, Ebrahim S, Davey Smith G. Meta-analysis of *MTHFR* 677C→T polymorphism and coronary heart disease: Does totality of evidence support causal role for homocysteine and preventive potential of folate? *BMJ* 2005; 331:1053.

47. Girelli D, Martinelli N, Pizzolo F, Friso S, Olivieri O, Stranieri C, Trabetti E, et al. The interaction between *MTHFR* 677 C→T genotype and folate status is a determinant of coronary atherosclerosis risk. *J Nutr* 2003; 133:1281–85.

48. Mager A, Lalezari S, Shohat T, Birnbaum Y, Adler Y, Magal N, Shohat M. Methylenetetrahydrofolate reductase genotypes and early-onset coronary artery disease. *Circulation* 1999; 100:2406–10.

49. Rallidis LS, Gialeraki A, Komporozos C, Vavoulis P, Pavlakis G, Travlou A, Lekakis I, Kremastinos DT. Role of methylenetetrahydrofolate reductase 677C→T polymorphism in the development of premature myocardial infarction. *Atherosclerosis* 2008; 200:115–20.

50. Gemmati D, Serino ML, Trivellato C, Fiorini S, Scapoli GL. C677T substitution in the methylenetetrahydrofolate reductase gene as a risk factor for venous thrombosis and arterial disease in selected patients. *Haematologica* 1999; 84:824–28.

51. Cronin S, Furie KL, Kelly PJ. Dose-related association of MTHFR 677T allele with risk of ischemic stroke: Evidence from a cumulative meta-analysis. *Stroke* 2005; 36:1581–87.

52. Casas JP, Bautista LE, Smeeth L, Sharma P, Hingorani AD. Homocysteine and stroke: Evidence on a causal link from mendelian randomisation. *Lancet* 2005; 365:224–32.

53. Ray JG, Shmorgun D, Chan WS. Common C677T polymorphism of the methylenetetrahydrofolate reductase gene and the risk of venous thromboembolism: Meta-analysis of 31 studies. *Pathophysiol Haemost Thromb* 2002; 32:51–58.

54. Den Heijer M, Lewington S, Clarke R. Homocysteine, MTHFR and risk of venous thrombosis: A meta-analysis of published epidemiological studies. *J Thromb Haemost* 2005; 3:292–99.

55. Chen J, Giovannucci E, Kelsey K, Rimm EB, Stampfer MJ, Colditz GA, Spiegelman D, Willett WC, Hunter DJ. A methylenetetrahydrofolate reductase polymorphism and the risk of colorectal cancer. *Cancer Res* 1996; 56:4862–64.

56. Ma J, Stampfer MJ, Giovannucci E, Artigas C, Hunter DJ, Fuchs C, Willett WC, Selhub J, Hennekens CH, Rozen R. Methylenetetrahydrofolate reductase polymorphism, dietary interactions, and risk of colorectal cancer. *Cancer Res* 1997; 57:1098–102.

57. Crott JW, Mason JB. *MTHFR* polymorphisms and colorectal neoplasia. In: Ueland PM, Rozen R, eds., *MTHFR Polymorphisms and Disease*. Georgetown, TX: Landes Bioscience, 2005:179–96.

58. Blount BC, Mack MM, Wehr CM, MacGregor JT, Hiatt RA, Wang G, Wickramasinghe SN, Everson RB, Ames BN. Folate deficiency causes uracil misincorporation into human DNA and chromosome breakage: Implications for cancer and neuronal damage. *Proc Natl Acad Sci USA* 1997; 94:3290–95.

59. Huang Y, Han S, Li Y, Mao Y, Xie Y. Different roles of MTHFR C677T and A1298C polymorphisms in colorectal adenoma and colorectal cancer: A meta-analysis. *J Hum Genet* 2007; 52:73–85.

60. Le Marchand L, Donlon T, Hankin JH, Kolonel LN, Wilkens LR, Seifried A. B-vitamin intake, metabolic genes, and colorectal cancer risk (United States). *Cancer Causes Control* 2002; 13:239–48.

61. Toffoli G, Gafa R, Russo A, Lanza G, Dolcetti R, Sartor F, Libra M, Viel A, Boiocchi M. Methylenetetrahydrofolate reductase 677 C→T polymorphism and risk of proximal colon cancer in north Italy. *Clin Cancer Res* 2003; 9:743–48.

62. Boccia S, Hung R, Ricciardi G, Gianfagna F, Ebert MP, Fang JY, Gao CM, et al. Meta- and pooled analyses of the methylenetetrahydrofolate reductase C677T and A1298C polymorphisms and gastric cancer risk: A huge-GSEC review. *Am J Epidemiol* 2008; 167:505–16.

63. Sun L, Sun YH, Wang B, Cao HY, Yu C. Methylenetetrahydrofolate reductase polymorphisms and susceptibility to gastric cancer in Chinese populations: A meta-analysis. *Eur J Cancer Prev* 2008; 17:446–52.

64. Muntjewerff JW, Kahn RS, Blom HJ, den Heijer M. Homocysteine, methylenetetrahydrofolate reductase and risk of schizophrenia: A meta-analysis. *Mol Psychiatry* 2006; 11:143–49.

65. Gilbody S, Lewis S, Lightfoot T. Methylenetetrahydrofolate reductase (MTHFR) genetic polymorphisms and psychiatric disorders: A HuGE review. *Am J Epidemiol* 2007; 165:1–13.

66. Nelen WL, Blom HJ, Steegers EA, den Heijer M, Eskes TK. Hyperhomocysteinemia and recurrent early pregnancy loss: A meta-analysis. *Fertil Steril* 2000; 74:1196–99.
67. Kosmas IP, Tatsioni A, Ioannidis JP. Association of C677T polymorphism in the methylenetetrahydrofolate reductase gene with hypertension in pregnancy and pre-eclampsia: A meta-analysis. *J Hypertens* 2004; 22:1655–62.
68. Schwahn BC, Rozen R. Methylenetetrahydrofolate reductase polymorphisms: Pharmacogenetic effects. In: Ueland PM, Rozen R, eds., *MTHFR Polymorphisms and Disease.* Georgetown, TX: Landes Bioscience, 2005:197–205.
69. Brown NM, Pratt VM, Buller A, Pike-Buchanan L, Redman JB, Sun W, Chen R, et al. Detection of 677CT/1298AC "double variant" chromosomes: Implications for interpretation of MTHFR genotyping results. *Genet Med* 2005; 7:278–82.
70. Weisberg IS, Jacques PF, Selhub J, Bostom AG, Chen Z, Curtis Ellison R, Eckfeldt JH, Rozen R. The 1298A→C polymorphism in methylenetetrahydrofolate reductase (MTHFR): In vitro expression and association with homocysteine. *Atherosclerosis* 2001; 156:409–15.
71. Parle-McDermott A, Mills JL, Kirke PN, O'Leary VB, Swanson DA, Pangilinan F, Conley M, et al. Analysis of the MTHFR 1298A→C and 677C→T polymorphisms as risk factors for neural tube defects. *J Hum Genet* 2003; 48:190–93.
72. Relton CL, Wilding CS, Laffling AJ, Jonas PA, Burgess T, Binks K, Tawn EJ, Burn J. Low erythrocyte folate status and polymorphic variation in folate-related genes are associated with risk of neural tube defect pregnancy. *Mol Genet Metab* 2004; 81:273–81.
73. Hanson NQ, Aras O, Yang F, Tsai MY. C677T and A1298C polymorphisms of the methylenetetrahydrofolate reductase gene: Incidence and effect of combined genotypes on plasma fasting and post-methionine load homocysteine in vascular disease. *Clin Chem* 2001; 47:661–66.
74. Ray JG, Langman LJ, Vermeulen MJ, Evrovski J, Yeo EL, Cole DE. Genetics University of Toronto Thrombophilia Study in Women (GUTTSI): Genetic and other risk factors for venous thromboembolism in women. *Curr Control Trials Cardiovasc Med* 2001; 2:141–49.
75. Chen Z, Karaplis AC, Ackerman SL, Pogribny IP, Melnyk S, Lussier-Cacan S, Chen MF, et al. Mice deficient in methylenetetrahydrofolate reductase exhibit hyperhomocysteinemia and decreased methylation capacity, with neuropathology and aortic lipid deposition. *Hum Mol Genet* 2001; 10:433–43.
76. Celtikci B, Leclerc D, Lawrance AK, Deng L, Friedman HC, Krupenko NI, Krupenko SA, et al. Altered expression of methylenetetrahydrofolate reductase modifies response to methotrexate in mice. *Pharmacogenet Genom* 2008; 18:577–89.
77. Schwahn BC, Chen Z, Laryea MD, Wendel U, Lussier-Cacan S, Genest JJ, Mar M-H, et al. Homocysteine-betaine interactions in a murine model of 5,10-methylenetetrahydrofolate reductase deficiency. *FASEB J* 2003; 17:512–14.
78. Li D, Pickell L, Liu Y, Wu Q, Cohn JS, Rozen R. Maternal methylenetetrahydrofolate reductase deficiency and low dietary folate lead to adverse reproductive outcomes and congenital heart defects in mice. *Am J Clin Nutr* 2005; 82:188–95.
79. Schwahn BC, Wang XL, Mikael LG, Wu Q, Cohn J, Jiang H, Maclean KN, Rozen R. Betaine supplementation improves the atherogenic risk factor profile in a transgenic mouse model of hyperhomocysteinemia. *Atherosclerosis* 2007; 195:e100–07.
80. Schwahn BC, Laryea MD, Chen Z, Melnyk S, Pogribny I, Garrow T, James SJ, Rozen R. Betaine rescue of an animal model with methylenetetrahydrofolate reductase deficiency. *Biochem J* 2004; 382:831–40.
81. Ghandour H, Chen Z, Selhub J, Rozen R. Mice deficient in methylenetetrahydrofolate reductase exhibit tissue-specific distribution of folates. *J Nutr* 2004; 134:2975–78.

82. Li D, Karp N, Wu Q, Wang XL, Melnyk S, James SJ, Rozen R. Mefolinate (5-methyltetrahydrofolate), but not folic acid, decreases mortality in an animal model of severe methylenetetrahydrofolate reductase deficiency. *J Inherit Metab Dis* 2008; 31:403–11.
83. Virdis A, Iglarz M, Neves MF, Amiri F, Touyz RM, Rozen R, Schiffrin EL. Effect of hyperhomocystinemia and hypertension on endothelial function in methylenetetrahydrofolate reductase-deficient mice. *Arterioscler Thromb Vasc Biol* 2003; 23:1352–57.
84. Neves MF, Endemann D, Amiri F, Virdis A, Pu Q, Rozen R, Schiffrin EL. Small artery mechanics in hyperhomocysteinemic mice: Effects of angiotensin II. *J Hypertens* 2004; 22:959–66.
85. Mikael LG, Genest J Jr, Rozen R. Elevated homocysteine reduces apolipoprotein A-I expression in hyperhomocysteinemic mice and in males with coronary artery disease. *Circ Res* 2006; 98:564–71.
86. Knock E, Deng L, Wu Q, Leclerc D, Wang XL, Rozen R. Low dietary folate initiates intestinal tumors in mice, with altered expression of G2-M checkpoint regulators polo-like kinase 1 and cell division cycle 25c. *Cancer Res* 2006; 66:10349–56.
87. Mikael LG, Rozen R. Homocysteine modulates the effect of simvastatin on expression of ApoA-I and NF-κB/iNOS. *Cardiovasc Res* 2008; 80:151–58.
88. Roy M, Leclerc D, Wu Q, Gupta S, Kruger WD, Rozen R. Valproic acid increases expression of methylenetetrahydrofolate reductase (MTHFR) and induces lower teratogenicity in MTHFR deficiency. *J Cell Biochem* 2008; 105:467–76.
89. Chen LH, Liu M-L, Hwang H-Y, Chen L-S, Korenberg J, Shane B. Human methionine synthase. cDNA cloning, gene localization, and expression. *J Biol Chem* 1997; 272:3628–34.
90. Olteanu H, Munson T, Banerjee R. Differences in the efficiency of reductive activation of methionine synthase and exogenous electron acceptors between the common polymorphic variants of human methionine synthase reductase. *Biochemistry* 2002; 41:13378–85.
91. van der Put NM, van der Molen EF, Kluijtmans LA, Heil SG, Trijbels JM, Eskes TK, Van Oppenraaij-Emmerzaal D, Banerjee R, Blom HJ. Sequence analysis of the coding region of human methionine synthase: Relevance to hyperhomocysteinaemia in neural-tube defects and vascular disease. *QJM* 1997; 90:511–17.
92. Theodoratou E, Farrington SM, Tenesa A, McNeill G, Cetnarskyj R, Barnetson RA, Porteous ME, Dunlop MG, Campbell H. Dietary vitamin B6 intake and the risk of colorectal cancer. *Cancer Epidemiol Biomarkers Prev* 2008; 17:171–82.
93. Koushik A, Kraft P, Fuchs CS, Hankinson SE, Willett WC, Giovannucci EL, Hunter DJ. Nonsynonymous polymorphisms in genes in the one-carbon metabolism pathway and associations with colorectal cancer. *Cancer Epidemiol Biomarkers Prev* 2006; 15:2408–17.
94. Chen J, Stampfer MJ, Ma J, Selhub J, Malinow MR, Hennekens CH, Hunter DJ. Influence of a methionine synthase (D919G) polymorphism on plasma homocysteine and folate levels and relation to risk of myocardial infarction. *Atherosclerosis* 2001; 154:667–72.
95. Ma J, Stampfer MJ, Christensen B, Giovannucci E, Hunter DJ, Chen J, Willett WC, et al. A polymorphism of the methionine synthase gene: Association with plasma folate, vitamin B12, homocyst(e)ine, and colorectal cancer risk. *Cancer Epidemiol Biomarkers Prev* 1999; 8:825–29.
96. Klerk M, Lievers KJ, Kluijtmans LA, Blom HJ, den Heijer M, Schouten EG, Kok FJ, Verhoef P. The 2756A→G variant in the gene encoding methionine synthase: Its relation with plasma homocysteine levels and risk of coronary heart disease in a Dutch case-control study. *Thromb Res* 2003; 110:87–91.
97. Gueant-Rodriguez RM, Juilliere Y, Candito M, Adjalla CE, Gibelin P, Herbeth B, Van Obberghen E, Gueant JL. Association of MTRRA66G polymorphism (but not of

MTHFR C677T and A1298C, MTRA2756G, TCN C776G) with homocysteine and coronary artery disease in the French population. *Thromb Haemost* 2005; 94:510–15.

98. Ulvik A, Vollset SE, Hansen S, Gislefoss R, Jellum E, Ueland PM. Colorectal cancer and the methylenetetrahydrofolate reductase 677C→T and methionine synthase 2756A→G polymorphisms: A study of 2,168 case-control pairs from the JANUS cohort. *Cancer Epidemiol Biomarkers Prev* 2004; 13:2175–80.

99. Zhu H, Wicker NJ, Shaw GM, Lammer EJ, Hendricks K, Suarez L, Canfield M, Finnell RH. Homocysteine remethylation enzyme polymorphisms and increased risks for neural tube defects. *Mol Genet Metab* 2003; 78:216–21.

100. van der Linden IJ, den Heijer M, Afman LA, Gellekink H, Vermeulen SH, Kluijtmans LA, Blom HJ. The methionine synthase reductase 66A→G polymorphism is a maternal risk factor for spina bifida. *J Mol Med* 2006; 84:1047–54.

101. Zhang G, Dai C. Gene polymorphisms of homocysteine metabolism-related enzymes in Chinese patients with occlusive coronary artery or cerebral vascular diseases. *Thromb Res* 2001; 104:187–95.

102. Ulrich CM, Curtin K, Potter JD, Bigler J, Caan B, Slattery ML. Polymorphisms in the reduced folate carrier, thymidylate synthase, or methionine synthase and risk of colon cancer. *Cancer Epidemiol Biomarkers Prev* 2005; 14:2509–16.

103. Hazra A, Wu K, Kraft P, Fuchs CS, Giovannucci EL, Hunter DJ. Twenty-four non-synonymous polymorphisms in the one-carbon metabolic pathway and risk of colorectal adenoma in the Nurses' Health Study. *Carcinogenesis* 2007; 28:1510–19.

104. Bosco P, Gueant-Rodriguez RM, Anello G, Romano A, Namour B, Spada RS, Caraci F, Tringali G, Ferri R, Gueant JL. Association of IL-1 RN*2 allele and methionine synthase 2756 AA genotype with dementia severity of sporadic Alzheimer's disease. *J Neurol Neurosurg Psychiatry* 2004; 75:1036–38.

105. Beyer K, Lao JI, Latorre P, Ariza A. Age at onset: An essential variable for the definition of genetic risk factors for sporadic Alzheimer's disease. *Ann N Y Acad Sci* 2005; 1057:260–78.

106. Swanson DA, Liu ML, Baker PJ, Garrett L, Stitzel M, Wu J, Harris M, Banerjee R, Shane B, Brody LC. Targeted disruption of the methionine synthase gene in mice. *Mol Cell Biol* 2001; 21:1058–65.

107. Dayal S, Devlin AM, McCaw RB, Liu M-L, Arning E, Bottiglieri T, Shane B, Faraci FM, Lentz SR. Cerebral vascular dysfunction in methionine synthase-deficient mice. *Circulation* 2005; 112:737–44.

108. Yamada K, Gravel RA, Toraya T, Matthews RG. Human methionine synthase reductase is a molecular chaperone for human methionine synthase. *Proc Natl Acad Sci USA* 2006; 103:9476–81.

109. Wilson A, Platt R, Wu Q, Leclerc D, Christensen B, Yang H, Gravel RA, Rozen R. A common variant in methionine synthase reductase combined with low cobalamin (vitamin B12) increases risk for spina bifida. *Mol Genet Metab* 1999; 67:317–23.

110. Shi M, Caprau D, Romitti P, Christensen K, Murray JC. Genotype frequencies and linkage disequilibrium in the CEPH human diversity panel for variants in folate pathway genes MTHFR, MTHFD, MTRR, RFC1, and GCP2. *Birth Defects Res A Clin Mol Teratol* 2003; 67:545–49.

111. Olteanu H, Wolthers KR, Munro AW, Scrutton NS, Banerjee R. Kinetic and thermodynamic characterization of the common polymorphic variants of human methionine synthase reductase. *Biochemistry* 2004; 43:1988–97.

112. Wolthers KR, Scrutton NS. Protein interactions in the human methionine synthase-methionine synthase reductase complex and implications for the mechanism of enzyme reactivation. *Biochemistry* 2007; 46:6696–709.

113. Brown CA, McKinney KQ, Kaufman JS, Gravel RA, Rozen R. A common polymorphism in methionine synthase reductase increases risk of premature coronary artery disease. *J Cardiovasc Risk* 2000; 7:197–200.

114. Brilakis ES, Berger PB, Ballman KV, Rozen R. Methylenetetrahydrofolate reductase (*MTHFR*) 677C→T and methionine synthase reductase (MTRR) 66A→G polymorphisms: Association with serum homocysteine and angiographic coronary artery disease in the era of flour products fortified with folic acid. *Atherosclerosis* 2003; 168:315–22.

115. Barbosa PR, Stabler SP, Trentin R, Carvalho FR, Luchessi AD, Hirata RD, Hirata MH, Allen RH, Guerra-Shinohara EM. Evaluation of nutritional and genetic determinants of total homocysteine, methylmalonic acid and S-adenosylmethionine/S-adenosylhomocysteine values in Brazilian childbearing-age women. *Clin Chim Acta* 2008; 388:139–47.

116. Gaughan DJ, Kluijtmans LA, Barbaux S, McMaster D, Young IS, Yarnell JW, Evans A, Whitehead AS. The methionine synthase reductase (MTRR) A66G polymorphism is a novel genetic determinant of plasma homocysteine concentrations. *Atherosclerosis* 2001; 157:451–56.

117. Verkleij-Hagoort AC, van Driel LM, Lindemans J, Isaacs A, Steegers EA, Helbing WA, Uitterlinden AG, Steegers-Theunissen RP. Genetic and lifestyle factors related to the periconception vitamin B12 status and congenital heart defects: A Dutch case-control study. *Mol Genet Metab* 2008; 94:112–19.

118. van Beynum IM, Kouwenberg M, Kapusta L, den Heijer M, van der Linden IJ, Daniels O, Blom HJ. MTRR 66A→G polymorphism in relation to congenital heart defects. *Clin Chem Lab Med* 2006; 44:1317–23.

119. Shi Q, Zhang Z, Li G, Pillow PC, Hernandez LM, Spitz MR, Wei Q. Polymorphisms of methionine synthase and methionine synthase reductase and risk of lung cancer: A case-control analysis. *Pharmacogenet Genomics* 2005; 15:547–55.

120. Elmore CL, Wu X, Leclerc D, Watson ED, Bottiglieri T, Krupenko NI, Krupenko SA, et al. Metabolic derangement of methionine and folate metabolism in mice deficient in methionine synthase reductase. *Mol Genet Metab* 2007; 91:85–97.

121. Deng L, Elmore CL, Lawrance AK, Matthews RG, Rozen R. Methionine synthase reductase deficiency results in adverse reproductive outcomes and congenital heart defects in mice. *Mol Genet Metab* 2008; 94:336–42.

122. Hum DW, MacKenzie RE. Expression of active domains of a human folate-dependent trifunctional enzyme in *Escherichia coli. Protein Eng* 1991; 4:493–500.

123. Hol FA, van der Put NM, Geurds MP, Heil SG, Trijbels FJ, Hamel BC, Mariman EC, Blom HJ. Molecular genetic analysis of the gene encoding the trifunctional enzyme MTHFD (methylenetetrahydrofolate-dehydrogenase, methenyltetrahydrofolate-cyclo-hydrolase, formyltetrahydrofolate synthetase) in patients with neural tube defects. *Clin Genet* 1998; 53:119–25.

124. Brody LC, Conley M, Cox C, Kirke PN, McKeever MP, Mills JL, Molloy AM, et al. A polymorphism, R653Q, in the trifunctional enzyme methylenetetrahydrofolate dehydrogenase/methenyltetrahydrofolate cyclohydrolase/formyltetrahydrofolate synthetase is a maternal genetic risk factor for neural tube defects: Report of the Birth Defects Research Group. *Am J Hum Genet* 2002; 71:1207–15.

125. Chen J, Kyte C, Valcin M, Chan W, Wetmur JG, Selhub J, Hunter DJ, Ma J. Polymorphisms in the one-carbon metabolic pathway, plasma folate levels and colorectal cancer in a prospective study. *Int J Cancer* 2004; 110:617–20.

126. Parle-McDermott A, Mills JL, Kirke PN, Cox C, Signore CC, Kirke S, Molloy AM, et al. MTHFD1 R653Q polymorphism is a maternal genetic risk factor for severe abruptio placentae. *Am J Med Genet A* 2005; 132:365–68.

127. Parle-McDermott A, Pangilinan F, Mills JL, Signore CC, Molloy AM, Cotter A, Conley M, et al. A polymorphism in the MTHFD1 gene increases a mother's risk of having an unexplained second trimester pregnancy loss. *Mol Hum Reprod* 2005; 11:477–80.

128. De Marco P, Merello E, Calevo MG, Mascelli S, Raso A, Cama A, Capra V. Evaluation of a methylenetetrahydrofolate-dehydrogenase 1958G→A polymorphism for neural tube defect risk. *J Hum Genet* 2006; 51:98–103.

129. van der Linden IJ, Heil SG, Kouwenberg IC, den Heijer M, Blom HJ. The methylenetetrahydrofolate dehydrogenase (MTHFD1) 1958G→A variant is not associated with spina bifida risk in the Dutch population. *Clin Genet* 2007; 72:599–600.

130. Cheng J, Zhu WL, Dao JJ, Li SQ, Li Y. Relationship between polymorphism of methylenetetrahydrofolate dehydrogenase and congenital heart defect. *Biomed Environ Sci* 2005; 18:58–64.

131. Wang L, Ke Q, Chen W, Wang J, Tan Y, Zhou Y, Hua Z, et al. Polymorphisms of MTHFD, plasma homocysteine levels, and risk of gastric cancer in a high-risk Chinese population. *Clin Cancer Res* 2007; 13:2526–32.

132. Christensen KE, Rohlicek CV, Andelfinger GU, Michaud J, Bigras JL, Richter A, Mackenzie RE, Rozen R. The MTHFD1 p.Arg653Gln variant alters enzyme function and increases risk for congenital heart defects. *Hum Mutat* 2009; 30:212–20.

133. Kohlmeier M, da Costa KA, Fischer LM, Zeisel SH. Genetic variation of folate-mediated one-carbon transfer pathway predicts susceptibility to choline deficiency in humans. *Proc Natl Acad Sci USA* 2005; 102:16025–30.

134. Parle-McDermott A, Kirke PN, Mills JL, Molloy AM, Cox C, O'Leary VB, Pangilinan F, et al. Confirmation of the R653Q polymorphism of the trifunctional C1-synthase enzyme as a maternal risk for neural tube defects in the Irish population. *Eur J Hum Genet* 2006; 14:768–72.

135. Scala I, Granese B, Sellitto M, Salome S, Sammartino A, Pepe A, Mastroiacovo P, Sebastio G, Andria G. Analysis of seven maternal polymorphisms of genes involved in homocysteine/folate metabolism and risk of Down syndrome offspring. *Genet Med* 2006; 8:409–16.

136. Stevens VL, McCullough ML, Pavluck AL, Talbot JT, Feigelson HS, Thun MJ, Calle EE. Association of polymorphisms in one-carbon metabolism genes and postmenopausal breast cancer incidence. *Cancer Epidemiol Biomarkers Prev* 2007; 16:1140–47.

137. Oterino A, Valle N, Pascual J, Bravo Y, Munoz P, Castillo J, Ruiz-Alegria C, Sanchez-Velasco P, Leyva-Cobian F, Cid C. Thymidylate synthase promoter tandem repeat and MTHFD1 R653Q polymorphisms modulate the risk for migraine conferred by the MTHFR T677 allele. *Mol Brain Res* 2005; 139:163–68.

138. Krajinovic M, Lemieux-Blanchard E, Chiasson S, Primeau M, Costea I, Moghrabi A. Role of polymorphisms in MTHFR and MTHFD1 genes in the outcome of childhood acute lymphoblastic leukemia. *Pharmacogenomics J* 2004; 4:66–72.

139. Woeller CF, Anderson DD, Szebenyi DM, Stover PJ. Evidence for small ubiquitin-like modifier-dependent nuclear import of the thymidylate biosynthesis pathway. *J Biol Chem* 2007; 282:17623–31.

140. Herbig K, Chiang EP, Lee LR, Hills J, Shane B, Stover PJ. Cytoplasmic serine hydroxymethyltransferase mediates competition between folate-dependent deoxyribonucleotide and S-adenosylmethionine biosyntheses. *J Biol Chem* 2002; 277:38381–89.

141. Heil SG, Van der Put NM, Waas ET, den Heijer M, Trijbels FJ, Blom HJ. Is mutated serine hydroxymethyltransferase (SHMT) involved in the etiology of neural tube defects? *Mol Genet Metab* 2001; 73:164–72.

142. Girgis S, Nasrallah IM, Suh JR, Oppenheim E, Zanetti KA, Mastri MG, Stover PJ. Molecular cloning, characterization and alternative splicing of the human cytoplasmic serine hydroxymethyltransferase gene. *Gene* 1998; 210:315–24.

143. van den Donk M, Visker MH, Harryvan JL, Kok FJ, Kampman E. Dietary intake of B-vitamins, polymorphisms in thymidylate synthase and serine hydroxymethyltransferase 1, and colorectal adenoma risk: A Dutch case-control study. *Cancer Lett* 2007; 250:146–53.

144. Engel SM, Olshan AF, Siega-Riz AM, Savitz DA, Chanock SJ. Polymorphisms in folate metabolizing genes and risk for spontaneous preterm and small-for-gestational age birth. *Am J Obstet Gynecol* 2006; 195:1231 e1–11.
145. Hishida A, Matsuo K, Hamajima N, Ito H, Ogura M, Kagami Y, Taji H, Morishima Y, Emi N, Tajima K. Associations between polymorphisms in the thymidylate synthase and serine hydroxymethyltransferase genes and susceptibility to malignant lymphoma. *Haematologica* 2003; 88:159–66.
146. Cheng CW, Yu JC, Huang CS, Shieh JC, Fu YP, Wang HW, Wu PE, Shen CY. Polymorphism of cytosolic serine hydroxymethyltransferase, estrogen and breast cancer risk among Chinese women in Taiwan. *Breast Cancer Res Treat* 2008; 111:145–55.
147. Fu TF, Hunt S, Schirch V, Safo MK, Chen BH. Properties of human and rabbit cytosolic serine hydroxymethyltransferase are changed by single nucleotide polymorphic mutations. *Arch Biochem Biophys* 2005; 442:92–101.
148. Lim U, Peng K, Shane B, Stover PJ, Litonjua AA, Weiss ST, Gaziano JM, et al. Polymorphisms in cytoplasmic serine hydroxymethyltransferase and methylenetetrahydrofolate reductase affect the risk of cardiovascular disease in men. *J Nutr* 2005; 135:1989–94.
149. MacFarlane AJ, Liu X, Perry CA, Flodby P, Allen RH, Stabler SP, Stover PJ. Cytoplasmic serine hydroxymethyltransferase regulates the metabolic partitioning of methylenetetrahydrofolate but is not essential in mice. *J Biol Chem* 2008; 283:25846–53.
150. Horie N, Aiba H, Oguro K, Hojo H, Takeishi K. Functional analysis and DNA polymorphism of the tandemly repeated sequences in the 5'-terminal regulatory region of the human gene for thymidylate synthase. *Cell Struct Funct* 1995; 20:191–97.
151. Ulrich CM, Bigler J, Velicer CM, Greene EA, Farin FM, Potter JD. Searching expressed sequence tag databases: Discovery and confirmation of a common polymorphism in the thymidylate synthase gene. *Cancer Epidemiol Biomarkers Prev* 2000; 9:1381–85.
152. Ulrich CM, Bigler J, Bostick R, Fosdick L, Potter JD. Thymidylate synthase promoter polymorphism, interaction with folate intake, and risk of colorectal adenomas. *Cancer Res* 2002; 62:3361–64.
153. Nief N, Le Morvan V, Robert J. Involvement of gene polymorphisms of thymidylate synthase in gene expression, protein activity and anticancer drug cytotoxicity using the NCI-60 panel. *Eur J Cancer* 2007; 43:955–62.
154. Mandola MV, Stoehlmacher J, Muller-Weeks S, Cesarone G, Yu MC, Lenz HJ, Ladner RD. A novel single nucleotide polymorphism within the 5' tandem repeat polymorphism of the thymidylate synthase gene abolishes USF-1 binding and alters transcriptional activity. *Cancer Res* 2003; 63:2898–904.
155. Wang L, Miao X, Tan W, Lu X, Zhao P, Zhao X, Shan Y, Li H, Lin D. Genetic polymorphisms in methylenetetrahydrofolate reductase and thymidylate synthase and risk of pancreatic cancer. *Clin Gastroenterol Hepatol* 2005; 3:743–51.
156. Kawakami K, Salonga D, Park JM, Danenberg KD, Uetake H, Brabender J, Omura K, Watanabe G, Danenberg PV. Different lengths of a polymorphic repeat sequence in the thymidylate synthase gene affect translational efficiency but not its gene expression. *Clin Cancer Res* 2001; 7:4096–101.
157. Calascibetta A, Cabibi D, Martorana A, Sanguedolce G, Rausa L, Feo S, Dardanoni G, Sanguedolce R. Thymidylate synthase gene promoter polymorphisms are associated with TSmRNA expressions but not with microsatellite instability in colorectal cancer. *Anticancer Res* 2004; 24:3875–80.
158. Chen J, Hunter DJ, Stampfer MJ, Kyte C, Chan W, Wetmur JG, Mosig R, Selhub J, Ma J. Polymorphism in the thymidylate synthase promoter enhancer region modifies the risk and survival of colorectal cancer. *Cancer Epidemiol Biomarkers Prev* 2003; 12:958–62.
159. Brown KS, Kluijtmans LA, Young IS, McNulty H, Mitchell LE, Yarnell JW, Woodside JV, et al. The thymidylate synthase tandem repeat polymorphism is not associated with

homocysteine concentrations in healthy young subjects. *Hum Genet* 2004; 114:182–85.
160. Iacopetta B, Grieu F, Joseph D, Elsaleh H. A polymorphism in the enhancer region of the thymidylate synthase promoter influences the survival of colorectal cancer patients treated with 5-fluorouracil. *Br J Cancer* 2001; 85:827–30.
161. Villafranca E, Okruzhnov Y, Dominguez MA, Garcia-Foncillas J, Azinovic I, Martinez E, Illarramendi JJ, et al. Polymorphisms of the repeated sequences in the enhancer region of the thymidylate synthase gene promoter may predict downstaging after preoperative chemoradiation in rectal cancer. *J Clin Oncol* 2001; 19:1779–86.
162. Tsuji T, Hidaka S, Sawai T, Nakagoe T, Yano H, Haseba M, Komatsu H, et al. Polymorphism in the thymidylate synthase promoter enhancer region is not an efficacious marker for tumor sensitivity to 5-fluorouracil-based oral adjuvant chemotherapy in colorectal cancer. *Clin Cancer Res* 2003; 9:3700–04.
163. Ott K, Vogelsang H, Marton N, Becker K, Lordick F, Kobl M, Schuhmacher C, et al. The thymidylate synthase tandem repeat promoter polymorphism: A predictor for tumor-related survival in neoadjuvant treated locally advanced gastric cancer. *Int J Cancer* 2006; 119:2885–94.
164. Huang ZH, Hua D, Li LH. The polymorphisms of TS and MTHFR predict survival of gastric cancer patients treated with fluorouracil-based adjuvant chemotherapy in Chinese population. *Cancer Chemother Pharmacol* 2009; 63:911–18.
165. Chen M, Rahman L, Voeller D, Kastanos E, Yang SX, Feigenbaum L, Allegra C, Kaye FJ, Steeg P, Zajac-Kaye M. Transgenic expression of human thymidylate synthase accelerates the development of hyperplasia and tumors in the endocrine pancreas. *Oncogene* 2007; 26:4817–24.
166. Chango A, Emery-Fillon N, de Courcy GP, Lambert D, Pfister M, Rosenblatt DS, Nicolas JP. A polymorphism (80G→A) in the reduced folate carrier gene and its associations with folate status and homocysteinemia. *Mol Genet Metab* 2000; 70:310–15.
167. Whetstine JR, Gifford AJ, Witt T, Liu XY, Flatley RM, Norris M, Haber M, Taub JW, Ravindranath Y, Matherly LH. Single nucleotide polymorphisms in the human reduced folate carrier: Characterization of a high-frequency G/A variant at position 80 and transport properties of the His27 and Arg27 carriers. *Clin Cancer Res* 2001; 7:3416–22.
168. Morin I, Devlin AM, Leclerc D, Sabbaghian N, Halsted CH, Finnell R, Rozen R. Evaluation of genetic variants in the reduced folate carrier and in glutamate carboxypeptidase II for spina bifida risk. *Mol Genet Metab* 2003; 79:197–200.
169. Shaw GM, Zhu H, Lammer EJ, Yang W, Finnell RH. Genetic variation of infant reduced folate carrier (A80G) and risk of orofacial and conotruncal heart defects. *Am J Epidemiol* 2003; 158:747–52.
170. O'Leary VB, Pangilinan F, Cox C, Parle-McDermott A, Conley M, Molloy AM, Kirke PN, Mills JL, Brody LC, Scott JM. Reduced folate carrier polymorphisms and neural tube defect risk. *Mol Genet Metab* 2006; 87:364–69.
171. Pei L, Zhu H, Ren A, Li Z, Hao L, Finnell RH, Li Z. Reduced folate carrier gene is a risk factor for neural tube defects in a Chinese population. *Birth Defects Res A Clin Mol Teratol* 2005; 73:430–33.
172. Pei L, Zhu H, Zhu J, Ren A, Finnell RH, Li Z. Genetic variation of infant reduced folate carrier (A80G) and risk of orofacial defects and congenital heart defects in China. *Ann Epidemiol* 2006; 16:352–56.
173. Baslund B, Gregers J, Nielsen CH. Reduced folate carrier polymorphism determines methotrexate uptake by B cells and CD4+ T cells. *Rheumatology (Oxford)* 2008; 47:451–53.
174. De Marco P, Calevo MG, Moroni A, Merello E, Raso A, Finnell RH, Zhu H, Andreussi L, Cama A, Capra V. Reduced folate carrier polymorphism (80A→G) and neural tube defects. *Eur J Hum Genet* 2003; 11:245–52.

175. Shaw GM, Lammer EJ, Zhu H, Baker MW, Neri E, Finnell RH. Maternal periconceptional vitamin use, genetic variation of infant reduced folate carrier (A80G), and risk of spina bifida. *Am J Med Genet* 2002; 108:1–6.

176. Coppede F, Marini G, Bargagna S, Stuppia L, Minichilli F, Fontana I, Colognato R, Astrea G, Palka G, Migliore L. Folate gene polymorphisms and the risk of Down syndrome pregnancies in young Italian women. *Am J Med Genet A* 2006; 140:1083–91.

177. Eklof V, Van Guelpen B, Hultdin J, Johansson I, Hallmans G, Palmqvist R. The reduced folate carrier (RFC1) 80G→A and folate hydrolase 1 (FOLH1) 1561C→T polymorphisms and the risk of colorectal cancer: A nested case-referent study. *Scand J Clin Lab Invest* 2007; 21:1–9.

178. Laverdiere C, Chiasson S, Costea I, Moghrabi A, Krajinovic M. Polymorphism G80A in the reduced folate carrier gene and its relationship to methotrexate plasma levels and outcome of childhood acute lymphoblastic leukemia. *Blood* 2002; 100:3832–34.

179. Imanishi H, Okamura N, Yagi M, Noro Y, Moriya Y, Nakamura T, Hayakawa A, et al. Genetic polymorphisms associated with adverse events and elimination of methotrexate in childhood acute lymphoblastic leukemia and malignant lymphoma. *J Hum Genet* 2007; 52:166–71.

180. Zhao R, Russell RG, Wang Y, Liu L, Gao F, Kneitz B, Edelmann W, Goldman ID. Rescue of embryonic lethality in reduced folate carrier-deficient mice by maternal folic acid supplementation reveals early neonatal failure of hematopoietic organs. *J Biol Chem* 2001; 276:10224–28.

181. Ma DW, Finnell RH, Davidson LA, Callaway ES, Spiegelstein O, Piedrahita JA, Salbaum JM, et al. Folate transport gene inactivation in mice increases sensitivity to colon carcinogenesis. *Cancer Res* 2005; 65:887–97.

182. Gelineau-van Waes J, Heller S, Bauer LK, Wilberding J, Maddox JR, Aleman F, Rosenquist TH, Finnell RH. Embryonic development in the reduced folate carrier knockout mouse is modulated by maternal folate supplementation. *Birth Defects Res A Clin Mol Teratol* 2008; 82:494–507.

183. Lawrance AK, Deng L, Brody LC, Finnell RH, Shane B, Rozen R. Genetic and nutritional deficiencies in folate metabolism influence tumorigenicity in Apcmin/+ mice. *J Nutr Biochem* 2007; 18:305–12.

184. Tsai G, Dunham KS, Drager U, Grier A, Anderson C, Collura J, Coyle JT. Early embryonic death of glutamate carboxypeptidase II (NAALADase) homozygous mutants. *Synapse* 2003; 50:285–92.

185. Devlin AM, Ling EH, Peerson JM, Fernando S, Clarke R, Smith AD, Halsted CH. Glutamate carboxypeptidase II: A polymorphism associated with lower levels of serum folate and hyperhomocysteinemia. *Hum Mol Genet* 2000; 9:2837–44.

186. Lievers KJ, Kluijtmans LA, Boers GH, Verhoef P, den Heijer M, Trijbels FJ, Blom HJ. Influence of a glutamate carboxypeptidase II (GCPII) polymorphism (1561C→T) on plasma homocysteine, folate and vitamin B(12) levels and its relationship to cardiovascular disease risk. *Atherosclerosis* 2002; 164:269–73.

187. Melse-Boonstra A, Lievers KJ, Blom HJ, Verhoef P. Bioavailability of polyglutamyl folic acid relative to that of monoglutamyl folic acid in subjects with different genotypes of the glutamate carboxypeptidase II gene. *Am J Clin Nutr* 2004; 80:700–04.

188. Bacich DJ, Ramadan E, O'Keefe DS, Bukhari N, Wegorzewska I, Ojeifo O, Olszewski R, et al. Deletion of the glutamate carboxypeptidase II gene in mice reveals a second enzyme activity that hydrolyzes N-acetylaspartylglutamate. *J Neurochem* 2002; 83:20–29.

189. Ou X, Yang H, Ramani K, Ara AI, Chen H, Mato JM, Lu SC. Inhibition of human betaine-homocysteine methyltransferase expression by S-adenosylmethionine and methylthioadenosine. *Biochem J* 2007; 401:87–96.

190. Heil SG, Lievers KJ, Boers GH, Verhoef P, den Heijer M, Trijbels FJ, Blom HJ. Betaine-homocysteine methyltransferase (BHMT): Genomic sequencing and relevance

to hyperhomocysteinemia and vascular disease in humans. *Mol Genet Metab* 2000; 71:511–19.

191. Weisberg IS, Park E, Ballman KV, Berger P, Nunn M, Suh DS, Breksa AP 3rd, Garrow TA, Rozen R. Investigations of a common genetic variant in betaine-homocysteine methyltransferase (BHMT) in coronary artery disease. *Atherosclerosis* 2003; 167:205–14.

192. Morin I, Platt R, Weisberg I, Sabbaghian N, Wu Q, Garrow TA, Rozen R. Common variant in betaine-homocysteine methyltransferase (BHMT) and risk for spina bifida. *Am J Med Genet A* 2003; 119:172–76.

193. Zhu H, Curry S, Wen S, Wicker NJ, Shaw GM, Lammer EJ, Yang W, Jafarov T, Finnell RH. Are the betaine-homocysteine methyltransferase (BHMT and BHMT2) genes risk factors for spina bifida and orofacial clefts? *Am J Med Genet A* 2005; 135:274–77.

194. Ananth CV, Elsasser DA, Kinzler WL, Peltier MR, Getahun D, Leclerc D, Rozen RR. Polymorphisms in methionine synthase reductase and betaine-homocysteine S-methyltransferase genes: Risk of placental abruption. *Mol Genet Metab* 2007; 91:104–10.

195. Xu X, Gammon MD, Zeisel SH, Lee YL, Wetmur JG, Teitelbaum SL, Bradshaw PT, Neugut AI, Santella RM, Chen J. Choline metabolism and risk of breast cancer in a population-based study. *FASEB J* 2008; 22:2045–52.

196. Xu X, Gammon MD, Wetmur JG, Bradshaw PT, Teitelbaum SL, Neugut AI, Santella RM, Chen J. B-vitamin intake, one-carbon metabolism, and survival in a population-based study of women with breast cancer. *Cancer Epidemiol Biomarkers Prev* 2008; 17:2109–16.

197. Ji C, Shinohara M, Vance D, Than TA, Ookhtens M, Chan C, Kaplowitz N. Effect of transgenic extrahepatic expression of betaine-homocysteine methyltransferase on alcohol or homocysteine-induced fatty liver. *Alcohol Clin Exp Res* 2008; 32:1049–58.

198. Johnson WG, Stenroos ES, Spychala JR, Chatkupt S, Ming SX, Buyske S. New 19 bp deletion polymorphism in intron-1 of dihydrofolate reductase (DHFR): A risk factor for spina bifida acting in mothers during pregnancy? *Am J Med Genet A* 2004; 124A:339–45.

199. Gellekink H, Blom HJ, van der Linden IJ, den Heijer M. Molecular genetic analysis of the human dihydrofolate reductase gene: Relation with plasma total homocysteine, serum and red blood cell folate levels. *Eur J Hum Genet* 2007; 15:103–09.

200. van der Linden IJ, Nguyen U, Heil SG, Franke B, Vloet S, Gellekink H, den Heijer M, Blom HJ. Variation and expression of dihydrofolate reductase (DHFR) in relation to spina bifida. *Mol Genet Metab* 2007; 91:98–103.

201. Xu X, Gammon MD, Wetmur JG, Rao M, Gaudet MM, Teitelbaum SL, Britton JA, Neugut AI, Santella RM, Chen J. A functional 19-base pair deletion polymorphism of dihydrofolate reductase (DHFR) and risk of breast cancer in multivitamin users. *Am J Clin Nutr* 2007; 85:1098–102.

202. Parle-McDermott A, Pangilinan F, Mills JL, Kirke PN, Gibney ER, Troendle J, O'Leary VB, et al. The 19-bp deletion polymorphism in intron-1 of dihydrofolate reductase (DHFR) may decrease rather than increase risk for spina bifida in the Irish population. *Am J Med Genet A* 2007; 143:1174–80.

5 Folate in Pregnancy and Lactation

Tsunenobu Tamura, Mary Frances Picciano, and Michelle Kay McGuire

CONTENTS

I. INTRODUCTION

The historical discovery by Dr. Lucy Wills in the 1930s that pregnancy-related anemia could be successfully treated with a folate-rich yeast extract provided the first evidence of the now well-established role of folate for optimal maternal health and fetal development [1]. Indeed, results from this and countless subsequent studies have been responsible for the long-held recommendation that women consume sufficient folate during pregnancy [2]. The role of folate as a one-carbon source for the biosynthesis of DNA and RNA and metabolism of key amino acids is the primary basis for the increase in folate requirements during pregnancy enabling both maternal and fetal cell proliferation and growth [3].

The focus as to the importance of folate nutrition during pregnancy has shifted from its role in preventing megaloblastic anemia to that of decreasing the risk of neural tube defects (NTDs). As such, periconceptional folic acid supplementation is now recommended not only to treat or prevent pregnancy-induced folate deficiency but also to correct abnormal folate metabolism or subtle folate inadequacy that may result in abnormal fetal development. These discoveries and recommendations have led to the mandatory addition of folic acid to selected foods in an increasing number of countries, including the United States and Canada [4]. In addition to the recognized role of folate during gestation for normal fetal growth and development, the continuing need for optimal folate intake during breastfeeding provides the impetus for understanding maternal folate status and requirements during lactation. The primary focus of this chapter is on the physiological need for folate during pregnancy and possible relationships between folate status and pregnancy complications and/or impaired fetal growth with a synopsis of the importance of folate during lactation.

II. IMPORTANCE OF FOLATE IN PREGNANCY

Folate is a coenzyme required for a myriad of chemical reactions related to one-carbon transfers such as biosynthesis of thymidylate and purines, building blocks of DNA and RNA. Thus, folate is critical for the production and maintenance of cells—especially during crucial periods of rapid growth and development, including pregnancy with the associated increases in both fetal and maternal tissue growth.

A. PHYSIOLOGICAL CHANGES INFLUENCING FOLATE REQUIREMENTS IN PREGNANCY

Many researchers have documented physiological changes influencing maternal folate requirements and status during pregnancy, including a decrease in serum and red blood cell (RBC) folate concentrations in women not consuming folic acid supplements [2,4–8]. Data also suggest that, even in healthy women, RBC folate concentration decreases during pregnancy [2,4,6]. It is possible that these decreases in blood folate concentrations represent healthy, physiological responses to pregnancy in most women. However, in those with inadequate folate intake and/or polymorphisms of folate-related protein genes, decreasing circulating folate may have detrimental consequences. Possible causes of the observed decrease in circulating maternal blood folate concentration include increased fetal and uteroplacental folate demand, dilution of folate resulting from blood-volume expansion, increased folate catabolism and clearance, decreased folate absorption, hormonal influences, and inadequate folate intake [2,3].

1. Hemodilution and Fluctuations in Blood Folate Concentrations

Bruinse et al. [5] determined the influence of blood-volume expansion on circulating folate concentration during pregnancy. Results indicate that *serum* folate decreased by 42%, whereas *total* circulating folate decreased by only 28%, suggesting that the pregnancy-related decline in serum folate cannot be explained solely by an effect of pregnancy-induced hemodilution.

2. Intestinal Folate Absorption (Bioavailability)

Studies designed to determine whether decreased folate absorption contributes to decreasing blood folate concentrations in pregnancy have provided mixed results. Chanarin et al. [9] reported that peak serum folate concentration after consumption of a folic acid supplement was lower in pregnant than in nonpregnant women, whereas Landon and Hytten [10] found no difference between pregnant and nonpregnant women in terms of folate bioavailability. Clearly, further studies are needed to ascertain the influence of pregnancy on folate bioavailability.

3. Folate Catabolism

Excretion of folate catabolites in late pregnancy has been documented as being higher than that in nonpregnant women [11]. In contrast, in mid-pregnancy urinary folate catabolites were not found to be increased [12]. Furthermore, no differences were detected in urinary stable-isotope-labeled folates or their catabolites between women in the second trimester and nonpregnant women [13]. These findings suggest that the observed increase in folate catabolism may be specific to late pregnancy.

4. Folate Clearance

Chanarin et al. [9] reported that after intravenous folic acid injection, folate clearance was higher in pregnant than in nonpregnant women, accelerated as pregnancy progressed, and was greater in women with megaloblastic anemia than in those without anemia. Similarly, Landon and Hytten [14] estimated 24-hour urinary folate excretion in pregnancy and postpartum periods to be 32 and 8 nmol/day, respectively. Collectively, these data support greater folate clearance (rapid uptake by cells and/or increased urinary excretion) in pregnant than in nonpregnant women.

B. PLACENTAL FOLATE TRANSPORT AND METABOLISM

Although nutrient transfer across the placenta must be effective to optimize fetal growth and development, the mechanism for placental folate transfer is not well established. In one of the few studies related to this topic, Landon et al. [15] determined placental transport of intravenously administered tritium-labeled folic acid in women scheduled for elective pregnancy termination at 12 to 18 weeks of gestation. Analysis of tritium-labeled folates at 24 hours after injection indicated that about 0.45% and 0.1% of the injected dose was found in the placenta and fetal liver, respectively, as labeled reduced folates. These data suggest rapid metabolism of tritium-labeled folic acid to reduced folates before they are transferred to the fetus. In another study, Baker et al. [16] found a positive association among maternal plasma, cord plasma, and placental tissue folate concentrations, suggesting that transplacental folate delivery is highly dependent on maternal plasma folate concentration. However, Wallace et al. [8] reported that relatively high cord blood folate concentration may be maintained at the expense of maternal folate stores in pregnant women with chronically low folate intake. Limited data also suggest that although smoking is associated with decreased circulating folate concentrations in pregnant women, transfer of folate from maternal to fetal circulation in the first trimester was not observed to be altered by smoking [17,18]. Additional research is needed to understand placental folate transfer and how it may be affected by factors such as gestational age, smoking, and maternal folate status.

Although the mechanisms by which folate is transferred from maternal to fetal circulation are unknown, chorionic folate receptors are clearly involved. Henderson et al. [19] reported that 5-methyltetrahydrofolate (5-methyl-THF) is rapidly bound to folate receptors in the placenta and transferred to the intervillous blood where its concentration is about three times that of the maternal blood. This allows for folate to ultimately move into the fetal circulation against a concentration gradient. Bisseling et al. [20] reported that the transport of 5-methyl-THF from the maternal to the fetal compartments in concentrations greater than typical physiological concentrations was not saturable. Delineating the mechanisms by which folate is passively and actively transported into placental tissue and eventually the fetus is essential for understanding the relationship between maternal and fetal folate homeostasis. Once within the placental cells, however, folate appears to be actively metabolized and used. For example, activities of folate-related enzymes have been detected in the placenta [21–25]. These enzymes include dihydrofolate reductase (DHFR), folate conjugase, methionine synthase, 5,10-methylene-THF reductase (MTHFR), and serine hydroxymethyltransferase (SHMT).

C. Fetal Folate Metabolism

Once transported across the placenta, folates are released into the fetal circulation and subsequently metabolized. Research findings indicate that fetal and newborn blood folate concentrations are markedly elevated compared with maternal circulation, again indicating active placental folate transport. Nonetheless, hepatic storage of folate in the fetus appears to be limited [26], suggesting that the fetus acquires and uses folate differently than adults. It could be argued that the liver does not function as a storage site of folate during intrauterine life, although this organ is considered to be one of the major storage sites in later life.

Because of ethical considerations, the ontogeny of folate-dependent enzymes in utero has not been studied extensively in humans. Gaull et al. [27], however, reported that methionine synthase activity of fetal tissues is higher than in adult tissues, whereas that of SHMT is similar. Kalnitsky et al. [28] reported that activities of hepatic MTHFR and methionine synthase tend to be higher in pre-term infants than in full-term infants and young children. The relative activities of fetal hepatic formiminotransferase and 5,10-methylene-THF dehydrogenase are higher in full-term infants and young children than in preterm infants [28]. The significance of these developmental changes in enzyme activities to fetal growth and development is currently unknown.

III. MATERNAL FOLATE STATUS AND PREGNANCY COMPLICATIONS

Although the mechanisms by which folate is transferred from the pregnant woman to her growing fetus have not been delineated, adequate maternal folate status has long been known to be important to optimal fetal growth and development. Further, various pregnancy complications have been associated with folate deficiency, although findings are equivocal. Nonetheless, considerable evidence supports deleterious effects of folate deficiency on a variety of pregnancy complications, some of which are described here.

A. PLACENTAL ABRUPTION

Researchers have long reported an association between folate deficiency and placental abruption (a premature detachment of the placenta) [29], although the data are somewhat inconsistent [30]. Nonetheless, because of the possible vasculotoxicity of hyperhomocysteinemia [31], interest in a potential relationship between homocysteine (Hcy) and placental abruption was renewed in the 1990s, and most studies conducted thus far have indicated a weak, but positive, association between hyperhomocysteinemia and risk for placental abruption [32].

Risk of placental abruption has more recently been associated with various polymorphisms of folate-related genes [33,34]. For example, Parle-McDermott et al. [34] reported that having the 1958G→A variant of the 10-formyl-THF synthetase gene places a woman at increased risk. Although associations between placental abruption and altered folate or Hcy metabolism appear weak, it is plausible that there are interactions between lifestyle factors (e.g., maternal folate status) and gene polymorphisms that complicate the relationship.

B. PREECLAMPSIA

Early studies did not support an association between folate deficiency and risk for preeclampsia (hypertension and proteinuria) or pregnancy-induced hypertension [35]. However, interest in this area renewed recently as researchers investigated the premise that placental vasculopathy secondary to hyperhomocysteinemia may be the underlying cause of preeclampsia. Indeed, recent findings have indicated that plasma Hcy concentration in women with preeclampsia is higher than in that women without preeclampsia [32,36]. A meta-analysis published in 2005 involving 25 studies, however, indicated that hyperhomocysteinemia as the *causative* factor is not compelling [37], suggesting that elevated Hcy is only a surrogate of some metabolic event that responds to preeclampsia.

Also of interest is the relationship between plasma folate and risk for preeclampsia, as well as whether folic acid supplementation reduces its incidence. Results from several studies, however, indicate that plasma folate concentrations are similar between women with and without preeclampsia [36,38]. Table 5.1 shows the results of studies where both plasma/serum folate and Hcy concentrations were measured more than once during pregnancy in patients with preeclampsia [39–41]. It is apparent that the findings in the literature are not consistent; therefore, it is difficult to draw a firm conclusion. Although the reason for this discrepancy is unknown, it may be because of the difference in the gestational time points when determinations of folate and Hcy were made between the studies.

Wen et al. [42] carried out a large prospective cohort study to assess the relation between voluntary intake of folic acid–containing dietary supplements and risk for preeclampsia. After adjusting for confounding factors, women consuming supplements were 63% less likely to experience preeclampsia than women not taking supplements. With regard to the effect of folic acid fortification, Ray and Mamdani [43] reported no difference in risk for preeclampsia before and after food folic acid fortification in Canada.

As with many other aspects of the relationship between maternal folate status and risk for poor pregnancy outcome, polymorphisms in folate-related enzyme genes have been implicated to be associated with preeclampsia. Since the maternal *MTHFR* 677C→T variant was first reported in 1997 to be associated with

TABLE 5.1

Plasma Total Homocysteine and Plasma/Serum Folate Concentrations in Women with Preeclampsia and Controls in Studies in Which More Than One Analysis Was Made

Investigator	Gestational Age at Blood Drawing	Plasma/Serum Folate (nmol/L)[a]		Plasma Homocysteine (μmol/L)	
		Preeclampsia	Controls	Preeclampsia	Controls
Laivuori et al. [39]	29–39 weeks	11 ± 7 (22)[b]	14 ± 6 (16)[b]	6.7 ± 1.9 (22)[b]	3.8 ± 0.8 (16)[b]
mean ± SD (n)	delivery	11 ± 8 (14)[b]	8 ± 3 (11)[b]	9.1 ± 2.2 (14)[b]	8.2 ± 2.0 (11)[b]
Hogg et al. [40]	26 weeks	30 ± 19 (16)	34 ± 20 (409)	5.2 ± 1.3 (16)	4.6 ± 1.4 (409)
mean ± SD (n)	37 weeks	26 ± 22 (16)	33 ± 21 (409)	6.6 ± 2.1 (16)[b]	5.3 ± 1.7 (409)[b]
Herrmann et al. [41]	24–34 weeks	18 ± 2 (37)[b]	33 ± 3 (41)[b]	10.4 ± 0.9 (37)[b]	5.7 ± 0.3 (41)[b]
geometric mean ±	35–38 weeks	16 ± 2 (38)[b]	33 ± 5 (18)[b]	10.4 ± 1.1 (38)[b]	6.1 ± 0.3 (18)[b]
SE (n)	>38 weeks	17 ± 1 (33)[b]	25 ± 3 (64)[b]	9.9 ± 0.6 (33)[b]	7.7 ± 0.8 (33)[b]

[a] All folate values were converted to nmol/L (some were initially reported in ng/mL).

[b] These numbers in the same row are significantly different with *P* values < .05.

preeclampsia [44], many groups have evaluated this association. However, studies to date have provided limited evidence to support an increased risk for preeclampsia in most women with this variant [45]. One study suggesting an effect was conducted by Hernandez-Diaz et al. [46], who reported that women with the *MTHFR* 677TT genotype have increased risk for preeclampsia, and that the observed risk may be attenuated when folic acid supplements are consumed. Further, in a meta-analysis involving 32 studies published before 2003, Kosmas et al. [47] found that earlier studies relating 677C→T variants of MTHFR to preeclampsia tended to indicate stronger associations than did later studies; however, the reason for this change over time is unknown. Analysis of fetal and neonatal *MTHFR* 677C→T polymorphisms also indicated no association with preeclampsia [48]. Together, these studies indicate that the 677C→T variant of MTHFR is not likely to be associated with preeclampsia, but if a relationship does exist, it is probably modified by other genetic and/or lifestyle factors.

C. SPONTANEOUS ABORTIONS AND STILLBIRTHS

Although factors associated with spontaneous abortion (loss before 20-week gestation) or stillbirth (born dead after 20 weeks) are poorly understood, their etiologies are multifactorial, and folate status may be involved [3]. As with other relationships, data are also inconsistent. For example, George et al. [49] reported that women with lower plasma folate concentrations (<4.9 nmol/L) were at greater risk for miscarriage than those with higher plasma folate concentrations, particularly when fetal chromosomal anomalies existed. Chanarin et al. [50], however, found that RBC folate concentrations were similar between women who had miscarried and those who had not. Other researchers [51] have also reported no association between folate status and spontaneous abortion. Some, but not all, data indicate that elevated plasma Hcy concentration may be related to increased risk for early pregnancy loss [52,53], although studies to investigate the relation between folic acid supplementation and early pregnancy loss have not supported such an association [54,55]. It remains unclear whether a relationship exists between maternal folate status and risk for early pregnancy loss.

Discrepancies in conclusions from epidemiological studies may, in part, be the result of differences in the prevalence of various folate-related gene polymorphisms in the populations studied. For example, Isotalo et al. [56] found that the combination of 677CT/1298CC or 677TT/1298CC *MTHFR* genotypes in the fetus was associated with an increased risk for spontaneous abortion. Zetterberg et al. [57] also reported an increased risk for spontaneous abortion for combined fetal 677TT/CT *MTHFR* and 776GG/CG transcobalamin genotypes. The findings of Volcik et al. [58] indicate that the 677CT/1298CC *MTHFR* genotype did not affect fetal viability, a finding confirmed by others [59]. Recently, Parle-McDermott et al. [59] found that women with the 1958AA genotype for the 10-formyl-THF synthetase enzyme had a 64% increased risk for pregnancy loss compared with either the 1958AG or 1958GG genotypes. However, in this study, they found no evidence that MTHFR variants were associated with pregnancy loss. These inconsistencies warrant further studies designed to evaluate interactions between maternal nutritional status and genetic variants on risk for miscarriage because this may have important implications for genetic and nutritional counseling.

Some, but not all, data also suggest an inverse relation between folate status and risk for stillbirth [60,61]. Vollset et al. [62], studying a large Norwegian cohort of women at increased risk for stillbirth, found that those in the highest quartile for plasma Hcy concentration were at higher risk for stillbirth than those in the lowest quartile. However, about 80% of the pregnancies took place more than 10 years before the blood sample used for Hcy assay was collected, bringing into question the issue of causality. Only a few research groups have evaluated whether risk for stillbirth is associated with *MTHFR* 677C→T variants, and findings are equivocal. Nurk et al. [63], however, reported that the presence of the 677CT or 677TT *MTFHR* variants strengthened the association between factor V Leiden (the most common cause of inherited thrombophilia) and risk of stillbirth. Clearly, further studies are needed to understand the potential for genetic variations to independently and interactively influence the risk of stillbirth.

D. MATERNAL FOLATE STATUS AND FETAL GROWTH AND DEVELOPMENT

1. Fetal Growth

Because folate is critical for adequate growth, several researchers have examined the relationships among maternal folate status or folate intake during pregnancy and birth weight [64–68]. For example, Lindblad et al. [69] investigated the relationship between maternal or fetal circulating folate and risk for fetal-growth restriction (FGR). They reported that in full-term, but not preterm, deliveries with FGR, maternal and cord blood folate concentrations were half of those in deliveries of normal birth weight infants.

However, it is possible that Hcy may be inversely associated with fetal growth. In 1992, Burke et al. [70] first noted the possible relation between elevated Hcy concentration and FGR. Vollset et al. [62] later reported that risk of FGR was higher in pregnant women in the highest quartile of Hcy concentration compared with the lowest quartile. Although others have reported similar findings [32,71], there are conflicting data [62,72]. Most recently, Takimoto et al. [7] studied 94 pregnant Japanese women and concluded that a 1.0 μmol/L increase in plasma Hcy in the third trimester corresponded to a 151 g decrease in birth weight. Whether an increase in Hcy is causally linked to poor fetal growth cannot be ascertained from these data.

The relationship between FGR risk and maternal or fetal *MTHFR* polymorphisms is also controversial. For example, Kupferminc et al. [73] reported an increased risk for FGR in women with the 677TT genotype, and Nurk et al. [33] found marginal associations between risk for FGR, low birth weight (<2,500 g), or very low birth weight (<1,500 g) infants and the presence of the 677C→T or 1298A→C variant. Similarly, Relton et al. [74] determined the presence of five polymorphisms in folate-related genes in mothers and infants from 998 pregnancies and investigated whether the presence of these gene variants was related to birth weight. After controlling for infant gender and gestational age at birth, they found no independent associations with birth weight. However, either the maternal homozygous or heterozygous genotype for the *MTHFR* 677C→T variant and the infant polymorphism involving a 68–base pair insertion of the cystathionine-β-synthase (*CBS*) gene were related to birth weight when found in association with low maternal RBC folate concentration. Again, this suggests that gene–nutrient interactions are important. Engel et al. [75] provided additional evidence for a complex relationship between gene polymorphisms and birth weight as they reported an interaction between dietary folate intake and the homozygous or heterozygous variants of the cytosolic *SHMT1* 1420C→T gene only in African American women—an example of a three-way interaction.

In contrast, Gebhardt et al. [76] reported that *MTHFR* 677CT, 1298AC, or both genotypes for the *MTHFR* variants were not related to FGR, a finding similar to that of others [77]. However, as previously discussed, the relationship between folate-related polymorphisms and FGR is likely modified by a variety of factors that are known to affect fetal growth. In summary, there is no firm consensus about whether maternal folate metabolism influences risk for FGR.

2. Folic Acid Supplementation, Fortification, and Fetal Growth

The relationship between folic acid supplementation and fetal growth has also received significant scientific attention. Although some researchers have reported a positive effect of folic acid supplementation on fetal growth as assessed by birth weight, others have not [78–83]. These disparate results are likely because of differences in maternal prepregnancy and periconceptional folate status, such that only folate-inadequate women are likely to respond favorably to supplementation. Other possible reasons include race, maternal size, socioeconomic status, and dietary habits.

Nonetheless, the apparent magnitude of "effect" on fetal growth in some studies is noteworthy. For example, an impressive increase in birth weight (300 g) was demonstrated in Bantu women whose diet consisted mainly of maize meal with infrequent vegetable consumption, whereas no effect was seen in white women whose diet habitually contained folate-rich vegetables and fruits [78]. Indeed, the overall findings of these epidemiological studies lead to the conclusion that adequate folate status promotes fetal growth. This conclusion is supported by a more recent report from an analysis of more than 5 million birth records in California showing small but significant reductions in rates of low and very low birth weight incidence, as well as preterm delivery, after initiation of the folic acid fortification program [84].

3. Preterm Delivery

The possibility that maternal folate nutrition and metabolism influence preterm delivery has also been examined. Biological plausibility for this association centers on the theory that elevated Hcy resulting from poor folate status along with the presence of the *MTHFR* 677C→T variant leads to decidual vasculopathy. As such, the relationship between the 677C→T variant and the risk for preterm delivery has been examined in several studies [85,86]; in only one was such an association found [86]. Johnson et al. [87], however, reported that a maternal 19-bp deletion polymorphism in intron I of the *DHFR* gene is a risk factor for preterm delivery. In addition, Bukowski et al. [88] found that the risk for preterm delivery between 20 and 28 weeks and 28 and 32 weeks of gestation was reduced by 70% and 50%, respectively, in women who took folic acid supplements. Clearly, more research is needed to delineate the putative role of folate intake and metabolism on preterm delivery.

4. Folate and Fetal Neurodevelopment

Mental retardation is one of the clinical signs of inborn errors of folate metabolism, although the mechanisms by which altered metabolism may cause impaired cognitive function are unknown. In fact, studies of the consequences of inadequate prenatal folate status on neurodevelopment of infants and children are scarce, and the two studies that did evaluate this connection yielded conflicting results [89,90]. This may be because of differences in the degree of maternal folate deficiency, age of children at assessment, and sensitivity and specificity of assessment tools. Recently, Wehby and Murray [91] analyzed the data reported by mothers in the 1988 National Maternal Infant Health study and its 1991 follow-up study in more than 6,700 mother–child pairs. They found that maternal use of folic acid supplements 3 months before becoming aware of pregnancy and/or during the following 3 months was associated with improved gross motor development at 3 years of age in African-American children. Further studies are warranted in this area, including evaluations of childhood neurodevelopment before and after initiation of the folic acid fortification program worldwide.

5. Maternal Body Weight, Folate, and Risk of Neural Tube Defects

In 1996, two independent research groups reported an interaction between maternal adiposity and folate intake on risk for NTDs [92,93]. This interaction was such that women with high body weight had increased risk regardless of folate intake, whereas risk in normal weight women was related to folate intake. Werler et al. [92] found a threefold increase in NTD risk among women with the highest body weight regardless of dietary folate intake. They also reported reduced risk of NTDs in women weighing 70 kg or less when they consumed more than 400 µg/day folate, whereas no such reduction was observed in heavier women. Shaw et al. [93] reported increased risk of NTD in women when body mass index was 29 kg/m^2 or higher, and that this relationship was independent of periconceptional folic acid supplementation. Since then, similar studies have been carried out by many researchers with similar findings. Based on these, Rasmussen et al. [94] conducted a meta-analysis and found that odds ratios for NTDs increase as maternal body mass index increases compared with normal weight women. Furthermore, Ray et al. [95] reported higher risk of NTDs with increasing maternal weight even after folic acid fortification was initiated.

Although the mechanism(s) driving this interaction is unknown, these findings suggest a possible difference in folate metabolism or placental folate transfer among pregnant women differing in adiposity [96]. Supporting this theory are data showing a negative correlation between body mass index and serum folate among women of child-bearing age [97]. As such, chronically low plasma folate concentrations in heavier women may be especially detrimental to fetal growth and development because plasma folate concentration may be one of the rate-limiting factors for placental folate transfer. Because the prevalence of obesity is increasing, the burden of pregnancies affected by NTDs or newborns with NTDs may be magnified in years to come.

E. MATERNAL FOLATE STATUS AND MULTIPLE BIRTHS

In 1994, Czeizel et al. [98] was the first to report in Hungary that the rate of multiple births in mothers consuming multivitamins containing folic acid was significantly higher than in those who consumed no folic acid supplements (3.8% vs. 2.7%, respectively).Similar findings were reported from Sweden and Hungary [99–101]. In contrast to these European studies, researchers in the United States reported at best a weak association between folic acid supplementation/fortification and risk for multiple births [102–107]. In addition, Li et al. [108] reported that folic acid supplementation was not associated with increased multiple births in China. Vollset et al. [109] and Haggarty et al. [110] in Norway and the United Kingdom, respectively, reported that if the association between folic acid supplementation or better folate status and twinning existed, it was likely confounded with in vitro fertilization (IVF) procedures. Similarly, Berry et al. [111] proposed a model to evaluate the association between use of folic acid and twinning, suggesting that the use of IVF is a strong confounder in this relationship, in turn leading to a possible false association. Considering all the findings of these studies, it appears questionable that the association between twinning and high folic acid intake exists.

IV. IMPORTANCE OF FOLATE DURING LACTATION

Human milk feeding is considered the "gold standard" for healthy, full-term infants [112]. As such, exclusive breastfeeding for the first 6 months has been endorsed by the American Academy of Pediatrics, as has continued breastfeeding for at least the first year of life [113]. Not surprisingly, maternal nutritional requirements for producing milk adequate in all the essential nutrients, including folate, are high. In this section, data concerning milk folate content, its relationship to folate status, and folate requirements of lactating women are reviewed.

A. FOLATE CONTENT OF HUMAN MILK

Historically, the folate concentration of human milk has been difficult to measure largely because of issues related to assay methods. More recent application of the trienzyme extraction method permits more reliable estimation, and folate concentrations of human milk obtained by this method are presented in Table 5.2 [114–118].

1. Characterization of Human Milk Folates

A large fraction of human milk folate exists as reduced forms of polyglutamates having at least four glutamyl residues, and 20% to 40% of folate exists as 5-methyl-THF [119–121]. The presence of reduced polyglutamyl folates in milk indicates that the mammary epithelium is capable of both interconversion of folates and polyglutamate synthesis.

Milk folate is bound to folate-binding proteins, which may be involved in regulating its secretion into the alveolar lumen [122]. A positive relationship has been reported between milk folate and folate-binding protein concentrations, with binding capacity being in excess of about 68 nmol/L. This excess capacity may aid in

TABLE 5.2

Milk Folate Contents by Microbiological Assay after the Trienzyme Extraction Method

Investigators	Country	Stage of Lactation (mo)	Maternal Folic Acid Supplementation (μg/d)	Number of Samples Assayed	Mean ± SD (nmol/L)
Lim et al. [114]	United	3	None	42	205 ± 8
	States	6		42	185 ± 8
Mackey and	United	3	None	21	224 ± 12
Picciano [115]	States	6		21	187 ± 12
	United	3	1,000	21	186 ± 10
	States	6		21	182 ± 12
Villalpando et al. [116]	Mexico	<1	None	68	108 ± 32
Khambalia et al. [117]	Mexico	<1	None	68	103
		3	400	68	155
		5	400	68	144
Han et al. [118]	Korea	1	None	17	281 ± 112
		2		18	365 ± 207
		4		20	328 ± 159
		5		20	288 ± 185
		6		20	201 ± 86

concentrating folates for secretion against a concentration gradient [123] because milk folate concentration is typically 5- to 10-fold higher than that of maternal plasma [123,124]. Additionally, the presence of protein-bound folates in milk may enhance intestinal absorption of folate by the infant [125,126].

2. Factors Related to Milk Folate Concentration

Milk folate content is dependent on several factors. For example, its concentration is generally lower in foremilk than in hindmilk and lower in the morning or early afternoon than in the late afternoon [125,126]. Reports of fluctuations in milk folate concentration with the progression of lactation are not consistent, with some researchers reporting a gradual increase [126] and others reporting no change [127]. It is possible that these apparent discrepancies are influenced by differences in maternal folate status, sample collection procedures, and assay methodologies.

B. MATERNAL FOLATE STATUS IN LACTATION

Maternal plasma folate concentration generally decreases below that typical at parturition in women not consuming folic acid supplements during lactation [5,9,20,67]. For example, Bruinse et al. [5] reported that total circulating folate decreases as pregnancy progresses and remains low during lactation in women not receiving supplements.

They also found that serum folate was lower in women who breastfed for 6 weeks or more compared with those who did not. Smith et al. [125] reported that RBC folate concentrations decreased from 6 to 12 weeks of lactation in mothers without folic acid supplementation, although serum folate remained unchanged. Similarly, Andersson et al. [128] found that, within 6 days after parturition, plasma Hcy increased rapidly, and its return to prepregnancy concentrations did not occur until 35 weeks postpartum. These findings may indicate that folate status can deteriorate during prolonged lactation, especially when folic acid supplements are not consumed. Ramlau-Hansen et al. [129] reported lower Hcy concentration in folic acid–supplemented lactating women compared with those consuming no supplements.

As with pregnancy, some evidence suggests that maintenance of adequate milk folate concentration may occur at the expense of maternal folate status during lactation. For example, Metz et al. [130] monitored the effect of folic acid supplementation in two lactating women with megaloblastic anemia. Within 4 days of initiation of the therapy, milk folate increased; however, even after 10 days maternal serum folate and reticulocyte counts remained at baseline values. These data indicate that folate was taken up by secretory mammary epithelial cells preferentially over the hematopoietic system.

Because some evidence suggests that lactating women may benefit from folic acid supplementation, several investigators have studied the effects of folic acid supplements on maternal folate status and milk folate concentration. For example, Mackey and Picciano [115] examined the effect of folic acid supplementation (1 mg/day) in lactating women already consuming approximately 380 µg/day dietary folate. Results suggested that plasma Hcy concentration was within the normal range throughout the study but was slightly increased from 3 to 6 months postpartum in both folic acid–supplemented women and those not receiving supplements. However, plasma and RBC folate decreased during the study period in subjects not receiving supplements. Similarly, Willoughby and Jewell [131] reported that 300 µg/day of folic acid supplementation in addition to dietary folate intake helped maintain adequate folate status during lactation.

V. FOLATE AND THE DEVELOPMENTAL ORIGINS OF ADULT HEALTH AND DISEASE HYPOTHESIS

The "Developmental Origins of Health and Disease (DOHaD)" hypothesis is based on growing epidemiological and experimental data suggesting that adult health is influenced by conditions before birth, during infancy, and in early childhood. This emerging theory has provided researchers with a new paradigm to study and conceptualize the relation of the early nutritional environment to risk of chronic disease in adulthood. For example, data from animal experiments indicate that malnutrition in early life can result in biochemical, physiological, and morphological alterations years later [132]. One of the proposed mechanisms of DOHaD is epigenetic modification secondary to altered methylation of DNA. Interestingly, folate emerges as perhaps the most influential single nutrient in terms of DNA methylation in this regard.

Among studies conducted with animal models, the most impressive have investigated the effect of maternal dietary supplementation of methylation-related nutrients (including folic acid) during pregnancy on coat color and obese phenotypes in off-spring of the agouti mouse. For example, Wolff et al. [133,134] studied the effect of feeding a "methyl-supplemented" diet containing additional folic acid, vitamin B12, betaine, and choline to various allelic combinations of two strains of agouti mice during pregnancy. The investigators recorded effects of the dietary intervention on the immediate offspring and 20 years later were still observing effects in subsequent generations. They hypothesized that these intergenerational effects may be mediated via changes in methyl metabolism.

Aside from this unique model, however, there are only limited experiments that have evaluated the effect of differential folate intake during early life on long-term health, and these have often been performed by altering maternal intakes of not only folic acid but also other dietary components such as protein or fish oil [135,136]. Therefore, in terms of folate nutrition, the data are often difficult to interpret. To our knowledge, there has been only a single human study concerning the potential for early folate status to influence long-term health and disease. In this epidemiological investigation, researchers evaluated the relationship between maternal folate status in the second trimester and later insulin sensitivity or anthropometry of the children [137]. Children born to mothers with higher RBC folate concentrations during gestation had a higher rate of insulin resistance and adiposity at 6 years of age. Well-designed, long-term prospective human studies are warranted to better test the DOHaD hypothesis—specifically as it relates to folate nutrition—in humans.

VI. SUMMARY

In summary, adequate folate nutritional status is important during all phases of the human reproductive cycle, and there appear to be a variety of well-orchestrated, homeostatic mechanisms by which most pregnant women and their growing fetuses obtain adequate amounts of this vitamin. However, there are clearly some situations in which poor folate status, folate-related polymorphisms, or a combination of factors results in poor pregnancy outcomes. The well-documented influence of folic acid supplementation on reducing the risk for NTD has prompted folic acid fortification programs internationally. However, targeted folic acid supplementation during pregnancy and lactation in at-risk populations may be warranted in the future as scientists learn more about how folate intake, allelic variation, other environmental and lifestyle factors, and perhaps even epigenetics, interactively play a role in folate metabolism.

REFERENCES

1. Wills L. Treatment of "pernicious anaemia of pregnancy" and "tropical anaemia" with special reference to yeast extract as a curative agent. *BMJ* 1931; 1:1059–64.
2. Chanarin I. *The Megaloblastic Anemias.* Oxford, UK: Blackwell Scientific Publications, 1979.
3. Tamura T, Picciano MF. Folate and human reproduction. *Am J Clin Nutr* 2006; 83:993–1016.
4. Food Standards: Amendment of Standards of Identity for Enriched Grain Products to Require Addition of Folic Acid. Final Rule. 21 CFR Parts 136, 137, and 139. *Fed Reg* 1996: 8781–89.

5. Bruinse HW, van der Berg H, Haspels AA. Maternal serum folacin levels during and after normal pregnancy. *Eur J Obstet Gynecol Reprod Biol* 1985; 20:153–58.

6. Qvist I, Abdulla M, Jagerstad M, Svensson S. Iron, zinc and folate status during pregnancy and two months after delivery. *Acta Obstet Gynecol Scand* 1986; 65:15–22.

7. Takimoto H, Mito N, Umegaki K, Ishiwaki A, Kusama K, Abe S, Yamawaki M, Fukuoka H, Ohta C, Yoshiike N. Relationship between dietary folate intakes, maternal plasma total homocysteine and B-vitamins during pregnancy and fetal growth in Japan. *Eur J Nutr* 2007; 46:300–06.

8. Wallace JMW, Bonham MP, Strain JJ, Duffy EM, Robson PJ, Ward M, McNulty H, et al. Homocysteine concentration, related B vitamins, and betaine in pregnant women recruited to the Seychelles Child Development Study. *Am J Clin Nutr* 2008; 87:391–97.

9. Chanarin I, MacGibbon BM, O'Sullivan WJ, Mollin DL. Folic acid deficiency in pregnancy. The pathogenesis of megaloblastic anaemia of pregnancy. *Lancet* 1959; 274:634–39.

10. Landon MJ, Hytten FE. Plasma folate levels following an oral load of folic acid during pregnancy. *J Obstet Gynaecol Br Commonw* 1972; 79:577–83.

11. McPartlin J, Weir DG, Halligan A, Darling M, Scott JM. Accelerated folate breakdown in pregnancy. *Lancet* 1993; 341:148–49.

12. Caudill MA, Gregory JF, Hutson AD, Bailey LB. Folate catabolism in pregnant and nonpregnant women with controlled folate intakes. *J Nutr* 1998; 128:204–08.

13. Gregory JF 3rd, Caudill MA, Opalko FJ, Bailey LB. Kinetics of folate turnover in pregnant women (second trimester) and nonpregnant controls during folic acid supplementation: Stable-isotopic labeling of plasma folate, urinary folate and folate catabolites shows subtle effects of pregnancy on turnover of folate pools. *J Nutr* 2001; 131:1928–37.

14. Landon MJ, Hytten FE. The excretion of folate in pregnancy. *J Obstet Gynaecol Br Commonw* 1971; 78:769–75.

15. Landon MJ, Eyre DH, Hytten FE. Transfer of folate to the fetus. *Br J Obstet Gynaecol* 1975; 82:12–19.

16. Baker H, Frank O, Deangelis B, Feingold S, Kaminetzky HA. Role of placenta in maternal-fetal vitamin transfer in humans. *Am J Obstet Gynecol* 1981; 141:792–96.

17. Stark KD, Pawlosky RJ, Sokol RJ, Hannigan JH, Salem N Jr. Maternal smoking is associated with decreased 5-methyltetrahydrofolate in cord plasma. *Am J Clin Nutr* 2007; 85:796–802.

18. Jauniaux E, Johns J, Gulbis B, Spasic-Boskovic O, Burton GJ. Transfer of folic acid inside the first-trimester gestational sac and the effect of maternal smoking. *Am J Obstet Gynecol* 2007; 197:58.e1–.e6.

19. Henderson GI, Perez T, Schenker S, Mackins J, Antony AC. Maternal-to-fetal transfer of 5-methyltetrahydrofolate by the perfused human placental cotyledon: Evidence for a concentrative role by placental folate receptors in fetal folate delivery. *J Lab Clin Med* 1995; 126:184–203.

20. Bisseling TM, Steegers EAP, van den Heuvel JJM, Siero HLM, van de Water FM, Walker AJ, Steegers-Theunissen RPM, Smits P, Russel FGM. Placental folate transport and binding are not impaired in pregnancies complicated by fetal growth restriction. *Placenta* 2004; 25:588–93.

21. Jarabak J, Bachur NR. A soluble dihydrofolate reductase from human placenta: Purification and properties. *Arch Biochem Biophys* 1971; 142:417–25.

22. Landon MJ. Placental [gamma]-glutamyl carboxypeptidase. *Int J Biochem* 1972; 3:387–88.

23. Utley CS, Marcell PD, Allen RH, Antony AC, Kolhouse JF. Isolation and characterization of methionine synthetase from human placenta. *J Biol Chem* 1985; 260: 13656–65.

24. Daly SF, Molloy AM, Mills JL, Lee YJ, Conley M, Kirke PN, Weir DG, Scott JM. The influence of 5,10 methylenetetrahydrofolate reductase genotypes on enzyme activity in placental tissue. *Br J Obstet Gynaecol* 1999; 106:1214–18.

25. Lewis RM, Godfrey KM, Jackson AA, Cameron IT, Hanson MA. Low serine hydroxymethyltransferase activity in the human placenta has important implications for fetal glycine supply. *J Clin Endocrinol Metab* 2005; 90:1594–98.

26. Iyengar L, Apte SV. Nutrient stores in human foetal livers. *Br J Nutr* 1972; 27:313–17.

27. Gaull GE, Von Berg W, Raiha NC, Sturman JA. Development of methyltransferase activities of human fetal tissues. *Pediatr Res* 1973; 7:527–33.

28. Kalnitsky A, Rosenblatt D, Zlotkin S. Differences in liver folate enzyme patterns in premature and full term infants. *Pediatr Res* 1982; 16:628–31.

29. Hibbard BM, Hibbard ED, Hwa TS, Tan P. Abruptio placentae and defective folate metabolism in Singapore women. *J Obstet Gynaecol Br Commonw* 1969; 76:1003–07.

30. Pritchard JA, Cunningham FG, Pritchard SA, Mason RA. On reducing the frequency of severe abruptio placentae. *Am J Obstet Gynecol* 1991; 165:1345–51.

31. Green R, Jacobsen DW. Clinical implications of hyperhomocysteinemia. In: Bailey LB, ed., *Folate in Health and Disease*. New York: Marcel Dekker, 1995:75–122.

32. Steegers-Theunissen RP, Van Iersel CA, Peer PG, Nelen WL, Steegers EA. Hyperhomocysteinemia, pregnancy complications, and the timing of investigation. *Obstet Gynecol* 2004; 104:336–43.

33. Nurk E, Tell GS, Refsum H, Ueland PM, Vollset SE. Associations between maternal methylenetetrahydrofolate reductase polymorphisms and adverse outcomes of pregnancy: The Hordaland Homocysteine Study. *Am J Med* 2004; 117:26–31.

34. Parle-McDermott A, Mills JL, Kirke PN, Cox C, Signore CC, Kirke S, Molloy AM, et al. MTHFD1 R653Q polymorphism is a maternal genetic risk factor for severe abruptio placentae. *Am J Med Genet A* 2005; 132:365–68.

35. Whalley PJ, Scott DE, Pritchard JA. Maternal folate deficiency and pregnancy wastage. 3. Pregnancy-induced hypertension. *Obstet Gynecol* 1970; 36:29–31.

36. Powers RW, Majors AK, Kerchner LJ, Conrad KP. Renal handling of homocysteine during normal pregnancy and preeclampsia. *J Soc Gynecol Invest* 2004; 11:45–50.

37. Mignini LE, Latthe PM, Villar J, Kilby MD, Carroli G, Khan KS. Mapping the theories of preeclampsia: The role of homocysteine. *Obstet Gynecol* 2005; 105:411–25.

38. Cotter AM, Molloy AM, Scott JM, Daly SF. Elevated plasma homocysteine in early pregnancy: A risk factor for the development of nonsevere preeclampsia. *Am J Obstet Gynecol* 2003; 189:391–94.

39. Laivuori H, Kaaja R, Turpeinen U, Viinikka L, Ylikorkala O. Plasma homocysteine levels elevated and inversely related to insulin sensitivity in preeclampsia. *Obstet Gynecol* 1999; 93:489–93.

40. Hogg BB, Tamura T, Johnston KE, DuBard MB, Goldenberg RL. Second-trimester plasma homocysteine levels and pregnancy-induced hypertension, preeclampsia, and intrauterine growth restriction. *Am J Obstet Gynecol* 2000; 183:805–09.

41. Herrmann W, Isber S, Obeid R, Herrmann M, Jouma M. Concentrations of homocysteine, related metabolites and asymmetric dimethylarginine in preeclamptic women with poor nutritional status. *Clin Chem Lab Med* 2005; 43:1139–46.

42. Wen SW, Chen X-K, Rodger M, White RR, Yang Q, Smith GN, Sigal RJ, Perkins SL, Walker MC. Folic acid supplementation in early second trimester and the risk of preeclampsia. *Am J Obstet Gynecol* 2008; 198:45.e1–.e7.

43. Ray JG, Mamdani MM. Association between folic acid food fortification and hypertension or preeclampsia in pregnancy. *Arch Intern Med* 2002; 162:1776–77.

44. Grandone E, Margaglione M, Colaizzo D, Cappucci G, Paladini D, Martinelli P, Montanaro S, Pavone G, Di Minno G. Factor V Leiden, C > T MTHFR polymorphism and genetic susceptibility to preeclampsia. *Thromb Haemost* 1997; 77:1052–54.

45. Also-Rallo E, Lopez-Quesada E, Urreizti R, Vilaseca MA, Lailla JM, Balcells S, Grinberg D. Polymorphisms of genes involved in homocysteine metabolism in preeclampsia and in uncomplicated pregnancies. *Eur J Obstet Gynecol Reprod Biol* 2005; 120:45–52.
46. Hernandez-Diaz S, Wu XF, Hayes C, Werler MM, Ashok TD, Badovinac R, Kelsey KT, Mitchell AA. Methylenetetrahydrofolate reductase polymorphisms and the risk of gestational hypertension. *Epidemiology* 2005; 16:628–34.
47. Kosmas IP, Tatsioni A, Ioannidis JP. Association of C677T polymorphism in the methylenetetrahydrofolate reductase gene with hypertension in pregnancy and pre-eclampsia: A meta-analysis. *J Hypertens* 2004; 22:1655–62.
48. Vefring H, Lie RT, Ødegård R, Mansoor MA, Nilsen ST. Maternal and fetal variants of genetic thrombophilias and the risk of preeclampsia. *Epidemiology* 2004; 15: 317–22.
49. George L, Mills JL, Johansson AL, Nordmark A, Olander B, Granath F, Cnattingius S. Plasma folate levels and risk of spontaneous abortion. *JAMA* 2002; 288:1867–73.
50. Chanarin I, Rothman D, Ward A, Perry J. Folate status and requirement in pregnancy. *BMJ* 1968; 2:390–94.
51. Ronnenberg AG, Venners SA, Xu X, Chen C, Wang L, Guang W, Huang A, Wang X. Preconception B-vitamin and homocysteine status, conception, and early pregnancy loss. *Am J Epidemiol* 2007; 166:304–12.
52. Wouters MG, Boers GH, Blom HJ, Trijbels FJ, Thomas CM, Borm GF, Steegers-Theunissen RP, Eskes TK. Hyperhomocysteinemia: A risk factor in women with unexplained recurrent early pregnancy loss. *Fertil Steril* 1993; 60:820–25.
53. Ronnenberg AG, Goldman MB, Chen D, Aitken IW, Willett WC, Selhub J, Xu X. Preconception folate and vitamin B(6) status and clinical spontaneous abortion in Chinese women. *Obstet Gynecol* 2002; 100:107–13.
54. Czeizel AE, Dudas I, Metneki J. Pregnancy outcomes in a randomised controlled trial of periconceptional multivitamin supplementation. Final report. *Arch Gynecol Obstet* 1994; 255:131–39.
55. Gindler J, Li Z, Berry RJ, Zheng J-C, Correa A, Sun X-M, Wong L-Y, et al. Folic acid supplements during pregnancy and risk of miscarriage. *Lancet* 2001; 358:796–800.
56. Isotalo PA, Wells GA, Donnelly JG. Neonatal and fetal methylenetetrahydrofolate reductase genetic polymorphisms: An examination of C677T and A1298C mutations. *Am J Hum Genet* 2000; 67:986–90.
57. Zetterberg H, Zafiropoulos A, Spandidos DA, Rymo L, Blennow K. Gene-gene interaction between fetal MTHFR 677C>T and transcobalamin 776C>G polymorphisms in human spontaneous abortion. *Hum Reprod* 2003; 18:1948–50.
58. Volcik KA, Blanton SH, Northrup H. Examinations of methylenetetrahydrofolate reductase C677T and A1298C mutations—and in utero viability. *Am J Hum Genet* 2001; 69:1150–53.
59. Parle-McDermott A, Pangilinan F, Mills JL, Signore CC, Molloy AM, Cotter A, Conley M, et al. A polymorphism in the MTHFD1 gene increases a mother's risk of having an unexplained second trimester pregnancy loss. *Mol Hum Reprod* 2005; 11:477–80.
60. Giles C. An account of 335 cases of megaloblastic anaemia of pregnancy and the puerperium. *J Clin Pathol* 1966; 19:1–11.
61. Varadi S, Abbott D, Elwis A. Correlation of peripheral white cell and bone marrow changes with folate levels in pregnancy and their clinical significance. *J Clin Pathol* 1966; 19:33–36.
62. Vollset SE, Refsum H, Irgens LM, Emblem BM, Tverdal A, Gjessing HK, Monsen ALB, Ueland PM. Plasma total homocysteine, pregnancy complications, and adverse pregnancy outcomes: The Hordaland Homocysteine Study. *Am J Clin Nutr* 2000; 71:962–68.

63. Nurk E, Tell GS, Refsum H, Ueland PM, Vollset SE. Factor V Leiden, pregnancy complications and adverse outcomes: The Hordaland Homocysteine Study. *QJM* 2006; 99:289–98.

64. Baker H, Thind IS, Frank O, DeAngelis B, Caterini H, Louria DB. Vitamin levels in low-birth-weight newborn infants and their mothers. *Am J Obstet Gynecol* 1977; 129:521–24.

65. Tamura T, Goldenberg RL, Freeberg LE, Cliver SP, Cutter GR, Hoffman HJ. Maternal serum folate and zinc concentrations and their relationships to pregnancy outcome. *Am J Clin Nutr* 1992; 56:365–70.

66. Chanarin I, Rothman D, Perry J, Stratfull D. Normal dietary folate, iron, and protein intake, with particular reference to pregnancy. *BMJ* 1968; 2:394–97.

67. Lowenstein L, Cantlie G, Ramos O, Brunton L. The incidence and prevention of folate deficiency in a pregnant clinic population. *Can Med Assoc J* 1966; 95:797–806.

68. Chanarin I, Rothman D. Further observations on the relation between iron and folate status in pregnancy. *BMJ* 1971; 2:81–84.

69. Lindblad B, Zaman S, Malik A, Martin H, Ekström AM, Amu S, Holmgren A, Norman M. Folate, vitamin B12, and homocysteine levels in South Asian women with growth-retarded fetuses. *Acta Obstet Gynecol Scand* 2005; 84:1055–61.

70. Burke G, Robinson K, Refsum H, Stuart B, Drumm J, Graham I. Intrauterine growth retardation, perinatal death, and maternal homocysteine levels. *N Engl J Med* 1992; 326:69–70.

71. Murphy MM, Scott JM, Arija V, Molloy AM, Fernandez-Ballart JD. Maternal homocysteine before conception and throughout pregnancy predicts fetal homocysteine and birth weight. *Clin Chem* 2004; 50:1406–12.

72. Ronnenberg AG, Goldman MB, Chen D, Aitken IW, Willett WC, Selhub J, Xu X. Preconception homocysteine and B vitamin status and birth outcomes in Chinese women. *Am J Clin Nutr* 2002; 76:1385–91.

73. Kupferminc MJ, Eldor A, Steinman N, Many A, Bar-Am A, Jaffa A, Fait G, Lessing JB. Increased frequency of genetic thrombophilia in women with complications of pregnancy. *N Engl J Med* 1999; 340:9–13.

74. Relton CL, Pearce MS, Burn J, Parker L. An investigation of folate-related genetic factors in the determination of birthweight. *Paediatr Perinat Epidemiol* 2005; 19:360–67.

75. Engel SM, Olshan AF, Siega-Riz AM, Savitz DA, Chanock SJ. Polymorphisms in folate metabolizing genes and risk for spontaneous preterm and small-for-gestational age birth. *Am J Obstet Gynecol* 2006; 195:1231.e1–.e11.

76. Gebhardt GS, Scholtz CL, Hillermann R, Odendaal HJ. Combined heterozygosity for methylenetetrahydrofolate reductase (MTHFR) mutations C677T and A1298C is associated with abruptio placentae but not with intrauterine growth restriction. *Eur J Obstet Gynecol Reprod Biol* 2001; 97:174–77.

77. Glanville T, Yates Z, Ovadia L, Walker JJ, Lucock M, Simpson NA. Fetal folate C677T methylenetetrahydrofolate reductase gene polymorphism and low birth weight. *J Obstet Gynaecol* 2006; 26:11–14.

78. Baumslag N, Edelstein T, Metz J. Reduction of incidence of prematurity by folic acid supplementation in pregnancy. *BMJ* 1970; 1:16–17.

79. Iyengar L. Folic acid requirements of Indian pregnant women. *Am J Obstet Gynecol* 1971; 111:13–16.

80. Fletcher J, Gurr A, Fellingham FR, Prankerd TA, Brant HA, Menzies DN. The value of folic acid supplements in pregnancy. *J Obstet Gynaecol Br Commonw* 1971; 78:781–85.

81. Agarwal KN, Agarwal DK, Mishra KP. Impact of anaemia prophylaxis in pregnancy on maternal haemoglobin, serum ferritin & birth weight. *Indian J Med Res* 1991; 94:277–80.

82. Rolschau J, Kristoffersen K, Ulrich M, Grinsted P, Schaumburg E, Foged N. The influence of folic acid supplement on the outcome of pregnancies in the county of Funen in Denmark: Part I. *Eur J Obstet Gynecol Reprod Biol* 1999; 87:105–10.

83. Giles PF, Harcourt AG, Whiteside MG. The effect of prescribing folic acid during pregnancy on birth-weight and duration of pregnancy. A double-blind trial. *Med J Aust* 1971; 2:17–21.

84. Shaw GM, Carmichael SL, Nelson V, Selvin S, Schaffer DM. Occurrence of low birthweight and preterm delivery among California infants before and after compulsory food fortification with folic acid. *Public Health Rep* 2004; 119:170–73.

85. Scholl TO, Hediger ML, Schall JI, Khoo CS, Fischer RL. Dietary and serum folate: Their influence on the outcome of pregnancy. *Am J Clin Nutr* 1996; 63:520–25.

86. Valdez LL, Quintero A, Garcia E, Olivares N, Celis A, Rivas F. Thrombophilic polymorphisms in preterm delivery. *Blood Cells Mol Dis* 2004; 33:51–56.

87. Johnson WG, Scholl TO, Spychala JR, Buyske S, Stenroos ES, Chen X. Common dihydrofolate reductase 19-base pair deletion allele: A novel risk factor for preterm delivery. *Am J Clin Nutr* 2005; 81:664–68.

88. Bukowski R, Malone FD, Porter F, Nybery DA, Comstock C, Hankins G, Eddleman K, et al. Preconceptional folate prevents preterm delivery. Abstract. *Am J Obstet Gynecol* 2007; 197:S3.

89. Gross RL, Newberne PM, Reid JVO. Adverse effects on infant development associated with maternal folic acid deficiency. *Nutr Rep Int* 1974; 10:241–48.

90. Tamura T, Goldenberg RL, Chapman VR, Johnston KE, Ramey SL, Nelson KG. Folate status of mothers during pregnancy and mental and psychomotor development of their children at five years of age. *Pediatrics* 2005; 116:703–08.

91. Wehby G, Murray J. The effects of prenatal use of folic acid and other dietary supplements on early child development. *Matern Child Health J* 2008; 12:180–87.

92. Werler MM, Louik C, Shapiro S, Mitchell AA. Prepregnant weight in relation to risk of neural tube defects. *JAMA* 1996; 275:1089–92.

93. Shaw GM, Velie EM, Schaffer D. Risk of neural tube defect-affected pregnancies among obese women. *JAMA* 1996; 275:1093–96.

94. Rasmussen SA, Chu SY, Kim SY, Schmid CH, Lau J. Maternal obesity and risk of neural tube defects: A metaanalysis. *Am J Obstet Gynecol* 2008; 198:611–19.

95. Ray JG, Wyatt PR, Vermeulen MJ, Meier C, Cole DEC. Greater maternal weight and the ongoing risk of neural tube defects after folic acid flour fortification. *Obstet Gynecol* 2005; 105:261–65.

96. Goldenberg RL, Tamura T. Prepregnancy weight and pregnancy outcome. *JAMA* 1996; 275:1127–28.

97. Mojtabai R. Body mass index and serum folate in childbearing age women. *Eur J Epidemiol* 2004; 19:1029–36.

98. Czeizel AE, Metneki J, Dudas I. Higher rate of multiple births after periconceptional vitamin supplementation. *N Engl J Med* 1994; 330:1687–88.

99. Ericson A, Kallen B, Aberg A. Use of multivitamins and folic acid in early pregnancy and multiple births in Sweden. *Twin Res* 2001; 4:63–66.

100. Källén B. Use of folic acid supplementation and risk for dizygotic twinning. *Early Hum Dev* 2004; 80:143–51.

101. Czeizel AE, Vargha P. Periconceptional folic acid/multivitamin supplementation and twin pregnancy. *Am J Obstet Gynecol* 2004; 191:790–94.

102. Werler MM, Cragan JD, Wasserman CR, Shaw GM, Erickson JD, Mitchell AA. Multivitamin supplementation and multiple births. *Am J Med Genet* 1997; 71:93–96.

103. Shaw GM, Carmichael SL, Nelson V, Selvin S, Schaffer DM. Food fortification with folic acid and twinning among California infants. *Am J Med Genet* 2003; 119A:137–40.

104. Waller DK, Tita ATN, Annegers JF. Rates of twinning before and after fortification of foods in the US with folic acid, Texas, 1996 to 1998. *Paediatr Perinat Epidemiol* 2003; 17:378–83.
105. Kucik J, Correa A. Trends in twinning rates in Metropolitan Atlanta before and after folic acid fortification. *J Reprod Med* 2004; 49:707–12.
106. Lawrence JM, Watkins ML, Chiu V, Erickson JD, Petitti DB. Food fortification with folic acid and rate of multiple births, 1994–2000. *Birth Defects Res Part A Clin Mol Teratol* 2004; 70:948–52.
107. Signore C, Mills JL, Cox C, Trumble AC. Effects of folic acid fortification on twin gestation rates. *Obstet Gynecol* 2005; 105:757–62.
108. Li Z, Gindler J, Wang H, Berry RJ, Li S, Correa A, Zheng JC, Erickson JD, Wang Y. Folic acid supplements during early pregnancy and likelihood of multiple births: A population-based cohort study. *Lancet* 2003; 361:380–84.
109. Vollset SE, Gjessing HK, Tandberg A, Ronning T, Irgens LM, Baste V, Nilsen RM, Daltveit AK. Folate supplementation and twin pregnancies. *Epidemiology* 2005; 16:201–05.
110. Haggarty P, McCallum H, McBain H, Andrews K, Duthie S, McNeill G, Templeton A, Haites N, Campbell D, Bhattacharya S. Effect of B vitamins and genetics on success of in-vitro fertilisation: Prospective cohort study. *Lancet* 2006; 367:1513–19.
111. Berry RJ, Kihlberg R, Devine O. Impact of misclassification of in vitro fertilisation in studies of folic acid and twinning: Modelling using population based Swedish vital records. *BMJ* 2005; 330:815–17.
112. Picciano MF. Nutrient composition of human milk. *Pediatr Clin North Am* 2001; 48:53–67.
113. Gartner LM, Morton J, Lawrence RA, Naylor AJ, O'Hare D, Schanler RJ, Eidelman AI. Breastfeeding and the use of human milk. *Pediatrics* 2005; 115:496–506.
114. Lim HS, Mackey AD, Tamura T, Wong SC, Picciano MF. Measurable human milk folate is increased by treatment with alpha-amylase and protease in addition to folate conjugase. *Food Chem* 1998; 63:401–07.
115. Mackey AD, Picciano MF. Maternal folate status during extended lactation and the effect of supplemental folic acid. *Am J Clin Nutr* 1999; 69:285–92.
116. Villalpando S, Latulippe ME, Rosas G, Irurita MJ, Picciano MF, O'Connor DL. Milk folate but not milk iron concentrations may be inadequate for some infants in a rural farming community in San Mateo, Capulhuac, Mexico. *Am J Clin Nutr* 2003; 78:782–89.
117. Khambalia A, Latulippe ME, Campos C, Merlos C, Villalpando S, Picciano MF, O'Connor DL. Milk folate secretion is not impaired during iron deficiency in humans. *J Nutr* 2006; 136:2617–24.
118. Han Y-H, Yon M, Han H-S, Kim K-Y, Tamura T, Hyun TH. Folate contents in human milk, and casein-based and soy-based formulas and folate status in Korean infants. *Br J Nutr* 2008; 101:1769–74.
119. O'Connor DL, Tamura T, Picciano MF. Pteroylpolyglutamates in human milk. *Am J Clin Nutr* 1991; 53:930–34.
120. Selhub J. Determination of tissue folate composition by affinity chromatography followed by high-pressure ion pair liquid chromatography. *Anal Biochem* 1989; 182:84–93.
121. Brown CM, Smith AM, Picciano MF. Forms of human milk folacin and variation patterns. *J Pediatr Gastroenterol Nutr* 1986; 5:278–82.
122. Selhub J, Arnold R, Smith AM, Picciano MF. Milk folate binding protein (FBP): A secretory protein for folate? *Nutr Res* 1984; 4:181–87.
123. Smith AM, Picciano MF, Deering RH. Folate intake and blood concentrations of term infants. *Am J Clin Nutr* 1985; 41:590–98.
124. Tamura T, Yoshimura Y, Arakawa T. Human milk folate and folate status in lactating mothers and their infants. *Am J Clin Nutr* 1980; 33:193–97.

125. Smith AM, Picciano MF, Deering RH. Folate supplementation during lactation: Maternal folate status, human milk folate content, and their relationship to infant folate status. *J Pediatr Gastroenterol Nutr* 1983; 2:622–28.

126. Picciano MF, West SG, Ruch AL, Kris-Etherton PM, Zhao G, Johnston KE, Maddox DH, Fishell VK, Dirienzo DB, Tamura T. Effect of cow milk on food folate bioavailability in young women. *Am J Clin Nutr* 2004; 80:1565–69.

127. Keizer SE, Gibson RS, O'Connor DL. Postpartum folic acid supplementation of adolescents: Impact on maternal folate and zinc status and milk composition. *Am J Clin Nutr* 1995; 62:377–84.

128. Andersson A, Hultberg B, Brattstrom L, Isaksson A. Decreased serum homocysteine in pregnancy. *Eur J Clin Chem Clin Biochem* 1992; 30:377–79.

129. Ramlau-Hansen CH, Moller UK, Henriksen TB, Nexo E, Moller J. Folate and vitamin B12 in relation to lactation: A 9-month postpartum follow-up study. *Eur J Clin Nutr* 2005; 60:120–28.

130. Metz J, Zalusky R, Herbert V. Folic acid binding by serum and milk. *Am J Clin Nutr* 1968; 21:289–97.

131. Willoughby ML, Jewell FG. Folate status throughout pregnancy and in postpartum period. *BMJ* 1968; 4:356–60.

132. Gluckman PD, Hanson MA. Living with the past: Evolution, development, and patterns of disease. *Science* 2004; 305:1733–36.

133. Wolff GL, Kodell RL, Moore SR, Cooney CA. Maternal epigenetics and methyl supplements affect agouti gene expression in Avy/a mice. *FASEB J* 1998; 12:949–57.

134. Wolff GL. Influence of maternal phenotype on metabolic differentiation of agouti locus mutants in the mouse. *Genetics* 1978; 88:529–39.

135. Joshi S, Rao S, Golwilkar A, Patwardhan M, Bhonde R. Fish oil supplementation of rats during pregnancy reduces adult disease risks in their offspring. *J Nutr* 2003; 133:3170–74.

136. Lillycrop KA, Phillips ES, Jackson AA, Hanson MA, Burdge GC. Dietary protein restriction of pregnant rats induces and folic acid supplementation prevents epigenetic modification of hepatic gene expression in the offspring. *J Nutr* 2005; 135:1382–86.

137. Yajnik CS, Deshpande SS, Jackson AA, Refsum H, Rao S, Fisher DJ, Bhat DS, et al. Vitamin B12 and folate concentrations during pregnancy and insulin resistance in the offspring: The Pune Maternal Nutrition Study. *Diabetologia* 2008; 51:29–38.

6 Folate Status and Birth Defect Risk
Epidemiological Perspective

Charlotte A. Hobbs, Gary M. Shaw, Martha M. Werler, and Bridget Mosley

CONTENTS

I. INTRODUCTION

The majority of structural birth defects result from a complex interplay between environmental exposures, lifestyle factors, and genetic and epigenetic processes [1–4]. Most defects are isolated, affecting only one organ system, and have no identified teratogenic, chromosomal, or genetic etiology [5,6]. The complex mechanistic processes involved in normal and abnormal human embryological development remain only vaguely understood. Fortunately, within the complex orchestration of human development, factors that are both protective and harmful to the developing fetus have been identified. It is well established that maternal folic acid intake during the periconceptional period reduces the risk of neural tube defects (NTDs) [7,8] and orofacial clefts [9,10]. There is limited, but still compelling, evidence to indicate that folic acid supplementation also reduces the occurrence of some cardiac defects and that alterations in folate-related mechanisms perturb cardiogenesis. There is insufficient but suggestive evidence of an association between maternal folate status and other birth defects, specifically limb defects [11,12], abdominal wall defects [13,14], and urogenital defects [15].

Multiple epidemiological studies [7,8,16–23], including randomized controlled trials and observational studies, provide compelling evidence to demonstrate that folic acid reduces the occurrence of NTDs. By the early 1990s, the weight of the cumulative evidence resulted in general recommendations for women of child-bearing age, a national education campaign, and recommendations for mandatory folic acid fortification of enriched cereal grain products in the United States. In 1992, the US Public Health Service recommended that all women of child-bearing age who were capable of becoming pregnant take a daily 400 μg supplement of folic acid [24]. This was the first of a series of recommendations from professional associations including the American College of Obstetricians and Gynecologists [25], the March of Dimes [26], the American Academy of Pediatrics [27], and the Institute of Medicine [28]. In 1996, the Food and Drug Administration announced a plan to mandate fortification of enriched cereal grain products with folic acid by January 1, 1998 [29].

Although the mechanism by which maternal folate status is protective is not well understood, converging evidence stresses the importance of folate to the developing fetus. In animal models of birth defects, exposure to punitive or protective factors is carefully administered by the investigator while controlling for other potentially confounding or modifying effects. In contrast, epidemiological studies of human populations are subject to multiple factors that are extraneous to the primary factor of interest (e.g., folate status), making interpretation of findings related to birth defect risk challenging. This chapter summarizes the human observational data linking folate intake and status with risk for birth defects, with a primary focus on NTDs, orofacial clefts, and congenital heart defects (CHDs). Data presented in this chapter link the basic mechanisms discussed in the subsequent chapter with observations in human populations related to folate and birth defect risk.

II. FOLATE AND NEURAL TUBE DEFECTS

The birth prevalence of NTDs varies from approximately 0.8 per 1,000 births [10] in areas of the United States to 13.8 per 1,000 births in north-central China [30]. Worldwide, it is estimated that 300,000 or more children with NTDs [31] are born each year. Within the United States, the prevalence of NTDs varies by race/ethnicity, as illustrated by the rank order of NTDs (i.e., Mexican Americans > non-Hispanic whites > non-Hispanic blacks) [32–35].

The development and closure of the neural tube are usually completed within 28 days postconception. Closure occurs at several discontinuous sites, and clinical types of NTDs differ depending on the site at which closure fails to take place normally [36]. Anencephaly and spina bifida are the most common and severe forms of NTDs. Infants with anencephaly are stillborn or die shortly after birth, whereas many infants with spina bifida survive, although often with severe, life-long disabilities. Many infants born with spina bifida have no other structural birth defect [37,38], and no single gene, chromosomal disorder, or teratogen has been identified [39,40]. Women who have had a previously affected pregnancy are 20 to 50 times more likely than women in the general population to have subsequent pregnancies affected by NTDs, with higher risks observed among populations not taking periconceptional folic acid [41,42].

Several comprehensive reviews of studies describe an association between NTDs and folate [43–45]. Compelling evidence from clinical trials and observational studies throughout the 1980s and 1990s demonstrated that maternal intake of folic acid reduced the occurrence and recurrence of NTDs (Table 6.1) [7,8,17–23,32,46]. More than 30 years ago, seminal work by Smithells et al. showed that diets and postpartum blood concentrations of women who had a fetus with an NTD were low for several micronutrients, particularly folate [47]. Subsequent small, nonrandomized trials in women who had previous NTD-affected pregnancies provided evidence that folic acid or multivitamins taken in the periconceptional period reduced recurrence risks [16,17,48–51].

A trial performed in Hungary demonstrated that a multivitamin supplement containing 0.8 mg of folic acid taken daily significantly reduced a woman's risk of having a fetus with an NTD [20]. Mulinare et al. [18] found that periconceptional use of multivitamins resulted in 60% protection from NTDs in infants. Bower and Stanley [52] also reported a 60% reduction in risk among Australian women whose folate intake from both dietary and supplemental sources in early pregnancy was more than 0.35 mg/day compared with women whose intake was less than 0.18 mg/day. Moore et al. [53] observed a 44% to 71% reduced risk of NTDs among women in the northeastern United States who took multivitamins containing folic acid during the second trimester of pregnancy. Werler et al. [21] found that periconceptional use of vitamins containing folic acid resulted in a 50% reduction in NTDs among women from New England and eastern Canada [21]. Shaw et al. [9] observed that, in general, California women who used folic acid–containing vitamins periconceptionally were approximately 25% to 50% less likely to have an NTD-affected pregnancy. However, this reduction in risk was particular to subsets of the population, primarily non-Hispanic women, women who did not seek early prenatal diagnosis, and women whose education did not exceed a high school diploma. The lack of an association for Hispanic women has since been observed elsewhere [54]. In contrast, Mills et al. [55] found no association between periconceptional multivitamin supplementation and NTDs among offspring of California and Illinois women.

Evidence also exists that folic acid supplementation reduces both *recurrence* [17,48] and *occurrence* of NTDs. The double-blind, placebo-controlled, randomized trial [7] rigorously conducted by the Medical Research Council among women from 13 countries showed that supplementation with 4 mg/day of folic acid resulted in a threefold reduction in NTD recurrence risk. The trials, taken in composite, argue that supplementation of folic acid in the dose range of approximately 0.4 mg/day [17,48] to 5 mg/day [50] prevents NTD births among most women who have previously had NTD-affected pregnancies.

In a community intervention in areas of north and south China where women were asked to take a pill containing 400 µg/day of folic acid, Berry et al. [8] observed a substantial reduction in NTD occurrence. The risk reduction was 85% in north China, where NTD prevalence was high (4.8 per 1,000 pregnancies), and the risk reduction was 40% in south China, where NTD prevalence was low (1.0 per 1,000 pregnancies).

TABLE 6.1

Selected Studies Examining the Relationship between Folic Acid and Neural Tube Defects

Study Type	Year	Finding	Reference
Randomized trials	2002	Maternal intake of low levels (100 µg) of folic acid–fortified cereal lowered homocysteine to levels similar to those consuming cereal fortified at higher folic acid levels	Venn et al. [65]
	1992	Multivitamin supplements containing 0.8 mg of folic acid reduced the risk of NTD occurrence	Czeizel and Dudas [20]
	1991	Multivitamin supplements containing 4.0 mg of folic acid reduced the risk of NTD recurrence by 72%	MRC Vitamin Study [7]
	1981	Similar risks of NTD recurrence were observed between those allocated for folic acid tablets and those given placebo; however, a reduction in NTD risk was found among tablet users when compliance with the allocated treatment was taken into account	Laurence et al. [16]
Nonrandomized trials	1981	Periconceptional multivitamin supplement users reduced recurrent risk of NTDs significantly compared with nonusers	Smithells et al. [48]
	1980	Women counseled about a "healthy diet" had lower NTD recurrence rates compared with women not counseled, although the relative risk was not significant	Laurence et al. [46]
Cohort	2003	Increased doses of total maternal dietary folate intake resulted in 77% lower NTD occurrence risk	Moore et al. [53]
	1999	Periconceptional folic acid supplements reduced occurrence risk of NTDs by 79% in northern China and 16% in southern China	Berry et al. [8]
	1989	A 73% reduction in occurrence risk of NTDs was observed among multivitamin users compared with nonusers	Milunsky et al. [19]
	1983	Recurrent NTD rates were lower among fully supplemented women compared with unsupplemented women, 0.7% vs. 4.7%, respectively	Smithells et al. [17]
Case–control	2008	Since folic acid fortification in the United States, no significant protective effects of maternal folate intake on NTD risk were observed	Mosley et al. [60]
	2006	Higher maternal homocysteine levels and a metabolic profile consistent with reduced methylation and increased oxidative stress were observed among cases vs. controls	Zhao et al. [73]
	2004	Nine of 12 mothers who delivered infants with NTDs exhibited folate-receptor autoantibodies compared with 2 of 20 control mothers	Rothenberg et al. [74]

TABLE 6.1 (continued)
Selected Studies Examining the Relationship between Folic Acid and Neural Tube Defects

Study Type	Year	Finding	Reference
	2000	Maternal use of folic acid antagonist medication was associated with higher risk of heart defects and oral clefts; multivitamin use decreased this risk	Hernandez-Diaz et al. [61]
	2000	Periconceptional folic acid supplement use was rare among Hispanic Mexican-Americans for both NTD cases (5.4%) and controls (3.2%)	Suarez et al. [54]
	1999	Among nonusers of supplements, no significant association was observed between dietary folate and NTDs	Shaw et al. [77]
	1999	Periconceptional intake of zinc was associated with reduced risk of NTDs and was not modified by folate intake	Velie et al. [76]
	1997	Increasing maternal intake of methionine was associated with reduced risk of NTDs even after controlling for folate intake	Shaw et al. [75]
	1996	Maternal folic acid supplement use was associated with a reduced risk of NTDs with multiple birth defects by 60%	Khoury et al. [23]
	1996	Folate intake had little effect on altering the association between maternal prepregnancy body weight and NTD risk	Werler et al. [82]
	1995	Women with lower plasma folate and red blood cell folate levels were estimated to be at higher risk for NTDs	Daly et al. [63]
	1995	Lower maternal dietary folate was associated with an increase risk of NTDs among Newfoundland women	Friel et al. [79]
	1995	Higher homocysteine levels were observed among women with NTD-affected pregnancies vs. control women; vitamin B12 modified the association	Mills et al. [67]
	1994	Mean values for basal homocysteine and homocysteine following a methionine load were significantly higher among women who previously had an NTD infant vs. control women	Steegers-Theunissen et al. [66]
	1993	Daily maternal use of periconceptional folic acid supplements reduces risk of NTDs by 60%	Werler et al. [21]
	1989	Maternal dietary folate intake early in pregnancy was associated with a reduced risk of isolated NTDs	Bower and Stanley [52]
	1989	Maternal use of periconceptional supplements containing folic acid was not associated with a reduced risk of NTDs	Mills et al. [55]
	1988	Maternal periconceptional multivitamin use reduced the risk of NTDs by 60%	Mulinare et al. [18]

continued

TABLE 6.1 (continued)

Selected Studies Examining the Relationship between Folic Acid and Neural Tube Defects

Study Type	Year	Finding	Reference
	1976	Maternal red blood cell folate was significantly lower in NTD case mothers compared with control mothers	Smithells et al. [47]
Ecological	2008	Among a California birth population, a decrease in NTD prevalence occurred before folic acid fortification, and no further decrease was observed after fortification	Chen et al. [58]
	2005	Using surveillance program data, anencephaly and spina bifida prevalence decreased 16% and 34%, respectively, in the period following folic acid fortification in the United States	Canfield et al. [14]
	2005	The decrease in prevalence of anencephaly and spina bifida since fortification was more pronounced among births to Hispanic and white women than African American women	Williams et al. [35]
	2003	No significant decline in the prevalence of trisomy 21 was observed in a Canadian population following folic acid fortification	Ray et al. [64]
	2002	Using surveillance program data, anencephaly and spina bifida prevalence decreased 16% and 31%, respectively, in the period following folic acid fortification in the United States	Williams et al. [56]
	2001	Using birth certificate data, anencephaly and spina bifida prevalence decreased 11% and 23%, respectively, in the period following folic acid fortification in the United States	Honein et al. [10]
Cross-sectional	2007	Serum folate and red blood cell folate increased among the US population since folic acid fortification	Pfeiffer et al. [57]

By the 1990s, sufficient evidence led to multiple clinical and public health interventions and recommendations. Beginning in 1992, in response to mounting evidence, multiple professional medical organizations in the United States recommended that all women of child-bearing age who are capable of becoming pregnant should consume 400 µg of synthetic folic acid daily [24]. The Food and Drug Administration mandated that all enriched cereal grain products contain 140 µg of folic acid per 100 g of grain by January 1998 [29].

Currently, investigations in which the impact of mandatory fortification has been evaluated are limited to ecological and case–control studies. Four ecological studies [10,14,56,57] found that NTD prevalence decreased since folic acid fortification has been in place. An 11% to 20% reduction in the occurrence of anencephaly and a 21% to 34% reduction in the occurrence of spina bifida were observed when comparing the pre- versus postfortification time eras [10]. In contrast, a decrease in NTD prevalence associated with fortification was not observed in one recent study from California [58]. Food fortification with folic acid has been effective in increasing both serum and red blood cell (RBC) folate concentrations among women of child-bearing age [59]. These increased blood folate concentrations are attributed to fortification of food rather than to increased use of vitamin supplements among these women [57]. This fortification has coincided with decreases in prevalence of 19% for overall NTDs [10] and of 16% for anencephaly [56].

The National Birth Defects Prevention Study is a population-based, case–control study of birth defects in the United States. In this ongoing study conducted among pregnancies conceived after mandatory folic acid fortification, no significant association was observed between NTDs and maternal folic acid supplement use or dietary folate intake [60]. These results suggest that folic acid fortification reduced the occurrence of folic acid–sensitive NTDs in the United States. Further discussion of the impact of fortification on population groups may be found in Chapter 8.

Additional evidence indicating the importance of folate in NTD risk reduction was provided by Hernandez-Diaz et al. [61], who observed that periconceptional intake of folic acid antagonist medications, including trimethoprim, triamterene, sulfasalazine, phenytoin, phenobarbital, primidone, or carbamazepine, may double the risk of NTD-affected pregnancies. Moreover, these investigators reported that some NTD risks associated with folate antagonists were attenuated in the presence of supplemental folic acid intake.

Some epidemiological studies have measured biomarkers in maternal serum either during or following pregnancy. Smithell et al.'s landmark findings [47] of low maternal serum folate concentration among women carrying fetuses affected by NTDs were observed in subsequent studies [62,63]. Other folate-related components in maternal serum have also been measured, e.g., vitamin B12 [64] and homocysteine (Hcy). Folic acid intakes as low as 100 μg, consumed daily in fortified breakfast cereal, have been reported to lower blood Hcy concentrations by 16% while increasing serum folate concentrations by 28% [65]. Elevated plasma Hcy concentration has been observed in mothers who gave birth to children with NTDs [66–69]. It has been proposed that elevated maternal Hcy concentration may disrupt embryogenesis by either a direct embryotoxic effect [70] or through indirect effects, such as a disruption of methylation, accumulation of S-adenosylhomocysteine (SAH), or an increase in oxidative stress [71]. During transsulfuration, Hcy is irreversibly condensed with serine to cystathionine by the B6-dependent enzyme cystathionine-β-synthase (CBS), and subsequently to cysteine, γ-glutamylcysteine (GluCys), and ultimately to glutathione [72]. Zhao et al. [73] evaluated the relationship between NTDs and maternal alterations in plasma concentrations of biomarkers. Mothers of offspring with NTDs had increased SAH, adenosine, Hcy, and oxidized glutathione concentrations relative to that of control subjects. However, the controls exhibited higher plasma S-adenosylmethionine (SAM) concentrations. These results indicated that women whose pregnancies were affected by NTDs demonstrated lower methylation capacity and higher oxidative stress.

Evidence for a potential mechanism that may further elucidate the association between NTDs and folate was identified in a study [74]. Investigators obtained serum from 12 women who were or had been pregnant with a fetus with an NTD and from

24 control women who were pregnant, nulligravid, or had previous unaffected pregnancies. Serum from women with affected pregnancies was more likely to contain autoantibodies that bind to folate receptors, thus potentially blocking cellular uptake of folate.

Multiple genetic epidemiological studies have reported on the association between NTDs and functional single nucleotide polymorphisms in folate-related pathways, and some have investigated the interaction between folate intake and common genetic variants. The reader is referred to Chapter 4 for a complete discussion of this topic. Further analysis of relevant genetic and environmental factors is required to define the basis for these observed alterations.

The underlying mechanism by which folic acid contributes to reduction in NTD risks or other malformation risks is only partially understood and is described in Chapter 7. Also unknown is why a substantial proportion of women who take folic acid supplements in the periconceptional period still deliver offspring with NTDs. Other nutrients and nutrition-related factors influence NTD risks. For example, increased intakes of methionine [75], zinc [76], dairy products [77], and vitamin B12 [78] have been associated with reduced NTD risks, whereas increased intake of sweets [79], diabetes, hyperinsulinemia [80], and prepregnancy obesity [81–83] have been associated with elevated NTD risks. These unexplained observations have served to direct research inquiries toward genetic variation in folate metabolism and transport as potential underlying mechanisms.

III. FOLATE AND OROFACIAL CLEFTS

Orofacial clefts are among the most common congenital malformations. Worldwide occurrence of orofacial clefts is 15.21 per 10,000 births [84]. The neural tube cells important in formation of the lip and palate are undoubtedly the critical cell population that is highly responsive to maternal folic acid supplementation [7]. These cells share an embryological origin with the cranial neural crest cells that are the principal contributor to the cartilage and bones of the face, including most of the tissues involved in lip and palate closure. Neural crest cells disperse throughout the embryo and are also important in formation of other body systems.

A recent meta-analysis by Badovinac et al. [85] identified all English-language studies published between 1958 and 2004, which included one randomized controlled trial, four cohort studies, and 12 case–control studies in which the association between folic acid intake and risk of cleft lip with or without cleft palate was investigated (Figures 6.1 and 6.2). In both controlled trials and observational studies, folic acid–containing supplements taken during pregnancy were found to reduce the risk of cleft lip with or without cleft palate. However, folic acid supplements were not consistently associated with the risk of cleft palate alone. Several lines of evidence reviewed in this meta-analysis and elsewhere support an association between maternal use of a vitamin supplement with folic acid in early pregnancy and a reduced risk for offspring with orofacial clefts.

A large, rigorously conducted, population-based case–control study in California observed as much as a 50% reduction in the *occurrence* risk for cleft lip among offspring of women who used folic acid–containing vitamins in early

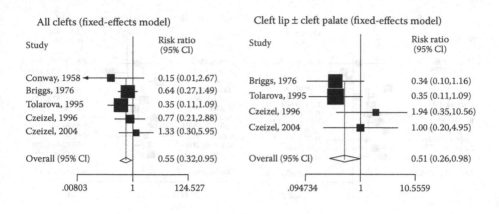

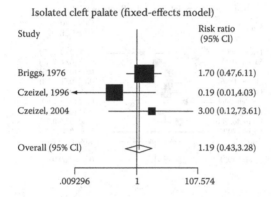

FIGURE 6.1 Results of meta-analysis on five prospective studies on folic acid–containing supplement consumption during pregnancy and risk for oral clefts. (Reprinted from Badovinac RL, et al. *Birth Defects Res A Clin Mol Teratol* 2007; 79:8–15. Copyright 2007 John Wiley & Sons Inc. With permission of Wiley-Liss, Inc., a subsidiary of John Wiley & Sons, Inc.)

pregnancy [9]. In a number of other epidemiological investigations [86,87], including the premier intervention trial conducted in China by the Centers for Disease Control and Prevention [8], reductions in risk of cleft lip with and without cleft palate but not in cleft palate alone have been reported. Early literature findings suggested an association between maternal vitamin use and reduced *recurrence* risk [88–91].

In the National Birth Defects Prevention Study, neither folic acid supplement use nor dietary folate was found to significantly reduce the risk of orofacial clefts among pregnancies conceived between 1997 and 2000 [92]. A recently published population-based case–control study by Wilcox et al. [93] describes maternal intake of folic acid supplements, multivitamins, and dietary folates among 573 infants with facial clefts and 763 controls born between 1996 and 2001 in Norway. Folic acid supplementation (≥400 μg/day) was associated with a reduced risk of isolated cleft lip with or without cleft palate. Independent from supplements, dietary folate was not found to be

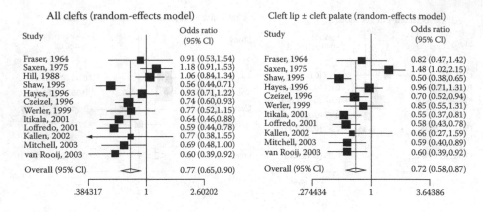

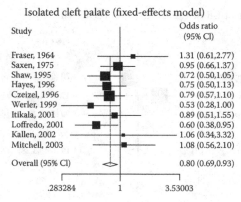

FIGURE 6.2   Results of meta-analysis of 12 case–control studies on folic acid–containing supplement consumption during pregnancy and risk for oral clefts. (Reprinted from Badovinac RL, et al. *Birth Defects Res A Clin Mol Teratol* 2007; 79:8–15. Copyright 2007 John Wiley & Sons Inc. With permission of Wiley-Liss, Inc., a subsidiary of John Wiley & Sons, Inc.)

statistically different between cases and controls. Folic acid supplementation among women with folate-rich diets appeared to provide the most protection.

Hernandez-Diaz et al. [61] demonstrated that women who had offspring with oral clefts were more likely to report taking a folic acid antagonist at some time during the second or third month of pregnancy. Other investigators have noted associations between maternal anticonvulsant use and clefting [94,95].

As with NTD studies, some investigators have measured biomarkers in maternal serum either during or following pregnancies among case and control women. In a clinic-based study conducted at the University of Nijmegen in the Netherlands, an oral methionine loading test was performed on 35 mothers of children with orofacial clefts and 56 control mothers whose infants had no malformations. Cases had higher mean Hcy concentrations than controls for both the fasting and methionine after-load tests. However, case mothers had higher mean serum concentrations of folate but lower vitamin B6 status [96]. In other studies [97,98], lower vitamin B12 and B6 but similar folate and Hcy concentrations were found among mothers of children with orofacial clefts compared with mothers of healthy children.

IV. FOLATE AND CONGENITAL HEART DEFECTS

CHDs, the most common birth defects in the United States, occur in 11 per 1,000 live US births [99] and are substantially more prevalent among stillbirths and miscarriages [100]. Annually, heart defects account for 6,000 total deaths and one-tenth of infant deaths, and only 15% of heart defects can be attributed to a known cause [99]. Several lines of evidence support an association between maternal use of a vitamin with folic acid in early pregnancy and a reduced risk for offspring with some heart defects, especially ventricular septal defects and conotruncal defects (tetralogy of Fallot and D-transposition of the great arteries). Botto et al. [99] provide an excellent review of studies investigating the association between CHDs and folic acid supplements (Table 6.2). Shaw et al. [11] in a large, rigorously conducted, population-based case–control study in California, observed a 30% reduction in the *occurrence* risk for conotruncal defects among the offspring of women who used folic acid–containing vitamins in early pregnancy. Botto et al. [101] observed an even greater reduction of risk in an Atlanta case–control study. A follow-up study also found a much reduced risk associated with periconceptional vitamin use and heart defects, particularly conotruncal defects [5]. In a randomized clinical trial in which women were given a daily supplement containing 12 vitamins, including 0.8 mg of folic acid versus a supplement with only trace elements, the frequency of CHDs was reduced by 50% with risk for conotruncal defects especially affected [102]. Two subsequent case–control studies, however, did not observe lower risks [12,103].

The use of folic acid antagonists during pregnancy has been reported to increase the risk of having an infant with a CHD. Among 3,870 women who had infants with CHDs, 63 (1.6%) reported taking a folic acid antagonist during the second or third month after their last menstrual period [61] compared with 68 (0.8%) of the control women. Indirect evidence has been reported that indicates that folic acid supplements can decrease the negative impact of folate antagonists on CHD risk [61]. Similar indirect evidence also exists for folic acid and the amelioration of CHD risk associated with febrile illnesses [104].

Some studies have investigated the association between blood concentrations of folate-related metabolites, especially Hcy, and CHD risk [105,106]. Using a case–control design, Hobbs et al. [107] examined a maternal folate-related metabolic risk profile for nonsyndromic CHDs, which provided evidence that Hcy, SAH, and methionine were the most important biomarkers predictive of CHD status.

V. FOLATE AND OTHER BIRTH DEFECTS

There are far fewer reports of the relationship between folic acid use in pregnancy and the occurrence of birth defects other than NTDs, heart defects, and oral clefts. The following is a brief overview of other birth defects for which there have been some reports of an association with maternal folic acid supplement use and risk.

TABLE 6.2
Studies on Multivitamin Supplements and Congenital Heart Defects, 1992–2000

Type of Study	Authors and Year	Population-Based?	Study Participants	Exposure	Heart Defects (Overall)	Outflow Tract Defects	Ventricular Septal Defects
					Relative Risk (95% Confidence Interval)		
Randomized clinical trial	Czeizel [102]	—	2,471 women on MV supplements; 2,391 on trace elements	MV pill with 0.8 mg of folic acid	0.42 (0.19–0.98)	048 (0.04–5.34)	0.24 (0.05–1.14)
Case–control	Shaw et al. [11]	Yes	207 with OTD, 481 controls	MV supplements	—	0.70 (0.46–1.1)	—
Case–control	Scanlon et al. [103]	Yes	126 with OTD, 679 controls	MV supplements with folic acid	—	0.97 (0.6–1.6)	—
Case–control	Botto et al. [5,101]	Yes	958 with heart defects, 3,029 controls	MV supplements	0.76 (0.60–0.97)	0.46 (0.24–0.86)	0.61 (0.38–0.99)
Case–control	Werler et al. [12]	No	157 with OTD, 186 with VSD, 521 controls	MV supplements	—	1.00 (0.70–1.50)	1.20 (0.80–1.80)

MV, multivitamin; OTD, outflow tract defects; VSD, ventricular septal defects.

Source: Reprinted from Botto LD, et al. *Am J Med Genet A* 2003; 121A:95–101. Copyright 2003 Wiley-Liss, Inc. A Wiley Company. With permission of John Wiley & Sons, Inc.

A. Urinary Tract Defects

Defects of the urinary tract encompass a wide range of anomalies such as renal agenesis, cystic kidneys, and obstructions anywhere from the nephrons to the opening of the urethra. Three studies, one of which included a targeted subgroup that included defects of the kidney, ureters, bladder, and urethra provided evidence for reduced risks associated with early pregnancy use of multivitamins, which are likely, but not necessarily, to include folic acid [12,15,108]. Supporting a folic acid effect, rather than the effect of another nutrient or group of nutrients, is a positive association for use of folic acid–antagonizing medication in early pregnancy and urinary tract defects in offspring. Studies that have examined trends in prevalences of these defects before and after folic acid fortification of the cereal grain supply in the United States show increases in obstructive genitourinary defects [14,109] and a decrease in renal agenesis in prenatal surveillance areas [14].

B. Limb Reduction

Studies that have focused on limb reductions provide some evidence of a decreased risk associated with prepregnancy or early pregnancy multivitamin supplementation [11,12,110]. Limb reduction defects can be classified into several different subtypes, which are heterogenous with respect to epidemiological characteristics and presumably their etiologies [111,112]. Hence, it is important for studies of folic acid supplementation to consider subtypes. In the three studies that estimated risks for subtypes of limb reductions, no consistent pattern was observed [11,108,110]. Risk estimates for upper, but not lower, limb reductions were reported to decrease slightly after folic acid fortification [14].

C. Trisomy 21

Trisomy 21 is most often caused by nondisjunction during meiosis, but only advanced maternal age has been identified as a risk factor. Multivitamin use in the periconceptional period was not associated with trisomy 21 in the United States [113]. There is a suggestion from a Hungarian study that high-dose folic acid (6 mg/day) might reduce this risk; intervention trials in that same country found that a lower dose of 0.6 to 0.8 mg of folic acid was not associated with a reduction in risk [114]. Since folic acid fortification, no change in the prevalence of trisomy 21 has been reported in Canada [64] compared with a slight increase and a small decrease in two separate studies in the United States [13,14]. The relationship between trisomy 21 and maternal polymorphisms in the folate pathway has been examined in a number of studies, with inconsistent results across a range of alleles and study populations [115].

D. Omphalocele

Omphalocele, an abdominal wall defect, often occurs with other structural defects, including NTDs, raising the possibility that the observed findings represent the underlying protective effect on NTDs, with or without omphalocele. The defect was observed to occur less frequently in offspring whose mothers took multivitamins in early pregnancy [116], whose births were after folic acid fortification [13,14], or whose mothers were homozygous for cysteine at the 677 locus of the methylenetetra-hydrofolate reductase gene [117]. Reduced risk estimates for multivitamin use were observed, albeit without statistical significance, regardless of whether the omphalo-cele occurred in the absence or presence of NTDs or other midline defects [116].

E. ANOPHTHALMIA AND MICROPHTHALMIA

Normal eye development requires the interaction of several embryonic tissues, including the neuroectoderm and neural crest cells [118]. Consequently, disruption to neu-roepithelium predictably results in anophthalmia and microphthalmia. Evaluating the possible relationships between NTDs, inadequate blood folate concentrations, and neuroepithelial development may indicate the important role that adequate maternal folate status may play in preventing eye malformation. A recent observation indicated that anophthalmia and microphthalmia were 11 and three times, respectively, more likely to co-occur with folate-responsive anomalies, namely, cleft lip and cleft palate [119].

VI.   INCONCLUSIVE STUDIES ON FOLATE AND BIRTH DEFECTS

Reports of reduced risks, which were subsequently countered with reports of no association, have been published for multivitamin or folic acid use and anal atre-sia/stenosis [120,121] and pyloric stenosis [12,108,121,122]. The vast majority of observational studies of multivitamin use and these selected birth defects were con-ducted in the United States before folic acid fortification of the food supply. As with NTDs, oral clefts, and cardiovascular defects, contemporary studies with null find-ings could mean either that folic acid intake through the food supply is effectively preventive or that there is no underlying association. In other words, these prefort-ification studies are a valuable and vanishing resource for evaluating the effects of multivitamins on birth defect risks in North American populations. The ecological studies that compare rates of birth defects before and after fortification [10,123] can support observational findings, as has been the case for NTDs, but their potential for confounding and other sources of bias is high, especially when evaluating non-NTD birth defects.

VII.   SUMMARY AND CONCLUSIONS

The most common and severe forms of NTDs are anencephaly and spina bifida, and the prevalence of NTDs varies from less than 1 per 1,000 births in the United States to nearly 14 per 1,000 births in China. Women who previously delivered infants with NTDs are at greater risk to have subsequent affected pregnancies.

The association between maternal folate status and the risk of infant birth defect is not fully understood; however, women who receive 400 µg/day of folic acid peri-conceptionally have a reduced risk of delivering a child with an NTD. In addition, maternal intake of particular minerals, dairy products, or vitamins may relate to reduced NTDs. The research in this area is ongoing.

Within the United States, the Food and Drug Administration required cereal and grain products to be folic acid–fortified by 1998, following which the NTD incidence rates decreased in some subpopulations. The National Birth Defects Prevention Study, initiated by Congress and administered through the Centers for Disease Control and Prevention, is an ongoing surveillance of birth defects within 10 registries throughout the United States in an attempt to identify birth defect risk factors.

The biological mechanism by which naturally occurring folate and synthetic folic acid are protective is not fully understood; however, folate is only one component of a complex metabolic pathway consisting of multiple metabolites, enzymes, and micronutrients. Few studies have investigated the impact of folate while controlling for the effects of supplement use and other micronutrients. New technologies and strategies for investigating biomarkers, genetic variants, and epigenetic phenomena will be essential to further understand the complex relationship between folate and birth defects.

REFERENCES

1. Brender JD, Suarez L. Paternal occupation and anencephaly. *Am J Epidemiol* 1990; 131:517–21.
2. Dansky LV, Finnell RH. Parental epilepsy, anticonvulsant drugs, and reproductive outcome: Epidemiologic and experimental findings spanning three decades; 2: Human studies. *Reprod Toxicol* 1991; 5:301–35.
3. Carmichael SL, Shaw GM. Maternal life event stress and congenital anomalies. *Epidemiology* 2000; 11:30–35.
4. Hobbs CA, Sherman SL, Yi P, Hopkins SE, Torfs CP, Hine RJ, Pogribna M, Rozen R, James SJ. Polymorphisms in genes involved in folate metabolism as maternal risk factors for Down syndrome. *Am J Hum Genet* 2000; 67:623–30.
5. Botto LD, Mulinare J, Erickson JD. Occurrence of congenital heart defects in relation to maternal multivitamin use. *Am J Epidemiol* 2000; 151:878–84.
6. Hobbs CA, Cleves MA, Simmons CJ. Genetic epidemiology and congenital malformations: From the chromosome to the crib. *Arch Pediatr Adolesc Med* 2002; 156:315–20.
7. MRC Vitamin Study Research Group. Prevention of neural tube defects: Results of the Medical Research Council Vitamin Study. *Lancet* 1991; 338:131–37.
8. Berry RJ, Li Z, Erickson JD, Li S, Moore CA, Wang H, Mulinare J, et al. Prevention of neural-tube defects with folic acid in China. China–U.S. Collaborative Project for Neural Tube Defect Prevention. *N Engl J Med* 1999; 341:1485–90.
9. Shaw GM, Lammer EJ, Wasserman CR, O'Malley CD, Tolarova MM. Risks of orofacial clefts in children born to women using multivitamins containing folic acid periconceptionally. *Lancet* 1995; 346:393–96.
10. Honein MA, Paulozzi LJ, Mathews TJ, Erickson JD, Wong LY. Impact of folic acid fortification of the US food supply on the occurrence of neural tube defects. *JAMA* 2001; 285:2981–86.
11. Shaw GM, O'Malley CD, Wasserman CR, Tolarova MM, Lammer EJ. Maternal periconceptional use of multivitamins and reduced risk for conotruncal heart defects and limb deficiencies among offspring. *Am J Med Genet* 1995; 59:536–45.
12. Werler MM, Hayes C, Louik C, Shapiro S, Mitchell AA. Multivitamin supplementation and risk of birth defects. *Am J Epidemiol* 1999; 150:675–82.
13. Simmons CJ, Mosley BS, Fulton-Bond CA, Hobbs CA. Birth defects in Arkansas: Is folic acid fortification making a difference? *Birth Defects Res A Clin Mol Teratol* 2004; 70:559–64.

14. Canfield MA, Collins JS, Botto LD, Williams LJ, Mai CT, Kirby RS, Pearson K, Devine O, Mulinare J. Changes in the birth prevalence of selected birth defects after grain fortification with folic acid in the United States: Findings from a multi-state population-based study. *Birth Defects Res A Clin Mol Teratol* 2005; 73:679–89.
15. Li DK, Daling JR, Mueller BA, Hickok DE, Fantel AG, Weiss NS. Periconceptional multivitamin use in relation to the risk of congenital urinary tract anomalies. *Epidemiology* 1995; 6:212–18.
16. Laurence KM, James N, Miller MH, Tennant GB, Campbell H. Double-blind randomised controlled trial of folate treatment before conception to prevent recurrence of neural-tube defects. *BMJ (Clin Res Ed)* 1981; 282:1509–11.
17. Smithells RW, Nevin NC, Seller MJ, Sheppard S, Harris R, Read AP, Fielding DW, Walker S, Schorah CJ, Wild J. Further experience of vitamin supplementation for prevention of neural tube defect recurrences. *Lancet* 1983; 1:1027–31.
18. Mulinare J, Cordero JF, Erickson JD, Berry RJ. Periconceptional use of multivitamins and the occurrence of neural tube defects. *JAMA* 1988; 260:3141–45.
19. Milunsky A, Jick H, Jick SS, Bruell CL, MacLaughlin DS, Rothman KJ, Willett W. Multivitamin/folic acid supplementation in early pregnancy reduces the prevalence of neural tube defects. *JAMA* 1989; 262:2847–52.
20. Czeizel AE, Dudas I. Prevention of the first occurrence of neural-tube defects by periconceptional vitamin supplementation. *N Engl J Med* 1992; 327:1832–35.
21. Werler MM, Shapiro S, Mitchell AA. Periconceptional folic acid exposure and risk of occurrent neural tube defects. *JAMA* 1993; 269:1257–61.
22. Shaw GM, Schaffer D, Velie EM, Morland K, Harris JA. Periconceptional vitamin use, dietary folate, and the occurrence of neural tube defects. *Epidemiology* 1995; 6:219–26.
23. Khoury MJ, Shaw GM, Moore CA, Lammer EJ, Mulinare J. Does periconceptional multivitamin use reduce the risk of neural tube defects associated with other birth defects? Data from two population-based case-control studies. *Am J Med Genet* 1996; 61:30–36.
24. Recommendations for the use of folic acid to reduce the number of cases of spina bifida and other neural tube defects. *MMWR Recomm Rep* 1992; 41:1–7.
25. Take Folic Acid before You're Pregnant. March of Dimes. http://www.marchofdimes.com/hbhb_syndication/18613_769.asp. Updated December 2008.
26. Nutrition during Pregnancy. American College of Obstetricians and Gynecologists Committee on Patient Education. http://www.acog.org/publications/patient_education/bp001.cfm. Updated June 2008.
27. Folic acid for the prevention of neural tube defects. American Academy of Pediatrics. Committee on Genetics. *Pediatrics* 1999; 104:325–27.
28. Institute of Medicine. *Dietary Reference Intake: Folate, Other B Vitamins, and Choline.* Washington, DC: National Academy Press, 1998.
29. Department of Health and Human Services, Food and Drug Administration. *Food Standards: Amendment of Standards of Identity for Enriched Grain Products to Require Addition of Folic Acid.* 21 CFR Parts 136,137,139, 8781–8797. 1996. 91N-100S.
30. Li Z, Ren A, Zhang L, Ye R, Li S, Zheng J, Hong S, Wang T, Li Z. Extremely high prevalence of neural tube defects in a 4-county area in Shanxi Province, China. *Birth Defects Res A Clin Mol Teratol* 2006; 76:237–40.
31. *Global Burden of Disease: A Comprehensive Assessment of Mortality and Disability from Diseases, Injuries, and Risk Factors in 1990 and Projected to 2020.* Cambridge, MA: Harvard School of Public Health, 1996.
32. Shaw GM, Jensvold NG, Wasserman CR, Lammer EJ. Epidemiologic characteristics of phenotypically distinct neural tube defects among 0.7 million California births, 1983–1987. *Teratology* 1994; 49:143–49.
33. Hendricks KA, Simpson JS, Larsen RD. Neural tube defects along the Texas-Mexico border, 1993–1995. *Am J Epidemiol* 1999; 149:1119–27.

34. Canfield MA, Honein MA, Yuskiv N, Xing J, Mai CT, Collins JS, Devine O, et al. National estimates and race/ethnic-specific variation of selected birth defects in the United States, 1999–2001. *Birth Defects Res A Clin Mol Teratol* 2006; 76:747–56.
35. Williams LJ, Rasmussen SA, Flores A, Kirby RS, Edmonds LD. Decline in the prevalence of spina bifida and anencephaly by race/ethnicity: 1995–2002. *Pediatrics* 2005; 116:580–86.
36. O'Rahilly R, Muller F. The two sites of fusion of the neural folds and the two neuropores in the human embryo. *Teratology* 2002; 65:162–70.
37. Khoury MJ, Erickson JD, James LM. Etiologic heterogeneity of neural tube defects: Clues from epidemiology. *Am J Epidemiol* 1982; 115:538–48.
38. Simpson JL, Mills J, Rhoads GG, Cunningham GC, Conley MR, Hoffman HJ. Genetic heterogeneity in neural tube defects. *Ann Genet* 1991; 34:279–86.
39. Rasmussen SA, Frias JL. Genetics of syndromic neural tube defects. In: Wyszynski DF, ed., *Neural Tube Defects: From Origin to Treatment*. New York: Oxford University Press, 2006:185–97.
40. Dunlevy LP, Chitty LS, Burren KA, Doudney K, Stojilkovic-Mikic T, Stanier P, Scott R, Copp AJ, Greene ND. Abnormal folate metabolism in foetuses affected by neural tube defects. *Brain* 2007; 130:1043–49.
41. Elwood JM, Little J, Elwood JH. Epidemiology and control of neural tube defects. In: Kelsey JL, Marmot MG, Stolley PD, Vessey MP, eds., *Monographs in Epidemiology and Biostatistics*. Oxford, UK: Oxford University Press, 1992.
42. Saul RA. Genetic counseling and interpretation of risk figures. In: Wyszynski DF, ed., *Neural Tube Defects: From Origin to Treatment*. New York: Oxford University Press, 2006:330–332.
43. Kalter H. Folic acid and human malformations: A summary and evaluation. *Reprod Toxicol* 2000; 14:463–76.
44. Lumley J, Watson L, Watson M, Bower C. Periconceptional supplementation with folate and/or multivitamins for preventing neural tube defects. *Cochrane Database Syst Rev* 2001; CD001056.
45. Green NS. Folic acid supplementation and prevention of birth defects. *J Nutr* 2002; 132:2356S–60S.
46. Laurence KM, James N, Miller M, Campbell H. Increased risk of recurrence of pregnancies complicated by fetal neural tube defects in mothers receiving poor diets, and possible benefit of dietary counselling. *BMJ* 1980; 281:1592–94.
47. Smithells RW, Sheppard S, Schorah CJ. Vitamin dificiencies and neural tube defects. *Arch Dis Child* 1976; 51:944–50.
48. Smithells RW, Sheppard S, Schorah CJ, Seller MJ, Nevin NC, Harris R, Read AP, Fielding DW. Apparent prevention of neural tube defects by periconceptional vitamin supplementation. *Arch Dis Child* 1981; 56:911–18.
49. Seller MJ, Nevin NC. Periconceptional vitamin supplementation and the prevention of neural tube defects in south-east England and Northern Ireland. *J Med Genet* 1984; 21:325–30.
50. Vergel RG, Sanchez LR, Heredero BL, Rodriguez PL, Martinez AJ. Primary prevention of neural tube defects with folic acid supplementation: Cuban experience. *Prenat Diagn* 1990; 10:149–52.
51. Holmes-Siedle M, Dennis J, Lindenbaum RH, Galliard A. Long term effects of periconceptional multivitamin supplements for prevention of neural tube defects: A seven to 10 year follow up. *Arch Dis Child* 1992; 67:1436–41.
52. Bower C, Stanley FJ. Dietary folate as a risk factor for neural-tube defects: Evidence from a case-control study in Western Australia. *Med J Aust* 1989; 150:613–19.
53. Moore LL, Bradlee ML, Singer MR, Rothman KJ, Milunsky A. Folate intake and the risk of neural tube defects: An estimation of dose-response. *Epidemiology* 2003; 14:200–05.

54. Suarez L, Hendricks KA, Cooper SP, Sweeney AM, Hardy RJ, Larsen RD. Neural tube defects among Mexican Americans living on the US-Mexico border: Effects of folic acid and dietary folate. *Am J Epidemiol* 2000; 152:1017–23.

55. Mills JL, Rhoads GG, Simpson JL, Cunningham GC, Conley MR, Lassman MR, Walden ME, Depp OR, Hoffman HJ. The absence of a relation between the periconceptional use of vitamins and neural-tube defects. National Institute of Child Health and Human Development Neural Tube Defects Study Group. *N Engl J Med* 1989; 321:430–35.

56. Williams LJ, Mai CT, Edmonds LD, Shaw GM, Kirby RS, Hobbs CA, Sever LE, Miller LA, Meaney FJ, Levitt M. Prevalence of spina bifida and anencephaly during the transition to mandatory folic acid fortification in the United States. *Teratology* 2002; 66:33–39.

57. Pfeiffer CM, Johnson CL, Jain RB, Yetley EA, Picciano MF, Rader JI, Fisher KD, Mulinare J, Osterloh JD. Trends in blood folate and vitamin B-12 concentrations in the United States, 1988–2004. *Am J Clin Nutr* 2007; 86:718–27.

58. Chen BH, Carmichael SL, Selvin S, Abrams B, Shaw GM. NTD prevalences in central California before and after folic acid fortification. *Birth Defects Res A Clin Mol Teratol* 2008; 82:547–52.

59. Folate status in women of childbearing age--United States, 1999. *MMWR Morb Mortal Wkly Rep* 2000; 49:962–65.

60. Mosley BS, Cleves MA, Siega-Riz AM, Shaw GM, Canfield MA, Waller DK, Werler MM, Hobbs CA, National Birth Defects Prevention Study. Neural tube defects and maternal folate intake among pregnancies conceived after folic acid fortification in the U.S. *Am J Epidemiol* 2009; 169:9–17.

61. Hernandez-Diaz S, Werler MM, Walker AM, Mitchell AA. Folic acid antagonists during pregnancy and the risk of birth defects. *N Engl J Med* 2000; 343:1608–14.

62. Yates JR, Ferguson-Smith MA, Shenkin A, Guzman-Rodriguez R, White M, Clark BJ. Is disordered folate metabolism the basis for the genetic predisposition to neural tube defects? *Clin Genet* 1987; 31:279–87.

63. Daly LE, Kirke PN, Molloy A, Weir DG, Scott JM. Folate levels and neural tube defects. Implications for prevention. *JAMA* 1995; 274:1698–702.

64. Ray JG, Meier C, Vermeulen MJ, Cole DE, Wyatt PR. Prevalence of trisomy 21 following folic acid food fortification. *Am J Med Genet A* 2003; 120A:309–13.

65. Venn BJ, Mann JI, Williams SM, Riddell LJ, Chisholm A, Harper MJ, Aitken W, Rossaak JI. Assessment of three levels of folic acid on serum folate and plasma homocysteine: A randomised placebo-controlled double-blind dietary intervention trial. *Eur J Clin Nutr* 2002; 56:748–54.

66. Steegers-Theunissen RP, Boers GH, Trijbels FJ, Finkelstein JD, Blom HJ, Thomas CM, Borm GF, Wouters MG, Eskes TK. Maternal hyperhomocysteinemia: A risk factor for neural-tube defects? *Metabolism* 1994; 43:1475–80.

67. Mills JL, McPartlin JM, Kirke PN, Lee YJ, Conley MR, Weir DG, Scott JM. Homocysteine metabolism in pregnancies complicated by neural-tube defects. *Lancet* 1995; 345:149–51.

68. van der Put NM, Blom HJ. Neural tube defects and a disturbed folate dependent homocysteine metabolism. *Eur J Obstet Gynecol Reprod Biol* 2000; 92:57–61.

69. van der Put NM, van Straaten HW, Trijbels FJ, Blom HJ. Folate, homocysteine and neural tube defects: An overview. *Exp Biol Med* (Maywood) 2001; 226:243–70.

70. Rosenquist TH, Ratashak SA, Selhub J. Homocysteine induces congenital defects of the heart and neural tube: Effect of folic acid. *Proc Natl Acad Sci USA* 1996; 93:15227–32.

71. Chern CL, Huang RF, Chen YH, Cheng JT, Liu TZ. Folate deficiency-induced oxidative stress and apoptosis are mediated via homocysteine-dependent overproduction of hydrogen peroxide and enhanced activation of NF-kappaB in human Hep G2 cells. *Biomed Pharmacother* 2001; 55:434–42.

72. Finkelstein JD. The metabolism of homocysteine: Pathways and regulation. *Eur J Pediatr* 1998; 157(Suppl 2):S40–S44.
73. Zhao W, Mosley BS, Cleves MA, Melnyk S, James SJ, Hobbs CA. Neural tube defects and maternal biomarkers of folate, homocysteine, and glutathione metabolism. *Birth Defects Res A Clin Mol Teratol* 2006; 76:230–36.
74. Rothenberg SP, da Costa MP, Sequeira JM, Cracco J, Roberts JL, Weedon J, Quadros EV. Autoantibodies against folate receptors in women with a pregnancy complicated by a neural-tube defect. *N Engl J Med* 2004; 350:134–42.
75. Shaw GM, Velie EM, Schaffer DM. Is dietary intake of methionine associated with a reduction in risk for neural tube defect-affected pregnancies? *Teratology* 1997; 56:295–99.
76. Velie EM, Block G, Shaw GM, Samuels SJ, Schaffer DM, Kulldorff M. Maternal supplemental and dietary zinc intake and the occurrence of neural tube defects in California. *Am J Epidemiol* 1999; 150:605–16.
77. Shaw GM, Todoroff K, Schaffer DM, Selvin S. Periconceptional nutrient intake and risk for neural tube defect-affected pregnancies. *Epidemiology* 1999; 10:711–16.
78. Suarez L, Hendricks K, Felkner M, Gunter E. Maternal serum B12 levels and risk for neural tube defects in a Texas-Mexico border population. *Ann Epidemiol* 2003; 13:81–88.
79. Friel JK, Frecker M, Fraser FC. Nutritional patterns of mothers of children with neural tube defects in Newfoundland. *Am J Med Genet* 1995; 55:195–99.
80. Hendricks KA, Nuno OM, Suarez L, Larsen R. Effects of hyperinsulinemia and obesity on risk of neural tube defects among Mexican Americans. *Epidemiology* 2001; 12:630–35.
81. Shaw GM, Velie EM, Schaffer D. Risk of neural tube defect-affected pregnancies among obese women. *JAMA* 1996; 275:1093–96.
82. Werler MM, Louik C, Shapiro S, Mitchell AA. Prepregnant weight in relation to risk of neural tube defects. *JAMA* 1996; 275:1089–92.
83. Waller DK, Shaw GM, Rasmussen SA, Hobbs CA, Canfield MA, Siega-Riz AM, Gallaway MS, Correa A. Prepregnancy obesity as a risk factor for structural birth defects. *Arch Pediatr Adolesc Med* 2007; 161:745–50.
84. World Health Organization. *Typical Orofacial Clefts—Cumulative Data by Register.* World Health Organization, 2007. Available at http://www.who.int/genomics/anomalies/cumulative_data/en/print.html; accessed June 26, 2008.
85. Badovinac RL, Werler MM, Williams PL, Kelsey KT, Hayes C. Folic acid-containing supplement consumption during pregnancy and risk for oral clefts: A meta-analysis. *Birth Defects Res A Clin Mol Teratol* 2007; 79:8–15.
86. Khoury MJ, Cordero JF, Mulinare J, Opitz JM. Selected midline defect associations: A population study. *Pediatrics* 1989; 84:266–72.
87. Itikala PR, Watkins ML, Mulinare J, Moore CA, Liu Y. Maternal multivitamin use and orofacial clefts in offspring. *Teratology* 2001; 63:79–86.
88. Conway H. Effect of supplemental vitamin therapy on the limitation of incidence of cleft lip and cleft palate in humans. *Plast Reconstr Surg Transplant Bull* 1958; 22:450–53.
89. Briggs RM. Vitamin supplementation as a possible factor in the incidence of cleft lip/palate deformities in humans. *Clin Plast Surg* 1976; 3:647–52.
90. Tolarova M. Periconceptional supplementation with vitamins and folic acid to prevent recurrence of cleft lip. *Lancet* 1982; 2:217.
91. Tolarova M. Orofacial clefts in Czechoslovakia. Incidence, genetics and prevention of cleft lip and palate over a 19-year period. *Scand J Plast Reconstr Surg Hand Surg* 1987; 21:19–25.
92. Shaw GM, Carmichael SL, Laurent C, Rasmussen SA. Maternal nutrient intakes and risk of orofacial clefts. *Epidemiology* 2006; 17:285–91.

93. Wilcox AJ, Lie RT, Solvoll K, Taylor J, McConnaughey DR, Abyholm F, Vindenes H, Vollset SE, Drevon CA. Folic acid supplements and risk of facial clefts: National population based case-control study. *BMJ* 2007; 334:464.
94. Speidel BD, Meadow SR. Maternal epilepsy and abnormalities of the fetus and newborn. *Lancet* 1972; 2:839–43.
95. Hill L, Murphy M, McDowall M, Paul AH. Maternal drug histories and congenital malformations: Limb reduction defects and oral clefts. *J Epidemiol Community Health* 1988; 42:1–7.
96. Wong WY, Eskes TK, Kuijpers-Jagtman AM, Spauwen PH, Steegers EA, Thomas CM, Hamel BC, Blom HJ, Steegers-Theunissen RP. Nonsyndromic orofacial clefts: Association with maternal hyperhomocysteinemia. *Teratology* 1999; 60:253–57.
97. van Rooij IA, Swinkels DW, Blom HJ, Merkus HM, Steegers-Theunissen RP. Vitamin and homocysteine status of mothers and infants and the risk of nonsyndromic orofacial clefts. *Am J Obstet Gynecol* 2003; 189:1155–60.
98. Munger RG, Sauberlich HE, Corcoran C, Nepomuceno B, Daack-Hirsch S, Solon FS. Maternal vitamin B-6 and folate status and risk of oral cleft birth defects in the Philippines. *Birth Defects Res A Clin Mol Teratol* 2004; 70:464–71.
99. Botto LD, Mulinare J, Erickson JD. Do multivitamin or folic acid supplements reduce the risk for congenital heart defects? Evidence and gaps. *Am J Med Genet A* 2003; 121A:95–101.
100. Tennstedt C, Chaoui R, Korner H, Dietel M. Spectrum of congenital heart defects and extracardiac malformations associated with chromosomal abnormalities: Results of a seven year necropsy study. *Heart* 1999; 82:34–39.
101. Botto LD, Khoury MJ, Mulinare J, Erickson JD. Periconceptional multivitamin use and the occurrence of conotruncal heart defects: Results from a population-based, case-control study. *Pediatrics* 1996; 98:911–17.
102. Czeizel AE. Periconceptional folic acid containing multivitamin supplementation. *Eur J Obstet Gynecol Reprod Biol* 1998; 78:151–61.
103. Scanlon KS, Ferencz C, Loffredo CA, Wilson PD, Correa-Villasenor A, Khoury MJ, Willett WC. Preconceptional folate intake and malformations of the cardiac outflow tract. Baltimore-Washington Infant Study Group. *Epidemiology* 1998; 9:95–98.
104. Botto LD, Lynberg MC, Erickson JD. Congenital heart defects, maternal febrile illness, and multivitamin use: A population-based study. *Epidemiology* 2001; 12:485–90.
105. Kapusta L, Haagmans ML, Steegers EA, Cuypers MH, Blom HJ, Eskes TK. Congenital heart defects and maternal derangement of homocysteine metabolism. *J Pediatr* 1999; 135:773–74.
106. Wenstrom KD, Johanning GL, Johnston KE, DuBard M. Association of the C677T methylenetetrahydrofolate reductase mutation and elevated homocysteine levels with congenital cardiac malformations. *Am J Obstet Gynecol* 2001; 184:806–12.
107. Hobbs CA, Cleves MA, Melnyk S, Zhao W, James SJ. Congenital heart defects and abnormal maternal biomarkers of methionine and homocysteine metabolism. *Am J Clin Nutr* 2005; 81:147–53.
108. Czeizel AE. The primary prevention of birth defects: Multivitamins or folic acid? *Int J Med Sci* 2004; 1:50–61.
109. Gordon TE, Leeth EA, Nowinski CJ, MacGregor SN, Kambich M, Silver RK. Geographic and temporal analysis of folate-sensitive fetal malformations. *J Soc Gynecol Invest* 2003; 10:298–301.
110. Yang Q, Khoury MJ, Olney RS, Mulinare J. Does periconceptional multivitamin use reduce the risk for limb deficiency in offspring? *Epidemiology* 1997; 8:157–61.
111. Lin S, Marshall EG, Davidson GK, Roth GB, Druschel CM. Evaluation of congenital limb reduction defects in upstate New York. *Teratology* 1993; 47:127–35.

112. Wasserman CR, Shaw GM, O'Malley CD, Tolarova MM, Lammer EJ. Parental cigarette smoking and risk for congenital anomalies of the heart, neural tube, or limb. *Teratology* 1996; 53:261–67.

113. Botto LD, Mulinare J, Yang Q, Liu Y, Erickson JD. Autosomal trisomy and maternal use of multivitamin supplements. *Am J Med Genet A* 2004; 125A:113–16.

114. Czeizel AE, Puho E. Maternal use of nutritional supplements during the first month of pregnancy and decreased risk of Down's syndrome: Case-control study. *Nutrition* 2005; 21:698–704.

115. Zintzaras E. Maternal gene polymorphisms involved in folate metabolism and risk of Down syndrome offspring: A meta-analysis. *J Hum Genet* 2007; 52:943–53.

116. Botto LD, Mulinare J, Erickson JD. Occurrence of omphalocele in relation to maternal multivitamin use: A population-based study. *Pediatrics* 2002; 109:904–08.

117. Mills JL, Druschel CM, Pangilinan F, Pass K, Cox C, Seltzer RR, Conley MR, Brody LC. Folate-related genes and omphalocele. *Am J Med Genet A* 2005; 136:8–11.

118. Moore KL, Persaud TVN. *The Developing Human: Clinically Oriented Embryology.* 7th ed. Philadelphia: Saunders/Elsevier, 2003.

119. Shaw GM, Carmichael SL, Yang W, Harris JA, Lammer EJ. Congenital malformations in births with orofacial clefts among 3.6 million California births, 1983–1997. *Am J Med Genet A* 2004; 125A:250–56.

120. Myers MF, Li S, Correa-Villasenor A, Li Z, Moore CA, Hong SX, Berry RJ. Folic acid supplementation and risk for imperforate anus in China. *Am J Epidemiol* 2001; 154:1051–56.

121. Correa A, Botto L, Liu Y, Mulinare J, Erickson JD. Do multivitamin supplements attenuate the risk for diabetes-associated birth defects? *Pediatrics* 2003; 111:1146–51.

122. Czeizel AE. Prevention of congenital abnormalities by periconceptional multivitamin supplementation. *BMJ* 1993; 306:1645–48.

123. De Wals P, Tairou F, Van Allen MI, Uh SH, Lowry RB, Sibbald B, Evans JA, et al. Reduction in neural-tube defects after folic acid fortification in Canada. *N Engl J Med* 2007; 357:135–42.

7 Folate-Related Birth Defects

Embryonic Consequences of Abnormal Folate Transport and Metabolism

Deeann Wallis, Johnathan L. Ballard, Gary M. Shaw, Edward J. Lammer, and Richard H. Finnell

CONTENTS

I. INTRODUCTION

Birth defects are a global problem that affect approximately 6% of all births [1]. In the United States, birth defects are the leading cause of hospitalizations [2], medical expenditures [3], and death in the first year of life [4]. Worldwide, at least 3.3 million children under the age of 5 years die each year because of a serious birth defect [1]. Indeed, birth defects are one, if not the leading, health care concern for the youngest members of our societies.

Folate is a key nutrient required for proper embryonic development. Population-based studies of human pregnancies consistently show that periconceptional folic acid supplementation has a significant protective effect for embryos during early development, resulting in a significant reduction in developmental defects of the craniofacies, the neural tube, and the heart. A common link among these three major folate-sensitive anatomical regions is that normal development of each structure depends on a set of multipotent cells that originate in the mid-dorsal region of the neural epithelium (Figure 7.1). These neural crest cells have a high demand for folate to support cellular growth, differentiation, and migration. Limiting the transport of folate to embryonic tissues through nutritional folate deficiency, exposure to folate antagonists or antibodies to folate receptors, or through genetic alterations, results in serious structural malformations. Transport defects also have far-reaching

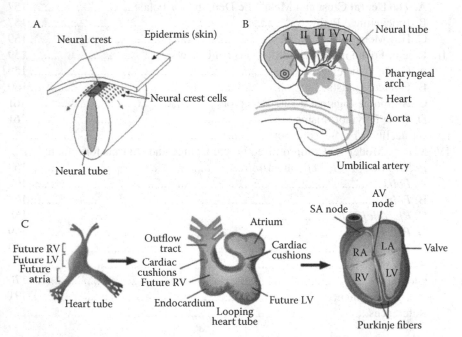

FIGURE 7.1   Neural crest cells. A, the origin of neural crest cells from the dorsal-most region of the neural tube. B, migration of neural crest cells into the pharyngeal arches (which later form the head, face, and neck) and the heart. C, embryonic heart development. Cardiac neural crest plays a role in forming the septa and outflow tract.

implications for cellular metabolism that encompass the biosynthesis of DNA, proteins, and lipids, as well as the homeostasis of key metabolites such as homocysteine (Hcy) and methionine. Animal models of neural crest cell–dependent embryonic malformations that use directed mutagenesis and teratogenic exposures have focused on the consequences of restricting the import of folates into neural crest cells and the subsequent perturbations in folate-using metabolic pathways. These animal models have allowed us to start defining the functions of specific genes implicated in these transport pathways, such as *Folr1*, *Folr2*, *Rcf1/Slc19A1*, and *Pcft/Hcp1*.

In this chapter, the role of intracellular folate transport and its impact on normal embryonic development are reviewed. This topic is approached by a comprehensive analysis of the nutritional benefit of folate on selected "folate-sensitive" birth defects. The specific defects that are the focus of the chapter are cleft lip with or without cleft palate, neural tube defects (NTDs), and selected congenital heart defects (CHDs).

A. THE NEURAL CREST AND METABOLIC DEMAND FOR FOLATE

These three major folate-responsive birth defects all share a commonality in that neural crest cells are involved in the development of these seemingly diverse structures (Figure 7.1). Premigratory neural crest cells are virtually indistinguishable from the dorsal-most presumptive neurons of the neural fold, both anatomically and functionally (Figure 7.1A) [5]. It is these cells that participate in neural tube closure. Migrating neural crest cells also contribute significantly to the development of the face as they are the principal contributor to the facial cartilage and bones, including most of the tissues directly involved in lip and palate closure (Figure 7.1B) [6–9]. Additionally, the embryology of heart development is a complex process that involves migration of cells from the neural crest into the developing heart primordia. In fact, normal septation of the cardiac outflow tract requires migration of neural crest cells from the posterior rhombencephalon to the branchial arches and developing conotruncal endocardial cushions (Figure 7.1C) [10]. Disruptions in any of the differentiation, specification, migratory, or developmental events may result in birth defects of neural crest cell origin such as cleft lip with or without cleft palate, NTDs, and CHDs.

Presumptive neural tissue has an unusually high requirement for folates. The most telling evidence that neural crest cells have a high demand for folates that, unlike most other embryonic tissue, neural crest cells express very high levels of the message for folate receptors [11–15]. It has been clearly demonstrated that mRNA for *Folr1*, the murine ortholog of the human *FRα* (described later in this chapter), is expressed in neuroepithelial cells of both the neural plate and contiguous areas that would include presumptive cranial neural crest cells [12,13,15].

B. BIOCHEMICAL PATHWAYS

Folate is a water-soluble B vitamin that must be obtained through the diet as it cannot be synthesized de novo by the human body. 5-Methyltetrahydrofolate (5-methyl-THF) is its physiologically active form whose major metabolic role is to carry one-carbon units. These reactions (reviewed in other chapters) include the conversion of serine to glycine, catabolism of histidine, synthesis of thymidylate, remethylation of Hcy to methionine, and purine synthesis. Hence disruptions of folate and folate pathways have diverse implications for cellular metabolism.

Hcy feeds into two separate biochemical pathways: de novo methionine biosynthesis and transsulfuration to cystathionine (Figure 7.2). Of these reactions, the Hcy remethylation cycle bears particular importance on our discussion as it has been repeatedly linked to birth defects. During the remethylation cycle, methylenetetrahydrofolate reductase (MTHFR) catalyzes the irreversible reduction of 5,10-MTHF to 5-methyl-THF, the requisite methyl donor for conversion of Hcy to methionine. Through regulating the usage of 5,10-MTHF, MTHFR also regulates the supply of this substrate for purine synthesis via thymidylate synthase [16]. Methionine synthase (MTR) catalyzes the remethylation of Hcy to methionine with the help of methylcobalamin as an intermediate methyl carrier. MTR plays a critical role in maintaining adequate intracellular methionine and Hcy concentrations as well as the folate pool. The cobalamin cofactor of MTR becomes oxidized over time, and the enzyme becomes inactivated. Regeneration of the functional enzyme requires reductive methylation catalyzed by methionine synthase reductase (MTRR). Because MTRR is the key enzyme in the reductive methylation reaction of MTR, the function

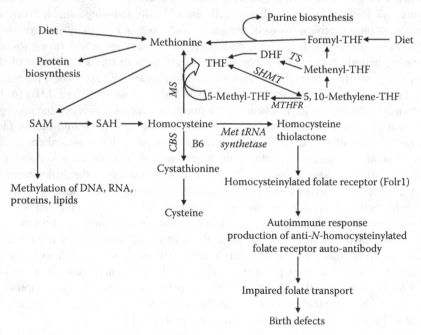

FIGURE 7.2 Homocysteine remethylation cycle with implications for consequences of abnormal folate transport. 5-methyl THF, 5-methyl tetrahydrofolate; 5,10-methylene THF, 5,10-methylene tetrahydrofolate; CBS, cystathionine B-synthase; DHF, dihydrofolate; Formyl THF, formyl tetrahydrofolate; Met tRNA, methionine transfer RNA; Methenyl THF, methenyl tetrahydrofolate; MS, methionine synthase; MTHFR, methylenetetrahydrofolate; SHMT, serine hydroxymethyl transferase; THF, tetrahydrofolate; TS, thymidylate synthase; SAH, S-adenosylhomocysteine; SAM, S-adenosylmethionine. (Reprinted from Taparia S, Gelineau-van Waes J, Rosenquist TH, Finnell RH, *Clin Chem Lab Med* 2007; 45:1717–27. With permission.)

of MTR partly depends on the normal function of MTRR. Methionine is a precursor of S-adenosylmethionine (SAM), which serves as the principal methyl donor for methylation reactions of DNA, proteins, lipids, and other organic and inorganic compounds [17] (Figure 7.2). SAM is then converted to S-adenosylhomocysteine (SAH), which is then hydrolyzed back to Hcy. Therefore, the SAM/SAH ratio, concentration of Hcy, and specific dietary factors such as folate are all important determinants of one-carbon metabolism.

C. HCY METABOLISM

Because of Hcy's pivotal role in folate metabolism, cellular metabolism, and potentially as a contributor to birth defect risks, efforts have been made to more clearly define its contributions during development. Hcy can be converted into Hcy-thiolactone by methionyl-tRNA synthetase, which prevents translational incorporation of Hcy into proteins [18] (Figure 7.2). Hcy-thiolactone is amino reactive and can homocysteinylate proteins at lysine residues, thereby disrupting their function [19]. Homocysteinylated proteins are readily detectable in human serum [20]. Hcy is also readily oxidized, principally as a consequence of auto-oxidation. During oxidation of the sulfhydryl group, superoxide and hydrogen peroxide (H_2O_2) are generated [21]. Although reactive oxygen species molecules are essential for many cellular reactions, partially reduced oxygen species shed from a variety of cellular housekeeping reactions can have significant adverse consequences for the cell. Oxidative stress induces the expression of metallothionein and important antioxidant enzymes, such as superoxide dismutase, that can nevertheless lead to enhanced accumulation of reactive species and the promotion of further oxidative damage. In addition to inducing H_2O_2 and its precursor, superoxide, Hcy further compromises the cell's ability to enzymatically detoxify these radicals. Additionally, hyperhomocysteinemia also increases the sensitivity of mitochondria to oxidative stress–induced toxicity. Further, hyperhomocysteinemia both decreases glutathione peroxidase (GPX) mRNA expression and inactivates GPX function. This enzyme is largely responsible for the dismutation of toxic H_2O_2 to molecular oxygen and water.

II. ROLE OF FOLATE IN SUSCEPTIBILITY TO BIRTH DEFECTS

Several different lines of evidence suggest a role for folate in these aforementioned birth defects involving neural crest cells. These lines of evidence include periconceptional vitamin usage, folate deficiency, folate agonists, antibodies against folate receptors, and polymorphisms in genes related to folate and folate pathways. Chapter 6 provides comprehensive details regarding the association between vitamin usage and birth defects; thus, we refer the reader to that chapter for those details. The other lines of evidence are explored in detail below.

A. FOLATE DEFICIENCY

Experimental animal studies create additional biological plausibility for a relationship between folic acid and reduced risk for human birth defects. Such defects, including orofacial clefts and cardiovascular anomalies, were observed among the offspring of female mice and rats maintained on folate-deficient diets [22–24]. Further, folic acid added to the in vitro medium promotes palatal fusion [25]. Most recently, the Finnell laboratory and others have demonstrated that mouse embryos lacking genes important for folate transport and/or metabolism (*Folr1*, *Folr2*, *Rfc1*, and *Mthfr*) develop congenital malformations spontaneously or are more susceptible to developing such malformations when exposed to environmental contaminants [11,26–29]. These mice are discussed further below.

Mechanistically, folate deficiency leads to a decrease in SAM and an increase in Hcy concentration. Further, dietary deficiencies in folate have been observed to decrease genome-wide methylation both in humans and in animal models, and methylation is corrected when a folate-replete diet is restored (reviewed in Choi and Mason [30]). Hyperhomocysteinemia and DNA hypomethylation contribute to the development of complex congenital disorders [31]. It has been suggested that maternal hyperhomocysteinemia is associated with an increased risk of NTDs. Significantly elevated plasma Hcy and reduced folate concentrations were found in mothers of NTD-affected children [32–35]. Interestingly, maternal hyperhomocysteinemia is associated with an increased risk of CHDs, partially because of low folate and vitamin B12 status [36]. Indeed, maternal hyperhomocysteinemia was significantly associated with a 4.4-fold increased risk of having a child with a CHD [37].

Overall, folate deficiency can compromise genomic integrity and disrupt the normal methylation states of genes. This demonstrates the importance of proper maternal nutrition to transcriptional competence [38]. When we consider that changes in the patterns of gene expression occur during development in response to the dynamic physiological needs of the rapidly growing embryo, nutritional status may directly alter the transcriptional response of a gene encoding a critical protein involved in embryogenesis. This concept highlights the role of folate in proper embryonic development.

B. FOLATE AGONISTS

Additional evidence in support of a role for folate in the etiology of selected birth defects comes from observations in both animal and human studies in which in utero exposures to folate agonists result in malformations. Orofacial clefts have been observed in the offspring of experimental animals treated with folate antimetabolites [39,40]. Hernandez-Diaz et al. [41] demonstrated an increased risk among mothers who used folic acid antagonist medications to deliver children with oral clefts. This risk was reduced if the mother took multivitamin supplements containing folic acid along with dihydrofolate reductase inhibitors (folic acid antagonists) [41]. There are also reports of an association between maternal anticonvulsant use and adverse pregnancy outcomes [42]. Most frontline anticonvulsants are known folate antagonists [43–46]. Other investigators have previously noted associations between maternal anticonvulsant use and clefting [47–49]. Reduction in the bioavailability of folate to the fetus has been proposed as one of their potential underlying teratogenic mechanisms of action. However, to date, there is no evidence that folic acid supplementation helps to reduce the risk of these birth defects in mothers taking antiepileptic drugs, so additional mechanisms must also be involved [50–52].

C.   Antibodies against Folate Receptors

Evidence has emerged that maternal immunological responses can have a substantive impact on embryonic development. When antibodies to rat placenta, kidney, heart, and other tissues are generated and administered to pregnant rats, they bind to the yolk sac and embryonic tissue and are believed to contribute to congenital abnormalities and embryonic death [53,54]. It was postulated that the antibodies binding to the yolk sac impaired the delivery of nutrients to the embryo [54,55]. Further studies provided evidence that monospecific antibodies to folate receptors, also known as folate-binding proteins, can bind in vivo to the membrane-bound receptors on embryonic and extraembryonic tissues, inducing resorptions and developmental defects by blocking cellular uptake of folate [56]. Additionally, large doses of antiserum may cause immune-mediated damage to embryonic tissues [56]. Rothenberg et al. [55] reported the presence of autoantibodies to the folate receptor in 75% of mothers who had given birth to infants affected with an NTD but in only 10% of mothers with nonmalformed infants. This discrepancy in frequency resulted in an odds ratio of 27.0 (95% confidence interval [CI], 3.0–325.1). This extremely provocative, albeit small, study suggests that maternal autoantibodies that bind to the folate receptor and thus block the intracellular uptake of folate by targeting epithelial cells may cause human malformations. These observations could explain the beneficial effect of periconceptional folic acid supplementation. The lack of folate available to the developing embryo secondary to a defective or blocked folate receptor has been demonstrated to increase the risk for folate-responsive congenital anomalies in experimental animal model systems [11,15,27,28,57].

Homocysteinylation of the folate receptor may contribute to the generation of these autoantibodies against the folate receptor. As mentioned previously, methionyl-tRNA synthetase can convert Hcy to Hcy-thiolactone, which can then form N-homocysteinylated protein adducts that can result in altered protein function. These adducts may also be recognized as neo-self antigens and induce an autoimmune response [58]. Thus, a homocysteinylated folate receptor and antibodies with specificity against the homocysteinylated folate receptor could be involved in the causation of selected birth defects. This is an attractive hypothesis as it provides a potential explanation for the observed increase in occurrence of birth defects associated with low folate status, especially because serum antihomocysteinylated protein autoantibodies are directly correlated with plasma total Hcy concentration [58,59].

D.   Gene Polymorphisms

A final line of evidence that implicates the role of folate in birth defects is that polymorphisms in folate transport or metabolism genes have been implicated as risk factors for the complex folate-responsive birth defects discussed in this chapter. Finnell and others [60–71] have investigated the role that polymorphisms in genes participating in folate metabolism and transport play in contributing to risk for specific birth defects.

The *MTHFR* gene and its polymorphisms have been studied extensively and are considered by many to be an established genetic risk factor for NTDs and recurrent early fetal loss, as previously reviewed [69]. The best-characterized *MTHFR* genetic polymorphism is the 677C → T transition that affects the predicted catalytic domain of the MTHFR protein. Homozygosity for the 677T variant predisposes individuals to the development of hyperhomocysteinemia, especially during times of folate insufficiency [72–74]. In 1998, a second common polymorphism in the *MTHFR* gene (1298A → C) was discovered, leading to a glutamate-to-alanine substitution in the presumed regulatory domain of the protein. Individuals who are either heterozygous 1298AC or homozygous 1298CC showed decreased enzyme activity, although their plasma Hcy concentrations were not altered significantly [73,75]. Heterozygosity for both variants in humans has been associated with a 50% to 60% reduction in enzyme activity, elevated Hcy, and reduced folate concentrations [75,76]. Mills et al. [71] observed an increased risk for clefting among individuals who were homozygous for the 677C → T transition. However, other investigators [61,68,70] did not observe an association, either alone or in combination with low maternal folate intake. Interestingly, some evidence for the reverse effect (i.e., lower risk for clefting for those with the TT genotype) has also been observed; in the subset of families in which mothers took less than 400 µg of folic acid, the *MTHFR* T allele was protective for the maternal genotype (LRT *P* = .037, one copy .60, 95% CI 0.39–0.92; two copies .44, 95% CI 0.21–0.95) [77]. Alternatively, an association between TT genotype and spina bifida has been reported [62]. In fact, an association for the two *MTHFR* polymorphisms (677C → T and 1298A → C) and NTDs has been observed in many studies in various populations [34,35,78–84]. Other enzymes in the Hcy remethylation pathway, MTR and MTRR, have modest association with NTD risk [66].

Shaw et al. [62] have investigated the folate transporter, reduced folate carrier (RFC1) [60], and identified a gene–nutrient interaction for NTD risk between RFC1 and periconceptional folic acid use. There is recent evidence from human epidemiological studies demonstrating an association between the 80A → G RFC1 polymorphism and increased risk for NTDs and conotruncal heart defects [60,63,85–87], supporting this hypothesis. We have also observed evidence of a gene–nutrient interaction for risk of clefting in a study in which maternal supplemental folic acid intake and infant transforming growth factor–α genotypes were investigated [88].

The published literature for specific variants is plagued by weak and imprecise estimates of association, as well as a lack of consistent replication across studies. Moreover, it is often unclear whether associations that have been observed reflect genetic effects that are mediated via the maternal genotype, genetic effects that are mediated via the embryonic genotype, or maternal–embryonic genotype interactions [89–91]. Such genetic variation could explain why the body of scientific evidence is replete with varying risk reductions among population subgroups who took folic acid vitamin supplements and obtained clinically adequate amounts of folate from their diets [48]. Hence, definitive conclusions regarding the precise role of specific gene variants are precluded at this time. Nevertheless, there is evidence that mothers of human fetuses with NTDs and CHDs typically exhibit normal folate concentrations [78,92–97], indicating that the etiology is unlikely to be based solely on maternal folate deficiency and suggesting that genetic variation of fetal folate metabolism and/or transport may underlie the beneficial effect of maternal folate supplementation.

III. INTRACELLULAR FOLATE TRANSPORT

Mammalian cells harvest folate from the diet and circulating blood via several different folate transport systems (Table 7.1). The primary mechanisms for folate delivery into the cell are through carrier-mediated, receptor-mediated, and transport-mediated processes. Carrier mediated involves the reduced folate carrier 1 (Rfc1); receptor mediated occurs through folate receptors 1, 2 and 3 (Folr1, Folr2, and Folr3); and transport mediated occurs through the proton-coupled folate transporter(Pcft). These three transport systems are distinguished by their unique patterns of tissue expression, divergent specificities for oxidized versus reduced folates, and differing protein structures and mechanisms for the transmembrane transport of folates. The major route of folate transport into mammalian cells is Rfc1, which is a bidirectional transporter characterized by 12 transmembrane domains (reviewed in Matherly and Goldman [98] and Sirotnak and Tolner [99]). Rfc1 is expressed in multiple tissue types [100,101] and preferentially transports reduced forms of folates. Whereas Rfc1 is fairly ubiquitous, folate receptors are highly localized and are expressed in specific tissues and cellular populations [102,103]. Binding of folates to their receptors is a highly regulated process, thus making *Folr*s excellent candidate genes for conferring susceptibility to congenital defects such as CHDs and NTDs. Murine folate receptor 1 (*Folr1*) is a membrane-bound protein with high binding affinity for 5-methyl-THF. Because most embryonic cells do not express *Folr1* [104], the presence of these receptors in neuroepithelial and neural crest cells [12,13] suggests a critical role for *Folr1*-mediated folate transport in the normal morphogenetic events involved in neural tube closure and neural crest cell–mediated migrations and transformations that regulate development of the cardiac outflow tract [11,26,27]. Murine folate receptor 2 (*Folr2*), on the other hand, has a broader distribution; however, it has a relatively low expression and reduced binding affinity compared with Folr1 [105]. Pcft/heme carrier protein (Hcp1) is a recently discovered intestinal transporter involved in heme and folate uptake in intestinal epithelia [106,107].

IV. MURINE MODELS OF COMPROMISED FOLATE UPTAKE AND BIOTRANSFORMATION: *FOLR1, FOLR2, RFC1, PCFT,* AND *MTHFR*

A. *FOLR1*

Folr1 (previously referred to as *folbp1*, folate-binding protein 1) was genetically ablated in a mouse model by the Finnell laboratory [11]. *Folr1*^{−/−} (knockout) embryos have severe morphogenetic abnormalities and die in utero by embryonic day (E) 10. Histological examination of transverse sections of gestational day (E) 8.5 nullizygous embryos revealed dramatic defects in the neuroepithelium (Figure 7.3). In the cephalic neural tube, neither the forebrain nor the optic vesicles were formed (Figures 7.3A and 7.3B). The neuroepithelium was only one to two cells thick. Perhaps most significantly, the migration of neural crest cells was altered, as only small aggregates of cells were identified within the mesenchyme in the region of the first branchial arch. Furthermore, there was no evidence of neural cell condensations lateral to the alar plate where the trigeminal ganglia normally develop. At the level of the otic placode, the neural tube remained widely flared and thinned (Figures 7.3C and 7.3D).

TABLE 7.1

Folate Transport Systems

System	Synonyms	Description
Reduced folate carrier 1 (Rfc1)	Solute carrier family 19, member 1 (Slc19a1) Folate transporter (Folt) Intestinal folate carrier (Ifc1)	A major route of bidirectional folate transport characterized by 12 transmembrane domains, preferentially transports reduced folates, highly expressed in placenta, yolk sac, neural tube, craniofacial region, limb buds, heart, brush border of the small and large intestine, basolateral membrane of renal tubular epithelium, hepatocytes, choroid plexus, and retinal pigment epithelium
Folate receptors		
Folate receptor 1, adult (Folr1)	Folate receptor (Folr) Folate-binding protein, adult (Fbp) Folate receptor, α Ovarian cancer–associated antigen (Mov18)	A membrane-bound protein with high binding affinity for folic acid, highly expressed in the placenta, yolk sac membrane, dorsal neural tube, choroid plexus, ependymal cells, and peripheral edge of the retina; the GPI-anchored Folr1 internalizes folate via endocytosis and is localized in unique sphingolipid-enriched plasma membrane microdomains known as lipid rafts
Folate receptor 2, fetal (Folr2)	Folate-binding protein, placental Folate receptor, β	A high-affinity receptor for folic acid and several reduced folic acid derivatives; also mediates delivery of 5-methyl-THF to the interior of cells; expressed in placenta, spleen, bone marrow, and thymus; 68% and 79% sequence homology with the Folr1 and Folr3 proteins, respectively
Folate receptor 3 (Folr3)	Folate receptor, γ	A GPI membrane–anchored protein with 23-residue amino-terminal signal peptide, 16 conserved cysteine residues, and 3 potential N-linked glycosylation sites with 71% and 79% amino acid sequence homology to Folr1 and Folr2, respectively; expressed in the immune system and reproductive tissues
Proton-coupled folate transporter (Pcft)	Heme carrier protein 1 (Hcp1) Folate receptor 4 (Folr4) Solute carrier family 46, member 1 (Slc46a1)	Responsible for intestinal absorption of folate and reduced folates; 12 transmembrane domains and intracellular N and C termini; expressed in brush-border membrane, apical cytoplasm of duodenum, brain, breast, kidney, liver, prostate, spleen, retina, and retinal pigment epithelium

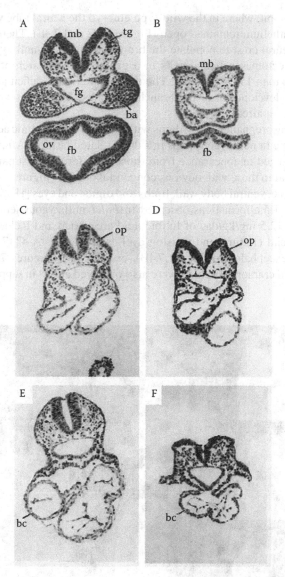

FIGURE 7.3 Histological comparison of the developing neural tube of wild-type (A, C, E) and *Folbp1*^{-/-} (B, D, F) embryos. A, B, frontal sections of the forebrain at the level of the first branchial arch. The neuroepithelium is thin, and the first branchial arch and trigeminal ganglia are absent. C, D, frontal sections at the level of the otic placode reveal thin neuroepithelium and a poorly developed otic pit. E, F, frontal sections caudal to the otic pit. The magnification of the sections was ×120. ba, first branchial arch; bc, bulbus cordis; fb, forebrain; fg, foregut; mb, midbrain; op, otic placode; ov, optic vesicle; tg, trigeminal ganglion. (Reprinted from Piedrahita JA, Oetama B, Bennett GD, van Waes J, Kamen BA, Richardson J, Lacey SW, Anderson RG, Finnell RH, *Nat Genet* 1999; 23:228–32. With permission.)

Caudal to the otic pit, where in the wild-type embryo the neural tube was closed, the mutant neuroepithelium remained open (Figure 7.3E and 7.3F). There was a failure of the cranial neural crest to populate the branchial arches in nullizygous embryos. The number of ectomesenchymal cells in a given branchial arch of a nullizygous embryo was less than 15% of normal. The magnitude of this deficit at E8.5 predicts that subsequent development of the branchial arches and the nascent conotruncus will be severely impaired.

Supplementing pregnant *Folr1*$^{+/-}$ dams with 5-fomyl-THF (folinic acid) rescues the normal phenotype in nullizygous pups in a dose-related fashion. After supplementation, the pups ranged in appearance from those that, for the most part, appeared to be grossly normal to those with obvious congenital defects (Figure 7.4) of the neural tube, lip and palate, ventral body wall, limbs and digits, and eyes [11,15,26,27,57,108–110]. Craniofacial malformations observed in *Folr1* nullizygous fetuses (E18) supplemented with 12.5 mg/kg/day of folinic acid are varied and include cleft lip and palate, craniofacial clefting, and missing eyelids (Figure 7.4A–C, 7.4F, and 7.4G). NTDs such as encephalocele (Figure 7.4B), exencephaly (Figures 7.4D and 7.4E), iniencephaly, and craniorachischisis were also observed at E18 in supplemented *Folr1*

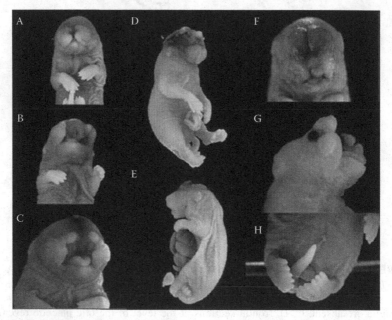

FIGURE 7.4 *Folr1*$^{-/-}$ embryos demonstrate various congenital malformations. A, unilateral midline cleft lip and palate; B, encephalocele and cleft lip and palate; C, bilateral craniofacial clefting; D, exencephaly and omphalocele; E, exencephaly and gastroschisis; F, encephalocele and cleft lip; G, side view of craniofacial cleft in which the *Folr1*$^{-/-}$ embryo has missing eyelids; H, *Folr1*$^{-/-}$ embryo with polydactyly. (Reprinted from Taparia S, Gelineau-van Waes J, Rosenquist TH, Finnell RH, *Clin Chem Lab Med* 2007; 45:1717–27. With permission.)

pups. Additional malformations of *Folr1⁻/⁻* pups include abdominal wall defects such as omphalocele (Figure 7.4D), gastroschisis (Figure 7.4E), and polydactyly (Figure 7.4H).

Cardiovascular phenotypes in *Folr1⁻/⁻* nullizygous mice resemble the phenotypes observed as a consequence of the physical ablation or reduction in neural crest cell precursors observed in chick embryo studies [110]. Gross examination of the hearts from *Folr1⁻/⁻* embryos revealed that they were smaller in overall size compared with wild-type hearts, especially the ventricular chambers (Figure 7.5). There is a wide range of conotruncal heart defects in partially rescued *Folr1⁻/⁻* fetuses, particularly defects of the outflow tract, aortic arch artery abnormalities, and isolated dextrocardia [108,110]. All nullizygous fetuses had ventricular septal defects (VSDs) in the experimental group of dams supplemented with 6.25 mg/kg/day of oral folinic acid [110]. Outflow tract anomalies included transposition of the great arteries (Figures 7.5A and 7.5E), wherein the pulmonary trunk arises from the left ventricle and the aorta arises from the right ventricle, overriding aorta (Figure 7.5F), and double-outlet right ventricle (DORV) (Figures 7.5C and 7.5G), characterized by the pulmonary trunk and the aorta both arising from the right ventricle. Less than 10% of the *Folr1⁻/⁻* hearts exhibited a DORV and a bulging of the pericardial sac. Aortic arch abnormalities included persistent truncus arteriosus (Figure 7.5B), right-sided aortic arch, right-sided ductus arteriosus, and right-sided descending aorta with or without a retroesophageal right subclavian artery, coarctation of aortic arch, or interrupted aortic arch.

Biochemically, *Folr1* heterozygotes (*Folr1⁺/⁻*) and null (*Folr1⁻/⁻*) mice have decreased plasma folate concentrations as compared with wild-type mice of comparable developmental stage. Thus, the *Folr1* gene ablation causes an effective reduction in circulating and tissue folate stores [111]. The plasma folate concentration in unsupplemented *Folr1* null mice is one-third that observed in wild-type mice [26]. Plasma folate concentration of *Folr1⁻/⁻* mice supplemented with 5-methyl-THF is

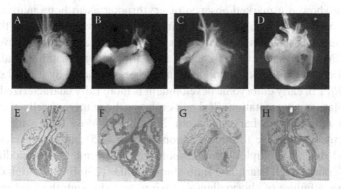

FIGURE 7.5 Outflow track defects in *Folr1* nullizygotes. A, E, transposition of great arteries, interrupted aortic arch; B, persistent truncus arteriosus, dextrocardia; C, G, double-outlet right ventricle; F, overriding aorta; D, H, normal heart. (Reprinted from Zhu H, Wlodarczyk BJ, Scott M, Yu W, Merriweather M, Gelineau-van Waes J, Schwartz RJ, Finnell RH, *Birth Defects Res A Clin Mol Teratol* 2007; 79:257–68. With permission.)

no different from the concentrations found in mice receiving folinic acid [26]. On a folate-replete diet, the plasma concentrations of Hcy in nonpregnant wild-type and *Folr1*$^{+/-}$ dams were the same, but when shifted to a folate-deficient diet, the plasma Hcy values were significantly higher than the corresponding value obtained from dams on a folate-sufficient diet [11].

B. *FOLR2*

Genetic inactivation of the *Folr2* gene (previously referred to as *folbp2*, folate-binding protein 2) did not adversely affect embryonic development, and all nullizygous pups were grossly normal [11]. However, in studies of environmental teratogens, *Folr2* null embryos were extremely sensitive to in utero arsenic exposure, which led to congenital malformations [112]. *Folr2* nullizygous embryos had a significantly higher rate of exencephaly on arsenic exposure compared with wild-type littermates, and this was further exacerbated by folate deficiency. They also displayed other defects, such as omphalocele, gastroschisis, craniofacial clefts, acephalostomia, and microphthalmia [112]. Further, we identified that they have much higher valproic acid (VPA)-induced frequencies of embryonic lethality and exencephaly than did the wild-type control mice [113]. Folate supplementation of wild-type, but not *Folr2*$^{-/-}$, dams reduced embryonic lethality of VPA-treated wild-type embryos when compared on a folate-deficient diet.

C. *RFC1/SLC19A1*

Two research groups have made an *Rfc1* knockout mouse [111,114]. Zhao et al. [114] found that although *Rfc*-null embryos died in utero before E9.5, near-normal development could be sustained in *Rfc1*$^{-/-}$ embryos examined at E18.5 by supplementation of pregnant *Rfc1*$^{+/-}$ dams with 1 mg daily subcutaneous injections of folic acid. About 10% of these animals went on to live birth but died within 12 days. These *Rfc1*$^{-/-}$ mice showed a marked absence of erythropoiesis in bone marrow, spleen, and liver along with lymphoid depletion in the splenic white pulp and thymus. In addition, there was some impairment of renal and seminiferous tubule development. These data indicate that in the absence of *Rfc1* function, neonatal animals die as a result of failure of hematopoietic organs. In studies conducted by Finnell et al. [29], the role of *Rfc1* in early embryonic development is more fully characterized. Without maternal folate supplementation, *Rfc1* null embryos die in utero shortly after implantation. *Rfc1* null embryos harvested from dams on low-dose folic acid (25 mg/kg/day subcutaneous) survive to mid-gestation (E9.5–E10.5) but are developmentally delayed and display multiple "folate-responsive" malformations, including severe NTDs and craniofacial, heart, and limb abnormalities [29]. Examination of the placenta reveals a failure of chorioallantoic fusion, and although the fetal vasculature appears to form normally, there is a pronounced absence of erythropoiesis, with very few nucleated fetal red blood cells (RBC) present in either the fetal blood vessels or the yolk sac blood islands. Furthermore, fetal trophoblasts fail to invade the maternal decidua, and the neural tube also fails to close in most of the observed *Rfc1* nullizygotes as compared with wild-type embryos. Maternal folate supplementation with a high dose of folic acid (50 mg/kg/day subcutaneous) results in survival or "rescue" of 22% of *Rfc1* null fetuses until term (E18.5), although these offspring are often pale and small relative to their wild-type littermates and display a range of malformations of the craniofacies, heart, lungs, and skin. The cardiac malformations are characterized by membranous VSDs, muscular VSD, thin myocardial wall, and VSD with overriding aorta. *Rcf1* knockout mice also exhibit pale and underdeveloped lungs. *Rcf1* nullizygous embryos have an open eyelid defect, and the cornea is thickened and malformed [29]. Visceral yolk sacs of *Rcf1* nullizygous embryos at E9.5 also showed differences in expression of Folr1 as compared with wild-type embryos [29]. The *Rcf1* heterozygous mice do not present with decreased plasma folate concentration as compared with wild-type mice [111].

D. *Pcft/Hcp1*

Targeted inactivation of *Pcft* (also known as SLC46A1) is a newly developed knockout mouse model that is undergoing phenotypic analysis in our laboratory. Finnell et al. (unpublished data) have determined that homozygous mice die within 6 weeks of birth, shortly after being weaned. *Pcft* was initially determined to be a heme transporter; its primary function is still a matter of contention between several research groups that are studying this gene/protein. It is expected that the function of the protein will be conclusively determined in the Finnell laboratory with this model. Oral supplementation of *Pcft*$^{-/-}$ pups with folinic acid had no effect, but intraperitoneal injections (44 mg/kg) with folinic acid reversed hematopoietic phenotypes. Oral supplementation with 5-methyl-THF also reversed hematopoietic phenotypes in nullizygous animals. Phenotypes in unsupplemented nullizygous mice include macrocytic normochromic anemia and thrombocytopenia, as indicated by abnormally large and less mature RBC progenitors, extramedullary erythropoiesis of the spleen, elevated percentage of early erythroblasts, reduced iron storage, and fewer and less mature megakaryocytes. Our results suggest that Pcft has a critical role in dietary folate uptake. Further, this deficiency can be overcome by bypassing Pcft via intraperitoneal injections or via reduced folate carrier uptake of 5-methyl-THF.

E. *Mthfr*

Mthfr nullizygous mice lack functional activity of MTHFR, whereas the heterozygotes have activity of this enzyme reduced by 30% to 40% [115]. Mthfr knockout mice also exhibit hyperhomocysteinemia and global hypomethylation of DNA. Because of these features, the Mthfr-deficient mice provide a good model for a subgroup of humans, with the common polymorphism in *MTHFR* causing decreased activity of MTHFR. Plasma total Hcy concentrations in heterozygous and homozygous knockout mice are 1.6- and 10-fold higher than those in wild-type littermates, respectively. Both heterozygous and homozygous knockouts have significantly decreased SAM concentrations, significantly increased SAH concentrations, or both. The heterozygous knockout mice appear normal, whereas the homozygotes are smaller and show developmental retardation with cerebellar pathology. Abnormal lipid deposition in the proximal portion of the aorta was observed in older heterozygotes and homozygotes, alluding to an atherogenic effect of hyperhomocysteinemia in the mutant mice. Interestingly, *Mthfr* expression during neural tube closure in a VPA-resistant mouse strain (LM/Bc) was found to be significantly higher than that in a VPA-sensitive strain (SWV) [116].

V. SUMMARY

In conclusion, several lines of evidence support an association between maternal use of a multivitamin with folic acid in early pregnancy and a reduced risk for offspring with selected birth defects. The underlying process by which folic acid facilitates this reduced risk is unknown. The working hypothesis is that folate intake prevents defects by compensating for individual genetic susceptibility in several distinct areas. For example, transient elevation in maternal serum folate from supplementation could overcome a range of metabolic inefficiencies and be responsible for the preventive effects of folate intake during the periconceptional period. A search for a genetic explanation for decreased folate status has gained considerable scientific attention. If a putative genetic defect were severe enough to eliminate folate through these systems, it is possible that it would be embryo lethal, and none of the fetuses would survive to term with such elevated folate requirements. However, the risk reduction for NTDs, clefts, or conotruncal heart defects is unlikely to be explained by a simple maternal vitamin deficiency or by a simple maternal absorption deficiency [78,92,93,117–122]. Evidence points toward disordered folate metabolism in some individuals with malformations, with the metabolic error affecting uptake and/or metabolism of folate by fetal cells, which can in turn adversely affect gene expression critical to normal embryogenesis [123]. Thus, the epidemiological and clinical evidence suggests that genetic variation of fetal, or possibly maternal, folate metabolism may underlie some of the risk reduction associated with maternal folate supplementation. It is also possible that maternal immune functions are disrupted by elevated concentrations of Hcy-thiolactone secondary either to a variety of folate pathway gene variants that elevate Hcy concentrations or inhibit its remethylation, or nutritional deficiencies. These have been shown to specifically impact folate transport, and we hypothesize those maternal conditions that promote high plasma Hcy result in the homocysteinylation of the folate receptor (FR), leading to impaired folate binding and uptake, as well as the formation of (folate receptor) autoantibodies. These FR autoantibodies cause embryonic damage by preventing the uptake of folate into fetal tissues, thereby altering gene expression patterns of critical developmentally regulated genes much like that which has been demonstrated in mouse models in which folate transport has been genetically inhibited [15,27,57,108,124]. Clearly, understanding just how folic acid benefits developing embryos is a complex undertaking and will be open to controversial scientific explanations for years to come.

GLOSSARY

Alar plate A neural structure in the embryonic nervous system, part of the dorsal side of neural tube, that involves the communication of general somatic and general visceral sensory impulses. It later becomes a sensory region and part of the spinal cord.

Anophthalmia Absence of the eye, as a result of a congenital malformation of the globe.

Brachycephaly A short head, one that is short in diameter from front to back, caused by the coronal suture fusing prematurely, causing a shortened front-to-back diameter of the skull.

Coarctation A narrowing of the aorta between the upper-body artery branches and the branches to the lower body.

Craniorachischisis The most severe NTD, characterized by anencephaly confluent with spina bifida open from the cervical to the lumbar region.

Dextrocardia Situation of the heart on the right side of the body.

Ectomesenchymal Derived from the neural crest.

Encephalocele NTD characterized by sac-like protrusions of the brain and the membranes that cover it through openings in the skull.

Exencephaly Anterior NTD wherein the brain is located outside of the skull.

Gastroschisis: Abdominal wall defect in which the intestines and sometimes other organs develop outside the fetal abdomen through an opening in the abdominal wall.

Iniencephaly NTD that combines extreme retroflexion (backward bending) of the head with severe defects of the spine.

Malocclusion Misalignment of teeth.

Micrognathia Abnormally small lower jaw.

Omphalocele Abdominal wall defect in which the intestines, liver, and occasionally other organs remain outside the abdomen in a sac because of a defect in the development of the muscles of the abdominal wall.

Otic pit Embryonic rudiment of the internal ear.

Polydactyly Extra fingers.

Trigeminal ganglion A sensory ganglion of the trigeminal nerve responsible for sensation in the face-activating muscles of the mandible.

Truncus arteriosus A complex malformation in which only one artery arises from the heart and forms the aorta and pulmonary artery.

ACKNOWLEDGMENTS

The work was supported in part by National Institutes of Health (NIH) Grants DE016315 (to RHF), HL085859 and NS050249 (GMS), and HL66398 (THR). Additional support was provided by the Centers of Excellence (Award Number U59/CCU913241), the Texas Institute for Genomic Medicine, and the Margaret M. Alkek Foundation. Its contents are solely the responsibility of the authors and do not necessarily represent the official views of the National Institute of Environmental Health Sciences, NIH, or the Centers for Disease Control and Prevention.

REFERENCES

1. Christianson A, Howson CP, Modell B. *March of Dimes Global Report on Birth Defects*. White Plains, NY: March of Dimes Research Foundation, 2006.

2. Yoon PW, Olney RS, Khoury MJ, Sappenfield WM, Chavez GF, Taylor D. Contribution of birth defects and genetic diseases to pediatric hospitalizations. A population-based study. *Arch Pediatr Adolesc Med* 1997; 151:1096–103.
3. Waitzman NJ, Romano PS, Scheffler RM. Estimates of the economic costs of birth defects. *Inquiry* 1994; 31:188–205.
4. Martin JA, Kochanek KD, Strobino DM, Guyer B, MacGillivray I. Annual summary of vital statistics—2003. *Pediatrics* 2005; 115:619–34.
5. Scherson T, Serbedzija G, Fraser S, Bronner-Fraser M. Regulative capacity of the cranial neural tube to form neural crest. *Development* 1993; 118:1049–62.
6. Noden DM. An analysis of migratory behavior of avian cephalic neural crest cells. *Dev Biol* 1975; 42:106–30.
7. Noden DM. The control of avian cephalic neural crest cytodifferentiation. I. Skeletal and connective tissues. *Dev Biol* 1978; 67:296–312.
8. Noden DM. The control of avian cephalic neural crest cytodifferentiation. II. Neural tissues. *Dev Biol* 1978; 67:313–29.
9. Noden DM. The embryonic origins of avian cephalic and cervical muscles and associated connective tissues. *Am J Anat* 1983; 168:257–76.
10. Maschhoff KL, Baldwin HS. Molecular determinants of neural crest migration. *Am J Med Genet* 2000; 97:280–88.
11. Piedrahita JA, Oetama B, Bennett GD, van Waes J, Kamen BA, Richardson J, Lacey SW, Anderson RG, Finnell RH. Mice lacking the folic acid-binding protein Folbp1 are defective in early embryonic development. *Nat Genet* 1999; 23:228–32.
12. Barber RC, Bennett GD, Greer KA, Finnell RH. Expression patterns of folate binding proteins one and two in the developing mouse embryo. *Mol Genet Metab* 1999; 66:31–39.
13. Saitsu H, Ishibashi M, Nakano H, Shiota K. Spatial and temporal expression of folate-binding protein 1 (Fbp1) is closely associated with anterior neural tube closure in mice. *Dev Dyn* 2003; 226:112–17.
14. Shaw GM, O'Malley CD, Wasserman CR, Tolarova MM, Lammer EJ. Maternal periconceptional use of multivitamins and reduced risk for conotruncal heart defects and limb deficiencies among offspring. *Am J Med Genet* 1995; 59:536–45.
15. Tang LS, Finnell RH. Neural and orofacial defects in Folp1 knockout mice [corrected]. *Birth Defects Res A Clin Mol Teratol* 2003; 67:209–18.
16. Schwahn B, Rozen R. Polymorphisms in the methylenetetrahydrofolate reductase gene: Clinical consequences. *Am J Pharmacogenomics* 2001; 1:189–201.
17. Selhub J. Homocysteine metabolism. *Annu Rev Nutr* 1999; 19:217–46.
18. Jakubowski H. Molecular basis of homocysteine toxicity in humans. *Cell Mol Life Sci* 2004; 61:470–87.
19. Jakubowski H. Homocysteine thiolactone: Metabolic origin and protein homocysteinylation in humans. *J Nutr* 2000; 130:377S–81S.
20. Perna AF, Satta E, Acanfora F, Lombardi C, Ingrosso D, De Santo NG. Increased plasma protein homocysteinylation in hemodialysis patients. *Kidney Int* 2006; 69:869–76.
21. Loscalzo J. The oxidant stress of hyperhomocyst(e)inemia. *J Clin Invest* 1996; 98:5–7.
22. Nelson MM. Teratogenic effects of pteroylglutamic acid deficiency in the rat. *Ciba Foundation Symp Cong Malfs* 1960:134–57.
23. Nelson MM, Baird CD, Wright HV, Evans HM. Multiple congenital abnormalities in the rat resulting from riboflavin deficiency induced by the antimetabolite galactoflavin. *J Nutr* 1956; 58:125–34.
24. Warkany J, Nelson RC. Appearance of skeletal abnormalities in the offspring of rats reared on a deficient diet. *Science* 1940; 92:383–84.
25. Natsume N, Nagatsu Y, Kawai T. Direct effect of vitamins at the time of palatal fusion. *Plast Reconstr Surg* 1998; 102:2512–13.

26. Spiegelstein O, Mitchell LE, Merriweather MY, Wicker NJ, Zhang Q, Lammer EJ, Finnell RH. Embryonic development of folate binding protein-1 (Folbp1) knockout mice: Effects of the chemical form, dose, and timing of maternal folate supplementation. *Dev Dyn* 2004; 231:221–31.

27. Tang LS, Wlodarczyk BJ, Santillano DR, Miranda RC, Finnell RH. Developmental consequences of abnormal folate transport during murine heart morphogenesis. *Birth Defects Res A Clin Mol Teratol* 2004; 70:449–58.

28. Finnell RH, Spiegelstein O, Wlodarczyk B, Triplett A, Pogribny IP, Melnyk S, James JS. DNA methylation in Folbp1 knockout mice supplemented with folic acid during gestation. *J Nutr* 2002; 132:2457S–61S.

29. Gelineau-van Waes J, Heller S, Bauer LK, Wilberding J, Maddox JR, Aleman F, Rosenquist TH, Finnell RH. Embryonic development in the reduced folate carrier knockout mouse is modulated by maternal folate supplementation. *Birth Defects Res A Clin Mol Teratol* 2008; 82:494–507.

30. Choi SW, Mason JB. Folate status: Effects on pathways of colorectal carcinogenesis. *J Nutr* 2002; 132:2413S–18S.

31. McKay JA, Williams EA, Mathers JC. Folate and DNA methylation during in utero development and aging. *Biochem Soc Trans* 2004; 32:1006–07.

32. MRC Vitamin Study Research Group. Prevention of neural tube defects: Results of the Medical Research Council Vitamin Study. *Lancet* 1991; 338:131–37.

33. Czeizel AE, Dudas I. Prevention of the first occurrence of neural-tube defects by periconceptional vitamin supplementation. *N Engl J Med* 1992; 327:1832–35.

34. Whitehead AS, Gallagher P, Mills JL, Kirke PN, Burke H, Molloy AM, Weir DG, Shields DC, Scott JM. A genetic defect in 5,10 methylenetetrahydrofolate reductase in neural tube defects. *QJM* 1995; 88:763–66.

35. Mills JL, McPartlin JM, Kirke PN, Lee YJ, Conley MR, Weir DG, Scott JM. Homocysteine metabolism in pregnancies complicated by neural-tube defects. *Lancet* 1995; 345:149–51.

36. Verkleij-Hagoort AC, Verlinde M, Ursem NT, Lindemans J, Helbing WA, Ottenkamp J, Siebel FM, et al. Maternal hyperhomocysteinaemia is a risk factor for congenital heart disease. *BJOG* 2006; 113:1412–18.

37. Verkleij-Hagoort A, Bliek J, Sayed-Tabatabaei F, Ursem N, Steegers E, Steegers-Theunissen R. Hyperhomocysteinemia and MTHFR polymorphisms in association with orofacial clefts and congenital heart defects: A meta-analysis. *Am J Med Genet A* 2007; 143:952–60.

38. Friso S, Choi SW. Gene-nutrient interactions and DNA methylation. *J Nutr* 2002; 132:2382S–87S.

39. Jordan RL, Wilson JG, Schumacher HJ. Embryotoxicity of the folate antagonist methotrexate in rats and rabbits. *Teratology* 1977; 15:73–79.

40. Peer LA, Strean LP. Stress as an etiologic factor in the development of cleft palate. *Plast Reconstr Surg* 1956; 18:1–8.

41. Hernandez-Diaz S, Werler MM, Walker AH, Mitchell AA. Folic acid antagonists during pregnancy and the risk of birth defects. *N Engl J Med* 2000; 343:1608–14.

42. Anderson RC. Cardiac defects in children of mothers receiving anticonvulsant therapy during pregnancy. *J Pediatr* 1976; 89:318–19.

43. Dansky LV, Andermann E, Rosenblatt D, Sherwin AL, Andermann F. Anticonvulsants, folate levels, and pregnancy outcome: A prospective study. *Ann Neurol* 1987; 21:176–82.

44. Dansky LV, Finnell RH. Parental epilepsy, anticonvulsant drugs, and reproductive outcome: Epidemiologic and experimental findings spanning three decades; 2: Human studies. *Reprod Toxicol* 1991; 5:301–35.

45. Wegner C, Nau H. Diurnal variation of folate concentrations in mouse embryo and plasma: The protective effect of folinic acid on valproic-acid-induced teratogenicity is time dependent. *Reprod Toxicol* 1991; 5:465–71.

46. Wegner C, Nau H. Alteration of embryonic folate metabolism by valproic acid during organogenesis: Implications for mechanism of teratogenesis. *Neurology* 1992; 42:17–24.

47. Hill L, Murphy M, McDowall M, Paul AH. Maternal drug histories and congenital malformations: Limb reduction defects and oral clefts. *J Epidemiol Community Health* 1988; 42:1–7.

48. Shaw GM, Wasserman CR, O'Malley CD, Lammer EJ, Finnell RH. Orofacial clefts and maternal anticonvulsant use. *Reprod Toxicol* 1995; 9:97–98.

49. Speidel BD, Meadow SR. Maternal epilepsy and abnormalities of the fetus and newborn. *Lancet* 1972; 2:839–43.

50. Duncan S, Mercho S, Lopes-Cendes I, Seni MH, Benjamin A, Dubeau F, Andermann F, Andermann E. Repeated neural tube defects and valproate monotherapy suggest a pharmacogenetic abnormality. *Epilepsia* 2001; 42:750–53.

51. Kaneko S, Battino D, Andermann E, Wada K, Kan R, Takeda A, Nakane Y, et al. Congenital malformations due to antiepileptic drugs. *Epilepsy Res* 1999; 33:145–58.

52. Candito M, Naimi M, Boisson C, Rudigoz JC, Gaucherand P, Gueant JL, Luton D, Van Obberghen E. Plasma vitamin values and antiepileptic therapy: Case reports of pregnancy outcomes affected by a neural tube defect. *Birth Defects Res A Clin Mol Teratol* 2007; 79:62–64.

53. da Costa M, Rothenberg SP. Purification and characterization of folate binding proteins from rat placenta. *Biochim Biophys Acta* 1996; 1292:23–30.

54. da Costa M, Sequeira JM, Rothenberg SP, Weedon J. Antibodies to folate receptors impair embryogenesis and fetal development in the rat. *Birth Defects Res A Clin Mol Teratol* 2003; 67:837–47.

55. Rothenberg SP, da Costa MP, Sequeira JM, Cracco J, Roberts JL, Weedon J, Quadros EV. Autoantibodies against folate receptors in women with a pregnancy complicated by a neural-tube defect. *N Engl J Med* 2004; 350:134–42.

56. Sadasivan E, da Costa M, Rothenberg SP, Brink L. Purification, properties, and immunological characterization of folate-binding proteins from human leukemia cells. *Biochim Biophys Acta* 1987; 925:36–47.

57. Tang LS, Santillano DR, Wlodarczyk BJ, Miranda RC, Finnell RH. Role of Folbp1 in the regional regulation of apoptosis and cell proliferation in the developing neural tube and craniofacies. *Am J Med Genet C Semin Med Genet* 2005; 135:48–58.

58. Jakubowski H. Pathophysiological consequences of homocysteine excess. *J Nutr* 2006; 136:1741S–49S.

59. Undas A, Perla J, Lacinski M, Trzeciak W, Kazmierski R, Jakubowski H. Autoantibodies against N-homocysteinylated proteins in humans: Implications for atherosclerosis. *Stroke* 2004; 35:1299–304.

60. Shaw GM, Lammer EJ, Zhu H, Baker MW, Neri E, Finnell RH. Maternal periconceptional vitamin use, genetic variation of infant reduced folate carrier (A80G), and risk of spina bifida. *Am J Med Genet* 2002; 108:1–6.

61. Shaw GM, Rozen R, Finnell RH, Todoroff K, Lammer EJ. Infant C677T mutation in MTHFR, maternal periconceptional vitamin use, and cleft lip. *Am J Med Genet* 1998; 80:196–98.

62. Shaw GM, Rozen R, Finnell RH, Wasserman CR, Lammer EJ. Maternal vitamin use, genetic variation of infant methylenetetrahydrofolate reductase, and risk for spina bifida. *Am J Epidemiol* 1998; 148:30–37.

63. Shaw GM, Zhu H, Lammer EJ, Yang W, Finnell RH. Genetic variation of infant reduced folate carrier (A80G) and risk of orofacial and conotruncal heart defects. *Am J Epidemiol* 2003; 158:747–52.

64. Volcik KA, Blanton SH, Kruzel MC, Townsend IT, Tyerman GH, Mier RJ, Northrup H. Testing for genetic associations with the PAX gene family in a spina bifida population. *Am J Med Genet* 2002; 110:195–202.

65. Volcik KA, Shaw GM, Lammer EJ, Zhu H, Finnell RH. Evaluation of infant methyl-enetetrahydrofolate reductase genotype, maternal vitamin use, and risk of high versus low level spina bifida defects. *Birth Defects Res Part A Clin Mol Teratol* 2003; 67:154–57.

66. Zhu H, Wicker NJ, Shaw GM, Lammer EJ, Hendricks K, Suarez L, Canfield M, Finnell RH. Homocysteine remethylation enzyme polymorphisms and increased risks for neural tube defects. *Mol Genet Metab* 2003; 78:216–21.

67. Shaw GM, Todoroff K, Finnell RH, Lammer EJ, Leclerc D, Gravel RA, Rozen R. Infant methionine synthase variants and risk for spina bifida. *J Med Genet* 1999; 36:86–87.

68. Shaw GM, Todoroff K, Finnell RH, Rozen R, Lammer EJ. Maternal vitamin use, infant C677T mutation in MTHFR, and isolated cleft palate risk. *Am J Med Genet* 1999; 85:84–85.

69. Botto LD, Yang Q. 5,10-Methylenetetrahydrofolate reductase gene variants and congenital anomalies: A HuGE review. *Am J Epidemiol* 2000; 151:862–77.

70. Gaspar DA, Pavanello RC, Zatz M, Passos-Bueno MR, Andre M, Steman S, Wyszynski DF, Matiolli SR. Role of the C677T polymorphism at the MTHFR gene on risk to non-syndromic cleft lip with/without cleft palate: Results from a case-control study in Brazil. *Am J Med Genet* 1999; 87:197–99.

71. Mills JL, Kirke PN, Molloy AM, Burke H, Conley MR, Lee YJ, Mayne PD, Weir DG, Scott JM. Methylenetetrahydrofolate reductase thermolabile variant and oral clefts. *Am J Med Genet* 1999; 86:71–74.

72. Frosst P, Blom HJ, Milos R, Goyette P, Sheppard CA, Matthews RG, Boers GJ, et al. A candidate genetic risk factor for vascular disease: A common mutation in meth-ylenetetrahydrofolate reductase. *Nat Genet* 1995; 10:111–13.

73. van der Put NM, Gabreels F, Stevens EM, Smeitink JA, Trijbels FJ, Eskes TK, van den Heuvel LP, Blom HJ. A second common mutation in the methylenetetrahydrofo-late reductase gene: An additional risk factor for neural-tube defects? *Am J Hum Genet* 1998; 62:1044–51.

74. Jacques PF, Bostom AG, Williams RR, Ellison RC, Eckfeldt JH, Rosenberg IH, Selhub J, Rozen R. Relation between folate status, a common mutation in methylenetetrahydro-folate reductase, and plasma homocysteine concentrations. *Circulation* 1996; 93:7–9.

75. Weisberg I, Tran P, Christensen B, Sibani S, Rozen R. A second genetic polymorphism in methylenetetrahydrofolate reductase (MTHFR) associated with decreased enzyme activity. *Mol Genet Metab* 1998; 64:169–72.

76. Weisberg IS, Jacques PF, Selhub J, Bostom AG, Chen Z, Curtis Ellison R, Eckfeldt JH, Rozen R. The 1298A-->C polymorphism in methylenetetrahydrofolate reductase (MTHFR): In vitro expression and association with homocysteine. *Atherosclerosis* 2001; 156:409–15.

77. Boyles AL, Wilcox AJ, Taylor JA, Meyer K, Fredriksen A, Ueland PM, Drevon CA, Vollset SE, Lie RT. Folate and one-carbon metabolism gene polymorphisms and their associations with oral facial clefts. *Am J Med Genet A* 2008; 146A:440–49.

78. Kirke PN, Molloy AM, Daly LE, Burke H, Weir DG, Scott JM. Maternal plasma folate and vitamin B12 are independent risk factors for neural tube defects. *Q J Med* 1993; 86:703–08.

79. van der Put NM, Steegers-Theunissen RP, Frosst P, Trijbels FJ, Eskes TK, van den Heuvel LP, Mariman EC, den Heyer M, Rozen R, Blom HJ. Mutated methylenetetrahy-drofolate reductase as a risk factor for spina bifida. *Lancet* 1995; 346:1070–71.

80. van der Put NM, van den Heuvel LP, Steegers-Theunissen RP, Trijbels FJ, Eskes TK, Mariman EC, den Heyer M, Blom HJ. Decreased methylene tetrahydrofolate reductase activity due to the 677C-->T mutation in families with spina bifida offspring. *J Mol Med* 1996; 74:691–94.

81. Ou CY, Stevenson RE, Brown VK, Schwartz CE, Allen WP, Khoury MJ, Rozen R, Oakley GP Jr, Adams MJ Jr. 5,10 Methylenetetrahydrofolate reductase genetic polymorphism as a risk factor for neural tube defects. *Am J Med Genet* 1996; 63:610–14.

82. Grandone E, Corrao AM, Colaizzo D, Vecchione G, Di Girgenti C, Paladini D, Sardella L, et al. Homocysteine metabolism in families from southern Italy with neural tube defects: Role of genetic and nutritional determinants. *Prenat Diagn* 2006; 26:1–5.

83. Felix TM, Leistner S, Giugliani R. Metabolic effects and the methylenetetrahydrofolate reductase (MTHFR) polymorphism associated with neural tube defects in southern Brazil. *Birth Defects Res A Clin Mol Teratol* 2004; 70:459–63.

84. De Marco P, Calevo MG, Moroni A, Arata L, Merello E, Finnell RH, Zhu H, Andreussi L, Cama A, Capra V. Study of MTHFR and MS polymorphisms as risk factors for NTD in the Italian population. *J Hum Genet* 2002; 47:319–24.

85. De Marco P, Calevo MG, Moroni A, Merello E, Raso A, Finnell RH, Zhu H, Andreussi L, Cama A, Capra V. Reduced folate carrier polymorphism (80A-->G) and neural tube defects. *Eur J Hum Genet* 2003; 11:245–52.

86. Pei L, Zhu H, Ren A, Li Z, Hao L, Finnell RH. Reduced folate carrier gene is a risk factor for neural tube defects in a Chinese population. *Birth Defects Res A Clin Mol Teratol* 2005; 73:430–33.

87. Pei L, Zhu H, Zhu J, Ren A, Finnell RH, Li Z. Genetic variation of infant reduced folate carrier (A80G) and risk of orofacial defects and congenital heart defects in China. *Ann Epidemiol* 2006; 16:352–56.

88. Shaw GM, Wasserman CR, Murray JC, Lammer EJ. Infant TGF-alpha genotype, orofacial clefts, and maternal periconceptional multivitamin use. *Cleft Palate Craniofac J* 1998; 35:366–70.

89. Doolin MT, Barbaux S, McDonnell M, Hoess K, Whitehead AS, Mitchell LE. Maternal genetic effects, exerted by genes involved in homocysteine remethylation, influence the risk of spina bifida. *Am J Hum Genet* 2002; 71:1222–26.

90. Mitchell LE. Epidemiology of neural tube defects. *Am J Med Genet C Semin Med Genet* 2005; 135C:88–94.

91. Posey DL, Khoury MJ, Mulinare J, Adams MJ Jr, Ou CY. Is mutated MTHFR a risk factor for neural tube defects? *Lancet* 1996; 347:686–87.

92. Yates JR, Ferguson-Smith MA, Shenkin A, Guzman-Rodriguez R, White M, Clark BJ. Is disordered folate metabolism the basis for the genetic predisposition to neural tube defects? *Clin Genet* 1987; 31:279–87.

93. Economides DL, Ferguson J, Mackenzie IZ, Darley J, Ware II, Holmes-Siedle M. Folate and vitamin B12 concentrations in maternal and fetal blood, and amniotic fluid in second trimester pregnancies complicated by neural tube defects. *Br J Obstet Gynaecol* 1992; 99:23–25.

94. Mills JL, Tuomilehto J, Yu KF, Colman N, Blaner WS, Koskela P, Rundle WE, Forman M, Toivanen L, Rhoads GG. Maternal vitamin levels during pregnancies producing infants with neural tube defects. *J Pediatr* 1992; 120:863–71.

95. Molloy AM, Kirke P, Hillary I, Weir DG, Scott JM. Maternal serum folate and vitamin B12 concentrations in pregnancies associated with neural tube defects. *Arch Dis Child* 1985; 60:660–65.

96. van der Put NM, van Straaten HW, Trijbels FJ, Blom HJ. Folate, homocysteine and neural tube defects: An overview. *Exp Biol Med (Maywood)* 2001; 226:243–70.

97. Wald NJ, Hackshaw AD, Stone R, Sourial NA. Blood folic acid and vitamin B12 in relation to neural tube defects. *Br J Obstet Gynaecol* 1996; 103:319–24.

98. Matherly LH, Goldman DI. Membrane transport of folates. *Vitam Horm* 2003; 66:403–56.

99. Sirotnak FM, Tolner B. Carrier-mediated membrane transport of folates in mammalian cells. *Annu Rev Nutr* 1999; 19:91–122.

100. Maddox DM, Manlapat A, Roon P, Prasad P, Ganapathy V, Smith SB. Reduced-folate carrier (RFC) is expressed in placenta and yolk sac, as well as in cells of the developing forebrain, hindbrain, neural tube, craniofacial region, eye, limb buds and heart. *BMC Dev Biol* 2003; 3:6.

101. Wang Y, Zhao R, Russell RG, Goldman ID. Localization of the murine reduced folate carrier as assessed by immunohistochemical analysis. *Biochim Biophys Acta* 2001; 1513:49–54.
102. Elwood PC. Molecular cloning and characterization of the human folate-binding protein cDNA from placenta and malignant tissue culture (KB) cells. *J Biol Chem* 1989; 264:14893–901.
103. Ratnam M, Marquardt H, Duhring JL, Freisheim JH. Homologous membrane folate binding proteins in human placenta: Cloning and sequence of a cDNA. *Biochemistry* 1989; 28:8249–54.
104. Page ST, Owen WC, Price K, Elwood PC. Expression of the human placental folate receptor transcript is regulated in human tissues. Organization and full nucleotide sequence of the gene. *J Mol Biol* 1993; 229:1175–83.
105. Ross JF, Chaudhuri PK, Ratnam M. Differential regulation of folate receptor isoforms in normal and malignant tissues in vivo and in established cell lines. Physiologic and clinical implications. *Cancer* 1994; 73:2432–43.
106. Qiu A, Jansen M, Sakaris A, Min SH, Chattopadhyay S, Tsai E, Sandoval C, Zhao R, Akabas MH, Goldman ID. Identification of an intestinal folate transporter and the molecular basis for hereditary folate malabsorption. *Cell* 2006; 127:917–28.
107. Rouault TA. The intestinal heme transporter revealed. *Cell* 2005; 122:649–51.
108. Gelineau-van Waes J, Aleman F, Maddox J, Bauer L, Wilberding J, Rosenquist T, Finnell R. Folic acid prevents conotruncal malformations in Folbp1 knockout mice: Role of folate in cardiac neural crest cell survival and migration. In: Jansen G, Peters G, eds., *Chemistry and Biology of Pteridines and Folates.* Heilbronn, Germany: Kluwer Academic Publishers, 2007:483–502.
109. Spiegelstein O, Gould A, Wlodarczyk B, Tsie M, Lu X, Le C, Troen A, et al. Developmental consequences of in utero sodium arsenate exposure in mice with folate transport deficiencies. *Toxicol Appl Pharmacol* 2005; 203:18–26.
110. Zhu H, Wlodarczyk BJ, Scott M, Yu W, Merriweather M, Gelineau-van Waes J, Schwartz RJ, Finnell RH. Cardiovascular abnormalities in Folr1 knockout mice and folate rescue. *Birth Defects Res A Clin Mol Teratol* 2007; 79:257–68.
111. Ma DW, Finnell RH, Davidson LA, Callaway ES, Spiegelstein O, Piedrahita JA, Salbaum JM, et al. Folate transport gene inactivation in mice increases sensitivity to colon carcinogenesis. *Cancer Res* 2005; 65:887–97.
112. Wlodarczyk B, Spiegelstein O, Gelineau-van Waes J, Vorce RL, Lu X, Le CX, Finnell RH. Arsenic-induced congenital malformations in genetically susceptible folate binding protein-2 knockout mice. *Toxicol Appl Pharmacol* 2001; 177:238–46.
113. Spiegelstein O, Merriweather MY, Wicker NJ, Finnell RH. Valproate-induced neural tube defects in folate-binding protein-2 (Folbp2) knockout mice. *Birth Defects Res A Clin Mol Teratol* 2003; 67:974–78.
114. Zhao R, Russell RG, Wang Y, Liu L, Gao F, Kneitz B, Edelmann W, Goldman ID. Rescue of embryonic lethality in reduced folate carrier-deficient mice by maternal folic acid supplementation reveals early neonatal failure of hematopoietic organs. *J Biol Chem* 2001; 276:10224–28.
115. Chen Z, Karaplis AC, Ackerman SL, Pogribny IP, Melnyk S, Lussier-Cacan S, Chen MF, et al. Mice deficient in methylenetetrahydrofolate reductase exhibit hyperhomocysteinemia and decreased methylation capacity, with neuropathology and aortic lipid deposition. *Hum Mol Genet* 2001; 10:433–43.
116. Finnell RH, Wlodarczyk BC, Craig JC, Piedrahita JA, Bennett GD. Strain-dependent alterations in the expression of folate pathway genes following teratogenic exposure to valproic acid in a mouse model. *Am J Med Genet* 1997; 70:303–11.
117. Bower C, Stanley FJ, Croft M, de Klerk N, Davis RE, Nicol DJ. Absorption of pteroylpolyglutamates in mothers of infants with neural tube defects. *Br J Nutr* 1993; 69:827–34.

118. Bower C, Stanley FJ, Nicol DJ. Maternal folate status and the risk for neural tube defects. The role of dietary folate. *Ann N Y Acad Sci* 1993; 678:146–55.
119. Gardiki-Kouidou P, Seller MJ. Amniotic fluid folate, vitamin B12 and transcobalamins in neural tube defects. *Clin Genet* 1988; 33:441–48.
120. Lucock MD, Wild J, Schorah CJ, Levene MI, Hartley R. The methylfolate axis in neural tube defects: In vitro characterisation and clinical investigation. *Biochem Med Metab Biol* 1994; 52:101–14.
121. Weekes EW, Tamura T, Davis RO, Birch R, Vaughn WH, Franklin JC, Barganier C, Cosper P, Finley SC, Finley WH. Nutrient levels in amniotic fluid from women with normal and neural tube defect pregnancies. *Biol Neonate* 1992; 61:226–31.
122. Wild J, Schorah CJ, Sheldon TA, Smithells RW. Investigation of factors influencing folate status in women who have had a neural tube defect-affected infant. *Br J Obstet Gynaecol* 1993; 100:546–49.
123. Schorah CJ, Habibzadeh N, Wild J, Smithells RW, Seller MJ. Possible abnormalities of folate and vitamin B12 metabolism associated with neural tube defects. *Ann N Y Acad Sci* 1993; 678:81–91.
124. Gelineau-van Waes J, Maddox JR, Smith LM, van Waes M, Wilberding J, Eudy JD, Bauer LK, Finnell RH. Microarray analysis of E9.5 reduced folate carrier (RFC1; Slc19a1) knockout embryos reveals altered expression of genes in the cubilin-megalin multiligand endocytic receptor complex. *BMC Genomics* 2008; 9:156.
125. Taparia S, Gelineau-van Waes J, Rosenquist TH, Finnell RH. Importance of folate-homocysteine homeostasis during early embryonic development. *Clin Chem Lab Med* 2007; 45:1717–27.

8 Folic Acid Fortification

Neural Tube Defect Risk Reduction—A Global Perspective

*Robert J. Berry, Joseph Mulinare,
and Heather C. Hamner*

CONTENTS

I. INTRODUCTION

It became widely accepted in the early 1990s that adequate maternal consumption of folic acid before pregnancy and during the early weeks of gestation could prevent most, but not all, neural tube defects (NTDs). This acceptance resulted from the early stopping of both the British Medical Research Council (MRC) [1] and Hungarian [2] randomized controlled trials (RCTs) of vitamins to prevent NTDs in 1991 and 1992, respectively (see Section II, Recommendations to Prevent NTDs). In 1991, the Centers for Disease Control and Prevention (CDC) recommended that all women with a history of a previous NTD-affected pregnancy should consume 4,000 µg of folic acid daily to prevent the recurrence of an NTD-affected pregnancy [3]. In 1992, the US Public Health Service (USPHS) recommended that all women capable of becoming pregnant consume 400 µg of folic acid daily to prevent the first occurrence of an NTD-affected pregnancy [4]. In 1998, a similar recommendation from the Institute of Medicine (IOM) stated that women capable of becoming pregnant should consume 400 µg of folic acid daily from fortified foods, supplements, or both, in addition to consuming food folate from a varied diet [5].

In 1996, in an effort to ensure that women were consuming adequate folic acid and to assist in the prevention of NTDs, the United States became the first country (followed closely by Canada) to mandate fortification of all enriched cereal grain products* with folic acid [6]. Mandatory fortification was fully implemented in the United States and Canada by the start of 1998. Costa Rica [7] implemented wheat and corn flour fortification by 1998, and Chile followed in 2000 [8]. These mandatory fortification efforts have resulted in substantial reductions in the birth prevalence rate of NTDs in the United States, Canada, Costa Rica, and Chile [7–10]. More than 50 countries now implement mandatory flour fortification programs [11]. Mandatory folic acid fortification of a variety of products made from different flours is proving to be one of the most successful public health interventions ever in preventing serious birth defects of the brain and spine.

---

* *Enriched* implies that micronutrients have been added back to their original level after processing.

This chapter discusses existing recommendations, policies, and programs to fortify flour and other cereal grain products with folic acid and the effect folic acid has had on NTD birth prevalence rates, blood folate concentrations, and overall dietary intakes. Other chapters discuss other potential beneficial and adverse effects attributed to intake of folic acid from fortification programs.

II. RECOMMENDATIONS TO PREVENT NEURAL TUBE DEFECTS

In 1965, Hibbard et al. [12] first proposed that folate insufficiency might be involved in the causation of NTDs. A number of studies evaluating whether women's consumption of this vitamin had the potential for preventing NTDs began in the 1980s and early 1990s [13–22]. In 1991, the pivotal RCT, which was conducted by the British MRC, was stopped early because women with a history of a previous NTD-affected pregnancy who consumed 4,000 µg of folic acid daily reduced their risk of having another NTD-affected pregnancy by 70% [1]. In 1992, another RCT conducted in Hungary among women without a previous NTD-affected pregnancy was also stopped early because women who consumed a daily prenatal multivitamin containing 800 µg of folic acid reduced their risk of having an NTD-affected pregnancy by 100% [2]. These crucial studies led to key recommendations issued by the United States in 1991 [3], 1992 [4], and 1998 [5]. These recommendations have been the basis for the discussion and implementation of folic acid fortification programs in countries around the world.

A. UNITED STATES

1. Centers for Disease Control and Prevention

In 1991, the CDC issued a recommendation that all women with a history of a previous NTD-affected pregnancy should consume 4,000 µg of folic acid daily to prevent the recurrence of an NTD-affected pregnancy:

> Women who have had a pregnancy resulting in an infant or fetus with a neural tube defect should be advised to consult their physician as soon as they plan a pregnancy. Unless contraindicated, they should be advised to take 4 mg per day of folic acid starting at the time they plan to become pregnant [3].

2. United States Public Health Service

In 1992, the USPHS issued a recommendation targeting all women capable of becoming pregnant to prevent the first occurrence of an NTD-affected pregnancy:

> All women of childbearing age in the United States who are capable of becoming pregnant should consume 0.4 mg (400 µg) of folic acid per day for the purpose of reducing their risk of having a pregnancy affected with spina bifida or other NTDs [4].

3. Institute of Medicine

In 1998, after a thorough review of the available literature on folate, the IOM established the recommended Dietary Reference Intakes (DRIs) for folate for the US population [5]. The IOM also established a separate recommendation specifically targeted to women capable of becoming pregnant to reduce the risk of NTDs. This recommendation was similar to that made by the USPHS in 1992. The IOM recommendation stated:

> In particular, it is recommended that women capable of becoming pregnant consume 400 μg of folate daily from supplements, fortified foods, or both, in addition to consuming food folate from a varied diet [5].

B. CANADA, CENTRAL AMERICA, AND CHILE

In 1993, Health Canada and the Canadian Society of Obstetricians and Gynecologists recommended that all women planning a pregnancy or who were capable of becoming pregnant should consume 400 μg of folic acid daily [23,24]. "The Public Health Agency of Canada recommends that all women who could become pregnant take a daily multivitamin containing 0.4 mg of folic acid [25]." Some Central American countries were already fortifying flour when, in 1996, they agreed for the first time to establish uniform regional standards for fortification with iron and other micronutrients [26]. In 2000, the Chilean Ministry of Health mandated the addition of folic acid to wheat flour to reduce the risk of NTDs [8].

C. AUSTRALIA, NEW ZEALAND, UNITED KINGDOM, IRELAND, AND THE NETHERLANDS

During the past 5 years, food safety agencies from these countries have considered starting mandatory folic acid fortification programs (Food Standards Australia New Zealand [27], Food Standards Agency United Kingdom, the Scientific Advisory Committee on Nutrition [28], the Food Safety Authority of Ireland [29], and the Health Council of the Netherlands [30]) and have recommended that mandatory folic acid fortification programs be approved in their respective countries.

III. FORTIFICATION

Fortification, the process of increasing the level of nutrients normally present within an appropriate food vehicle, has been used around the world as a cost-effective nutrition intervention strategy to reach large numbers of a population to improve nutrition and prevent disease [31–33]. For example, in the United States, minerals such as iodine (used in iodized salt) and fluoride (used in water fluoridation) have produced dramatic reductions in the prevalence of goiter and dental caries, respectively [34]. Vitamins A, D, niacin, thiamin, and riboflavin have been added to various food products, such as milk and cereal grain products, within the United States with subsequent decreases in the rates of their respective deficiencies [33,35,36]. Fortification is a complex intervention and requires a thorough understanding of the population at risk and the deficiency or inadequacy that exists. Policy makers, public health professionals, nutritionists, and industry professionals need to consider several factors as they embark on implementing fortification programs.

A. FOOD VEHICLES THAT CAN BE FORTIFIED

In both mandatory* and voluntary† fortification programs, grain flour and enriched cereal grain products have been the primary vehicles that have been used to provide folic acid. Worldwide, more than 400 million metric tons of wheat and maize flours are milled annually by commercial roller mills and consumed as noodles, breads, pasta, and other flour products by people in nearly every nation of the world [37]. Besides flours made from wheat, maize, and other cereal grains, other foods such as rice, milk, and margarine have been used as vehicles to deliver folic acid to populations at risk [7,29]. Although high dietary consumption is a factor in determining an appropriate fortification vehicle, the food vehicle must also provide a stable platform for distribution, and the fortificant must not affect the taste, smell, consistency, or any other qualities of the food.

B. RECOMMENDATIONS TO DETERMINE THE LEVEL OF FOLIC ACID ADDED TO FLOUR

The level of folic acid added to wheat flour is primarily dependent on estimates of the per capita consumption of the food product(s) being considered as a vehicle. In 2005, a World Health Organization (WHO) Technical Consultation on folate and vitamin B12 deficiencies recommended that the level of folic acid that can be safely added to wheat flour should be based on three different per capita wheat flour consumption patterns (low, medium, or high) [38]. In 2008, the Flour Fortification Initiative (FFI) reviewed new information on wheat flour consumption patterns and added a fourth group for a few countries with very high per capita consumption (low, medium, high, very high) [39].

C. COST AND COST-EFFECTIVENESS OF ESTABLISHING A PROGRAM

In some countries, foods such as cereal grain flour, milk, and salt are already used as fortification vehicles for other micronutrients. These existing fortification programs could be expanded to include folic acid without incurring substantial costs. Extra costs would be minimal because no new machinery would need to be purchased [38,40,41]. In countries without an existing fortification program, the costs for purchasing premix containing the appropriate micronutrients, installing and maintaining the necessary equipment to fortify the vehicle, and training the workers involved in production and monitoring should be considered [38]. Industry might be required to update or modify its manufacturing methods and labeling processes, which could also add to the cost in the short term [42].

Fortification of wheat flour with folic acid has been a cost-effective intervention in Chile [40], where for every $1 spent on fortification, $11 was saved on provision of medical care to children with spina bifida. In the United States, because the observed decrease in NTD rates was greater than forecast, the economic gains were correspondingly larger. The net cost savings were estimated to be in the range of

---

* *Mandatory* fortification requires manufacturers to add specific micronutrients at a particular level as mandated by that country's policy for food fortification.
† *Voluntary* fortification allows manufacturers to choose to add specific micronutrients to foods as long as they are allowed by that country's policy for food fortification.

$88 million to $145 million per year, a direct medical cost savings of $40 for every dollar invested in folic acid fortification [43].

D. ESTABLISHMENT OF NEW PROGRAMS

A key aspect of establishing a new fortification program is the need for partnerships and collaborations between the public and private sectors. Such collaborations are essential to maintain the success of any fortification program over time. Another consideration is the need for policy or legislation to monitor compliance through quality control measures, which could affect the safety and effectiveness of the intended fortification effort.

IV. CURRENT FORTIFICATION POLICIES AND FORTIFICATION LEVELS

A. MANDATORY FORTIFICATION POLICIES

Each country that has established a mandatory fortification program has reviewed the current science and established the country's level of folic acid to be added to flour based on consumption patterns, target intakes, and safety issues (Table 8.1). These processes often took years to complete. Recently, WHO and the Food and Agriculture Organization (FAO) have jointly published guidelines for food fortification with micronutrients that contain information intended to make establishing fortification programs easier and faster [44].

1. United States

The US Food and Drug Administration (FDA) reviewed the evidence available regarding folic acid and the prevention of NTDs and determined that fortification of the food supply, as part of an overall strategy, was the most effective way to reach women of child-bearing age with folic acid [45]. Therefore, in 1996, the FDA mandated that by January 1, 1998 all enriched cereal grain products (e.g., flour, rice, breads, rolls and buns, pasta, corn grits, corn meal, farina, macaroni, and noodle products) be fortified with folic acid at 140 µg of folic acid per 100 g of flour [6]. Earlier, in 1993, the FDA had authorized a health claim on dietary supplements and conventional foods about the relation between folate and NTDs in women of child-bearing age [45]. Studies

---

TABLE 8.1

Folic Acid Fortification Levels of Wheat Flour in Countries with Mandatory Fortification Programs

Country	Implementation Date	Fortification Level
United States [6]	1998	140 µg/100 g
Canada [55]	1998	150 µg/100 g
Costa Rica [7]	1998	180 µg/100 g
Chile [8]	2000	220 µg/100 g
South Africa [57]	2003	150 µg/100 g

conducted after fortification estimated that the existing fortification levels would provide women of child-bearing age an average daily intake of 100 to 200 µg of folic acid [46–54].

2. Canada

In 1993, Canada began developing a folic acid fortification program similar to the one in the United States [23,24]. In 1996, Canada's Food and Drug Regulations amended the upper level of folic acid allowed in flour and pasta [55]. Mandatory fortification of enriched white flour, pasta, and cornmeal, but not rice, with folic acid was in place in 1998, using levels slightly higher than the United States [55]. White flour and cornmeal were fortified at 150 µg of folic acid per 100 g, and pasta was fortified at 200 to 270 µg of folic acid per 100 g of pasta to account for possible cooking losses [25]. Canada also allowed for small amounts of folic acid to be added to breakfast cereals [56].

3. Chile

Chile's program was designed to provide, on average, 400 µg of folic acid daily to women aged 15 to 44 years [8]. Considering the average intake of bread, it was determined that a fortification level of 220 µg of folic acid per 100 g of wheat flour would provide a folic acid intake of approximately 400 µg per day. Essentially, fortified bread provided the only large source of folic acid because other folic acid–fortified foods, such as breakfast cereals, are scarce, economically out of reach, and not culturally accepted, and there was little, if any, use of folic acid supplements among the Chilean population [41].

4. Other Countries

Costa Rica and South Africa have also implemented mandatory fortification programs. Costa Rica began fortifying wheat flour in 1998 at 150 µg/100 g of flour; in 1999, it increased the levels to 180 µg/100 g of flour. Since then, Costa Rica has used folic acid to fortify wheat and maize flour and rice (180 µg/100 g) and milk (40 µg/100 g) [7]. In 2003, the South African government set the level of folic acid fortification for wheat flour at 150 µg/100 g of flour and for maize meal at 221 µg/100 g of meal [57].

Benefits of mandatory programs include wide coverage of the entire population, less need for ongoing education programs, low cost to industry and consumers, and no required change in consumers' eating habits or reliance on their selecting and consuming fortified foods [42]. However, some studies have reported that fortification cannot reach certain subgroups of the population who do not consume the fortified product [58,59]. This situation could indicate the need to consider fortification of other food products with folic acid [38]. Other potential challenges of mandatory programs include obtaining widespread support from government agencies, scientific communities, industry, and consumers to move forward with fortification policies and a short-term increase in costs as described earlier.

B.   VOLUNTARY FORTIFICATION POLICIES

Some countries around the world have established policies and recommendations that allow voluntary folic acid fortification of specific food products in an effort to reduce the birth prevalence rate of NTDs. In Australia and New Zealand, wheat flour can be fortified up to 285 µg/100 g of flour if manufacturers choose to fortify [60]. Many countries in the European Union have recommendations regarding folic acid use to prevent NTD-affected pregnancies, and some have implemented voluntary fortification policies, whereas others are considering mandatory fortification policies [61]. The United Kingdom and Ireland have had long-standing voluntary fortification policies [62].

Benefits of voluntary fortification policies include allowing consumers to choose whether they want to purchase and eat fortified foods. This also reduces the potential cost to manufacturers from updating their equipment and labeling procedures. Potential problems with voluntary fortification include only reaching a select proportion of the population, relying on consumers to make the choice to buy fortified foods, and passing the costs of fortified foods on to the consumer (which could make fortified foods significantly more expensive than nonfortified foods and less available to those who might need them the most).

V. THE EFFECT OF FORTIFICATION PROGRAMS

Mandatory folic acid fortification policies have effectively reduced the birth prevalence rate of NTDs, increased blood folate concentrations, and increased overall dietary intake of folic acid [7–10,48,56,57,63–69].

Although some voluntary programs have also produced a slight increase in overall intake of folic acid as well as an increase in blood folate concentrations, they have not generally produced a reduction in the birth prevalence rate of NTDs [70,71]. One exception is a reduction in the birth prevalence rate of NTDs recently attributed to voluntary fortification in Australia [72–75].

The following section details the effect of mandatory fortification programs on birth prevalence rates of NTDs, blood folate concentrations, and dietary intakes of folic acid, as well as the limitations of these studies.

A. REDUCTION OF BIRTH PREVALENCE RATES OF NEURAL TUBE DEFECTS

1. United States

Several studies from within the United States have reported percent decreases in the overall birth prevalence rate of NTDs after 1998 when folic acid fortification was fully implemented [10,65]. Williams et al. [10] used 24 population-based state surveillance systems with and without prenatal ascertainment to estimate percent decreases of NTDs from prefortification (January 1995–December 1996) to postfortification (October 1998–December 1999). From all 24 systems, there was a reported 26% decrease [10], whereas the nine programs with prenatal ascertainment noted a 32% decrease. These decreases were higher than from two other published studies using birth certificate data. One study used data from 1995 to 1999 that included 45 states and Washington, DC [65]. This study reported a 19% decrease in the overall birth prevalence rate of NTDs. The second study, with additional birth certificate data from 1991 to 2005 from 47 states [67], reported a 23% decrease.

Individual trends for the specific NTDs spina bifida and anencephaly have also decreased. Williams et al. [10] reported a 31% reduction in spina bifida from all 24 population-based surveillance systems, the most dramatic reduction in overall birth prevalence rates since the implementation of mandatory fortification in the United States. Among the nine surveillance systems with prenatal ascertainment, a 40% decrease in spina bifida birth prevalence rates was observed [10]. Decreases in the birth prevalence rates of spina bifida ranging from 20% to 23% were reported based on birth certificate data [65,67]. Early in the fortification process the proportion of anencephaly cases appeared to decrease less than the proportion of spina bifida cases. From the 24 population-based surveillance systems an overall 16% decrease in anencephaly was observed, whereas a 19% decrease in anencephaly prevalence rates was observed from the nine surveillance systems with prenatal ascertainment [10]. Percent prevalence rate changes from birth certificates were variable, ranging from 11% to 21% [65,67]. More recently, Boulet et al. [76] reported a "catch up" of the decrease in prevalence rate for anencephaly through 2004. The reductions in prevalence for both spina bifida and anencephaly now appear to be about equal in the United States.

2. Canada

Using data from seven Canadian provinces that contributed to more than half of the total births in the country, De Wals et al. [9] reported an overall 46% reduction in all NTDs comparing prefortification (January 1993–September 1997) with postfortification (April 2000–December 2002). This was similar to the percentage reduction reported earlier for the province of Ontario (48%), from 11.3 to 5.8 per 10,000 births from prefortification (1994–1997) to postfortification (1998–2000), respectively, but was slightly higher than the percentage reduction in NTD birth prevalence rates reported earlier for the province of Quebec (32%), from 18.9 to 12.8 per 10,000 births from prefortification (1992–1997) to postfortification (1998–2000), respectively [56,69]. More dramatic reductions were reported in provinces with higher baseline birth prevalence rates of NTDs than in provinces with lower baseline rates [56]. For example, Nova Scotia reported larger decreases, with an overall 54% reduction in NTD birth prevalence rates from 25.5 to 11.7 per 10,000 births from prefortification (1991–1994) to postfortification (1998–2000), respectively [68]. In Newfoundland, a 78% decrease was observed after fortification [77].

Similar to the United States, birth prevalence rates of spina bifida decreased more than those for anencephaly from prefortification to postfortification in Canada. Among the seven provinces, there was a 53% decrease in spina bifida rates in contrast to a 38% decrease in anencephaly rates [9]. This same trend was observed in Quebec, where a 29% decrease in the birth prevalence rates of spina bifida was observed in contrast to a 12% decrease in anencephaly.

3. Chile

In 1999, a hospital surveillance system was implemented in nine public hospitals within Santiago with the assistance of the CDC and the Estudio Colaborativo Latino Americano de Malformaciones Congénitas (ECLAMC). Using data from these nine hospitals, Hertrampf and Cortes [8] reported a 40% decrease in the overall birth prevalence rate of NTDs from pre- to postfortification. Using data from other maternity hospitals within the ECLAMC surveillance system in Chile, Lopez-Camelo et al. [66] reported a 55% decrease in total NTDs from prefortification (1990–2000) to post-fortification (2001–2002); the decrease in the birth prevalence rate of spina bifida and anencephaly was 48% and 61%, respectively.

4. Summary

Mandatory fortification of flour with folic acid has proven to be one of the most suc-cessful public health interventions in preventing morbidity and mortality from NTDs. There has been a substantial reduction in the birth prevalence rate of NTDs in every country that has implemented mandatory fortification. Overall decreases have ranged from 19% to 78%, with reductions in the birth prevalence rates of spina bifida ranging from 20% to 57% (Table 8.2). Most decreases are within the expected range based on earlier RCTs [1,2]. The decrease in NTD rates postfortification are consistent with a predictive model [78], which was based on dose–response findings from Ireland [79]. The predictive model estimated a decrease in birth prevalence rates of NTDs of 18% to 22% with an increase in average daily intake of 100 µg of folic acid [78].

B. INCREASED BLOOD FOLATE CONCENTRATIONS POSTFORTIFICATION

Blood folate concentrations have been an important indicator of short- and long-term folate status for the population. Studies that measured serum or plasma folate concentrations have enabled researchers to track the effects of folic acid fortification on blood folate status. Table 8.3 provides information on serum folate concentrations, which indicate short-term changes in folate intake. Table 8.4 provides information on red blood cell (RBC) folate concentrations, which are less sensitive to short-term changes in folate intake and correlate better with folate stores. In the United States, blood folate concentrations have been collected on a nationally representative sample since 1976 [80]. Other countries have collected blood folate concentrations for specific segments of their population (e.g., women of child-bearing age) or on smaller segments of the total population (e.g., from hospitals or clinics) before and after fortification to estimate the effect of folic acid fortification.

1. United States

The National Health and Nutrition Examination Survey (NHANES) is a series of nationally representative surveys of the US population. Blood folate concentrations from NHANES III (1988–1994) represent the period before fortification, and those from NHANES 1999 and afterward represent the period after fortification. The mean concentration of serum folate from NHANES III was 5.0 ng/mL; it more than doubled to 11.9 ng/mL in NHANES 1999–2000, which was the first survey in the series after fortification [81]. Comparison of median serum folate concentrations from NHANES III with those from NHANES 1999–2004 revealed an overall increase of 7.5 ng/mL after fortification [82]. The mean concentration of RBC folate from NHANES III was 165.5 ng/mL and increased by 94.9 ng/mL to 260.4 ng/mL in NHANES 1999–2000 [81].

TABLE 8.2

Birth Prevalence Rates of Neural Tube Defects before and after Fortification in the United States, Canada, Chile, Costa Rica, and South Africa

Study	Prefortification Birth Prevalence Rate	Optional Fortification Birth Prevalence Rate	Postfortification Birth Prevalence Rate	Percent Decline[a]
United States				
Williams et al. [10]	January 1995–December 1996[b]	January 1997– September 1998[b]	October 1998–December 1999[b]	
24 population-based state surveillance systems with and without prenatal diagnosis				
Total neural tube defects	7.6	6.2	5.6	26%
Spina bifida	5.2	4.2	3.5	31%
Anencephaly	2.4	2.0	2.1	16%
Williams et al. [10]	January 1995–December 1996[c]	January 1997– September 1998[c]	October 1998–December 1999[c]	
Nine population-based state surveillance systems with prenatal diagnosis				
Total neural tube defects	10.9	8.8	7.4	32%
Spina bifida	6.7	5.4	4.0	40%
Anencephaly	4.2	3.4	3.4	19%
Honein et al. [65]	October 1995–December 1996[d]		October 1998–December 1999[d]	
Birth certificate data from 45 states and Washington, DC				
Total neural tube defects	3.78	NA	3.05	19%
Spina bifida	2.62	NA	2.02	23%
Anencephaly	1.16	NA	1.03	11%
Mathews [67]	1991–1995[d]	1996–1998[d]	1999–2005[d]	
Birth certificate data from 47 states				
Total neural tube defects	3.9	3.6	3.0	23%

continued

TABLE 8.2 (continued)
Birth Prevalence Rates of Neural Tube Defects before and after Fortification in the United States, Canada, Chile, Costa Rica, and South Africa

Study	Prefortification Birth Prevalence Rates	Optional Fortification Birth Prevalence Rates	Postfortification Birth Prevalence Rates	Percent Decline[a]
Spina bifida	2.5	2.5	2.0	20%
Anencephaly	1.4	1.2	1.1	21%
Canada				
De Wals et al. [9] Seven Canadian provinces	January 1993–September 1997c	October 1997–March 2000c	April 2000–December 2002c	
Total neural tube defects	15.8	10.9	8.6	46%
Spina bifida	8.6	5.7	4.0	53%
Anencephaly	5.2	3.8	3.2	38%
De Wals et al. [56] Province of Quebec	1992–1997e	NA	1998–2000e	32%
Total neural tube defects	18.9	NA	12.8	32%
Spina bifida	NA	NA	NA	NA
Anencephaly	NA	NA	NA	NA
Ray et al. [69] Province of Ontario	January 1994–December 1997e		January 1998–May 2000e	
Total neural tube defects	11.3	NA	5.8	48%
Spina bifida	7.5	NA	4.2	44%
Anencephaly	3.8	NA	1.6	58%
Persad et al. [68] Hospital records from Nova Scotia	1991–1994c	1995–1997c	1998–2000c	
Total neural tube defects	25.5	26.1	11.7	54%
Spina bifida	14.4	16.0	6.2	57%
Anencephaly	10.0	8.2	3.8	62%
Liu et al. [77] Newfoundland and Labrador Medical Genetics Program	1991–1997	NA	1998–2001	
Total neural tube defects	43.6	NA	9.6	78%
Spina bifida	NA	NA	NA	NA
Anencephaly	NA	NA	NA	NA

Chile

Hertrampf and Cortes [8]
Hospital-based surveillance system

	January 1999–December 2000[e]	January 2001–June 2002[e]	
Total neural tube defects	17.0	10.1	40%
Spina bifida	NA	NA	NA
Anencephaly	NA	NA	NA

Lopez-Camelo et al. [66] Hospital-based surveillance system

	1990–2000[e]	2001–2002[e]	
Total neural tube defects	17.5	7.9	55%
Spina bifida	9.3	4.8	48%
Anencephaly	8.2	3.2	61%

Costa Rica

Chen et al. [7]
Hospital-based surveillance system

	1996–1998[e]	1999–2000[e]	
Total neural tube defects	9.7	6.3	35%
Spina bifida	NA	NA	NA
Anencephaly	NA	NA	NA

South Africa

Sayed et al. [57]
Hospital-based surveillance system

	January 2003–June 2004[d]	October 2004–June 2005[d]	
Total neural tube defects	14.1	9.8	30%
Spina bifida	9.3	5.4	42%
Anencephaly	4.1	3.7	11%

[a] Percent decline is for prefortification vs. postfortification.
[b] Rates per 10,000 births (includes programs with and without prenatal ascertainment).
[c] Rates per 10,000 births (includes live birth, stillbirths, and termination of pregnancies).
[d] Rates per 10,000 live births.
[e] Rates per 10,000 births (includes live birth and stillbirths).

TABLE 8.3
Serum Folate Concentrations before and after Fortification in the United States, Canada, Chile, and Costa Rica

	Serum Folate Concentration		
	Prefortification	Postfortification	Absolute Difference
United States			
Lawrence et al. [84]	1994[a]	1998[a]	
HMO population in California			
Total population	12.6	18.7	+6.1
Jacques et al. [83]	January 1991–	September 1997–	
Framingham Offspring Study	December 1994[b]	March 1998[b]	
Study population (32–80 years) no supplement use	4.6	10.0	+5.4
Study population (32–80 years) supplement use	11.7	18.9	+7.2
CDC [85]			
National cross-sectional survey of US population (NHANES)	1988–1994[c]	1999–2000[c]	
Women (15–44 years)	4.8	13.0	+8.2
Dietrich et al. [81]			
National cross-sectional survey of US population (NHANES)	1988–1994[d]	1999–2000[d]	
Total population	5.0	11.9	+6.9
Women (20–39 years)	4.5	11.5	+7.0
Pfeiffer et al. [82]			
National cross-sectional survey of US population (NHANES)	1988–1994[c]	1999–2004[c]	
Total population	5.5	13.0	+7.5
Canada			
Liu et al. [77]	November 1997–	November 2000–	
Cross-sectional survey in Newfoundland	March 1998[e]	March 2001[e]	
Women (19–44 years)	6.0	8.0	+2.0
Chile			
Hertrampf et al. [64]	October 1999–	October 2000–	
Outpatient clinics in Santiago, Chile	December 1999[d]	December 2000[d]	
Women (22–37 years)	4.3	16.4	+12.1
Costa Rica			
Chen et al. [7]	1996[d]	2000[d]	
Hospital-based surveillance system			

TABLE 8.3 (continued)
Serum Folate Concentrations before and after Fortification in the United States, Canada, Chile, and Costa Rica

	Serum Folate Concentration		
	Prefortification	Postfortification	Absolute Difference
Women (15–44 years) in metropolitan areas	10.1	15.8	+5.7
Women (15–44 years) in rural areas	9.6	12.5	+2.9

[a] Median concentrations in ng/mL. Assays were done using automated chemiluminescence systems (ACS).

[b] Geometric mean concentrations in ng/mL. Assays were done using the microbiological assay.

[c] Median concentrations in ng/mL. Assays were done using the radioassay.

[d] Mean concentrations in ng/mL. Assays were done using the radioassay.

[e] Geometric mean concentrations in ng/mL. No information on type of assay used.

To convert from ng/mL to nmol/L multiply by the conversion factor of 2.266.

A prospective cohort study, the Framingham Offspring Study, reported slightly smaller increases (+5.4 ng/mL) in geometric mean serum folate concentrations from prefortification (1991–1994) to postfortification (1997–1998) among the population aged 32 to 80 years who did not report supplement use [83]. However, researchers did find similar increases in NHANES among the population aged 32 to 80 years who did report supplement use from pre- to postfortification (+7.2 ng/mL) [83]. In addition, a study in California had much higher baseline median serum folate concentrations (12.6 ng/mL) in 1994 but had similar increases in response to fortification in 1998 (+6.1 ng/mL) as reported in NHANES and the Framingham Offspring Study [84].

Differences between pre- and postfortification serum folate concentrations among women of child-bearing age were slightly higher than the total US population. Among women aged 20 to 39 years, the mean serum folate concentration increased by 7.0 ng/mL from NHANES III to NHANES 1999–2000 [81]. Among women aged 15 to 44 years, the median serum folate increased by 8.2 ng/mL during the same period [85].

2. Canada, Chile, and Costa Rica
Among women of childbearing age (18–42 years) who were patients in community-based medical centers in Ontario, Canada, the prefortification (1996–1997) geometric mean RBC folate concentrations were higher than those reported in the United States (232.6 ng/mL and increased to 327.1 ng/mL after fortification [1998–2000]) [86]. Canadian women had similar increases in RBC folate concentrations from prefortification to postfortification when compared with US women aged 20 to 39 years (+94.5 and 94.9 ng/mL, respectively) [81,85,86].

Because of the higher daily intake of folic acid associated with the Chilean fortification program, Chile had much larger increases in both serum folate and RBC folate concentrations from prefortification (1999) to postfortification (2000). Among women of child-bearing age who attended outpatient clinics, Hertrampf et al. [64] reported that serum folate concentration increased by 12.1 ng/mL from

TABLE 8.4
Red Blood Cell Folate Concentrations before and after Fortification in the United States, Canada, and Chile

Study	Red Blood Cell Folate Concentration		
	Prefortification	Postfortification	Absolute Difference
United States			
CDC [85]			
National cross-sectional survey of US population (NHANES)	1988–1994[a]	1999–2000[a]	
Women (15–44 years)	160	264	+104
Dietrich et al. [81]			
National cross-sectional survey of US population (NHANES)	1988–1994[b]	1999–2000[b]	
Total population	166	260	+95
Women (20–39 years)	150	245	+95
Pfeiffer et al. [82]			
National cross-sectional survey of US population (NHANES)	1988–1994[a]	1999–2004[a]	
Total population	174	269	+95
Canada			
Ray et al. [86] Community-based patients in Ontario	January 1996– December 1997[c]	January 1998– December 2000[c]	
Women (18–42 years)	233	327	+94
Liu et al. [77] Cross-sectional survey in Newfoundland	November 1997–March 1998[d]	November 2000– March 2001[d]	
Women (19–44 years)	276	361	+85
Chile			
Hertrampf et al. [64] Outpatient clinics in Santiago, Chile	October 1999– December 1999[b]	October 2000– December 2000[b]	
Women (22–37 years)	128	312	+184

[a] Median concentrations in ng/mL. Assays were done using the radioassay.
[b] Mean concentrations in ng/mL. Assays were done using the radioassay.
[c] Geometric mean concentrations in ng/mL. Assays were done using the radioassay.
[d] Geometric mean concentrations in ng/mL. No information provided on type of assay used.
    To convert from ng/mL to nmol/L, multiply by the conversion factor of 2.266.

prefortification to postfortification. Among this same group of women, RBC folate concentrations increased approximately +184.1 ng/mL from prefortification to post-fortification, an increase that was much higher than reported in the United States or Canada [64,81,85,86].

Serum folate concentrations in Costa Rica increased slightly less than in the United States from prefortification (1996) to postfortification (2000) [7]. Among women of child-bearing age (15–44 years) in a hospital-based surveillance system, Chen et al. found that urban areas had a more pronounced increase in serum folate concentrations after fortification when compared with women in rural areas (+5.7 and +2.9 ng/mL, respectively) [7], despite the fact that serum folate concentrations for urban and rural women did not appear to differ at baseline (10.1 ng/mL and 9.6 ng/mL, respectively) [7].

3. Summary

Blood folate concentrations have increased since fortification was implemented in the United States, Canada, Chile, and Costa Rica. In the United States, increases in serum folate concentrations have ranged from 5.4 to 8.2 ng/mL depending on the population studied [81–85]. Chile and Costa Rica have also reported dramatic increases in serum folate concentrations among women of child-bearing age [7,64]. Countries that have implemented folic acid fortification programs have also reported large increases in RBC folate concentrations after fortification began (~100 ng/mL or more) [81,82,85,86].

C. INCREASED DIETARY INTAKE OF FOLIC ACID FROM FORTIFICATION

Studies examining dietary intake of folic acid as a result of fortification have reported that overall intake has increased. In the United States, reports indicate an overall increase in the consumption of folic acid; however, data sources vary widely on the estimated amounts of additional intake of folic acid [48–54]. Chile has also reported increases in the overall dietary consumption of folic acid since fortification [8].

D. LIMITATIONS OF STUDIES OF THE EFFECTS OF FOLIC ACID FORTIFICATION

There are some limitations to the studies presented. First, data collection methods for birth defect surveillance systems vary within countries and among countries. In the United States, data from birth certificates raise a concern about validity and sensitivity for capturing all birth defects. However, birth defects that are apparent at birth are more likely to be documented, and the positive predictive value for both spina bifida and anencephaly are reported to be high [65,87]. Unfortunately, birth certificate data do not adequately capture trends of stillbirths or terminations. Although some surveillance systems report stillbirths and terminations, it is difficult to ascertain whether all possible NTDs are counted. Although data collection methods in Canada have many of the same issues as the United States in terms of capturing all births, terminations, and stillbirths, there was no indication that methods or procedures to identify birth defects changed from prefortification to postfortification periods [56]. In Chile, terminations of pregnancy are not expected to influence the ascertainment of NTDs because terminations are not routinely available [64].

Second, there is the possibility that birth prevalence rates of NTDs were already decreasing, and fortification did not change the downward trend. In the United States, Cragan et al. reported that there were some gradual decreases in both spina bifida and anencephaly within the United States before fortification [88]. Canada's reported percent decreases in NTD birth prevalence rates were greater than those in the United States; however, some of their baseline birth prevalence rates of NTDs were higher [9,77]. In Chile, surveillance data from ECLAMC were analyzed over a 21-year period, and no significant downward trends of NTD birth prevalence rates before fortification were reported [66].

Third, there are differences in the way that countries and programs measured blood folates. Many of the research studies examining the effect of folic acid fortification on blood folates used the radioassay that is now known to underestimate the true blood folate concentration by approximately 30% [82]. However, because both the pre- and postfortification concentrations were measured with the same assay within each study, the documented increases will have the same bias. Because of these methodological differences, comparisons between studies using different assays should be interpreted with caution.

Fourth, both blood folate concentrations and NTD birth prevalence rates have been reported to differ by race/ethnicity [82,85,89–91]. Non-Hispanic whites are reported to have higher concentrations of both serum and RBC folate concentrations than Hispanics, and non-Hispanic blacks have the lowest reported blood folate concentrations as well as the lowest NTD birth prevalence rate [82,85,89,90,92]. When comparing different populations within and between countries, it is important to take into consideration the racial/ethnic makeup of the population under observation.

Finally, it is difficult to link increases in blood folate concentrations directly or solely to fortification efforts. Women's reported dietary intake of folic acid could have varied over time, leading to a reduction in NTDs regardless of fortification efforts. One study reported that women's intake of folic acid is influenced most by consuming supplements containing folic acid [53]. In the United States, there was no indication of a significant change in the use of folic acid–containing supplements among women of child-bearing age that corresponds to the timing of fortification [93,94]. In one Canadian province, Quebec, the reported number of supplement products containing folic acid surged from 13 to 103 from 1992 to 1997. Nevertheless, the proportion of women of child-bearing age who reported consuming these supplements remained constant from prefortification to postfortification [56,95,96]. Chile has a limited number of available supplement products that contain folic acid; therefore, additional folic acid intake from consuming supplements containing folic acid is unlikely to be the explanation for the observed increases in blood folate concentrations [64].

Even with these limitations, the reduction in birth prevalence rates of NTDs, increases in blood folate concentrations, and increases in estimated daily dietary folic acid intake postfortification have been significant in the United States, Canada, Costa Rica, and Chile. Although the completeness of birth defects surveillance programs, natural variations in NTD birth prevalence rates, and variations in folic acid intake among women of child-bearing age could have resulted in an apparent reduction in NTDs associated with fortification, there was no evidence that these factors have had a significant effect from prefortification to postfortification.

VI. MINIMUM EFFECTIVE BLOOD FOLATE CONCENTRATION FOR NEURAL TUBE DEFECT PREVENTION

Currently, the minimum effective blood folate concentration for the maximum prevention of NTDs is unknown. Daly et al. [79] found that in a cohort study of the Irish population that although NTD risk was inversely associated with blood folate concentration, the risk continued to decrease in women with blood folate concentrations above the classical cut-offs for deficiency thus providing evidence that NTD-affected pregnancies occur among women who are not folate deficient. Increasing blood folates to those higher concentrations associated with maximum NTD risk reduction requires that women consume folic acid from supplements and/or fortified foods in addition to a healthy diet containing natural folates [97].

Findings from a prospective cohort community intervention trial in China might also provide a clue to how low the birth prevalence rate of NTDs can be reduced by folic acid. In this trial, women consumed 400 µg of folic acid daily with a 90% median compliance for pill taking; these women had no exposure to other vitamins from supplements [98]. Maternal use of periconceptional folic acid prevented NTDs in two regions of the country with very different birth prevalence rates of NTDs (much higher baseline birth prevalence rates of NTDs in the north than in the south). Among women in the northern region who consumed 400 µg of folic acid periconceptionally, the birth prevalence rate decreased 85%, from 48 to 7 in 10,000 pregnancies (>20 weeks gestation); in the southern region the rate decreased 40%, from 10 to 6 in 10,000 pregnancies (>20 weeks gestation). Despite the large differences in the baseline NTD birth prevalence rates, maternal use of 400 µg of folic acid resulted in similar postexposure birth prevalence rates in both the north and the south [99].

VII. OTHER POTENTIAL EFFECTS ASSOCIATED WITH FOLIC ACID FORTIFICATION

In the past several years several articles have been written describing potential adverse effects associated with consumption of folic acid and the strength of these findings varies greatly. These articles have prompted many reviews and commentaries that interpret the strength of these findings differently. Observational and ecological studies, hypotheses and opinions should not be used as evidence of cause and effect. Among the best sources of detailed, balanced information about the potential risks and benefits of folic acid fortification are several systematic reviews recently completed by national food safety agencies (FSANZ [27], FSA UK [28], FSA Ireland [29], and Health Council of the Netherlands [30]).

One major difficulty in assessing other potential effects that can be attributed to consumption of folic acid is teasing out the association between the different sources of folic acid (enriched cereal grain products, ready-to-eat products, or supplements) and any potential beneficial or harmful effects. For example, very high serum folate concentrations are primarily associated with the use of supplements containing folic acid [100,101]. It is important for researchers to differentiate folic acid intake attributable to voluntary consumption of supplements and ready-to-eat products from folic acid intake attributable to mandatory fortification of enriched cereal grain products. This is important when discussing the implications of implementing folic acid fortification programs in the developing world, where use of supplements containing folic acid and ready-to-eat breakfast cereals are uncommon. Current and future public health prevention strategies to fortify food with folic acid should be based on information taking into account the different dietary sources of folic acid.

VIII. SUMMARY

Countries that have implemented a folic acid fortification program specifically to prevent NTDs have documented dramatic increases in the blood folate concentrations and a concomitant decrease of NTD birth prevalence rates at a substantial cost savings in medical care. Even with the difference in data collection methods, fortification levels, folic acid–containing supplement use, and demographic and cultural characteristics, the overriding constant has been an increase in blood folate concentrations and a reduction in the birth prevalence rate of NTDs. Many countries have tried other approaches to decrease the occurrence of NTDs such as education campaigns to promote daily intake of folic acid among women of childbearing age as well as voluntary fortification programs. However, in 2005, evaluations of many of these programs revealed no detectable improvement in the national trends in the occurrence of NTDs [61,102]. After mandated fortification policies were in place in the United States, Canada, Chile, and Costa Rica, folic acid fortification resulted in increases in blood folate concentrations and fewer babies born with NTDs, indicating a tremendous public health achievement.

These successes have prompted action by international organizations. In April 2003, The Micronutrient Initiative, in collaboration with several other organizations, convened a group of knowledgeable scientists and policy experts to discuss ways to accelerate the global pace at which countries implement effective and sustainable programs to prevent folic acid–preventable birth defects [103]. In 2004, the FFI was formed to accelerate wheat flour fortification in roller mills throughout the world [37]. In December 2004, FFI, in collaboration with the CDC and the Mexican Institute of Public Health, convened a technical workshop, "Wheat Flour Fortification: Current Knowledge and Practical Applications," in Cuernavaca, Mexico [42]. Most recently in March 2008, the "Second Technical Workshop on Wheat Flour Fortification: Practical Recommendations for National Application," was convened in Stone Mountain, Georgia, with support from FFI, CDC, The Global Alliance for Improved Nutrition, and Cargill [39].

In 2006, WHO and the FAO published *Guidelines on Food Fortification with Micronutrients*, which is a useful document for those considering starting a food fortification program [44]. In 2005, WHO sponsored a technical consultation on folate and vitamin B12 deficiencies that provided guidance about developing fortification programs for folic acid and vitamin B12 [104]. Both of these documents are excellent sources of more detailed information about micronutrient fortification.

NTDs remain an important cause of perinatal morbidity and mortality worldwide. In 2006, the March of Dimes published prefortification country-specific estimates that more than 300,000 NTD-affected pregnancies occurred yearly worldwide [105]. Using these estimates, Bell and Oakley [106] calculated that of the more than 220,000 folic acid–preventable NTD-affected pregnancies worldwide, only 7% are prevented by fortifying wheat flour with folic acid. Mandatory folic acid fortification programs offer countries an intervention that can result in dramatic reductions in these numbers. With so many NTDs still occurring, this is clearly a great opportunity for more countries to establish mandatory fortification programs around the world. In the words of one folate expert, "Mandatory folic acid fortification may be the most important science driven intervention in nutrition and public health in decades [107]."

ACKNOWLEDGMENTS

The findings and conclusions in this report are those of the authors and do not necessarily represent the official position of the Centers for Disease Control and Prevention.

REFERENCES

1. MRC Vitamin Study Research Group. Prevention of neural tube defects: Results of the Medical Research Council Vitamin Study. *Lancet* 1991; 338:131–37.
2. Czeizel AE, Dudas I. Prevention of the first occurrence of neural-tube defects by periconceptional vitamin supplementation. *N Engl J Med* 1992; 327:1832–35.
3. Centers for Disease Control and Prevention. Use of folic acid for prevention of spina bifida and other neural tube defects—1983–1991. *MMWR Morb Mortal Wkly Rep* 1991; 40:513–16.
4. Centers for Disease Control and Prevention. Recommendations for the use of folic acid to reduce the number of cases of spina bifida and other neural tube defects. *MMWR Recomm Rep* 1992; 41:1–7.
5. Institute of Medicine. Folate. *Dietary Reference Intakes for Thiamin, Riboflavin, Niacin, Vitamin B6, Folate, Vitamin B12, Pantothenic Acid, Biotin, and Choline.* Washington, DC: National Academy Press, 1998:196–305.
6. Food and Drug Administration. Food standards: Amendment of standards of identity for enriched grain products to require addition of folic acid, Final rule. 21 CFR Parts 136, 137, and 139. *Fed Reg* 1996:8781–97.
7. Chen LT, Rivera MA. The Costa Rican experience: Reduction of neural tube defects following food fortification programs. *Nutr Rev* 2004; 62:S40–43.
8. Hertrampf E, Cortes F. Folic acid fortification of wheat flour: Chile. *Nutr Rev* 2004; 62:S44–48; discussion S49.
9. De Wals P, Tairou F, Van Allen MI, Uh SH, Lowry RB, Sibbald B, Evans JA, et al. Reduction in neural-tube defects after folic acid fortification in Canada. *N Engl J Med* 2007; 357:135–42.
10. Williams LJ, Mai CT, Edmonds LD, Shaw GM, Kirby RS, Hobbs CA, Sever LE, Miller LA, Meaney FJ, Levitt M. Prevalence of spina bifida and anencephaly during the transition to mandatory folic acid fortification in the United States. *Teratology* 2002; 66:33–39.
11. Centers for Disease Control and Prevention. Trends in wheat-flour fortification with folic acid and iron—Worldwide, 2004 and 2007. *MMWR Morb Mortal Wkly Rep* 2008; 57:8–10.

12. Hibbard BM, Hibbard ED, Jeffcoate TN. Folic acid and reproduction. *Acta Obstet Gynecol Scand* 1965; 44:375–400.
13. Smithells RW, Sheppard S. Possible prevention of neural-tube defects by periconceptional vitamin supplementation. *Lancet* 1980; 1:647.
14. Smithells RW, Sheppard S, Schorah CJ, Seller MJ, Nevin NC, Harris R, Read AP, Fielding DW. Apparent prevention of neural tube defects by periconceptional vitamin supplementation. *Arch Dis Child* 1981; 56:911–18.
15. Smithells RW, Nevin NC, Seller MJ, Sheppard S, Harris R, Read AP, Fielding DW, Walker S, Schorah CJ, Wild J. Further experience of vitamin supplementation for prevention of neural tube defect recurrences. *Lancet* 1983; 1:1027–31.
16. Laurence KM, Campbell H. Trial of folate treatment to prevent recurrence of neural tube defect. *Br Med J (Clin Res Ed)* 1981; 282:2131.
17. Milunsky A, Jick H, Jick SS, Bruell CL, MacLaughlin DS, Rothman KJ, Willett W. Multivitamin/folic acid supplementation in early pregnancy reduces the prevalence of neural tube defects. *JAMA* 1989; 262:2847–52.
18. Mulinare J, Cordero JF, Erickson JD, Berry RJ. Periconceptional use of multivitamins and the occurrence of neural tube defects. *JAMA* 1988; 260:3141–45.
19. Vergel RG, Sanchez LR, Heredero BL, Rodriguez PL, Martinez AJ. Primary prevention of neural tube defects with folic acid supplementation: Cuban experience. *Prenat Diagn* 1990; 10:149–52.
20. Bower C, Stanley FJ. Dietary folate as a risk factor for neural-tube defects: Evidence from a case-control study in Western Australia. *Med J Aust* 1989; 150:613–19.
21. Werler MM, Shapiro S, Mitchell AA. Periconceptional folic acid exposure and risk of occurrent neural tube defects. *JAMA* 1993; 269:1257–61.
22. Shaw GM, Schaffer D, Velie EM, Morland K, Harris JA. Periconceptional vitamin use, dietary folate, and the occurrence of neural tube defects. *Epidemiology* 1995; 6:219–26.
23. Health Canada. Folic acid: The vitamin that helps protect against neural tube (birth) defects. *Issues* April 1993.
24. SOGC Genetics Committee. Recommendation on the use of folic acid for the prevention of neural tube defects. *J Soc Obstet Gynaecol Can Supp* 1993; 15:41–46.
25. PHAC. *Folic Acid and Prevention of Neural Tube Defects: Information Update from PHAC—2008*. Available at http://www.phac-aspc.gc.ca/fa-af/fa-af08-eng.php; accessed June 18, 2008.
26. Pan American Health Organization. *Regional Meeting Report—Flour Fortification with Iron, Folic Acid, and Vitamin B12, Santiago, Chile [Report] 2003*. Available at http://www.paho.org/English/AD/FCH/NU/ChileRglReport_2004.pdf; accessed Nov 6, 2008.
27. Food Standards Australia New Zealand (FSANZ). *Final Assessment Report Proposal P295-Consideration for Mandatory Fortification with Folic Acid*, 2006. Available at http://www.foodstandards.gov.au/_srcfiles/FAR_P295_Folic_Acid_Fortification_%20 Att achs_1_6.pdf; accessed July 10, 2009.
28. SACN. *Folate and Disease Prevention*. Norwich, UK: The Stationary Office, 2006.
29. Food Safety Authority of Ireland. *Report of the National Committee on Folic Acid Food Fortification*. Available at http://www.fsai.ie/publications/reports/folic_acid.pdf; accessed August 21, 2008.
30. Health Council of the Netherlands. *Towards an Optimal Use of Folic Acid*. The Hague, the Netherlands: Health Council of the Netherlands, 2008: publication no. 2008/02E.
31. Darnton-Hill I, Webb P, Harvey PW, Hunt JM, Dalmiya N, Chopra M, Ball MJ, Bloem MW, de Benoist B. Micronutrient deficiencies and gender: Social and economic costs. *Am J Clin Nutr* 2005; 81:1198S–205S.

32. Mannar MG, Sankar R. Micronutrient fortification of foods—Rationale, application, and impact. *Indian J Pediatr* 2004; 71:997–1002.
33. Taucher SC. Services for the care and prevention of birth defects. Reduced report of a World Health Organization and March of Dimes Foundation meeting. *Rev Med Chile* 2007; 135:806–13.
34. Mertz W. Food fortification in the United States. *Nutr Rev* 1997; 55:44–49.
35. Hannon-Fletcher MP, Armstrong NC, Scott JM, Pentieva K, Bradbury I, Ward M, Strain JJ, et al. Determining bioavailability of food folates in a controlled intervention study. *Am J Clin Nutr* 2004; 80:911–18.
36. Richardson DP. Food fortification. *Proc Nutr Soc* 1990; 49:39–50.
37. Flour Fortification Initiative. *Flour Fortification Initiative Home Page.* Available at www.sph.emory.edu/wheatflour; accessed August 21, 2008.
38. Dary O. Establishing safe and potentially efficacious fortification contents for folic acid and vitamin B12. *Food Nutr Bull* 2008; 29:S214–24.
39. Flour Fortification Initiative. *Summary Report—Second Technical Workshop on Wheat Flour Fortification: Practical Recommendations for National Application, Stone Mountain, Georgia, USA.* Available at http://www.sph.emory.edu/wheatflour/atlanta08/Atlanta_Summary_Report_Oct%207.pdf; accessed October 17, 2008.
40. Llanos A, Hertrampf E, Cortes F, Pardo A, Grosse SD, Uauy R. Cost-effectiveness of a folic acid fortification program in Chile. *Health Policy* 2007; 83:295–303.
41. Hertrampf E, Cortes F. National food-fortification program with folic acid in Chile. *Food Nutr Bull* 2008; 29:S231–37.
42. Flour Fortification Initiative. *Report of the Workshop of Wheat Flour Fortification: Cuernavaca, Mexico.* Available at http://www.sph.emory.edu/wheatflour/CKPAFF/index.htm; accessed August 21, 2008.
43. Grosse SD, Waitzman NJ, Romano PS, Mulinare J. Reevaluating the benefits of folic acid fortification in the United States: Economic analysis, regulation, and public health. *Am J Public Health* 2005; 95:1917–22.
44. World Health Organization. *Food and Agriculture Organization. Guidelines on Food Fortification with Micronutrients. Geneva* World Health Organization and Food and Agriculture Organization of the United Nations, 2006.
45. Food and Drug Administration. Food labeling: Health claims and label statement; folate and neural tube defects. *Fed Reg* 1993:53254–95.
46. Lewis CJ, Crane NT, Wilson DB, Yetley EA. Estimated folate intakes: Data updated to reflect food fortification, increased bioavailability, and dietary supplement use. *Am J Clin Nutr* 1999; 70:198–207.
47. Yetley EA, Rader JI. Modeling the level of fortification and post-fortification assessments: U.S. experience. *Nutr Rev* 2004; 62:S50–59; discussion S60–61.
48. Boushey CJ, Edmonds JW, Welshimer KJ. Estimates of the effects of folic-acid fortification and folic-acid bioavailability for women. *Nutrition* 2001; 17:873–79.
49. Caudill MA, Le T, Moonie SA, Esfahani ST, Cogger EA. Folate status in women of childbearing age residing in Southern California after folic acid fortification. *J Am Coll Nutr* 2001; 20:129–34.
50. Choumenkovitch SF, Selhub J, Wilson PW, Rader JI, Rosenberg IH, Jacques PF. Folic acid intake from fortification in United States exceeds predictions. *J Nutr* 2002; 132:2792–98.
51. Quinlivan EP, Gregory JF 3rd. Effect of food fortification on folic acid intake in the United States. *Am J Clin Nutr* 2003; 77:221–25.
52. Quinlivan EP, Gregory JF 3rd. Reassessing folic acid consumption patterns in the United States (1999–2004): Potential effect on neural tube defects and overexposure to folate. *Am J Clin Nutr* 2007; 86:1773–79.

53. Yang QH, Carter HK, Mulinare J, Berry RJ, Friedman JM, Erickson JD. Race-ethnicity differences in folic acid intake in women of childbearing age in the United States after folic acid fortification: Findings from the National Health and Nutrition Examination Survey, 2001–2002. *Am J Clin Nutr* 2007; 85:1409–16.

54. Rader JI, Weaver CM, Angyal G. Total folate in enriched cereal-grain products in the United States following fortification. *Food Chem* 2000; 70:275–89.

55. Canada Gazette. Food and drugs regulations. SOR/96-527. *Canada Gazette* Part II 1996. Available at http://canadagazette.gc.ca/partII/1998/19981125/html/sor550-e. html; accessed September 27, 2008.

56. De Wals P, Rusen ID, Lee NS, Morin P, Niyonsenga T. Trend in prevalence of neural tube defects in Quebec. *Birth Defects Res A Clin Mol Teratol* 2003; 67:919–23.

57. Sayed AR, Bourne D, Pattinson R, Nixon J, Henderson B. Decline in the prevalence of neural tube defects following folic acid fortification and its cost-benefit in South Africa. *Birth Defects Res A Clin Mol Teratol* 2008; 82:211–16.

58. Berner LA, Clydesdale FM, Douglass JS. Fortification contributed greatly to vitamin and mineral intakes in the United States, 1989–1991. *J Nutr* 2001; 131:2177–83.

59. Imhoff-Kunsch B, Flores R, Dary O, Martorell R. Wheat flour fortification is unlikely to benefit the neediest in Guatemala. *J Nutr* 2007; 137:1017–22.

60. Oakley GP Jr, Weber MB, Bell KN, Colditz P. Scientific evidence supporting folic acid fortification of flour in Australia and New Zealand. *Birth Defects Res A Clin Mol Teratol* 2004; 70:838–41.

61. Busby A, Abramsky L, Dolk H, Armstrong B. Preventing neural tube defects in Europe: Population based study. *BMJ* 2005; 330:574–75.

62. Fletcher RJ, Bell IP, Lambert JP. Public health aspects of food fortification: A question of balance. *Proc Nutr Soc* 2004; 63:605–14.

63. Castilla EE, Orioli IM, Lopez-Camelo JS, Dutra Mda G, Nazer-Herrera J. Preliminary data on changes in neural tube defect prevalence rates after folic acid fortification in South America. *Am J Med Genet A* 2003; 123A:123–28.

64. Hertrampf E, Cortes F, Erickson JD, Cayazzo M, Freire W, Bailey LB, Howson C, Kauwell GP, Pfeiffer C. Consumption of folic acid-fortified bread improves folate status in women of reproductive age in Chile. *J Nutr* 2003; 133:3166–69.

65. Honein MA, Paulozzi LJ, Mathews TJ, Erickson JD, Wong LY. Impact of folic acid fortification of the US food supply on the occurrence of neural tube defects. *JAMA* 2001; 285:2981–86.

66. Lopez-Camelo JS, Orioli IM, da Graca Dutra M, Nazer-Herrera J, Rivera N, Ojeda ME, Canessa A, et al. Reduction of birth prevalence rates of neural tube defects after folic acid fortification in Chile. *Am J Med Genet A* 2005; 135:120–25.

67. Mathews TJ. *Trends in Spina Bifida and Anencephalus in the United States, 1991–2005. NCHS Health E-stats 2007.* Available at http://www.cdc.gov/nchs/products/pubs/pubd/ hestats/spine_anen.htm; accessed May 2, 2008.

68. Persad VL, Van den Hof MC, Dube JM, Zimmer P. Incidence of open neural tube defects in Nova Scotia after folic acid fortification. *CMAJ* 2002; 167:241–45.

69. Ray JG, Meier C, Vermeulen MJ, Boss S, Wyatt PR, Cole DE. Association of neural tube defects and folic acid food fortification in Canada. *Lancet* 2002; 360:2047–48.

70. Hickling S, Hung J, Knuiman M, Jamrozik K, McQuillan B, Beilby J, Thompson P. Impact of voluntary folate fortification on plasma homocysteine and serum folate in Australia from 1995 to 2001: A population based cohort study. *J Epidemiol Community Health* 2005; 59:371–76.

71. Hoey L, McNulty H, Askin N, Dunne A, Ward M, Pentieva K, Strain J, Molloy AM, Flynn CA, Scott JM. Effect of a voluntary food fortification policy on folate, related B vitamin status, and homocysteine in healthy adults. *Am J Clin Nutr* 2007; 86:1405–13.

72. Bower C, Ryan A, Rudy E, Miller M. Trends in neural tube defects in Western Australia. *Aust N Z J Public Health* 2002; 346:725–30.
73. Chan A, Pickering J, Haan E, Netting M, Burford A, Johnson A, Keane RJ. "Folate before pregnancy": The impact on women and health professionals of a population-based health promotion campaign in South Australia. *Med J Aust* 2001; 174:631–36.
74. Halliday JL, Riley M. Fortification of foods with folic acid. *N Engl J Med* 2000; 343:970–71; author reply 2.
75. Oddy WH, Miller M, Payne JM, Serna P, Bower CI. Awareness and consumption of folate-fortified foods by women of childbearing age in Western Australia. *Public Health Nutr* 2007; 10:989–95.
76. Boulet SL, Yang Q, Mai C, Kirby RS, Collins JS, Robbins JM, Meyer R, Canfield MA, Mulinare J. Trends in the postfortification prevalence of spina bifida and anencephaly in the United States. *Birth Defects Res A Clin Mol Teratol* 2008; 82:527–32.
77. Liu S, West R, Randell E, Longerich L, O'Connor KS, Scott H, Crowley M, Lam A, Prabhakaran V, McCourt C. A comprehensive evaluation of food fortification with folic acid for the primary prevention of neural tube defects. *BMC Pregnancy Childbirth* 2004; 4:20.
78. Wald NJ, Law MR, Morris JK, Wald DS. Quantifying the effect of folic acid. *Lancet* 2001; 358:2069–73.
79. Daly LE, Kirke PN, Molloy A, Weir DG, Scott JM. Folate levels and neural tube defects. Implications for prevention. *JAMA* 1995; 274:1698–702.
80. Senti FR, Pilch SM. Analysis of folate data from the second National Health and Nutrition Examination Survey (NHANES II). *J Nutr* 1985; 115:1398–402.
81. Dietrich M, Brown CJ, Block G. The effect of folate fortification of cereal-grain products on blood folate status, dietary folate intake, and dietary folate sources among adult non-supplement users in the United States. *J Am Coll Nutr* 2005; 24:266–74.
82. Pfeiffer CM, Johnson CL, Jain RB, Yetley EA, Picciano MF, Rader JI, Fisher KD, Mulinare J, Osterloh JD. Trends in blood folate and vitamin B-12 concentrations in the United States, 1988–2004. *Am J Clin Nutr* 2007; 86:718–27.
83. Jacques PF, Selhub J, Bostom AG, Wilson PW, Rosenberg IH. The effect of folic acid fortification on plasma folate and total homocysteine concentrations. *N Engl J Med* 1999; 340:1449–54.
84. Lawrence JM, Petitti DB, Watkins M, Umekubo MA. Trends in serum folate after food fortification. *Lancet* 1999; 354:915–16.
85. Centers for Disease Control and Prevention. Folate status in women of childbearing age, by race/ethnicity—United States, 1999–2000. *MMWR Morb Mortal Wkly Rep* 2002; 51:808–10.
86. Ray JG, Vermeulen MJ, Boss SC, Cole DE. Increased red cell folate concentrations in women of reproductive age after Canadian folic acid food fortification. *Epidemiology* 2002; 13:238–40.
87. Watkins ML, Edmonds L, McClearn A, Mullins L, Mulinare J, Khoury M. The surveillance of birth defects: The usefulness of the revised US standard birth certificate. *Am J Public Health* 1996; 86:731–34.
88. Cragan JD, Roberts HE, Edmonds LD, Khoury MJ, Kirby RS, Shaw GM, Velie EM, et al. Surveillance for anencephaly and spina bifida and the impact of prenatal diagnosis—United States, 1985–1994. *MMWR CDC Surveill Summ* 1995; 44:1–13.
89. Centers for Disease Control and Prevention. Folate status in women of childbearing age, by race/ethnicity—United States, 1999–2000, 2001–2002, and 2003–2004. *MMWR Morb Mortal Wkly Rep* 2007; 55:1377–80.
90. Ganji V, Kafai MR. Trends in serum folate, RBC folate, and circulating total homocysteine concentrations in the United States: Analysis of data from National Health and Nutrition Examination Surveys, 1988–1994, 1999–2000, and 2001–2002. *J Nutr* 2006; 136:153–58.

91. Williams LJ, Rasmussen SA, Flores A, Kirby RS, Edmonds LD. Decline in the prevalence of spina bifida and anencephaly by race/ethnicity: 1995–2002. *Pediatrics* 2005; 116:580–86.

92. Dowd JB, Aiello AE. Did national folic acid fortification reduce socioeconomic and racial disparities in folate status in the US? *Int J Epidemiol* 2008; 37:1059–66.

93. Centers for Disease Control and Prevention. Use of dietary supplements containing folic acid among women of childbearing age—US, 2005. *MMWR Morb Mortal Wkly Rep* 2005; 54:955–58.

94. Green-Raleigh K, Carter H, Mulinare J, Prue C, Petrini J. Trends in folic acid awareness and behavior in the United States: The Gallup Organization for the March of Dimes Foundation surveys, 1995–2005. *Matern Child Health J* 2006; 10:S177–82.

95. Morin P, De Wals P, Noiseux M, Niyonsenga T, St-Cyr-Tribble D, Tremblay C. Pregnancy planning and folic acid supplement use: Results from a survey in Quebec. *Prev Med* 2002; 35:143–49.

96. Morin P, De Wals P, St-Cyr-Tribble D, Niyonsenga T, Payette H. Pregnancy planning: A determinant of folic acid supplements use for the primary prevention of neural tube defects. *Can J Public Health* 2002; 93:259–63.

97. Cuskelly GJ, McNulty H, Scott JM. Effect of increasing dietary folate on red-cell folate: Implications for prevention of neural tube defects. *Lancet* 1996; 347:657–59.

98. Berry RJ, Li Z. Folic acid alone prevents neural tube defects: Evidence from the China study. *Epidemiology* 2002; 13:114–16.

99. Berry RJ, Li Z, Erickson JD, Li S, Moore CA, Wang H, Mulinare J, et al. Prevention of neural-tube defects with folic acid in China. China-U.S. Collaborative Project for Neural Tube Defect Prevention. *N Engl J Med* 1999; 341:1485–90.

100. Berry R, Carter H, Yang Q. Cognitive impairment in older Americans in the age of folic acid fortification. Letter. *Am J Clin Nutr* 2007; 86:265–67.

101. Yeung L, Yang Q, Berry RJ. Contributions of total daily intake of folic acid to serum folate concentrations. *JAMA* 2008; 300:2486–87.

102. Botto LD, Lisi A, Robert-Gnansia E, Erickson JD, Vollset SE, Mastroiacovo P, Botting B, et al. International retrospective cohort study of neural tube defects in relation to folic acid recommendations: Are the recommendations working? *BMJ* 2005; 330:571–73.

103. Oakley GP Jr, Bell KN, Weber MB. Recommendations for accelerating global action to prevent folic acid-preventable birth defects and other folate-deficiency diseases: Meeting of experts on preventing folic acid-preventable neural tube defects. *Birth Defects Res A Clin Mol Teratol* 2004; 70:835–37.

104. World Health Organization. *Folate and Vitamin B12 Deficiencies: Proceedings of a WHO Technical Consultation, October 18–21, 2005*. Boston: World Health Organization of the United Nations, 2008. *Food Nutr Bull* 2008 Jun; 29:no.2 (supplement)

105. Christianson A, Modell B, Howson C. *March of Dimes Global Report on Birth Defects: The Hidden Toll of Dying and Disabled Children*. White Plains, NY, 2006.

106. Bell KN, Oakley GP Jr. Tracking the prevention of folic acid-preventable spina bifida and anencephaly. *Birth Defects Res A Clin Mol Teratol*. 2006; 76:654–57.

107. Rosenberg IH. Science-based micronutrient fortification: Which nutrients, how much, and how to know? *Am J Clin Nutr* 2005; 82:279–80.

9 Folate and Cancer

Epidemiological Perspective

Jia Chen, Xinran Xu, Amy Liu, and Cornelia M. Ulrich

CONTENTS

I. INTRODUCTION

Previous chapters summarized biological and physiological mechanisms of folate and highlighted the critical role of folate in the etiology of human diseases, including cancer. Many of these results have been substantiated by epidemiological studies, which in turn help generate new hypotheses to be tested by experimental studies and, more importantly, aid the translation of laboratory findings into health policies and clinical care.

Human cancers are considered the result of genetic and epigenetic changes. Global hypomethylation, accompanied by promoter hypermethylation, is a common feature of tumor cells [1]. Global hypomethylation may induce chromosomal instability, reactivate transposons, promote loss of imprinting, and activate proto-oncogenes. Yet, reduced methylation may also protect against C→T mutations [2]. Promoter hypermethylation, on the other hand, is associated with the inactivation of genes in virtually all pathways protective of carcinogenesis (e.g., DNA repair, cell cycle control, inflammatory/stress response, detoxification, apoptosis). Folate-mediated one-carbon metabolism (FOCM) can impact both genetic and epigenetic procarcinogenic processes by playing critical roles in both DNA methylation and DNA synthesis [3]. A low methyl supply can induce DNA global hypomethylation and deficient conversion of deoxyuridine monophosphate (dUMP) to deoxythymidine monophosphate (dTMP), leading to uracil misincorporation into DNA. The repair activity by uracil glycosylases can lead to DNA strand breaks, resulting in enhanced mutagenesis and apoptosis. Because of the essential roles in these critical processes, folate metabolism not only is capable of influencing the pathogenesis of human cancers, but it has also been the target pathway for chemotherapy and chemoprevention of these diseases.

In this chapter, we summarize the epidemiological evidence for the association between folate status and genetic polymorphisms in folate metabolism in relation to cancer risk. We also discuss the role of folate in chemotherapy and cancer prevention, as well as increasing concerns that high intake of folate, especially from supplementation, may interfere with anticancer drugs and confer increased risk of cancers by promoting pre-existing lesions.

II. FOLATE INTAKE AND CANCER RISK: EPIDEMIOLOGICAL EVIDENCE

Associations of folate intake and cancer risk have been studied extensively in many cancer sites using both cohort and case–control study designs. Subsequent pooled and meta-analyses combining data from individual studies have also been performed for selected cancer sites. Whereas meta-analyses combine the published results of summary effects such as relative risk (RR) or odds ratio (OR), pooled analyses combine individual-level data that permit a full examination of effect modification within the data. It is important to note that these pooled or meta-analyses are performed retrospectively and are subject to inherent limitations such as study heterogeneity and publication bias. Nevertheless, these analyses offer increased power to detect associations, especially as the number of included studies increases.

In epidemiological studies, folate as an exposure of interest is often assessed from food frequency questionnaires or circulating biomarkers (i.e., plasma folate or red blood cell [RBC] folate concentration). Folate intake can be referred to as dietary intake (from food) or total intake (from food and supplements). Folate naturally found in foods is predominantly in the form of 5-methyl-tetrahydrofolate (5-methyl-THF); meanwhile, the fully unreduced (e.g., folic acid) and partially reduced (e.g., dihydrofolate [DHF]) forms are also found [4]. In contrast, folate in supplements and food fortification is the synthetic form, folic acid, which needs to be reduced before it can participate in cellular reactions [5]. Biomarkers of folate that are examined in epidemiological studies usually include RBC folate and serum/plasma folate concentrations. In addition to the use of biological folate in body fluids as a surrogate for folate exposure, total homocysteine (tHcy) concentration in plasma or serum is used as a functional marker of intracellular folate availability.

In this section, epidemiological evidence is grouped and considered by the strength of evidence. First, results from pooled analyses and meta-analyses are the primary focus, and cancer sites are discussed with these analysis results. Then, findings for cancer sites are summarized with cohort and case–control studies for which pooled or meta-analyses have not been carried out. Last, results of cancer sites that only have case–control study data, are presented.

A. POOLED ANALYSIS AND META-ANALYSIS ON FOLATE INTAKE AND CANCER RISK

Table 9.1 summarizes the results of six meta-analyses and one pooled analysis that were available as of March 2008 on folate intake and cancer risk. The cancer types include colorectal, breast, gastric, lung, esophageal, and pancreatic, among which colorectal and breast cancer have the most comprehensive data.

1. Colorectal Cancer

Colorectal cancer is the most intensively studied cancer site in terms of its risk association with folate consumption. Epidemiological evidence indicates a significant inverse relationship between dietary folate intake (folate from foods alone) and risk of colorectal neoplasia; however, the association is much attenuated with respect to total folate consumption (folate from foods and supplements). In a meta-analysis of seven cohort and nine case–control studies [6], the RR of colorectal cancer was 0.75 (95% confidence interval [CI], 0.64–0.89) for dietary folate and 0.95 (95% CI, 0.81–1.11) for total folate (high vs. low) in cohort studies. Combining the nine case–control studies, the overall RR associated with dietary folate (high vs. low) was 0.76 (95% CI, 0.60–0.96), although there was significant heterogeneity among

TABLE 9.1
Summary of Meta- and Pooled Analyses on Folate and Cancer Risk by Cancer Type

Cancer Type	Reference	Folate Measurement	No. of Studies Included	No. of Cases	No. of Controls[a]	Summary RR or OR	Comparison
Colorectal	Sanjoaquin et al. [6]	Dietary intake	5 cohort	2,394	177,689	0.75 (0.64–0.89)	High vs. low
		Total intake	3 cohort	2,689	175,059	0.95 (0.81–1.11)	High vs. low
		Dietary intake	7 case–control	6,166	9,676	0.76 (0.60–0.96)	High vs. low
		Total intake	3 case–control	958	1,499	0.81 (0.62–1.05)	High vs. low
Breast	Larsson et al. [13]	Dietary intake	8 cohort	8,367	302,959	0.97 (0.88–1.07)	200-µg/day increments
		Total intake	6 cohort	8,165	306,209	1.01 (0.97–1.05)	200-µg/day increments
		Dietary intake	13 case–control	8,558	10,812	0.80 (0.72–0.89)	200-µg/day increments
		Total intake	3 case–control	2,184	3,233	0.93 (0.81–1.07)	200-µg/day increments
		Blood levels	3 cohort	970	1,979	0.81 (0.59–1.10)	High vs. low
		Blood levels	2 case–control	269	366	0.41 (0.15–1.10)	High vs. low
	Lewis et al. [17]	Dietary intake	9 cohort	11,227	331,462	0.99 (0.98–1.01)	100-µg/day increments
		Dietary intake	13 case–control	8,566	10,834	0.91 (0.87–0.96)	100-µg/day increments
Gastric	Larsson et al. [23]	Dietary intake	2 cohort	438	64,556	1.01 (0.72–1.42)	Highest vs. lowest
		Dietary intake	9 case–control	3,205	5,574	0.88 (0.67–1.14)	Highest vs. lowest
Lung[b]	Cho et al. [25]	Dietary intake	8 cohort	3,155	430,281	0.88 (0.74–1.04)	Highest vs. lowest
		Total intake	5 cohort	1,734	430,281	1.02 (0.83–1.26)	Highest vs. lowest
Esophageal	Larsson et al. [23]	Dietary intake	7 case–control	1,496	3,747	0.62 (0.53–0.72)	Highest vs. lowest
Pancreatic	Larsson et al. [23]	Dietary intake	4 cohort and 1 case–control	722	253	0.52 (0.36–0.75)	Highest vs. lowest
		Dietary intake	4 cohort	618	210,315	0.49 (0.35–0.67)	Highest vs. lowest

[a] For cohort study, the numbers are total participants in the study.
[b] This is a pooled analysis.

these studies (P, heterogeneity $< .01$). For total folate, the RR was 0.81 (95% CI, 0.62–1.05). However, a concern is that these studies calculated "total folate" intake by adding up the micrograms of dietary folate with the micrograms derived from supplement use (synthetic folic acid). This is problematic because folic acid has 1.7-fold greater bioavailability. Using the crude approach of simply summing up can result in misclassification and bias risk estimates toward null effects. A more appropriate approach is to use dietary folate equivalents (DFE) as recommended by the Institute of Medicine [7,8], which allows for a combination of dietary and synthetic folic acid into a variable that accounts for this differential bioavailability.

Since publication of this meta-analysis in 2005, several prospective cohort studies have been published. Results from the Swedish Mammography Cohort, which followed 61,433 women from 1987 through 2004 with 805 cases, indicated an inverse association between dietary folate intake and risk of cancer only of the colon (RR, 0.61; 95% CI, 0.41–0.91), not rectum; this inverse association was more pronounced among smokers than nonsmokers [9]. In a randomized trial of disease prevention with aspirin and vitamin E (220 cases among 37,916 women with a 10-year average follow-up period) [10], dietary folate was inversely associated with colorectal cancer risk among women who were not taking supplements (RR, 0.46; 95% CI, 0.26–0.81); no apparent association was found with respect to total folate intake (micrograms, not DFE).

Besides folate consumption, folate concentration in serum or plasma provides an estimate of the physiological folate status of an individual that takes into account both lifestyle and genetic factors. In a nested case–control study within the prospective Physician's Health Study with a 12-year follow-up period (202 cases and 326 controls), baseline deficient plasma folate concentration (< 3 ng/ml) was associated with a marginal significantly increased risk of colorectal cancer (OR, 1.78; 95% CI, 0.93–3.42) [11]. However, in a recent report from the Northern Sweden Health and Disease Cohort (a nested case–control study of 226 cases and 437 controls), a bell-shaped association between plasma folate concentrations and risk of colorectal cancer was reported [12]. The OR for middle versus lowest quintile was 2.00 (95% CI, 1.13–3.56); in subjects with follow-up times greater than the median of 4.2 years, high plasma folate concentrations significantly increased the risk of colorectal cancer (highest vs. lowest: OR, 3.87; 95% CI, 1.52–9.87).

2. Breast Cancer

Although a number of cohort and case–control studies have suggested an inverse association between folate status and the risk of breast cancer, these results are far from conclusive. In a meta-analysis summarizing studies published between 1966 and 2006 [13], folate intake (both dietary and total) in increasing increments of 200 µg/day was not associated with the risk of breast cancer in eight prospective studies; however, an inverse association with dietary folate was observed in 13 case–control studies (OR, 0.80; 95% CI, 0.72–0.89). Data from several cohort studies, including the Nurses' Health Study, the Canadian National Breast Screening Study, and the Iowa Women's Health Study, also indicate that adequate folate intake could attenuate the elevated risk associated with moderate alcohol consumption [14–16]. In addition, there was an indication of inverse associations between blood folate concentrations and breast cancer risk, especially in case–control studies, although these associations failed to reach statistical significance.

Similar results were observed from another meta-analysis by Lewis et al. [17]. In this study, 13 case–control studies and nine cohort studies were included; some overlapped with the study by Larsson et al. [13]. Summary ORs for dietary folate were 0.91 (95% CI, 0.87–0.96) for the case–control studies and 0.99 (95% CI, 0.98–1.01) for the cohort studies with a 100-μg/day increase in folate intake. This study lends additional support that dietary folate (not total folate) may be moderately protective against breast cancer.

Results from subsequent cohort studies have been inconsistent or even conflicting. In a French cohort study (1,812 cases among 62,739 postmenopausal women with 9-year follow-up period), an inverse association was observed (RR, 0.78; 95% CI, 0.67–0.90) [18]. In a report from the Prostate, Lung, Colorectal, and Ovarian Cancer Screening Trial (691 cases among 25,400 women with a 10-year follow-up period), an increased risk of breast cancer was observed in postmenopausal women with folic acid supplemental use of 400 μg/day or more [19]. No apparent association between folate status and risk of breast cancer was observed in the Nurses' Health Study II, in which 90,663 premenopausal women were followed for 12 years with 1,032 documented breast cancer cases [20]. In the Malmö Diet and Cancer cohort study (392 cases among 11,699 women with 9.5-year follow-up period), a high folate intake (both dietary and total) was associated with an approximately 40% lower incidence of postmenopausal breast cancer [21].

Alcohol is known to be a folate antagonist. There is consistent evidence that lower folate intake in combination with high alcohol intake is associated with an increased risk of breast cancer [13]. This suggests that a more severe reduction of one-carbon status is needed to result in associations with breast cancer. The relationship between folate status and breast cancer is complex in that a nonlinear relationship may exist [22]. Although folate or one-carbon deficiency is thought to increase risk, there is also evidence that very high intake from diet and supplements may result in elevated risk [19]. This suggests an inverted U-shaped relationship, which requires further research [22].

3. Gastric Cancer

Evidence to date does not support an association between folate intake and gastric cancer risk. In a meta-analysis of nine case–control and two cohort studies (3,205 cases of gastric cancer) [23], no significant association was detected. However, heterogeneity related to geographical region may have contributed to this lack of association. The summary ORs for individuals in the highest category relative to the lowest category of dietary folate intake were 0.68 (95% CI, 0.58–0.80) in studies conducted in the United States ($n = 4$), 1.15 (95% CI, 0.91–1.45) in European studies ($n = 4$), and 0.89 (95% CI, 0.40–1.96) for studies conducted elsewhere ($n = 3$). There was no heterogeneity within the studies conducted in the United States or Europe.

With respect to biological folate status in relation to gastric cancer, the only report comes from a case–control study (247 cases and 631 controls) nested within the large European Prospective Investigation into Cancer and Nutrition cohort (> 500,000 participants) [24]. No association was found between plasma folate concentration and overall gastric cancer risk or by anatomical site (cardia/noncardia) or histological type (diffuse/intestinal).

4. Lung Cancer

Results from epidemiological studies currently do not provide strong evidence of the protective role of folate intake in lung cancer risk. A pooled analysis of eight prospective cohort studies was conducted [25]. A total of 3,206 incident cases of lung cancer (1,398 females and 1,808 males) were documented during 6 to 16 years of follow-up in these eight cohort studies. In the analyses adjusted for age only, both dietary and total folate intakes were significantly associated with reduction in lung cancer risk for comparison of the highest versus lowest quintiles of intake (dietary folate: RR, 0.61; 95% CI, 0.51–0.72; and total folate: RR, 0.73; 95% CI, 0.60–0.89). However, these inverse associations were substantially attenuated and did not reach statistical significance in multivariate analyses (dietary folate: RR, 0.88; 95% CI, 0.74–1.04; and total folate: RR, 1.02; 95% CI, 0.83–1.26). These results did not differ by gender, smoking habits, or cancer type. The same limitations regarding the calculation of "total folate" use apply, as discussed above for colorectal cancer. In the Vitamins and Lifestyle (VITAL) study ($n = 77,721$ men and women aged 50–76 years), daily use of supplemental folic acid for 10 years was not associated with risk of lung cancer; the association did not differ by smoking status or lung cancer morphology [26].

5. Esophageal Cancer

Epidemiological studies suggest that high dietary folate intake was associated with reduced risk of esophageal cancer. A meta-analysis of seven case–control studies [23] reported a reduction in risk for individuals in the highest relative to the lowest category of dietary folate intake; the summary ORs were 0.66 for esophageal squamous cell carcinoma (929 cases; 95% CI, 0.53–0.83), 0.50 for esophageal adenocarcinoma (501 cases; 95% CI, 0.39–0.65), and 0.62 for esophageal cancer (1,496 cases; 95% CI, 0.53–0.72). No heterogeneity was detected among these studies.

6. Pancreatic Cancer

Pancreatic cancer is a malignancy with very high mortality (median survival, 3 months) and few established risk factors. In a meta-analysis of four cohort and one case–control studies with a total of approximately 720 cases [13], a protective association between dietary folate and pancreatic cancer risk was observed (OR, 0.49; 95% CI, 0.35–0.67; high vs. low). No heterogeneity was detected among individual studies. Restricting the analysis to cohort studies yielded similar results (RR, 0.52; 95% CI, 0.36–0.75).

In a nested case–control study (126 cases and 247 controls) within the Alpha-Tocopherol, Beta-Carotene Cancer Prevention Study cohort of 29,133 Finnish male smokers, the highest serum folate concentration was associated with lower risk of pancreatic cancer (OR, 0.45; 95% CI, 0.24–0.82) [27]. However, data from a more recent case–control study (208 cases and 623 controls) nested in four large prospective cohorts did not support such an association. Comparing the highest with lowest quartiles of plasma folate concentration, the OR was 1.20 (95% CI, 0.76–1.91) [28].

B. Prospective Analyses on Folate and Cancer Risk

This section examines the evidence of folate–cancer relationships in which prospective studies and case–control studies, but no pooled or meta-analyses, have been conducted.

1. Ovarian Cancer

Results from prospective cohort studies in which folate status and ovarian cancer risk have been investigated are generally weak. Lack of association between dietary folate intake and risk of ovarian cancer has been reported from three cohort studies—the Canadian National Breast Screening Study (264 cases among 48,766 participants; RR, 0.75; 95% CI, 0.42–1.34) [29], the Nurses' Health Study (481 cases among 80,254 participants; RR, 1.21; 95% CI, 0.92–1.60) [30], and the Iowa Women's Health Study (147 cases among 27,205 participants) (RR, 1.73; 95% CI, 0.90–3.33) [31]. Results from these studies also suggested a reduced risk at relatively high levels of folate intake only among women consuming 4 g of alcohol or more per day. In a population-based cohort study, the Swedish Mammography Cohort (266 cases among 61,084 women) [32], dietary folate intake was inversely associated with total epithelial ovarian cancer risk with borderline significance (RR, 0.67; 95% CI, 0.43–1.04; P, trend = .08); this association was more profound among women who consumed more than 20 g of alcohol per week (RR, 0.26; 95% CI, 0.11–0.60; P, trend = .001).

2. Liver Cancer

In a high-risk Chinese cohort in which participants were hepatitis B surface antigen–positive (~400 cases among 90,836 participants) [33], a higher RBC folate concentration was associated with reduced risk of hepatocarcinoma (RR, 0.33; 95% CI, 0.13–0.86); however, the association with serum folate did not reach statistical significance (RR, 0.56; 95% CI, 0.21–1.50). It is commonly believed that RBC folate concentration reflects long-term folate status, whereas serum folate concentration may be subject to transient influences at the time of measurement.

3. Lymphoma

No significant association between dietary folate and risk of non-Hodgkin lymphoma was observed in two cohort studies [34,35]. There is an indication of lower risk of non-Hodgkin lymphoma associated with increasing folate intake from case–control studies [36,37]; however, no such association was observed in another case–control study [38].

C. Case–Control Analyses of Folate and Cancer Risk

In this section, the limited evidence related to folate consumption and cancer risk at the cancer sites for which only case–control studies have been carried out to date is briefly summarized.

1. Cervical Cancer

Case–control studies have not provided consistent results related to folate intake and risk of preinvasive cervical lesions or cervical cancer. Nonsignificant protective effects of folate intake were reported from two hospital-based case–control studies with approximately 100 cases in each [39,40] and several population-based studies with 200 to 300 cases in each [41–43]. This lack of association was also reported in other studies [44–47].

With respect to biomarkers of folate status, a low RBC folate concentration has been associated with increased risk of cervical cancer in a population tested extensively for high-risk human papillomaviruses (HPV) and cervical intraepithelial neoplasia [48] and may also enhance the effect of HPV infection for cervical dysplasia [49]. Meanwhile, no association between biomarkers of folate status and risk of cervical cancer was found in other studies [50–53]. Results from some small randomized trials have not generated convincing evidence for a protective effect of folate [54–57].

2. Leukemia

Data are sparse on folate–leukemia associations, perhaps because of the difficulty of measuring relevant folate intake in children and the rarity of adult leukemia. In a case–control study (83 cases and 166 controls) from Western Australia, a protective association between maternal folic acid supplementation during pregnancy and childhood acute lymphoblastic leukemia (ALL) was reported (OR, 0.37; 95% CI, 0.21–0.65) [58]. However, data from another case–control study (97 cases and 303 controls) conducted in New Zealand did not support such an association (OR, 1.1; 95% CI, 0.5–2.7) [59]. Nevertheless, several polymorphisms in folate-metabolizing enzymes have been associated with hematopoietic malignancies, as discussed later in this chapter.

3. Head and Neck Cancer

Few studies with limited sample sizes have been conducted on folate intake and risk of head and neck cancer. In two small case–control studies, a significantly lower concentration of serum folate was found in cases than in controls [60,61]. An inverse relationship between dietary folate and cancer risk was also reported in a case–control study (237 cases, 711 controls) [62]. Nevertheless, larger studies are warranted to confirm these associations.

4. Endometrial Cancer

Xu et al. [63] observed a significant reduction of cancer risk with high dietary folate intake in a case–control study (1,204 cases and 1,212 controls) (highest vs. lowest quartile of intake, OR, 0.6; 95% CI, 0.4–0.7), and the inverse association was more profound among non–B vitamin supplement users. A significant inverse association was also observed by McCann et al. [64] in a case–control study (232 cases and 639 controls) with an OR of 0.4 (95% CI, 0.2–0.7) for highest versus lowest quartile of intake. A nonsignificant reduction in risk was observed in another case–control study (368 cases and 713 controls) [65], whereas no association between dietary intake of folate-rich foods and cancer risk was found in a case–control study (399 cases and 296 controls) [66].

In summary, the association between folate and cancer risk has been most extensively studied for colorectal and breast cancer. Although the evidence supporting a protective role of folate in the prevention of colorectal cancer is strong, the association with breast cancer risk may be more complex and involve an interaction with alcohol intake as well as a nonlinear dose response. Seemingly inverse relationships between folate intake and risk of esophageal and pancreatic cancer should be further studied because few modifiable risk factors have been identified in these two cancers with high mortality rates. For other cancer sites, larger and well-designed studied are warranted to clarify folate–cancer associations.

III. GENETIC POLYMORPHISMS IN THE FOLATE METABOLISM PATHWAY AND ASSOCIATIONS WITH CANCER RISK

Accumulating evidence from molecular epidemiological studies has indicated that functional polymorphisms in FOCM can influence risk of cancer independently or jointly with dietary factors (folate, other B vitamins, and alcohol intake). This section provides an overview of functional genetic polymorphisms involved in FOCM genes and summarizes the results from epidemiological studies on cancer risk.

As illustrated in Figure 9.1, functioning of FOCM requires several micronutrients, including vitamins B12, B6, and riboflavin, as cofactors of various enzymes. It is important to consider that folate metabolism represents complex and interrelated metabolic reactions with many feedback mechanisms and other regulatory processes that ensure its robustness [67]. Accordingly, one may hypothesize that multiple disturbances within the pathway, or "stress" on the system, are needed to result in phenotypic effects. Such "stress" could be present under low intakes of folate or other nutrients or the presence of genetic polymorphisms with phenotypic changes of the enzymes involved in FOCM. Indeed, genetic polymorphisms in methylenetetrahydrofolate reductase (MTHFR) are most strongly associated with biomarkers, such as Hcy concentrations, when folate status is low. This provides a rationale for investigating gene–gene and gene–nutrient interactions within this complex system.

A. POLYMORPHISMS IN ONE-CARBON METABOLISM AND THEIR FUNCTIONAL IMPACT

Key enzymes involved in one-carbon metabolism are illustrated in Figure 9.1. They include MTHFR, thymidylate synthase (TS), methionine synthase (MTR), methionine synthase reductase (MTRR), serine hydroxymethyltransferase (SHMT), dihydrofolate reductase (DHFR), betaine-Hcy methyltransferase (BHMT), cystathionine-β-synthase (CBS), methylenetetrahydrofolate dehydrogenase (MTHFD1), reduced folate carrier (RFC1), and transcobalamin II (TCII).

An increasing number of genetic polymorphisms have been identified; their information is available on public databases such as the National Institutes of Health Database of Single Nucleotide Polymorphism (dbSNP). However, the number of "functional" polymorphisms, that is, those with confirmed phenotypic changes such as effects on activity or transcription of the protein, remains limited. Although results on tagging SNPs in one-carbon metabolism have started to emerge, most published studies have been on functional polymorphisms, that is, those with phenotypic effects, as indicated by biomarker measurements, or those that have been implicated in studies with disease endpoints (Table 9.2). These polymorphisms reside in key enzymes of the pathway; interruption of their functions may result in aberrant DNA

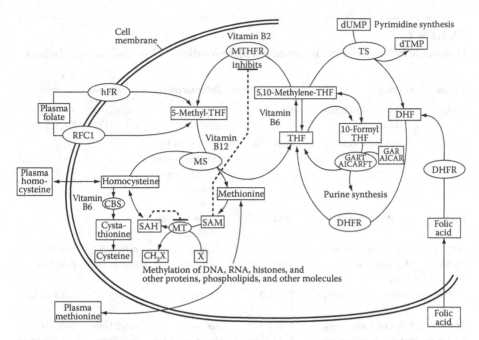

FIGURE 9.1 Overview of folate-mediated one-carbon metabolism (simplified), links to methylation reactions and nucleotide synthesis. AICAR, 5-aminoimidazole-4-carboxamide ribonucleotide; AICARFT, 5-amino-imidazole-4-carboxamide ribonucleotide transformylase; CBS, cystathionine-β-synthase; DHF, dihydrofolate; DHFR, dihydrofolate reductase; dTMP, deoxythymidine monophosphate; dUMP, deoxyuridine monophosphate; GAR, glycinamide ribonucleotide; GART, glycinamide ribonucleotide transformylase; hFR, human folate receptor; MS, methionine synthase; MT, methyltransferases; MTHFR, 5,10-methylenetetrahydrofolate reductase; RFC1 reduced folate carrier; SAH (AdoHcy), *S*-adenosylhomocysteine; SAM (AdoMet), *S*-adenosylmethionine; THF, tetrahydrofolate; TS, thymidylate synthase; X, a variety of substrates for methylation. (Modified from Ulrich CM, Robien K, McLeod HL, *Nat Rev Cancer* 2003; 3:912–20. With permission.)

synthesis or methylation (Figure 9.1). Several are nonsynonymous or reside in a regulatory region such as the 5′- or 3′-untranslated region (UTR), and they are generally common in human populations (> 5%). Although the biological effects of these polymorphisms are likely to be small or moderate at best, the underlying attributable risk cannot be neglected because of the high prevalence of these polymorphisms in the general population.

B. 5,10-METHYLENETETRAHYDROFOLATE REDUCTASE POLYMORPHISMS AND CANCER RISK

MTHFR is a pivotal enzyme in folate and Hcy metabolism, catalyzing the irreversible reduction of 5,10-methylene-THF to 5-methyl-THF. Its critical role in one-carbon metabolism provides strong biological rationale that inherited variability in the enzyme activity may influence cancer risk.

TABLE 9.2

Functional Polymorphisms Involved in Folate-Mediated One Carbon Metabolism

Genes	Enzyme	Chromosome	Polymorphism	rs Number	AA Change
MTHFR	5,10-methylene-THF reductase	1p36.3	677C→T	rs1801133	Ala222Val
			1298A→C	rs1801131	Glu429Ala
TS	Thymidylate synthase	18p11.32	5'-UTR 28-bp tandem repeat; 3'-UTR 6-bp deletion (1464del6)		
DHFR	Dihydrofolate reductase	5q11.2-q13.2	Intron 1–19-bp deletion		
MTR	Methionine synthase	1q43	2756A→G	rs1805087	Asp919Gly
MTRR	Methionine synthase reductase	5p15.3-p15.2	66A→G	rs1801394	Ile22Met
cSHMT	Serine hydroxymethyl-transferase	17p11.2	1420C→T	rs1979277	Leu474Phe
RFC1	Reduced folate carrier	21q22.3	80G→A	rs1051266	Arg27His
BHMT	Betaine-homocysteine methyltransferase	5q13.1-q15	742G→A	rs3733890	Arg239Gln
CBS	Cystathionine-β-synthase	21q22.3	31-bp VNTR		
MTHFD1	Methylene-THF dehydrogenase	14q24	401G→A	rs1950902	Arg134Lys
TCN2	Transcobalamin II	22q12.2	776C→G	rs1950902	Pro259Arg

The substrate of the MTHFR enzyme, 5,10-methylene-THF, is involved in the conversion of deoxyuridylate monophosphate to dTMP (for DNA synthesis). Low levels of 5,10-methylene-THF can result in misincorporation of uracil into DNA, leading to increased rates of point mutations and DNA/chromosome breakage [68]. A less active form of MTHFR should lead, all other factors being equal, to an accumulation of 5,10-methylene-THF and less uracil misincorporation, and thus a presumably lower cancer risk. Recent predictions from a mathematical simulation model of folate metabolism suggest such effects [69]. On the other hand, reduced MTHFR activity reduces the level of S-adenosylmethionine, the methyl donor for maintaining DNA methylation patterns, with possible impact on mutation rates and cancer risk [2,3,70].

Two SNPs of *MTHFR*, 677C→T (rs1801133) and 1298A→C (rs1801131), have been most extensively investigated in relation to cancer risk. The 677 variant homozygotes (677TT) have 70% lower enzyme activity compared with wild-type homozygotes (677CC), whereas heterozygotes retain 65% enzyme activity [71]. The functionality of the 1298A→C polymorphism is less well established. Individuals who are homozygous for the 1298 variant allele (CC) have about 60% activity compared with subjects carrying the 1298AA genotype in some studies [72]. The compound heterozygotes of the 677C→T and 1298A→C polymorphisms were shown to have similar phenotype as the 677TT genotype [72]; however, this phenotype may be partially explained by the fact that these two SNPs are in linkage disequilibrium [73]. Nevertheless, the two SNPs have been independently associated with folate and Hcy concentrations [74,75].

Table 9.3 summarizes the results from meta-analyses on the two *MTHFR* polymorphisms and cancer risk. Evidence of the reduced risk of colorectal cancer associated with the 677T allele is the strongest given the number of studies and the large sample sizes. The meta-analysis gave an estimate of about 20% lower risk for colorectal cancer for the *MTHFR* 677TT genotype compared with the 677CC genotype. Although there are fewer studies on the *MTHFR* 1298A→C polymorphism, the 1298C allele was associated with a comparable reduced risk. In contrast to colorectal cancer, an approximately 50% increased risk of gastric cancer was associated with the 677TT genotype from both pooled and meta-analyses. The 1298A→C polymorphism was not associated with gastric cancer risk. The difference in risk allele may suggest different etiological mechanisms of these diseases associated with one-carbon metabolism. Associations of *MTHFR* polymorphisms with risk of breast and lung cancer were also examined extensively. Although many individual studies reported significant findings, pooled and meta-analyses revealed no significant associations. In the case of ALL, results suggest that associations may differ by disease subtype (adult vs. childhood); nevertheless, these results conflict with the two meta-analyses that have been published. Although these two studies overlap with respect to individual studies that were included, an inverse relationship between the 677TT genotype and ALL was reported in adult ALL in one study [76] but in childhood ALL in the other [77]. No association with the 1298 polymorphism was found in either meta-analysis. A major limitation of the meta-analyses and pooled analyses performed on these polymorphisms to date is that they have not been able to take folate status (or one-carbon status in general) into account. Given the confirmed gene–diet interactions for *MTHFR*, solitary evaluation of the genetic factor is not very meaningful. In fact, combining results from study populations with divergent nutritional status may negate any effects.

C. SUMMARY OF STUDY RESULTS FOR OTHER POLYMORPHISMS AND CANCER RISK

1. Thymidylate Synthase

A polymorphic 28-bp tandem repeat is located in the 5′-UTR of the *TS* gene and functions as a *cis*-acting transcriptional enhancer element [78]. The *3R* allele was associated with approximately two to four times greater gene expression compared with the *2R* allele [79,80]. The *2R/2R* genotype was shown to be associated with reduced risk of colorectal cancer [81,82]. The *2R* allele was also associated with reduced risk of adult ALL [83]. With regard to breast cancer risk, the association was generally null. Within the 3′-UTR of the *TS* gene, a 6-bp deletion (1494del6) polymorphism was associated with reduced mRNA stability [84]. Some reports suggest

TABLE 9.3

Summary of Meta-Analysis Results of *MTHFR* Polymorphisms and Cancer Risk by Type

Cancer Type	Reference	SNP	No. Studies Included	Case/Control	Summary OR	P for Heterogeneity
Colorectal	Huang et al. [144]	C677T	23	10,131/15,362	0.93 (0.89–0.98) T vs. C allele	.22
					0.82 (0.75–0.89) TT vs. CC	
		A1298C	14	4,764/6,592	0.93 (0.85–1.01) C vs. A allele	.09
					0.80 (0.65–0.98) CC vs. AA	
	Hubner et al. [145]	C677T	25	12,243/17,688	0.83(0.75–0.93) TT vs. CC	.12
Breast	Lewis et al. [17]	C677T	17	6,373/8,434	1.04 (0.94–1.16) TT vs. CC	
	Zintzaras et al. [146]	C677T	18	5,476/7,336	1.02 (0.95–1.10) T vs. C allele	.08
		A1298C	10	3,768/5,276	0.97 (0.90–1.04) C vs. A allele	.21
Lung	Mao et al. [147]	C677T	8	5,111/6,415	1.12 (0.97–1.28) T vs. C allele	.0001
		A1298C	7	5,087/6,232	1.00 (0.92–1.08) C vs. A allele	.24
ALL[a]	Pereira et al. [76]	C677T	12	2,191/3,437	Childhood: 0.85 (0.70–1.04) TT vs. CC	.12
					Adult: 0.41 (0.24–0.72) TT vs. CC	.24
		A1298C	10	2,067/3,193	Childhood: 0.83 (0.55–1.25) CC vs. AA	.01
					Adult: 0.46 (0.03–7.46) CC vs. AA	
	Zintzaras et al. [77]	C677T	9	1,576/1,958	All: 0.88 (0.76–1.02) T vs. C allele	.09
					Childhood: 0.74 (0.57–0.96) T vs. C allele	.07
		A1298C	8	561/892	0.88 (0.72–1.07) C vs. A allele	.01
Gastric	Boccia et al. [148]	C677T	16 for meta	2,727/4,640	1.52 (1.31–1.77)	.37
			9 for pooled	1,540/2,577	1.49 (1.14–1.95) TT vs. CC	.06
		A1298C	7 for meta	1,223/2,015	0.94 (0.65–1.35)	
			5 for pooled	1,146/1,549	0.90 (0.69–1.34) CC vs. AA allele	.50
	Zintzaras [149]	C677T	8	1,584/2,785	1.27 (1.13–1.44) T vs. C allele	.12
		A1298C	4	760/1,624	1.00 (0.84–1.20) C vs. A allele	.47

a Acute lymphoblastic leukemia.

an interaction with nutrients to colorectal neoplasia [85]. However, the evidence of this polymorphism in relation to cancer risk is sparse, and the existing reports generally showed null results.

2. Methionine Synthase

The A2756G (Asp919Gly) polymorphism of *MTR* gene has been proposed to affect plasma Hcy concentrations [86,87]. This polymorphism has been investigated by several groups in relation to cancer risk. A reduced risk of colorectal cancer was associated with the 2756GG genotype in the Physician's Health Study [88] and a Norwegian cohort of more than 2,000 cases [89]. However, results from case–control studies were not consistent. With respect to breast cancer, one group found this SNP was associated with reduced risk [90], whereas null results were reported in other studies [91–93]. For other cancer sites, studies were generally of insufficient sample size to provide stable risk estimates for the rare homozygous variant genotype given the low frequency (< 5%). Because of the low allele frequency for this variant, statistical power for investigating gene–diet interactions has been generally insufficient [94].

3. Methionine Synthase Reductase

An association between the *MTR* A66G (Ile22Met) polymorphism and Hcy concentrations has been reported [95,96]; however, the functional impact of the variant has not been well defined [97]. One case–control study observed an elevated risk among whites with the GG genotype but not in people of other ethnicities [98]. In another case–control study, this polymorphism was not found to be associated with colorectal cancer risk, but it seems to interact with the association of folate and vitamin B6 in relation to colorectal cancer [99]. Among individuals with the AA genotype, vitamin B6 was associated with a decreased risk of colorectal cancer. A null association of this polymorphism with breast cancer risk was also reported in several studies [90–93].

4. Dihydrofolate Reductase

DHFR converts dihydrofolate into THF, and folic acid from supplements needs to be reduced by DHFR before participating in cellular reactions. A 19-bp polymorphism in intron 1 of the *DHFR* gene was identified with potential functionality [100]. One study found that although this 19-bp deletion polymorphism was not associated with breast cancer risk overall, the deletion allele was associated with increased breast cancer risk among multivitamin users [101]. A dose-dependent relationship between *DHFR* expression and the deletion genotype was observed. Compared with the 19-bp +/+ genotype, subjects with the −/− genotype had about fivefold higher mRNA levels [101].

5. Other Genes

There are many other sporadic reports on other polymorphisms of FOCM genes in relation to cancer risk, yet few researchers have performed systematic investigations. A number of positive findings are included here as examples. The *cSHMT* C1420T polymorphism was found to be associated with risk of esophageal [102] and ovarian [103] cancer in a case–control study, but no association with breast and lung cancer was found [92,104]. The *BHMT* G742A polymorphism was associated with risk of colorectal cancer [105]. The *RFC* G80A polymorphism has been studied in breast, gastric, colorectal, ovarian, and hematopoietic malignancies, but findings were generally null. The *MTHFD1* G401A polymorphism was found to be associated with a significant increased breast cancer risk among postmenopausal women in a case–control study [106]. Null associations with cancer risk were also reported for *TCNII* and *CBS* polymorphisms. However, some associations with these two genes have been found in specific studies. The *TCNII* Pro259 C776G polymorphism was associated with an overall increase in colorectal adenoma risk [107] and potential decrease in colorectal cancer risk among women [105]. Also, there is a weak inverse association between the *CBS* 844ins68 and colorectal carcinoma [98].

In summary, a large body of literature on genetic polymorphisms in relation to cancer risk lends support to the concept that genetic variability in FOCM plays a critical role in cancer etiology, especially in colorectal and gastric cancer. However, most epidemiological studies on FOCM polymorphisms have been limited in sample size. Larger and more systematic investigations that provide sufficient statistical power for investigating rarer variants and gene–gene and gene–diet interactions are needed. Another method of incorporating the extensive knowledge related to this pathway into the statistical analysis is through the use of a mathematical model of folate metabolism [108,109]. Initial result from the modeling has been promising, with model predictions consistent with experimental data [108–111]. This approach is a powerful tool to better understand gene–gene and gene–diet interactions in the FOCM pathway and biological mechanisms linking FOCM to carcinogenesis.

IV. FOLATE IN CHEMOTHERAPY

One major class of chemotherapeutic drugs for the treatment of cancers is characterized as antimetabolite/antifolate agents. These are designed to impair nucleotide synthesis and to disrupt normal cellular metabolism; consequently, they inhibit cell growth or induce cell death. These agents that target the folate-metabolic pathway can inhibit several intracellular folate-metabolizing enzymes. For example, 5-fluorouracil (5-FU), one of the most widely used chemotherapeutic drugs, inhibits TS; methotrexate (MTX), the mainstay for the treatment of ALL, targets primarily DHFR [112] (Figure 9.1). Both agents are able to induce cell cycle arrest and apoptosis by inhibiting the cell's ability to synthesize DNA and RNA. Although these antimetabolite/antifolate agents are widely used in cancer treatment, natural folate metabolites are used to modify the toxicity or efficacy of these drugs [113,114]. For example, folinic acid, a folic acid derivative, can maintain the vitamin activity of folic acid under MTX treatment because it does not require DHFR for its conversion, thereby allowing some DNA synthesis to occur in the presence of DHFR inhibition. Folinic acid is often administered along with MTX to "rescue" bone marrow and gastrointestinal mucosa cells from MTX treatment. Furthermore, folinic acid also enhances the inhibition of 5-FU on TS; thus, it is often used in combination with 5-FU in treating colon cancer.

However, there is considerable concern that nutritional folate intake, both from diet and in particular from high-dose supplements, may interfere with the efficacy of antifolate drugs (reviewed by Robien [115]). MTX, one of the classic antifolate drugs, has been widely used for several decades in the treatment of a variety of cancers, and the capacity of folate status to modify the clinical response of MTX in noncancerous outcomes has been well demonstrated [116–119]; nevertheless, the possible interaction between supplements and chemotherapeutic drugs has been rarely investigated. In the case of cancer treatment, a study of 71 children with non–B-cell acute lymphocytic leukemia receiving high-dose MTX reported that those who received a low dose of folinic acid had a lower risk of relapse compared with children receiving a high dose of folinic acid [120]. On the other hand, a clinical trial of adult patients receiving low-dose MTX for advanced or recurrent squamous cell head and neck cancer reported that patients receiving MTX alone had a statistically significant increase in overall toxicity compared with those receiving folinic acid at 24 hours after initiation of MTX [121]. It is not clear whether a reduction in toxicity may coincide with an abrogation in drug efficacy.

Several retrospective studies examined the effect of folate intake on outcomes of breast cancer chemotherapy. One study investigated the influence of folic acid supplements on chemotherapy-induced toxicity [122]. Toxicity was evaluated by measuring absolute neutrophil counts and the frequency and severity of oral mucositis. This small study included 49 breast cancer patients with multivitamin records and blood folate concentrations [122]. The decrease in neutrophil count caused by cytotoxic chemotherapy was shown to be ameliorated by the intake of folic acid–containing dietary supplements. Women with serum folate concentrations greater than 20 ng/mL exhibited a greater decrease in neutrophil count after chemotherapy than women with lower folate concentrations. This result suggests potential detrimental modulation of cytotoxic chemotherapy by excessive folic acid supplementation. However, these findings were not corroborated by the Iowa Women's Health Study, in which high folate intake was not associated with poor survival during a 14-year follow-up of 177 breast cancer cases treated with chemotherapy [123], although in this population-based setting no detailed information on treatment modalities and outcomes was available, which limits its clinical utility.

Use of antimetabolites/antifolates in chemotherapy could lead to drug resistance at many stages, from reduced drug transport to increased expression of target enzymes or by reducing metabolism of the drug [114]. Increased blood folate concentrations could theoretically facilitate drug resistance by a number of different mechanisms [114]. Data from in vitro studies support the conclusion that the cellular folate concentration is a determining factor in the sensitivity of cells to antifolates [124]. Folic acid in vitamin supplements or food fortification needs to be reduced by DHFR before it can act as a cofactor. As many antifolate drugs are inhibitors of DHFR, folic acid may compete with these drugs for the active site of the enzyme; thus, high folate concentration may result in up-regulation of DHFR activity, leading to drug resistance. Another mechanism of resistance may be mediated by proteins of the multidrug resistance family; these transporters may be up-regulated by exposure to elevated concentrations of folates and also trigger increased active transport of antifolate drugs out of the target cells [125].

In summary, folate metabolites may reduce toxicity and either abrogate or improve efficacy of antifolate-based chemotherapy [125]. Administering natural folate metabolites, such as folinic acid, may enhance the efficacy of antifolate therapy while reducing toxicity. To date, it is unknown whether the consumption of folic acid, in particular from vitamin supplements, interferes with the effectiveness of these drugs, affects toxicity, or possibly induces drug resistance. To develop clinical practice guidelines for the use of folic acid during antifolate therapy, we need more clinical and epidemiological studies that evaluate the types of folate (folic acid vs. folinic acid), timing, and dose. Some initial studies suggest that genetic polymorphisms in FOCM can also affect treatment outcomes [126,127]. Well-designed prospective studies are needed to evaluate the effects of folate status before treatment, dietary and supplemental folate intake during treatment, and genetic variation in the enzymes involved in folate metabolism on treatment-related toxicity and outcomes among patient populations receiving similar antifolate treatment regimens.

V. FOLATE IN CANCER PREVENTION

To date about 40 countries have adopted the policy of mandatory folic acid fortification. The primary aim of this policy has been to reduce the occurrence of neural tube defects [128]. These policies have been supported by purported benefits of folate in preventing cardiovascular disease [129–131] and possibly cognitive decline in aging populations [132]. In terms of cancer prevention, although a large body of evidence from cohort study or meta-analyses supports the chemopreventive role of folate against certain cancers, results from prevention trials are less convincing. More importantly, some evidence has begun to emerge that suggests folic acid may promote existing precancerous lesions, leading to increased risk of cancer. Although an inverse association of folate intake and cancer risk is suggested by epidemiological studies, folate antagonists, including MTX or 5-FU, demonstrate strong therapeutic efficacy in cancer treatment (see Section IV, Folates in Chemotherapy). This paradoxical observation suggests that the levels of folate exposure and the timing of exposure in relation to stage of tumorigenesis are critical in determining outcomes. This section focuses on the dual effects of folic acid in carcinogenesis, both from animal and epidemiological studies.

A. COLORECTAL CANCER

There is strong epidemiological evidence related to the inverse relationship between dietary folate intake and risk of colorectal cancer as discussed in Section II, Folate Intake and Cancer Risk: Epidemiological Evidence. Animal studies, on the other hand, generally support the causal relationship between folate deficiency and colorectal cancer risk, but they also demonstrate the importance of dosage and timing in the effects of folate on carcinogenesis [133]. For example, in a study using a mouse model of colorectal cancer (*APC/Min* mice), increasing dietary folate concentrations significantly reduced the number of ileal polyps in a dose-dependent manner at 3 months, but the association was reversed at 6 months [134]. In a more recent study exploring the timing of folic acid exposure in early life, folate depletion during pregnancy did not change intestinal tumor incidence; folate depletion after weaning, on the other hand, was shown to be protective against colorectal neoplasia in female mice [135]. These intriguing findings suggest that folic acid supplementation may enhance the development and progression of already existing, undiagnosed, premalignant and malignant lesions.

Nationwide fortification of enriched cereal grains with folic acid began in the United States and Canada in 1996 and 1997, respectively, and became mandatory in 1998. The rationale was to reduce the number of births complicated by NTDs. However, an ecological study suggests that both countries experienced a reversal of the downward trend in colorectal cancer incidence in the preceding decade [136]. Rates of colorectal cancer began to increase in 1996 in the United States and 1998 in Canada and peaked in 1998 and 2000, respectively. The rates have continued to exceed the pre-1996/1997 trends in both men and women. Changes in the rate of colorectal endoscopic procedures do not seem to account for this increased incidence of colorectal cancer [136]. Although these observations are derived from a study design (ecological study) that is prone to biases and does not prove causality, they are consistent with the recently suggested effects of folate on existing neoplasms, as shown in animal and clinical studies [133].

Recent findings from the Aspirin-Folate Polyp Prevention Study echo these concerns. This study was a double-blind, placebo-controlled, two-factor, randomized clinical trial of subjects with a recent history of colorectal adenomas. Folic acid supplementation in this trial not only showed no protection against adenoma recurrence but also conferred higher risks of having at least one advanced lesion during the 3 to 5-year follow-up period; folic acid was also associated with a higher risk of having three or more adenomas and of noncolorectal cancers [137]. Nevertheless, the study raised serious concerns not only about the lack of efficacy but also the potential adverse effects in colorectal cancer prevention and is consistent with a role of folate in promoting the growth of undetected preneoplastic lesions [138]. Making the field more complicated, the latest randomized, single-institution, double-blind, placebo-controlled trial demonstrated efficacy of folic acid in secondary chemoprevention of colorectal cancer [139]. In this study, high-dose (5 mg) supplementation of folic acid over a 3-year period was associated with a threefold lower incidence of recurring polyps. The unique aspect of this trial is the high dose (5 mg) compared with previous studies (0.4–1 mg). A recent modeling study suggests that folate fortification reduces colorectal cancer rates if started early in life but can increase rates if begun after age 20 [69]. Although these results did not establish convincing evidence for the role of folate in cancer prevention, they do draw attention on this very important and yet not well-studied topic. More well-designed studies are needed to clarify the role of timing and dose of the folate supplementation in cancer prevention.

B. BREAST CANCER

The paradoxical role of folate in colorectal carcinogenesis is, to some extent, mirrored in breast carcinogenesis. Although a number of cohort and case–control studies have suggested an inverse association between folate status and the risk of breast cancer, these results are far from conclusive (see Section II, Folate Intake and Cancer Risk: Epidemiological Evidence). Animal studies provide evidence for puzzling effects of folate in mammary tumorigenesis. To date, there are three animal studies, all using a well-established rat model of MNU-induced mammary tumor [140–142]. These studies collectively suggest that mild folate deficiency significantly inhibits mammary tumorigenesis, whereas folic acid supplementation does not alter the development or progression of the disease.

The earliest warning sign of detrimental effect of high-dose folic acid on breast cancer comes from a historic trial of folic acid supplementation conducted in the 1960s. In that trial, women who received 5 mg/day of folic acid had increased total cancer mortality (RR = 1.70; P = .02) and breast cancer mortality (RR = 2.02, P = .10) compared with women not taking supplements [143]. Recent results from the Prostate, Lung, Colorectal, and Ovarian Cancer Screening Trial (PLCO) also raised concerns over this adverse effect. In the PLCO trial of 77,376 women, a significant approximately 20% increased risk of breast cancer was observed for postmenopausal women with supplemental folic acid intake greater than 400 µg/day. In addition, although folate from food was not related to breast cancer risk, total folate, mainly from folic acid supplements, significantly increased the risk of breast cancer by 32% when comparing the highest versus lowest 20% intakes [19]. It is important to note that the PLCO recruitment period included the time when folic acid fortification was mandated and implemented in the United States, making it difficult to account for changes in folate status during the follow-up period.

Nevertheless, the precise role of folate in cancer prevention needs to be carefully studied and evaluated. Issues to be considered are the timing of the intervention during the multistep process of carcinogenesis, baseline levels in a given individual or population, the complexity of dietary interactions, dose–response effects, and the duration of the study.

VI. SUMMARY

In summary, the association between folate and cancer risk has been investigated in all major cancer sites; however, these studies very widely in terms of study design, sample size, and quality of the study. Among all the cancer sites, colorectal and breast cancers are the most extensively studied. Although the evidence supporting a protective role of folate in the prevention of colorectal cancer is strong, the association with breast cancer risk is more complex. Possible inverse relationships between folate intake and risk of esophageal and pancreatic cancer warrant further investigation as folate may be useful to prevent these two cancers with high mortality rates.

Existing results from epidemiological studies help us to understand the folate–cancer relationship for cancer prevention, treatment, and other aspects in the population level. It is important to bear in mind that folate may play a dual role in cancer development: It may provide protection early in carcinogenesis and in individuals with a low folate status, yet it may promote carcinogenesis if administered later and potentially at very high intakes. We need to evaluate this information carefully when developing public health recommendations and should be mindful that more folate is not better in all circumstances. More results are expected and will be translated to healthy guidance for the general population.

REFERENCES

1. Esteller M. Epigenetics in cancer. *N Engl J Med* 2008; 358:1148–59.
2. Ulrich CM, Curtin K, Samowitz W, Bigler J, Potter JD, Caan B, Slattery ML. MTHFR variants reduce the risk of G:C→A:T transition mutations within the p53 tumor suppressor gene in colon tumors. *J Nutr* 2005; 135:2462–67.
3. Stern LL, Mason JB, Selhub J, Choi SW. Genomic DNA hypomethylation, a characteristic of most cancers, is present in peripheral leukocytes of individuals who are homozygous for the C677T polymorphism in the methylenetetrahydrofolate reductase gene. *Cancer Epidemiol Biomarkers Prev* 2000; 9:849–53.
4. Combs GF. *The Vitamins: Fundamental Aspects in Nutrition and Health.* San Diego, CA: Academic Press, 1992.
5. Machlin LJ. *Handbook of Vitamins,* 2nd ed., revised and expanded ed. New York: M. Dekker, 1991.
6. Sanjoaquin MA, Allen N, Couto E, Roddam AW, Key TJ. Folate intake and colorectal cancer risk: A meta-analytical approach. *Int J Cancer* 2005; 113:825–28.
7. Sauberlich HE, Kretsch MJ, Skala JH, Johnson HL, Taylor PC. Folate requirement and metabolism in nonpregnant women. *Am J Clin Nutr* 1987; 46:1016–28.
8. Hannon-Fletcher MP, Armstrong NC, Scott JM, Pentieva K, Bradbury I, Ward M, Strain JJ, et al. Determining bioavailability of food folates in a controlled intervention study. *Am J Clin Nutr* 2004; 80:911–18.
9. Larsson SC, Giovannucci E, Wolk A. A prospective study of dietary folate intake and risk of colorectal cancer: Modification by caffeine intake and cigarette smoking. *Cancer Epidemiol Biomarkers Prev* 2005; 14:740–43.
10. Zhang SM, Moore SC, Lin J, Cook NR, Manson JE, Lee I, Buring JE. Folate, vitamin B6, multivitamin supplements, and colorectal cancer risk in women. *Am J Epidemiol* 2006; 163:108–15.
11. Ma J, Stampfer MJ, Giovannucci E, Artigas C, Hunter DJ, Fuchs C, Willett WC, Selhub J, Hennekens CH, Rozen R. Methylenetetrahydrofolate reductase polymorphism, dietary interactions, and risk of colorectal cancer. *Cancer Res* 1997; 57:1098–102.
12. Van Guelpen B, Hultdin J, Johansson I, Hallmans G, Stenling R, Riboli E, Winkvist A, Palmqvist R. Low folate levels may protect against colorectal cancer. *Gut* 2006; 55:1461–66.
13. Larsson SC, Giovannucci E, Wolk A. Folate and risk of breast cancer: A meta-analysis. *J Natl Cancer Inst* 2007; 99:64–76.
14. Zhang S, Hunter DJ, Hankinson SE, Giovannucci EL, Rosner BA, Colditz GA, Speizer FE, Willett WC. A prospective study of folate intake and the risk of breast cancer. *JAMA* 1999; 281:1632–37.
15. Sellers TA, Kushi LH, Cerhan JR, Vierkant RA, Gapstur SM, Vachon CM, Olson JE, Therneau TM, Folsom AR. Dietary folate intake, alcohol, and risk of breast cancer in a prospective study of postmenopausal women. *Epidemiology* 2001; 12:420–28.
16. Rohan TE, Jain MG, Howe GR, Miller AB. Dietary folate consumption and breast cancer risk. *J Natl Cancer Inst* 2000; 92:266–69.
17. Lewis SJ, Harbord RM, Harris R, Smith GD. Meta-analyses of observational and genetic association studies of folate intakes or levels and breast cancer risk. *J Natl Cancer Inst* 2006; 98:1607–22.
18. Lajous M, Romieu I, Sabia S, Boutron-Ruault MC, Clavel-Chapelon F. Folate, vitamin B12 and postmenopausal breast cancer in a prospective study of French women. *Cancer Causes Control* 2006; 17:1209–13.
19. Stolzenberg-Solomon RZ, Chang SC, Leitzmann MF, Johnson KA, Johnson C, Buys SS, Hoover RN, Ziegler RG. Folate intake, alcohol use, and postmenopausal breast cancer risk in the prostate, lung, colorectal, and ovarian cancer screening trial. *Am J Clin Nutr* 2006; 83:895–904.

20. Cho E, Holmes M, Hankinson SE, Willett WC. Nutrients involved in one-carbon metabolism and risk of breast cancer among premenopausal women. *Cancer Epidemiol Biomarkers Prev* 2007; 16:2787–90.

21. Ericson U, Sonestedt E, Gullberg B, Olsson H, Wirfalt E. High folate intake is associated with lower breast cancer incidence in postmenopausal women in the Malmo diet and cancer cohort. *Am J Clin Nutr* 2007; 86:434–43.

22. Ulrich CM. Folate and cancer prevention: A closer look at a complex picture. *Am J Clin Nutr* 2007; 86:271–73.

23. Larsson SC, Giovannucci E, Wolk A. Folate intake, MTHFR polymorphisms, and risk of esophageal, gastric, and pancreatic cancer: A meta-analysis. *Gastroenterology* 2006; 131: 1271–83.

24. Vollset SE, Igland J, Jenab M, Fredriksen A, Meyer K, Eussen S, Gjessing HK, et al. The association of gastric cancer risk with plasma folate, cobalamin, and methylenetetrahydro-folate reductase polymorphisms in the European prospective investigation into cancer and nutrition. *Cancer Epidemiol Biomarkers Prev* 2007; 16:2416–24.

25. Cho E, Hunter DJ, Spiegelman D, Albanes D, Beeson WL, van den Brandt PA, Colditz GA, et al. Intakes of vitamins A, C and E and folate and multivitamins and lung cancer: A pooled analysis of 8 prospective studies. *Int J Cancer* 2006; 118:970–78.

26. Slatore CG, Littman AJ, Au DH, Satia JA, White E. Long-term use of supplemental multivitamins, vitamin C, vitamin E, and folate does not reduce the risk of lung cancer. *Am J Respir Crit Care Med* 2008; 177:524–30.

27. Stolzenberg-Solomon RZ, Albanes D, Nieto FJ, Hartman TJ, Tangrea JA, Rautalahti M, Sehlub J, Virtamo J, Taylor PR. Pancreatic cancer risk and nutrition-related methyl-group availability indicators in male smokers. *J Natl Cancer Inst* 1999; 91:535–41.

28. Schernhammer E, Wolpin B, Rifai N, Cochrane B, Manson JA, Ma J, Giovannucci E, Thomson C, Stampfer MJ, Fuchs C. Plasma folate, vitamin B6, vitamin B12, and homo-cysteine and pancreatic cancer risk in four large cohorts. *Cancer Res* 2007; 67:5553–60.

29. Navarro Silvera SA, Jain M, Howe GR, Miller AB, Rohan TE. Dietary folate consumption and risk of ovarian cancer: A prospective cohort study. *Eur J Cancer Prev* 2006; 15:511–15.

30. Tworoger SS, Hecht JL, Giovannucci E, Hankinson SE. Intake of folate and related nutrients in relation to risk of epithelial ovarian cancer. *Am J Epidemiol* 2006; 163:1101–11.

31. Kelemen LE, Sellers TA, Vierkant RA, Harnack L, Cerhan JR. Association of folate and alcohol with risk of ovarian cancer in a prospective study of postmenopausal women. *Cancer Causes Control* 2004; 15:1085–93.

32. Larsson SC, Giovannucci E, Wolk A. Dietary folate intake and incidence of ovarian cancer: The Swedish mammography cohort. *J Natl Cancer Inst* 2004; 96:396–402.

33. Welzel TM, Katki HA, Sakoda LC, Evans AA, London WT, Chen G, O'Broin S, Shen F, Lin W, McGlynn KA. Blood folate levels and risk of liver damage and hepatocellular carcinoma in a prospective high-risk cohort. *Cancer Epidemiol Biomarkers Prev* 2007; 16:1279–82.

34. Lim U, Weinstein S, Albanes D, Pietinen P, Teerenhovi L, Taylor PR, Virtamo J, Stolzenberg-Solomon R. Dietary factors of one-carbon metabolism in relation to non-Hodgkin lymphoma and multiple myeloma in a cohort of male smokers. *Cancer Epidemiol Biomarkers Prev* 2006; 15:1109–14.

35. Zhang SM, Hunter DJ, Rosner BA, Giovannucci EL, Colditz GA, Speizer FE, Willett WC. Intakes of fruits, vegetables, and related nutrients and the risk of non-Hodgkin's lymphoma among women. *Cancer Epidemiol Biomarkers Prev* 2000; 9:477–85.

36. Koutros S, Zhang Y, Zhu Y, Mayne ST, Zahm SH, Holford TR, Leaderer BP, Boyle P, Zheng T. Nutrients contributing to one-carbon metabolism and risk of non-Hodgkin lymphoma subtypes. *Am J Epidemiol* 2008; 167:287–94.

37. Lim U, Schenk M, Kelemen LE, Davis S, Cozen W, Hartge P, Ward MH, Stolzenberg-Solomon R. Dietary determinants of one-carbon metabolism and the risk of non-Hodgkin's lymphoma: NCI-SEER case-control study, 1998–2000. *Am J Epidemiol* 2005; 162:953–64.

38. Polesel J, Dal Maso L, La Vecchia C, Montella M, Spina M, Crispo A, Talamini R, Franceschi S. Dietary folate, alcohol consumption, and risk of non-Hodgkin lymphoma. *Nutr Cancer* 2007; 57:146–50.

39. Wang JT, Ma XC, Cheng YY, Ding L, Zhou Q. A case-control study on the association between folate and cervical cancer. *Zhonghua Liu Xing Bing Xue Za Zhi* 2006; 27:424–27.

40. VanEenwyk J, Davis FG, Bowen PE. Dietary and serum carotenoids and cervical intraepithelial neoplasia. *Int J Cancer* 1991; 48:34–38.

41. Ziegler RG, Jones CJ, Brinton LA, Norman SA, Mallin K, Levine RS, Lehman HF, Hamman RF, Trumble AC, Rosenthal JF. Diet and the risk of in situ cervical cancer among white women in the United States. *Cancer Causes Control* 1991; 2:17–29.

42. Liu T, Soong S, Wilson N, Craig C, Cole P, Macaluso M, Butterworth C Jr. A case control study of nutritional factors and cervical dysplasia. *Cancer Epidemiol Biomarkers Prev* 1993; 2:525–30.

43. Kwasniewska A, Charzewska J, Tukendorf A, Semczuk M. Dietary factors in women with dysplasia colli uteri associated with human papillomavirus infection. *Nutr Cancer* 1998; 30:39–45.

44. Brock KE, Berry G, Mock PA, MacLennan R, Truswell AS, Brinton LA. Nutrients in diet and plasma and risk of in situ cervical cancer. *J Natl Cancer Inst* 1988; 80:580–85.

45. Hernandez BY, McDuffie K, Wilkens LR, Kamemoto L, Goodman MT. Diet and premalignant lesions of the cervix: Evidence for a protective role for folate, riboflavin, thiamin, and vitamin B12. *Cancer Causes Control* 2003; 14:859–70.

46. Kjellberg L, Hallmans G, Ahren AM, Johansson R, Bergman F, Wadell G, Angstrom T, Dillner J. Smoking, diet, pregnancy and oral contraceptive use as risk factors for cervical intra-epithelial neoplasia in relation to human papillomavirus infection. *Br J Cancer* 2000; 82:1332–38.

47. Thomson SW, Heimburger DC, Cornwell PE, Turner ME, Sauberlich HE, Fox LM, Butterworth CE. Correlates of total plasma homocysteine: Folic acid, copper, and cervical dysplasia. *Nutrition* 2000; 16:411–16.

48. Piyathilake CJ, Macaluso M, Brill I, Heimburger DC, Partridge EE. Lower red blood cell folate enhances the HPV-16–associated risk of cervical intraepithelial neoplasia. *Nutrition* 2007; 23:203–10.

49. Butterworth CE Jr, Hatch KD, Macaluso M, Cole P, Sauberlich HE, Soong SJ, Borst M, Baker VV. Folate deficiency and cervical dysplasia. *JAMA* 1992; 267:528–33.

50. Potischman N, Brinton LA, Laiming VA, Reeves WC, Brenes MM, Herrero R, Tenorio F, de Britton RC, Gaitan E. A case-control study of serum folate levels and invasive cervical cancer. *Cancer Res* 1991; 51:4785–89.

51. Yeo AS, Schiff MA, Montoya G, Masuk M, van Asselt-King L, Becker TM. Serum micronutrients and cervical dysplasia in southwestern American Indian women. *Nutr Cancer* 2000; 38:141–50.

52. Weinstein SJ, Ziegler RG, Frongillo EA Jr, Colman N, Sauberlich HE, Brinton LA, Hamman RF, et al. Low serum and red blood cell folate are moderately, but nonsignificantly associated with increased risk of invasive cervical cancer in U.S. women. *J Nutr* 2001; 131:2040–48.

53. Ziegler RG, Weinstein SJ, Fears TR. Nutritional and genetic inefficiencies in one-carbon metabolism and cervical cancer risk. *J Nutr* 2002; 132:2345S–49.

54. Butterworth C Jr, Hatch K, Gore H, Mueller H, Krumdieck C. Improvement in cervical dysplasia associated with folic acid therapy in users of oral contraceptives. *Am J Clin Nutr* 1982; 35:73–82.

55. Butterworth CE Jr, Hatch KD, Soong SJ, Cole P, Tamura T, Sauberlich HE, Borst M, Macaluso M, Baker V. Oral folic acid supplementation for cervical dysplasia: A clinical intervention trial. *Am J Obstet Gynecol* 1992; 166:803–09.

56. Childers J, Chu J, Voigt L, Feigl P, Tamimi H, Franklin E, Alberts D, Meyskens F Jr. Chemoprevention of cervical cancer with folic acid: A phase III Southwest Oncology Group Intergroup study. *Cancer Epidemiol Biomarkers Prev* 1995; 4:155–59.

57. Zarcone R, Bellini P, Carfora E, Vicinanza G, Raucci F. Folic acid and cervix dysplasia. *Minerva Ginecol* 1996; 48:397–400.

58. Thompson JR, Gerald PF, Willoughby ML, Armstrong BK. Maternal folate supplementation in pregnancy and protection against acute lymphoblastic leukaemia in childhood: A case-control study. *Lancet* 2001; 358:1935–40.

59. Dockerty JD, Herbison P, Skegg DC, Elwood M. Vitamin and mineral supplements in pregnancy and the risk of childhood acute lymphoblastic leukaemia: A case-control study. *BMC Public Health* 2007; 7:136.

60. Almadori G, Bussu F, Galli J, Cadoni G, Zappacosta B, Persichilli S, Minucci A, Giardina B, Maurizi M. Serum levels of folate, homocysteine, and vitamin B12 in head and neck squamous cell carcinoma and in laryngeal leukoplakia. *Cancer* 2005; 103:284–92.

61. Eleftheriadou A, Chalastras T, Ferekidou E, Yiotakis I, Kyriou L, Tzagarakis M, Ferekidis E, Kandiloros D. Association between squamous cell carcinoma of the head and neck and serum folate and homocysteine. *Anticancer Res* 2006; 26(3B):2345–48.

62. Suzuki T, Matsuo K, Hasegawa Y, Hiraki A, Wakai K, Hirose K, Saito T, Sato S, Ueda R, Tajima K. One-carbon metabolism-related gene polymorphisms and risk of head and neck squamous cell carcinoma: Case-control study. *Cancer Sci* 2007; 98:1439–46.

63. Xu W, Shrubsole MJ, Xiang Y, Cai Q, Zhao G, Ruan Z, Cheng J, Zheng W, Shu XO. Dietary folate intake, MTHFR genetic polymorphisms, and the risk of endometrial cancer among Chinese women. *Cancer Epidemiol Biomarkers Prev* 2007; 16:281–87.

64. McCann SE, Freudenheim JL, Marshall JR, Brasure JR, Swanson MK, Graham S. Diet in the epidemiology of endometrial cancer in western New York (United States). *Cancer Causes Control* 2000; 11:965–74.

65. Negri E, La Vecchia C, Franceschi S, Levi F, Parazzini F. Intake of selected micronutrients and the risk of endometrial carcinoma. *Cancer* 1996; 77:917–23.

66. Potischman N, Swanson CA, Brinton LA, McAdams M, Barrett RJ, Berman ML, Mortel R, Twiggs LB, Wilbanks GD, Hoover RN. Dietary associations in a case-control study of endometrial cancer. *Cancer Causes Control* 1993; 4:239–50.

67. Nijhout HF, Reed MC, Budu P, Ulrich CM. A mathematical model of the folate cycle: New insights into folate homeostasis. *J Biol Chem* 2004; 279:55008–16.

68. Blount BC, Mack MM, Wehr CM, MacGregor JT, Hiatt RA, Wang G, Wickramasinghe SN, Everson RB, Ames BN. Folate deficiency causes uracil misincorporation into human DNA and chromosome breakage: Implications for cancer and neuronal damage. *Proc Natl Acad Sci USA* 1997; 94:3290–95.

69. Luebeck EG, Moolgavkar SH, Liu AY, Boynton A, Ulrich CM. Does folic acid supplementation prevent or promote colorectal cancer? Results from model-based predictions. *Cancer Epidemiol Biomarkers Prev* 2008; 7:1360–67.

70. Davis CD, Uthus EO. DNA methylation, cancer susceptibility, and nutrient interactions. *Exp Biol Med* 2004; 229:988–95.

71. Frosst P, Blom HJ, Milos R, Goyette P, Sheppard CA, Matthews RG, Boers GJ, den Heijer M, Kluijtmans LA, van den Heuvel LP. A candidate genetic risk factor for vascular disease: A common mutation in methylenetetrahydrofolate reductase. *Nat Genet* 1995; 10:111–13.

72. Weisberg IS, Jacques PF, Selhub J, Bostom AG, Chen Z, Curtis Ellison R, Eckfeldt JH, Rozen R. The 1298A→C polymorphism in methylenetetrahydrofolate reductase (MTHFR): In vitro expression and association with homocysteine. *Atherosclerosis* 2001; 156:409–15.

73. Chen J, Gammon MD, Chan W, Palomeque C, Wetmur JG, Kabat GC, Teitelbaum SL, et al. One-carbon metabolism, MTHFR polymorphisms, and risk of breast cancer. *Cancer Res* 2005; 65:1606–14.

74. Bailey LB, Gregory JF 3rd. Polymorphisms of methylenetetrahydrofolate reductase and other enzymes: Metabolic significance, risks and impact on folate requirement. *J Nutr* 1999; 129:919–22.

75. Ulvik A, Ueland PM, Fredriksen A, Meyer K, Vollset SE, Hoff G, Schneede J. Functional inference of the methylenetetrahydrofolate reductase 677C>T and 1298A>C polymorphisms from a large-scale epidemiological study. *Hum Genet* 2007; 121:57–64.

76. Pereira TV, Rudnicki M, Pereira AC, Pombo-de-Oliveira MS, Franco RF. 5,10-methyl-enetetrahydrofolate reductase polymorphisms and acute lymphoblastic leukemia risk: A meta-analysis. *Cancer Epidemiol Biomarkers Prev* 2006; 15:1956–63.

77. Zintzaras E, Koufakis T, Ziakas PD, Rodopoulou P, Giannouli S, Voulgarelis M. A meta-analysis of genotypes and haplotypes of methylenetetrahydrofolate reductase gene polymorphisms in acute lymphoblastic leukemia. *Eur J Epidemiol* 2006; 21:501–10.

78. Kaneda S, Takeishi K, Ayusawa D, Shimizu K, Seno T, Altman S. Role in translation of a triple tandemly repeated sequence in the 5'-untranslated region of human thymidylate synthase mRNA. *Nucl Acids Res* 1987; 15:1259–70.

79. Horie N, Aiba H, Oguro K, Hojo H, Takeishi K. Functional analysis and DNA polymorphism of the tandemly repeated sequences in the 5'-terminal regulatory region of the human gene for thymidylate synthase. *Cell Struct Funct* 1995; 20:191–97.

80. Pullarkat ST, Stoehlmacher J, Ghaderi V, Xiong YP, Ingles SA, Sherrod A, Warren R, Tsao-Wei D, Groshen S, Lenz HJ. Thymidylate synthase gene polymorphism determines response and toxicity of 5-FU chemotherapy. *Pharmacogenomics J* 2001; 1:65–70.

81. Chen J, Hunter DJ, Stampfer MJ, Kyte C, Chan W, Wetmur JG, Mosig R, Selhub J, Ma J. Polymorphism in the thymidylate synthase promoter enhancer region modifies the risk and survival of colorectal cancer. *Cancer Epidemiol Biomarkers Prev* 2003; 12:958–62.

82. Ulrich CM, Curtin K, Potter JD, Bigler J, Caan B, Slattery ML. Polymorphisms in the reduced folate carrier, thymidylate synthase, or methionine synthase and risk of colon cancer. *Cancer Epidemiol Biomarkers Prev* 2005; 14:2509–16.

83. Skibola CF, Smith MT, Hubbard A, Shane B, Roberts AC, Law GR, Rollinson S, Roman E, Cartwright RA, Morgan GJ. Polymorphisms in the thymidylate synthase and serine hydroxymethyltransferase genes and risk of adult acute lymphocytic leukemia. *Blood* 2002; 99:3786–91.

84. Mandola MV, Stoehlmacher J, Zhang W, Groshen S, Yu MC, Iqbal S, Lenz HJ, Ladner RD. A 6 bp polymorphism in the thymidylate synthase gene causes message instability and is associated with decreased intratumoral TS mRNA levels. *Pharmacogenetics* 2004; 14:319–27.

85. Ulrich CM, Bigler J, Bostick R, Fosdick L, Potter JD. Thymidylate synthase promoter polymorphism, interaction with folate intake, and risk of colorectal adenomas. *Cancer Res* 2002; 62:3361–64.

86. Chen J, Stampfer MJ, Ma J, Selhub J, Malinow MR, Hennekens CH, Hunter DJ. Influence of a methionine synthase (D919G) polymorphism on plasma homocysteine and folate levels and relation to risk of myocardial infarction. *Atherosclerosis* 2001; 154:667–72.

87. Harmon DL, Shields DC, Woodside JV, McMaster D, Yarnell JW, Young IS, Peng K, Shane B, Evans AE, Whitehead AS. Methionine synthase D919G polymorphism is a significant but modest determinant of circulating homocysteine concentrations. *Genet Epidemiol* 1999; 17:298–309.

88. Ma J, Stampfer MJ, Christensen B, Giovannucci E, Hunter DJ, Chen J, Willett WC, et al. A polymorphism of the methionine synthase gene: Association with plasma folate,

vitamin B12, homocyst(e)ine, and colorectal cancer risk. *Cancer Epidemiol Biomarkers Prev* 1999; 8:825–29.

89. Ulvik A, Vollset SE, Hansen S, Gislefoss R, Jellum E, Ueland PM. Colorectal cancer and the methylenetetrahydrofolate reductase 677C→T and methionine synthase 2756A→G polymorphisms: A study of 2,168 case-control pairs from the JANUS cohort. *Cancer Epidemiol Biomarkers Prev* 2004; 13:2175–80.

90. Lissowska J, Gaudet MM, Brinton LA, Chanock SJ, Peplonska B, Welch R, Zatonski W, et al. Genetic polymorphisms in the one-carbon metabolism pathway and breast cancer risk: A population-based case-control study and meta-analyses. *Int J Cancer* 2007; 120:2696–703.

91. Shrubsole MJ, Gao Y, Cai Q, Shu XO, Dai Q, Jin F, Zheng W. MTR and MTRR polymorphisms, dietary intake, and breast cancer risk. *Cancer Epidemiol Biomarkers Prev* 2006; 15:586–88.

92. Xu X, Gammon MD, Zhang H, Wetmur JG, Rao M, Teitelbaum SL, Britton JA, Neugut AI, Santella RM, Chen J. Polymorphisms of one-carbon metabolizing genes and risk of breast cancer in a population-based study. *Carcinogenesis* 2007; 28:1504–09.

93. Justenhoven C, Hamann U, Pierl CB, Rabstein S, Pesch B, Harth V, Baisch C, et al. One-carbon metabolism and breast cancer risk: No association of MTHFR, MTR, and TYMS polymorphisms in the GENICA study from Germany. *Cancer Epidemiol Biomarkers Prev* 2005; 14:3015–18.

94. Goode EL, Potter JD, Bigler J, Ulrich CM. Methionine synthase D919G polymorphism, folate metabolism, and colorectal adenoma risk. *Cancer Epidemiol Biomarkers Prev* 2004; 13:157–62.

95. Wilson A, Platt R, Wu Q, Leclerc D, Christensen B, Yang H, Gravel RA, Rozen R. A common variant in methionine synthase reductase combined with low cobalamin (vitamin B12) increases risk for spina bifida. *Mol Genet Metab* 1999; 67:317–23.

96. Gaughan DJ, Kluijtmans LA, Barbaux S, McMaster D, Young IS, Yarnell JW, Evans A, Whitehead AS. The methionine synthase reductase (MTRR) A66G polymorphism is a novel genetic determinant of plasma homocysteine concentrations. *Atherosclerosis* 2001; 157:451–56.

97. Jacques PF, Bostom AG, Selhub J, Rich S, Ellison RC, Eckfeldt JH, Gravel RA, Rozen R, National Heart, Lung and Blood Institute, National Institutes of Health. Effects of polymorphisms of methionine synthase and methionine synthase reductase on total plasma homocysteine in the NHLBI family heart study. *Atherosclerosis* 2003; 166:49–55.

98. Le Marchand L, Donlon T, Hankin JH, Kolonel LN, Wilkens LR, Seifried A. B-vitamin intake, metabolic genes, and colorectal cancer risk (United States). *Cancer Causes Control* 2002; 13:239–48.

99. Otani T, Iwasaki M, Hanaoka T, Kobayashi M, Ishihara J, Natsukawa S, Shaura K, et al. Folate, vitamin B6, vitamin B12, and vitamin B2 intake, genetic polymorphisms of related enzymes, and risk of colorectal cancer in a hospital-based case-control study in Japan. *Nutr Cancer* 2005; 53:42–50.

100. Johnson WG, Stenroos ES, Spychala JR, Chatkupt S, Ming SX, Buyske S. New 19 bp deletion polymorphism in intron-1 of dihydrofolate reductase (DHFR): A risk factor for spina bifida acting in mothers during pregnancy? *Am J Med Genet A* 2004; 124:339–45.

101. Xu X, Gammon MD, Wetmur JG, Rao M, Gaudet MM, Teitelbaum SL, Britton JA, Neugut AI, Santella RM, Chen J. A functional 19-base pair deletion polymorphism of dihydrofolate reductase (DHFR) and risk of breast cancer in multivitamin users. *Am J Clin Nutr* 2007; 85:1098–102.

102. Wang Y, Guo W, He Y, Chen Z, Wen D, Zhang X, Wang N, Li Y, Ge H, Zhang J. Association of MTHFR C677T and SHMT(1) C1420T with susceptibility to ESCC and GCA in a high incident region of northern China. *Cancer Causes Control* 2007; 18:143–52.

103. Kelemen LE, Sellers TA, Schildkraut JM, Cunningham JM, Vierkant RA, Pankratz VS, Fredericksen ZS, et al. Genetic variation in the one-carbon transfer pathway and ovarian cancer risk. *Cancer Res* 2008; 68:2498–506.
104. Wang L, Lu J, An J, Shi Q, Spitz MR, Wei Q. Polymorphisms of cytosolic serine hydroxymethyltransferase and risk of lung cancer: A case-control analysis. *Lung Cancer* 2007; 57:143–51.
105. Koushik A, Kraft P, Fuchs CS, Hankinson SE, Willett WC, Giovannucci EL, Hunter DJ. Nonsynonymous polymorphisms in genes in the one-carbon metabolism pathway and associations with colorectal cancer. *Cancer Epidemiol Biomarkers Prev* 2006;15:2408–17.
106. Stevens VL, McCullough ML, Pavluck AL, Talbot JT, Feigelson HS, Thun MJ, Calle EE. Association of polymorphisms in one-carbon metabolism genes and postmenopausal breast cancer incidence. *Cancer Epidemiol Biomarkers Prev* 2007; 16:1140–47.
107. Hazra A, Wu K, Kraft P, Fuchs CS, Giovannucci EL, Hunter DJ. Twenty-four nonsynonymous polymorphisms in the one-carbon metabolic pathway and risk of colorectal adenoma in the Nurses' Health Study. *Carcinogenesis* 2007; 28:1510–19.
108. Ulrich CM, Nijhout HF, Reed MC. Mathematical modeling: Epidemiology meets systems biology. *Cancer Epidemiol Biomarkers Prev* 2006; 15:827–29.
109. Reed MC, Nijhout HF, Neuhouser ML, Gregory JF III, Shane B, James SJ, Boynton A, Ulrich CM. A mathematical model gives insights into nutritional and genetic aspects of folate-mediated one-carbon metabolism. *J Nutr* 2006; 136:2653–61.
110. Nijhout HF, Reed MC, Anderson DF, Mattingly JC, James SJ, Ulrich CM. Long-range allosteric interactions between the folate and methionine cycles stabilize DNA methylation reaction rate. *Epigenetics* 2006; 1:81–87.
111. Nijhout HF, Reed M, Lam S, Shane B, Gregory J, Ulrich C. In silico experimentation with a model of hepatic mitochondrial folate metabolism. *Theor Biol Med Model* 2006; 3:40.
112. Chabner B. *Cancer Chemotherapy and Biotherapy: Principles and Practice*, 3rd ed., Philadelphia: Lippincott-Raven Publishers, 2001.
113. Zhao R, Gao F, Goldman ID. Marked suppression of the activity of some, but not all, antifolate compounds by augmentation of folate cofactor pools within tumor cells. *Biochem Pharmacol* 2001; 61:857–65.
114. Zhao R, Goldman ID. Resistance to antifolates. *Oncogene* 2003; 22:7431–57.
115. Robien K. Folate during antifolate chemotherapy: What we know... and do not know. *Nutr Clin Pract* 2005; 20:411–22.
116. Khanna D, Park GS, Paulus HE, Simpson KM, Elashoff D, Cohen SB, Emery P, Dorrier C, Furst DE. Reduction of the efficacy of methotrexate by the use of folic acid: Post hoc analysis from two randomized controlled studies. *Arthritis Rheum* 2005; 52:3030–38.
117. Dervieux T, Furst D, Lein DO, Capps R, Smith K, Caldwell J, Kremer J. Pharmacogenetic and metabolite measurements are associated with clinical status in patients with rheumatoid arthritis treated with methotrexate: Results of a multicentred cross-sectional observational study. *Ann Rheum Dis* 2005; 64:1180–85.
118. Salim A, Tan E, Ilchyshyn A, Berth-Jones J. Folic acid supplementation during treatment of psoriasis with methotrexate: A randomized, double-blind, placebo-controlled trial. *Br J Dermatol* 2006; 154:1169–74.
119. Takacs P, Rodriguez L. High folic acid levels and failure of single-dose methotrexate treatment in ectopic pregnancy. *Int J Gynaecol Obstet* 2005; 89:301–02.
120. Borsi JD, Wesenberg F, Stokland T, Moe PJ. How much is too much? Folinic acid rescue dose in children with acute lymphoblastic leukaemia. *Eur J Cancer* 1991; 27:1006–09.
121. Browman G, Goodyear M, Levine M, Russell R, Archibald S, Young J. Modulation of the antitumor effect of methotrexate by low-dose leucovorin in squamous cell head and neck cancer: A randomized placebo-controlled clinical trial. *J Clin Oncol* 1990; 8:203–08.

122. Branda RF, Naud SJ, Brooks EM, Chen Z, Muss H. Effect of vitamin B12, folate, and dietary supplements on breast carcinoma chemotherapy-induced mucositis and neutropenia. *Cancer* 2004; 101:1058–64.
123. Sellers TA, Alberts SR, Vierkant RA, Grabrick DM, Cerhan JR, Vachon CM, Olson JE, Kushi LH, Potter JD. High-folate diets and breast cancer survival in a prospective cohort study. *Nutr Cancer* 2002; 44:139–44.
124. Chattopadhyay S, Tamari R, Min SH, Zhao R, Tsai E, Goldman ID. Commentary: A case for minimizing folate supplementation in clinical regimens with pemetrexed based on the marked sensitivity of the drug to folate availability. *Oncologist* 2007; 12:808–15.
125. Hooijberg JH, de Vries NA, Kaspers GJ, Pieters R, Jansen G, Peters GJ. Multidrug resistance proteins and folate supplementation: Therapeutic implications for antifolates and other classes of drugs in cancer treatment. *Cancer Chemother Pharmacol* 2006; 58:1–12.
126. Ulrich CM, Robien K, McLeod HL. Cancer pharmacogenetics: Polymorphisms, pathways and beyond. *Nat Rev Cancer* 2003; 3:912–20.
127. Robien K, Boynton A, Ulrich CM. Pharmacogenetics of folate-related drug targets in cancer treatment. *Pharmacogenomics* 2005; 6:673–89.
128. Bell KN, Oakley GP Jr. Tracking the prevention of folic acid-preventable spina bifida and anencephaly. *Birth Defects Res A Clin Mol Teratol* 2006; 76:654–57.
129. Wald DS, Wald NJ, Morris JK, Law M. Folic acid, homocysteine, and cardiovascular disease: Judging causality in the face of inconclusive trial evidence. *BMJ* 2006; 333:1114–17.
130. McCully KS. Homocysteine, vitamins, and vascular disease prevention. *Am J Clin Nutr* 2007; 86:1563S–68.
131. Wang X, Qin X, Demirtas H, Li J, Mao G, Huo Y, Sun N, Liu L, Xu X. Efficacy of folic acid supplementation in stroke prevention: A meta-analysis. *Lancet* 2007; 369:1876–82.
132. Durga J, van Boxtel MP, Schouten EG, Kok FJ, Jolles J, Katan MB, Verhoef P. Effect of 3-year folic acid supplementation on cognitive function in older adults in the FACIT trial: A randomised, double blind, controlled trial. *Lancet* 2007; 369:208–16.
133. Kim Y. Role of folate in colon cancer development and progression. *J Nutr* 2003;133:3731S–39.
134. Song J, Medline A, Mason JB, Gallinger S, Kim Y. Effects of dietary folate on intestinal tumorigenesis in the ApcMin mouse. *Cancer Res* 2000; 60:5434–40.
135. McKay JA, Williams EA, Mathers JC. Gender-specific modulation of tumorigenesis by folic acid supply in the apc mouse during early neonatal life. *Br J Nutr* 2008; 99:550–58.
136. Mason JB, Dickstein A, Jacques PF, Haggarty P, Selhub J, Dallal G, Rosenberg IH. A temporal association between folic acid fortification and an increase in colorectal cancer rates may be illuminating important biological principles: A hypothesis. *Cancer Epidemiol Biomarkers Prev* 2007; 16:1325–29.
137. Cole BF, Baron JA, Sandler RS, Haile RW, Ahnen DJ, Bresalier RS, McKeown-Eyssen G, et al. Folic acid for the prevention of colorectal adenomas: A randomized clinical trial. *JAMA* 2007; 297:2351–59.
138. Ulrich CM, Potter JD. Folate and cancer—Timing is everything. *JAMA* 2007; 297:2408–09.
139. Jaszewski R, Misra S, Tobi M, Ullah N, Naumoff JA, Kucuk O, Levi E, Axelrod BN, Patel BB, Majumdar AP. Folic acid supplementation inhibits recurrence of colorectal adenomas: A randomized chemoprevention trial. *World J Gastroenterol* 2008; 14:4492–98.
140. Baggott JE, Vaughn WH, Juliana MM, Eto I, Krumdieck CL, Grubbs CJ. Effects of folate deficiency and supplementation on methylnitrosourea-induced rat mammary tumors. *J Natl Cancer Inst* 1992; 84:1740–44.

141. Kotsopoulos J, Sohn K, Martin R, Choi M, Renlund R, Mckerlie C, Hwang SW, Medline A, Kim YJ. Dietary folate deficiency suppresses *N*-methyl-*N*-nitrosourea-induced mammary tumorigenesis in rats. *Carcinogenesis* 2003; 24:937–44.

142. Kotsopoulos J, Medline A, Renlund R, Sohn K, Martin R, Hwang SW, Lu S, Archer MC, Kim Y. Effects of dietary folate on the development and progression of mammary tumors in rats. *Carcinogenesis* 2005; 26:1603–12.

143. Charles D, Ness AR, Campbell D, Davey Smith G, Hall MH. Taking folate in pregnancy and risk of maternal breast cancer. *BMJ* 2004; 329:1375–76.

144. Huang Y, Han S, Li Y, Mao Y, Xie Y. Different roles of MTHFR C677T and A1298C polymorphisms in colorectal adenoma and colorectal cancer: A meta-analysis. *J Hum Genet* 2007; 52:73–85.

145. Hubner RA, Houlston RS. MTHFR C677T and colorectal cancer risk: A meta-analysis of 25 populations. *Int J Cancer* 2007; 120:1027–35.

146. Zintzaras E. Methylenetetrahydrofolate reductase gene and susceptibility to breast cancer: A meta-analysis. *Clin Genet* 2006; 69:327–36.

147. Mao R, Fan Y, Jin Y, Bai J, Fu S. Methylenetetrahydrofolate reductase gene polymorphisms and lung cancer: A meta-analysis. *J Hum Genet* 2008; 53:340–48.

148. Boccia S, Hung R, Ricciardi G, Gianfagna F, Ebert MPA, Fang J, Gao C, et al. Meta- and pooled analyses of the methylenetetrahydrofolate reductase C677T and A1298C polymorphisms and gastric cancer risk: A huge-GSEC review. *Am J Epidemiol* 2008; 167:505–16.

149. Zintzaras E. Association of methylenetetrahydrofolate reductase (MTHFR) polymorphisms with genetic susceptibility to gastric cancer: A meta-analysis. *J Hum Genet* 2006; 51:618–24.

10 Folate and Carcinogenesis
Basic Mechanisms

Eric Ciappio and Joel B. Mason

CONTENTS

I. INTRODUCTION

A large and growing body of both preclinical and clinical studies pertaining to colorectal neoplasms constitutes the most compelling evidence for a protective effect of folate against the development of cancer [1,2], although evidence is also accruing in this regard for cancers of the breast [3,4], lung [5], pancreas, esophagus [6], and others. Complicating the matter are observations of a paradoxical nature: that overly abundant intake of folate may instead increase the risk of developing cancer if administered in an inopportune setting, such as to an individual who has existing foci of precancerous or cancerous cells [7–11]. In retrospect, what appears to be a paradoxical effect, however, is entirely consistent with our understanding of the cellular effects of folate. The likelihood of a "dual effect" of folate is creating considerable consternation for those who translate scientific advances into public health

235

policy because it exposes the fact that folate may have divergent effects on different segments of the population. Regardless of public health implications, however, any discussion purporting to explain the mechanistic avenues by which folate modulates the risk of carcinogenesis must take these disparate observations into account.

The discussion that follows summarizes our present understanding of the cellular pathways by which the availability of folate and related nutrients may modulate carcinogenesis. By necessity the discussion is a speculative one because there does not yet exist definitive proof of how the effects are mediated. To date the sole biochemical function identified for folate is its ability to serve as a cofactor and/or substrate in the transfer of one-carbon units from one biochemical compound to another. In this role it serves as an essential component of the machinery for biological methylation and for the de novo biosynthesis of purines and thymidylate. Consequently, the integrity with which a cell maintains normal patterns of synthesis, repair, and methylation of its DNA is very dependent on the above-mentioned roles of the vitamin, a concept for which there is abundant evidence. Because aberrations in DNA methylation and DNA synthesis and repair are strongly implicated as avenues by which malignant transformation occurs [12,13], they constitute the basis for the prevailing theories as to how inadequate folate availability enhances carcinogenesis. Moreover, because premalignant and malignant cells generally have much higher rates of proliferation (and therefore DNA synthesis) than their normal counterparts (e.g., Shpitz et al. [14]), abundant availability of folate is thought to enhance their ability to proliferate. It is through this route that folate is proposed to possess a paradoxical enhancing effect when it is administered in abundant quantities to an individual who harbors an existing focus of neoplastic cells.

Although these prevailing theories are widely accepted, this is a rapidly evolving field and one in which our understanding is still rudimentary. Moreover, evidence continues to accrue that certain other factors modify folate's impact on cancer risk: habitual alcohol intake, age, genetic background, and the intake of other micronutrients in the one-carbon network each seem to play roles in this schema. In particular, the interactions with some of the other nutrients that play a role in one-carbon metabolism (vitamins B2, B6, and B12 and methionine and choline) are not surprising given the biochemical interconnectedness of these cofactors in the one-carbon metabolic network (Figure 10.1). Moreover, the potential import of including the other three B vitamins in our considerations is underscored by population-based surveys that demonstrate that "subclinical" deficiencies of these vitamins (i.e., values below normative values but in the absence of classical deficiency syndromes) continue to be surprisingly common in the adult populations of industrialized nations [15–17], as well as by an increasing number of clinical studies that have provided evidence for a relationship between cancer risk and inadequacies of vitamins B6 and B12 (e.g., Theodoratou et al. [18] and Wu et al. [19]).

II. MECHANISMS OF CANCER PROTECTION

The integral role of folate in DNA metabolism, both at the genetic and epigenetic levels, is the logical starting point in any discussion on the protective effects of folate, because aberrations in DNA synthesis, repair, and methylation are all heavily

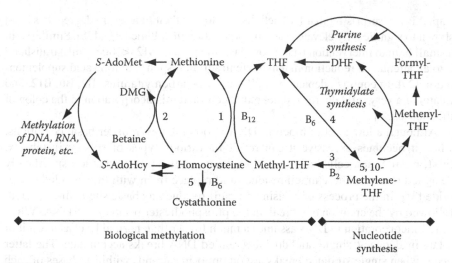

FIGURE 10.1 One-carbon metabolism in the cytosol of mammalian cells, emphasizing the interconversions of the different coenzymatic forms of folate. DHF, dihydrofolate; DMG, dimethylglycine; S-AdoHcy, S-adenosylhomocysteine; S-AdoMet, S-adenosylmethionine; THF, tetrahydrofolate; 1, methionine synthase; 2, betaine:homocysteine methyltransferase; 3, methylenetetrahydrofolate reductase; 4, serine hydroxymethyltransferase; 5, cystathionine-β-synthase.

implicated as seminal pathways through which cancers arise. There are a variety of potential mechanisms by which adequate folate status may bestow protection. Given the diversity of function that the various coenzymatic forms of folate play, it is entirely possible that protection reflects a combination of effects mediated through multiple pathways.

A. URACIL MISINCORPORATION AND DNA INTEGRITY

Folate, in the form of 5,10-methylenetetrahydrofolate (5,10-methylene-THF), is required for the synthesis of thymidine from uracil. Therefore, limited availability of folate causes an increase in the intracellular deoxyuridylate/deoxythymidylate (UTP/TTP) ratio and promotes the misincorporation of uracil into DNA, as has been reproducibly shown in cell culture, animal models, and intact humans [20–27]. However, the above-mentioned studies were performed in laboratory models of folate depletion and in individuals with flagrant folate deficiency; therefore, it remains to be demonstrated whether de novo thymidine synthesis among individuals who subsist in the lower range of folate status in the general population is sufficiently perturbed to produce substantial elevations of uracil in DNA.

Factors other than folate availability may act in conjunction with folate status in determining a tissue's susceptibility to uracil incorporation. One study in rodents showed that elder age enhances the colon's susceptibility to the uracil incorporation that develops as a result of folate inadequacy [22]. Also, because vitamin B12 deficiency produces a conditional deficiency of folate resulting from the methylfolate trap, it is not surprising that B12 deficiency alone, albeit of a severe degree, has been shown to significantly elevate uracil incorporation in colonic DNA [28]. Similarly, in a small human intervention trial, a low baseline plasma B12 (<400 pg/mL) translated into an attenuated reduction in leukocyte uracil in response to folic acid supplementation [29]. In contrast, depletion of all four one-carbon vitamins (B2, B6, B12, and folate) of a very mild degree did not enhance uracil misincorporation in the colon of the mouse [30].

Although a low level of uracil in DNA is observed even under basal conditions, when it becomes excessive it can result in various types of genetic instability. First, mammalian cells have several excision repair systems that are specifically designed to excise these uracil residues and replace them with the intended nucleotide [31]. In the process of excising a uracil residue an abasic site is first created, followed by the creation of a break in the phosphodiester backbone of DNA. When uracil incorporation in DNA assumes a much higher than normal level as a result of folate inadequacy, single- and double-stranded DNA breaks accumulate. The latter occur when single-stranded breaks are on opposing strands within 14 bases of each other [32]. Double-stranded breaks, in particular, are a highly mutagenic condition [32]. Gene deletions of tumor suppressor genes [33], chromosomal translocations [34–36], and gene amplification of oncogenes [37,38] have been observed to occur as a result of double-stranded breaks. Moreover, excessive strand breaks within the coding region of a gene can inhibit the expression of the gene by impairing the procession of RNA polymerase, and thereby transcription [39,40]. Consistent with this concept are several studies in animal models of one-carbon nutrient depletion in which the folate-deplete state has produced strand breaks in the coding regions of the colonic *Apc* and *p53* genes [30,41,42] accompanied by reductions in steady-state levels of mRNA of the corresponding genes. Whether the diminished gene expression in these studies is a direct consequence of strand breaks is not yet proven. It is also recognized that the accumulation of strand breaks in a gene caused by folate depletion does not invariably diminish mRNA levels. For example, in cultured human lymphocytes the induction of *p53* strand breaks was not accompanied by a reduction in *p53* mRNA [43].

Although diets deficient in several one-carbon nutrients or in folate alone have been shown to induce DNA strand breaks on a genomic level [44,45], there appears to be a high degree of specificity with regard to regions of the genome that are vulnerable to strand breakage. Even within a single gene, certain regions are far more likely to develop strand breaks than others as a result of folate depletion. For example, when the colonic *Apc* and *p53* genes were examined in rodent studies, it was the highly conserved regions (which are also the most frequent sites of mutations in human carcinogenesis) that were most susceptible to strand breakage [30,41]. In the case of the *Apc* gene, it was the "mutation cluster region" in exon 15, and in the case of p53 it corresponded to exons 5–8, which is the so-called "hypermutable region" where approximately 90% of *p53* mutations in human cancer occur. Concurrent depletion of all four of the one-carbon micronutrients, even though each inadequacy is minor in magnitude, amplifies the induction of strand breaks to an extent not observed with folate depletion alone [30]. Intuitively, one might speculate that the susceptibility of a particular locus to strand breaks would be defined by the vulnerability to uracil incorporation at that site; testing this hypothesis, however, awaits the development of an accurate means of determining site-specific uracil incorporation.

Two additional mechanisms by which uracil incorporation in DNA may result in genetic instability are described and depend on which of two avenues the incorporation has occurred (Figure 10.2). Cytosine residues in DNA are known to spontaneously undergo hydrolytic deamination via a nonenzymatic route, producing a U:G mispair; such an event is thought to occur 100 to 500 times/day/human cell. If DNA replication occurs before repair can be effected, a C:G to T:A transition mutation results [46]. Alternatively, as is the case with folate depletion, uracil may be inserted into a site where thymidine is intended, resulting in a U:A mispair. Although this is not an event that would likely produce a mutation, it is believed that such a mispair may distort the secondary structure of DNA, interfering with chromatin-associated proteins that depend on the conformation of DNA for proper function. Experimental folate deficiency in rodents has been shown to impair excision repair in the colon [47], but whether this is a consequence of excess uracil in DNA or other factors is not known.

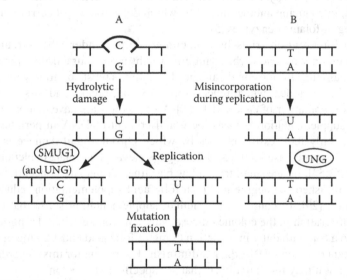

FIGURE 10.2 Compartment model for the repair of uracil residues in the mammalian genome. DNA regions temporarily present in single-stranded form as a result of replication or transcription are susceptible to hydrolytic deamination of cytosine residues (pathway A). The SMUG1 uracil-DNA glycosylase recognizes these U:G mispairs and repairs the lesion. If unrepaired, they give rise to U:A during subsequent replication, generating C to T transition mutations. The UNG uracil-DNA glycosylase appears to be mainly targeted to U:A base pairs, arising through incorporation of dUTP in place of TTP during DNA synthesis, a process accelerated by folate depletion (pathway B). *TDG* and *MBD4* genes encode for additional uracil glycosylases, the activity of which are less well defined. (Adapted from Barnes DE, Lindahl T, *Annu Rev Genet* 2004; 38:445–76. With permission.)

Thus, excessive uracil incorporation has become one of the prevailing hypotheses to explain how inadequate folate status initiates or promotes carcinogenesis. Although the induction of anomalies in biological methylation, especially DNA methylation, may also play a role (as discussed in Section II.B.2), recent animal data would suggest that the critical role that folate plays in DNA synthesis and repair is an even more important factor. Knock et al. [48] observed that the heightened susceptibility to intestinal tumorigenesis resulting from low folate that is evident in BALB/C mice compared with the more tumor-resistant C57/Bl6 strain concurred with an increased UTP/TTP ratio, indications of double-stranded DNA strand breaks and other DNA damage in the former strain. Moreover, correction of impaired methylation in the BALB/C strain with the administration of trimethylglycine (betaine) did not attenuate tumorigenesis. Similarly, by using rodents that possess gain-of-function and loss-of-function alterations in cytosolic serine hydroxymethyltransferase (cSHMT), a metabolic switch that controls the partitioning of folate coenzymes between the methylation and nucleotide synthesis arms of one-carbon metabolism [49], MacFarlane et al. [50] provided evidence that susceptibility to intestinal tumorigenesis paralleled the loss of coenzyme made available for nucleotide synthesis. In contrast, tumorigenesis was not concordant with the loss of substrate for biological methylation. Interestingly, folate depletion in colon cancer cells can alter the expression of cSHMT, introducing another means by which depletion might corrupt the normal partitioning of folate coenzymes [51].

Human intervention trials have begun to define under what circumstances supplementation with one-carbon vitamins might modify uracil incorporation and the accompanying chromosomal damage. The latter is most commonly measured by the micronucleus index, which reflects chromosomal breaks and losses and which is a putative biomarker of cancer risk [52]. Most such trials have demonstrated that folic acid supplementation reduces the uracil content of DNA in peripheral blood cells, but it only reduces the metrics by which chromosomal damage is assessed among those whose baseline level of damage is elevated by folate depletion or other factors [21,53,54]. In one small trial, a low baseline plasma B12 concentration (<400 pg/mL) diminished the degree to which folic acid supplementation reduced uracil incorporation [29]. In contrast, in a human supplementation study that examined uracil incorporation in the colonic mucosa, van den Donk et al. [55] reported that in response to a 6-month daily intervention (5 mg of folic acid and 1.25 mg of B12), the uracil content of colonic DNA did not diminish. The reason for this discordant result is unclear, but it may relate to effects that are specific to the colon.

B. BIOLOGICAL METHYLATION

Most cellular processes in which a compound acquires a methyl group use S-adenosylmethionine (S-AdoMet or SAM) as the methyl donor. The labile methyl group that enables S-AdoMet to serve that function is derived from its precursor, methionine, which in turn obtains that moiety from 5-methyltetrahydrofolate (5-methyl-THF), an essential factor in the de novo synthesis of methionine (Figure 10.1). The products of a methylation reaction mediated by S-AdoMet are the methylated target molecule and S-adenosylhomocysteine (S-AdoHcy or SAH) [56]. The latter is a potent inhibitor of nearly all S-AdoMet–dependent methyltransferases, with K_i values in the 2 to 6 µM range [57].

DNA, RNA, proteins, and phospholipids are among the molecules whose methylation is S-AdoMet dependent. Not surprisingly, inadequate delivery of one-carbon nutrients has been reported to produce low levels of methylation of each of these compounds in various experimental settings (e.g., Akesson et al. [58], Wainfan et al. [59], Balaghi and Wagner [60], Jacob et al. [61], and Ghandour et al. [62]). Abnormalities in DNA methylation, in particular, have been the focus of many studies that have explored pathways by which folate status modulates carcinogenesis because aberrations of DNA methylation are common in cancer and probably are in part causal in its development [12]. The following discussion is confined to the means by which folate modifies DNA methylation because explorations of the possible protransformational effects of abnormalities in protein, RNA, and phospholipid methylation produced by folate inadequacy are surprisingly few in number.

1. DNA Methylation and Cancer

Genomic methylation in mammalian cells occurs almost exclusively at the number 5 carbon of the pyrimidine ring of those cytosine residues that precede a guanine residue ("CpG sites"). About 50% to 70% of all CpG residues in the human genome of the adult are methylated [63]. CpG sites are concentrated in so-called "CpG islands," which are generally located in the 5'-untranslated region (UTR) of genes [12]. As a general rule, CpG islands are unmethylated under basal conditions, whereas the more scattered CpG sites within coding regions of genes tend to be heavily methylated. The conversion of cytosine to 5-methylcytosine is catalyzed by one of several DNA methyltransferases (DNMTs). DNMT1, a maintenance methyltransferase, copies the methylation pattern of the parental DNA strand onto the newly synthesized daughter strand during DNA replication. De novo methylation, most commonly observed during embryogenesis and in cancer cells, is preferentially mediated by DNMT3a and DNMT3b [12]. A DNMT2 has also been described, although whether it is primarily a DNA or RNA methyltransferase is unclear [64].

Science has yet to unravel the full meaning of the patterns of CpG methylation, but the fastidiousness with which the cell protects them makes it clear that the functions are important. Some patterns are set during embryogenesis or early in extrauterine life, and others seem to serve as lifelong mechanisms by which the organism reacts to the environment and regulates homeostasis. The latter function resides, at least in part, with the CpG islands in the 5'-UTR of many genes, regulating their expression. For many genes, transcription is enhanced by demethylation of the CpG islands in the 5'-UTR. In addition to controlling gene expression, DNA methylation has also been observed to be a determinant of genetic integrity, of chromatin organization, and of mutational susceptibility. For certain genes such as *p53*, nucleotide residues that are frequent sites for C to T transition mutations coincide with methylcytosine residues. This concordance is almost certainly linked in a causal manner, although by what mechanism remains a debate [65,66].

Two, seemingly paradoxical, abnormalities of DNA methylation common in epithelial cancers are overall *hypo*methylation of the genome on which is superimposed foci of CpG island *hyper*methylation. Why certain CpG islands are particularly susceptible to hypermethylation in the setting of neoplasia is unknown. Genomic hypomethylation is also commonly observed in dysplastic (i.e., premalignant) tissues and is often reported to be among the earliest of all molecular anomalies in carcinogenesis [66]. Moreover, when examined, the degree of genomic methylation has been shown to decrease incrementally with increasing grades of dysplasia (e.g., Kim et al. [67]). Site-specific hypermethylation in the early stages of carcinogenesis has not been as extensively examined but has been reported (e.g., Issa et al. [68]).

The evolution of cancer is perceived to largely be the consequence of gene-specific rather than genomic phenomena; thus, it is the abnormal hypermethylation of promoter regions that has been most frequently implicated in carcinogenesis [12]. Hypermethylation of CpG islands in the 5'-UTR of a number of tumor suppressor genes with concomitant silencing of expression of those genes has been observed in many cancers [69]. Alternatively, induction of hypomethylation at critical sites may abolish the constitutively suppressed expression of one allele of a critical gene (i.e., imprinting), a phenomenon that has been shown to promote dedifferentiation and tumorigenesis in the colorectum of laboratory animals [70]. Despite the greater importance ascribed to gene-specific phenomena, however, genomic hypomethylation is feasibly a causal mechanism in carcinogenesis. Genomic hypomethylation appears to make DNA more susceptible to mitotic recombination, thereby facilitating chromosomal breaks, translocations, and allelic loss [71,72].

2.   Effects of Folate and Other One-Carbon Nutrients on DNA Methylation

a.   Genomic Methylation

Folate depletion in cells [73], in intact animals [60], and in humans [61,74] produces genomic DNA hypomethylation under some experimental conditions and may produce site-specific hypermethylation as well [75]. This is reminiscent of the pattern that is present in epithelial cancers, and it is this similarity that lends credence to the concept that inadequate folate availability is promoting carcinogenesis through abnormalities in DNA methylation. As is true in cancer, the mechanisms underlying the induction of concurrent genomic hypomethylation and site-specific hypermethylation resulting from folate depletion are not well defined.

Nevertheless, changes in DNA methylation resulting from folate depletion have not been a consistently reproducible phenomenon. Inconsistencies between different studies may reflect the variable accuracies of different methodologies used to measure DNA methylation. However, other factors, such as age, are also determinants of methylation and therefore may confound the results of some studies. Moreover, both quantitative and qualitative changes in methylation that result from one-carbon nutrient depletion fluctuate during the course of depletion; therefore, the observed inconsistencies may instead reflect differences in the time points at which the biological system in question is sampled. For example, serial observations in laboratory rodents on a "methyl-deficient diet" (devoid of choline, B12, and folate) suggest that an initial wave of genomic hypomethylation, which increases incrementally over time, is accompanied by an up-regulation of DNA methyltransferase activity—perhaps as a compensatory response to the hypomethylation—and that this is followed by increased methylation at specific foci that presumably are receptive to the activity of enhanced methyltransferase activity [75]. Therefore, the chronology of sampling may explain why some investigators have observed no change, or even paradoxical increases, in genomic DNA methylation in various tissues in response to folate deprivation [8,76].

The means by which genomic hypomethylation is induced by folate depletion appears to be largely an increase in S-AdoHcy concentrations. Much less significant are limitations in S-AdoMet availability, as evidenced by experiments in animals whose synthesis of S-AdoMet is severely compromised by a genetically engineered loss of function [77]. A diminished SAM/SAH ratio, which many believe to be an effective index of the "methylation capability" of a biological system, is probably utilitarian only to the extent that it is a reflection of S-AdoHcy concentrations. In part, S-AdoHcy concentration is a better predictor of genomic DNA hypomethylation than S-AdoMet [78,79] because S-AdoMet concentrations are usually kept within a relatively narrow range by a feedback inhibition loop involving the enzyme methylene-THF reductase (MTHFR). Conversely, S-AdoHcy is a potent inhibitor of methyltransferases [72], and the accumulation of this compound is amplified by the thermodynamics of the hydrolysis of S-AdoHcy to homocysteine (i.e., the precursor is favored over the product, Figure 10.1). For example, a severe degree of folate deficiency in rats, resulting in approximately a 100-fold decrease in mucosal concentrations of folate in the colon and approximately a sixfold increase in colonic S-AdoHcy concentrations, was accompanied by no significant change in mucosal S-AdoMet [76]; similar results have been observed in cell culture [80]. However, even S-AdoHcy is sometimes a poor predictor of genomic DNA methylation (e.g., Kim et al. [81]). In sum, even though S-AdoMet and S-AdoHcy are partial determinants of genomic DNA methylation, their concentrations correlate with DNA methylation in a rather unpredictable fashion because other factors are significant determinants as well.

On a genomic level, the induction of hypomethylation by means of one-carbon nutrient depletion has been observed in both preclinical and clinical studies, although whether the effect occurs depends on the magnitude and duration of the depletion and whether depletion of more than one one-carbon nutrient is induced. Moreover, it is an effect that is often tissue-specific. The response to different degrees of folate depletion is exemplified by comparing two rodent studies [60,81] that followed very similar protocols, except the magnitude of folate depletion that was produced. In one of the studies, a severe folate deficiency was induced [60] and genomic hypomethylation was readily observed, whereas in the other study a more moderate level of depletion produced no evidence of hypomethylation [81]. The onset of genomic demethylation has not been precisely defined but is usually apparent within a matter of weeks. Tissues are idiosyncratic with regard to how readily they undergo hypomethylation in response to folate depletion. The colonic mucosa is a prime example. Notwithstanding observations made in cultured human colonocytes [26], the colonic mucosa of intact animals has repeatedly been observed to be highly resistant to the induction of hypomethylation with isolated folate depletion. [76]. Nevertheless, two factors have been identified in animal studies that appear to make the colon susceptible to the induction of hypomethylation. First, a synergistic effect is apparent when depletion of multiple one-carbon nutrients is induced. A mild, combined depletion of folate, B12, B6, and B2 has been observed to reduce genomic DNA methylation of the colonic mucosa in mice by approximately 50% even though folate depletion alone produced no effect [30]. Second, the genomic hypomethylation that has been described to accompany elder age in a wide variety of tissues [82] may sensitize the colonic mucosa to modulations by dietary folate [83], although this sensitizing effect has not invariably been observed [22].

A sustained inadequacy of dietary folate has been observed to produce genomic DNA hypomethylation in human subjects as well, although the number of intervention studies is small [61,74]. To date, the effect has been produced most convincingly under the highly controlled conditions of either having subjects reside within a metabolic unit or requiring that they obtain all their meals from such a unit. The results of two cross-sectional studies suggest that low folate status results in diminished genomic methylation in free-living subjects as well, but only when present in conjunction with the homozygous TT genotype of the common 677C→T polymorphism in the *MTHFR* gene [53,54]. Additional studies would be helpful to confirm whether the effects of limited folate intake on genomic DNA methylation in a free-living population are limited solely to individuals of this genotype. It is worth noting that genomic hypomethylation of white blood cell DNA was achieved in the subjects of both intervention studies at a point when mean plasma folate was approximately 9.0 to 13.7 nmol/L (≈4.1–6.3 ng/mL), a rather modest level of systemic depletion. It is likely that bone marrow, which is among the most rapidly proliferating organs in the body, is extremely sensitive to limited folate availability because of its extraordinarily high rates of DNA synthesis, and this may explain why induction of DNA hypomethylation was achieved in these two studies with such modest reductions in plasma folate. In fact, another tissue with an extraordinarily high rate of cell turnover—the colonic mucosa—has been shown to be particularly vulnerable to folate depletion [22], and this may be one reason why the data linking diminished folate intake and increased cancer risk are most compelling for the colorectum.

Detecting the effect of folate status on genomic DNA methylation in the general population is considerably more difficult than doing so in highly controlled metabolic unit studies, apparently because other factors are important determinants of DNA methylation as well. For example, three cross-sectional analyses would seem to indicate that in the absence of highly controlled restrictions on folate intake, little of the variance in genomic DNA methylation in ambulatory adult populations is determined by folate status [53,54,86]. However, a substantial effect was observed by Friso et al. [85] by taking into account a relevant nutrient–gene interaction: These investigators chose subjects by their specific 677C→T *MTHFR* genotype and demonstrated that the combination of the TT genotype and low folate status collectively defined those whose genomic DNA methylation was diminished.

Several intervention trials in humans indicate that supplementation with folic acid at supraphysiological doses may increase genomic DNA methylation, although null results have been reported as well. Cravo et al. [87] observed that, compared with a placebo arm, 10 mg/day of folic acid resulted in significant increases in genomic DNA methylation in normal rectal mucosa among subjects who had previously undergone removal of colonic adenomas or cancers. However, these investigators later reported that supplementation with 5 mg/day of folic acid led to a significant increase in colonic DNA methylation only among subjects who had one adenoma resected as compared with multiple [88]. Kim et al. [89] reported that, compared with placebo, treatment with 5 mg/day of folic acid significantly increased genomic DNA methylation in the colon of subjects with previously resected colorectal adenomas. Nevertheless, after 12 months of treatment the degree of methylation in the placebo group had increased and was nearly identical to the value observed with supplementation, an effect perhaps ascribable to nationwide folic acid fortification that was instituted during the course of the trial. In another placebo-controlled trial in which the level of supplementation was in a more physiological range (400 μg/day of folic acid), an increase in genomic methylation of blood leukocytes was accompanied by only a marginally significant increase ($P = .09$) in methylation of the colonic mucosa [90]. Two additional trials, using supplements containing 700 to 2,000 μg/day, failed to demonstrate an effect of folate supplementation on genomic methylation in lymphocytes [53,54]. Of note is that the two studies with null results were performed in young adults (mean ages, 25 years in Fenech et al. [54] and 42 years in Basten et al. [53]), whereas in the studies with positive results inclusion criteria required that subjects had a previous colonic adenoma, which translated into substantially older study populations (mean ages, 56–66 years). This may be important because age has been frequently observed to be a strong inverse determinant of genomic DNA methylation (e.g., Basten et al. [53] and Pufulete et al. [86]). Moreover, the presence of adenomas has been observed to be accompanied by a wide region of hypomethylation surrounding the neoplasm (a so-called "field defect") [87]. Therefore, one might reasonably infer that supplemental folic acid is only capable of increasing genomic DNA methylation in human tissues in situations where the basal level of methylation has been diminished by elder age and/or by other perturbations such as proximity to a neoplasm. This sensitizing effect of elder age recapitulates some recent observations in rodents [83].

b. Gene-Specific Methylation

Folate availability has also been shown to modify gene-specific methylation, although it is not yet known whether this effect exists in intact humans. As previously mentioned, gene-specific methylation is thought to be more relevant to the mechanisms by which carcinogenesis evolves than changes in genomic methylation. In the highly controlled environment of cell culture, folate depletion has been shown to induce hypermethylation of the promoter region of a putative tumor suppressor gene, H-cadherin, in conjunction with a severalfold decrease in expression of the gene [80]. An increase in site-specific methylation and gene repression caused by folate depletion appears counterintuitive but is consistent with the observation that folate depletion induces an increase in steady-state mRNA for DNMT1 in cultured human colonocytes [51] and that the quantities of DNMT1 and DNMT3a enzyme, as well as several species of methyl CpG binding proteins (which help mediate the repressor function of hypermethylated CpG islands), increase in the livers of animals when they are fed a diet deficient in methionine, choline, and folate [91]. Thus, the paradoxical increase in site-specific methylation that occurs in response to depletion of one-carbon nutrients may be the result of a compensatory up-regulation in the cellular machinery that is responsible for DNA methylation.

It is not yet clear whether folate status can modulate promoter methylation of critical genes in intact humans, although a few clinical observations are consistent with the concept. In a cross-sectional study of DNA from human head and neck cancers, low dietary folate intake was associated with a statistically significant 2.3-fold increased risk of hypermethylation of the *p16* tumor suppressor gene compared with tumor DNA from individuals with high folate intake [92]. Similarly, an analysis of the promoter methylation of six genes that are frequently hypermethylated in colon cancer and whose functions are thought to be "cancer-protective"—*O6-MGMT*, *hMLH1*, *p14ARF*, *p16INK4A*, *RASSF1A*, and *Apc*—were examined in colonic adenomas. There was a consistent trend, albeit not statistically significant, toward less promoter hypermethylation among those who habitually consumed higher amounts of folate (>212 μg/day) [93]. The same investigators reported findings from a placebo-controlled trial involving subjects with a history of colonic adenomas, and the results contrast somewhat with those of their cross-sectional analysis [55]. Those in the treatment group received 5 mg of folic acid and 1.25 mg of B12 each day for 6 months, and promoter methylation of the same six genes was assessed in colonic biopsies. There was a trend ($P = .08$) for a combined index of methylation, incorporating all six genes to be greater among the treated individuals versus the controls [55]. Clearly, the answer as to whether folate intake can modulate promoter methylation in humans awaits future studies. Nevertheless, to the extent to which these suggestive trends are real and that promoter methylation of these genes contributes to cancer risk, one might surmise that either too little or too much folate intake can be deleterious, which is consistent with the concept of a "dual effect" of folate.

The *p53* tumor suppressor gene has received considerable attention in this field because loss of its function is thought to play a seminal role in more than 85% of colorectal malignancies, but hypermethylation of its promoter region does not appear to be an avenue by which its expression is suppressed. Unlike many other tumor suppressor genes, the promoter region of *p53* contains no CpG islands. Instead, diminished *p53* function in colorectal carcinogenesis most often occurs when one allele undergoes a loss of heterozygosity event and the other undergoes a somatic mutation. This was substantiated by data from a rodent study in which the effect of severe folate deficiency on methylation at any of the 15 CpG sites in the p53 promoter region was examined [76]. A 40% reduction in expression of the colonic gene was observed but was not accompanied by any changes in CpG site methylation [76].

In sharp contrast, inducing hypomethylation at CpG sites in the coding region of *p53* via depletion of one-carbon nutrients has been a reproducible phenomenon and may have relevance to carcinogenesis. Although these scattered CpG sites are highly methylated under basal conditions, the "methyl-deficient diet" (i.e., deplete in methionine, choline, and folate), the isolated folate-deficient diet, and the combined folate/B12/B6/B2-deficient diet have each induced hypomethylation of the coding region, and this has been true when it has been examined in cultured colonocytes from human colon cancers and in the liver and colonic mucosa of rodents [30,42,44,45,73,76]. Most of these studies have examined the so-called "hypermutable region" of the *p53* gene (exons 5–8), where the vast majority of mutations in human cancer occur. The degree of hypomethylation induced in this region of the gene has been reported to be a function of the duration of the folate depletion [45]. Nevertheless, it has

TABLE 10.1

Other Possible Mechanisms by Which Folate (and Other One-Carbon Nutrients) Modulate Carcinogenesis

Mechanism	Pertinent References
Changes in methylation of RNA, protein	59, 62
Disturbances in mitochondrial DNA	102, 103
Facilitation of tumorigenic viruses	144–146
Impairment of cell-mediated immunity	147, 148
Secondary deficiency of choline	149, 150

yet to be demonstrated whether demethylation of CpG sites in the coding region of *p53* contributes to carcinogenesis. In fact, it is the methylation, not demethylation, of these sites that is thought to be responsible for the fact that they are "hotspots" for C→T transition mutations in human cancer because spontaneous deamination of methylcytosine results in the formation of thymidine [12].

C. OTHER MECHANISMS

Although perturbations in the integrity and methylation of nuclear DNA are the prevailing hypotheses at present, alternative or additional avenues through which one-carbon nutrients modulate carcinogenesis may exist. The observations supporting such alternative hypotheses are sparse at present. Moreover, for some, such as the impairment of cell-mediated immunity, the existing literature is dissuasive because effects are only observed with markedly severe (and thus clinically irrelevant) degrees of depletion. These mechanisms are presented in brief in Table 10.1, with selected relevant citations.

III. AGE AS A CODETERMINANT

The risk of several common cancers increases markedly with age. For example, the occurrence of colorectal cancer doubles every decade after the age of 40. Therefore, the question arises as to whether age might alter one-carbon metabolism in the colon, thereby creating a mechanistic avenue through which age mediates its effects on the risk of developing colorectal cancer. Supporting this concept was the observation that folate concentration in the colonic mucosa of the elder rodent was only about 60% of that observed in younger adults fed equivalent amounts of dietary folate [22], a differential that only disappeared when animals were fed a diet containing four times the basal requirement of the vitamin. This effect of age appeared to be a tissue-specific one because the difference between young and elder adults with regard to folate status was not as apparent in the blood. Interestingly, the effect of age was not solely a quantitative one. The proportion of total colonic folate that comprised methylfolates was markedly diminished in the elder animals compared with the young adults. Because it is plausible that the enhanced susceptibility of the colon to folate depletion is related to the extremely high state of proliferation of this tissue, it is germane that the epithelium of the elder colon of both the rat [94] and the human [95] proliferate even faster than that of the younger adult. Nevertheless, it is not yet known whether these quantitative and qualitative differences in the folate content of the rodent colon are a phenomenon in elderly humans as well.

Also in support of a mechanistic connection between elder age and folate metabolism are some select molecular alterations that occur in the aged colonic epithelium that are consistent with impairments in one-carbon metabolism. For example, genomic DNA methylation has been observed to decrease with age in most tissues [82]. Perhaps more importantly, hypermethylation of the 5'-UTR of many genes, including several of the tumor suppressor type, has been observed to increase progressively with elder age [96]. Included among the tissues in which this has been observed is the human colonic epithelium [97]. Thus, elder age, neoplastic transformation, and folate depletion share the commonality of being conditions in which genomic hypomethylation and site-specific hypermethylation occur. Might, therefore, each of these three factors magnify molecular effects produced by the other two?

Some studies in rodents indicate this synergy may exist. The elder colon of the rodent appears to be more susceptible to changes in both genetic and epigenetic aberrations that occur as a result of folate inadequacy. Only the elder colon is susceptible to the induction of uracil incorporation as a function of folate depletion [22]. Similarly, genomic and *p16* promoter methylation can be modulated by folate availability in the elder, but not young adult, colon [83]. Moreover, aging has been associated with diminished expression of certain tumor suppressor genes in the rodent colon, such as *p53* and insulin-like growth factor binding protein 3 (IGF-BP3) [98]. However, adequate folate intake abolishes this age-dependent phenomenon. Whether the effect of elder age as a major risk factor for colon cancer is in part conveyed by changes in colonic folate metabolism is a matter of speculation—but one that is ripe for investigation.

IV.   THE SEARCH FOR SPECIFIC SIGNALING PATHWAYS

Several cellular pathways have been implicated as the means by which folate inadequacy enhances carcinogenesis, but in no instance has definitive evidence of causality yet been established. However, in most of the studies that have explored pathways, investigators have chosen a priori to focus on a select set of genes. Therefore, their apparent importance in folate-related carcinogenesis may be as much a result of selection bias as the centrality of the roles they play.

To minimize such selection bias, genome-wide expression microarrays were used in a rodent study to screen for cellular pathways in the colon that are substantially altered by folate depletion and/or elder age [98]. The expression of nearly 200 genes, falling into several functional categories, was substantially and significantly altered by folate depletion. Although a discussion of all of them is beyond the scope of this chapter, some potentially important concepts were observed. For example, the number of genes whose expressions were substantially changed by depletion was reduced by about 50% in elder colon. Feasibly, this reflects an inadequate response to the folate-deplete state in the elder colon and might explain in part the elevated susceptibility to neoplasia observed in the elderly population. Moreover, it was of interest that diminished expression of *p53* and IGF-BP3 accompanied aging but only in the folate-deplete colon.

Interrogating the expression of a wide array of genes in cultured human colono-cytes exposed to folate depletion has also been reported [99,100], but the results are very difficult to interpret because they vary across cell lines. Nevertheless, reason-ably consistent protransformational changes in *Apc* and *β-catenin* (elements of the Wnt pathway) were noted in one study [99], as were changes in the expression of a downstream effector of the Wnt pathway, *cyclin D1*, in another [100]. Similarly, in both of these studies, decreases in *p53* expression were observed, as well as the expression of a downstream effector of *p53* that was down-regulated as well: *p21* in one study [99] and *MDM2* in the other [100]. Dysregulation of *Wnt-* and *p53*-mediated control of the cell cycle is thought to play a crucial role in the progres-sion of carcinogenesis in more than 80% of colorectal cancers, underscoring the potential functional importance of these observations. The means by which *Apc* and *p53* expression is modified by folate inadequacy in the colon does not appear to be through the induction of mutations [101]. Rather, it appears that such changes may be related more to impaired transcription as a result of the induction of DNA strand breaks, as discussed below.

The implication made by the above-mentioned gene expression studies—that perturbations in *p53-* and *Wnt*-mediated processes are playing a significant role—recapitulates the results of a number of rodent studies performed during the past 15 years. As early as 1995, DNA strand breaks in the coding region of *p53* were observed in the livers of "methyl-deficient" rodents [44], and subsequent studies with isolated folate deficiency extended these observations: DNA strand breaks in mutation-prone coding regions of the *p53* and *Apc* genes accrued over time in the colons of rodents and were accompanied by parallel decreases in gene expression [41]. Nevertheless, these two studies were performed with severe degrees of deficiency, limiting the extent to which the findings are relevant to human populations. However, a subsequent investigation in rodents indicated that even marginal degrees of one-carbon vitamin depletion have a great impact in the colonic epithelium when multiple inadequacies are present, producing effects that would otherwise not be observed with folate depletion alone. Combined marginal depletion of B2, B6, B12, and folate was effective in altering several elements of the Wnt signaling pathway in a protransformational manner and was accompanied by a 35% reduction in apoptosis, which is known to be controlled in part by Wnt signaling [30]. *Apc* strand breaks, and not promoter hypermethylation, appeared to be the proximal event responsible for this effect because all three methylation sites in the 5′-UTR of the rodent gene were unchanged by dietary perturbations. Similarly, diminished expression of *p53* and its downstream effector, MDM2, occurred as a result of the multiple depletion state [42]. That changes in both pathways were observed may not be just a coincidence because it is well known that there is considerable "cross-talk" between the Wnt signaling pathway and *p53*-mediated processes [104,105].

There has also been some interest in examining how altered one-carbon nutrient availability affects the expression of the cyclin-dependent kinase inhibitor 2A tumor suppressor gene (also commonly known as *p16* or *INK4a/ARF*), which exerts control over the G1 checkpoint of the cell cycle. This gene is commonly silenced in a variety of human neoplasms, including hepatocellular and colorectal cancers. Promoter hypermethylation appears to be the suppressive mechanism in a large proportion of instances [106], and a few preclinical and clinical observations suggest that this hypermethylation is influenced by the integrity of the biological methylation arm of one-carbon metabolism. In the methyl-deficient rodent model of hepatocellular carcinogenesis, methylation of the 5'-UTR of the *p16* gene (including the promoter region) increased incrementally with the stage of neoplastic transformation, although gene silencing only occurred with extensive degrees of methylation [107]. In human colorectal cancers, increased methylation of the *p16* gene was observed in the tumors of individuals whose MTHFR haplotype was one of diminished enzyme activity [108]. Because a remarkable increase in *p16* expression occurs in many tissues with aging as a result of regulatory factors other than methylation [109,110], it is not surprising that elder age was found to modify the relationship between folate availability and *p16* methylation/expression. Keyes et al. [83] observed that the methylation of the promoter region of the colonic *p16* gene (and to a lesser degree its expression) was modulated by changes in dietary folate intake in elder, but not younger, adult mice. However, in that study factors other than methylation appeared to exert primary control over expression of the gene in the elder animal because *p16* expression remained high even in the face of marked promoter methylation. The interrelationships between the *p16* gene, aging, folate status, and carcinogenesis are complex and warrant future attention.

Mutation of the Ki-*ras* proto-oncogene, which encodes for a membrane-bound guanosine triphosphate binding protein that assists in regulating the transmission of growth stimulatory signals from cell surface receptors to intracellular targets, is a common genetic event in the progression of small adenomas to larger ones that are more prone to malignant transformation. G→A transition mutations and G→T and G→C transversion mutations comprise the vast majority of mutational events. In a cross-sectional study of subjects harboring colorectal adenomas, stepwise increases in habitual dietary intake of folate were associated with stepwise decreases in both G→A transition mutations and G→T transversion mutations [111]. Likewise, in the Netherlands Cohort Study [112], the most robust observation was that increasing levels of dietary folate intake were associated with greater than a 10-fold reduction in G→A transition mutations in rectal cancers in women. From a mechanistic perspective, the most facile explanation for these epidemiological associations relates to the fact that C→T transition mutations (which result in G→A transitions in the opposing DNA strand) can be produced by either spontaneous deamination of methylcytosine [113] or by enzyme-mediated deamination of cytosine in the setting of low *S*-AdoMet concentrations [114]. Adequacy of intracellular folate may affect both the methylation status of cytosine and the intracellular concentrations of *S*-AdoMet, as described in earlier sections, thereby providing plausible explanations for the observed associations between folate intake and a reduction in Ki-*ras* mutations.

V.   THE *MTHFR* 677C→T POLYMORPHISM: WHAT DOES IT TELL US ABOUT MECHANISM?

The reaction catalyzed by MTHFR is a particularly critical one in one-carbon metabolism because it serves to partition cellular folates into those that are destined to serve biological methylation versus nucleotide synthesis and because it is unidirectional and therefore highly determinant in this partitioning process (Figure 10.1). In recognition of the importance of this partitioning, cells maintain tight control of the flux through the pathway via several regulators: *S*-AdoMet, by serving as an allosteric inhibitor of the enzyme, and indirectly by SHMT, by controlling the availability of precursors and products of the reaction [49]. Therefore, MTHFR sits as a virtual fulcrum in folate metabolism.

The fact that the common 677C→T polymorphism in *MTHFR* has repeatedly been associated with an altered risk of developing colorectal neoplasms and certain other cancers underscores the mechanistic import of this partitioning of folate coenzyme [115–117]. Other chapters in this book explore the epidemiological and clinical ramifications of this relationship. Apropos to this chapter, however, is the fact that the modulation of cancer risk can provide important clues as to the mechanisms by which folate availability modulates carcinogenesis.

Meta-analyses of the many clinical studies on this topic indicate that homozygosity for the *MTHFR* T allele is associated with a significant protective effect against colorectal cancer; in contrast, a protective effect on adenoma risk has been observed less consistently and is overall null [118,119]. Interestingly, in most of the studies that have examined the interaction between the TT genotype and folate status, the protective effect is attenuated among those with low plasma folate concentrations, and in some studies there is even a trend for homozygosity to become a significant risk factor among those with low folate status [116,120]. Moreover, what protective effect is conveyed by the TT genotype is largely lost among those who are moderate-to-heavy imbibers of alcohol [114,116]. The combination of the TT genotype and substantial alcohol intake appears to substantially enhance the risk of neoplastic transformation [116,120,121].

Although open to interpretation, the above-mentioned observations can reasonably be construed to imply the following:

1. The metabolic impairment created by the polymorphic form of the enzyme directs more folate coenzyme into thymidine and purine biosynthesis, which is biochemically important because biological methylation outcompetes for folate under basal conditions [122]. By directing more coenzyme toward purine and de novo thymidine synthesis, less uracil is incorporated into DNA, and conditions are optimized for DNA synthesis and repair.

   This may be the mechanism by which the TT polymorphism conveys protection against cancer. Experimental evidence in which human subjects possessing CC and TT genotypes are compared with stable isotopic labeling has demonstrated increased availability of formylated folates (a form readily interchangeable with 5,10-methylene-THF) in tissues, as well as enhanced de novo thymidine synthesis, substantiating this concept [123,124].

Mathematical modeling of one-carbon metabolism, although in its infancy, is consistent with these projections, predicting modest increases in thymidine and purine synthesis among those with the TT genotype [125].

This concept predicts that individuals with the TT variant genotype would have less uracil incorporation in their DNA. Such a prediction has been borne out by small cross-sectional studies [29,126,127]. In contrast, in another clinical study no effect of the TT genotype on the uracil content of lymphocyte DNA was observed [84]. The reason for these discordant results is unclear but may be related to the fact that subjects in these studies were not stratified by folate status, and the effect of the TT genotype might only be apparent under conditions of limited folate availability. Nevertheless, even under the highly controlled environment of cell culture (an ex vivo study in human lymphocytes), no effects of the TT genotype were observed under folate-deplete conditions [27,34]. In sum, the lack of consistent results makes it unclear whether the TT genotype is associated with a reduction in uracil incorporation into DNA.

2. If cellular folate concentrations are sufficiently low, the folate-deplete state, in concert with the redirection of flux conveyed by the TT genotype, produces profound enough perturbations in DNA methylation (or other methylation processes) to enhance carcinogenesis. This suggests that alterations in biological methylation also serve as an avenue by which folate can modulate carcinogenesis and might explain the loss of protection in individuals with the TT variant genotype that occurs with diminishing folate stores.

   A few clinical studies provide support for this hypothesis. One such study examined the two-way interaction between the TT genotype and folate status in the determination of genomic DNA methylation in immortalized human lymphocytes [84], and the second examined similar questions using DNA from circulating lymphocytes [85]. In both studies the level of genomic DNA methylation was similar in individuals with either the CC or TT genotype with adequate folate status. It was only when present in combination with low folate status that the TT genotype was associated with a reduction in genomic DNA methylation. Whether such an interaction similarly impacts gene-specific methylation is not well studied. In one clinical study the combination of low dietary folate intake and the TT genotype was associated with increased *p16* promoter methylation in head and neck cancers, albeit at a level of marginal statistical significance [92].

3. As mentioned above, the TT genotype impairs biological methylation, the manifestation of which becomes evident under conditions of limited folate availability. Similarly, although the impact of chronic and excessive alcohol consumption on one-carbon metabolism is multifaceted, one of the most prominent effects is the inhibition of methionine synthase [128], and thereby impairment of *S*-AdoMet-mediated methylation [129]. Thus, the clinical observations that indicate a synergy between alcohol intake and the TT genotype in promoting carcinogenesis are consistent with their known effects on biological methylation.

VI. PROCARCINOGENIC MECHANISMS

Neoplastic cells generally have a much faster rate of replication than their normal counterparts. This is true for both premalignant adenomas and frank malignancies of the colon [14]. Not surprisingly, rapidly proliferating cells appear to have an elevated requirement for folate, apparently to meet the demands imposed by increased DNA synthesis, and they meet these increased requirements by up-regulating processes that mediate the uptake and retention of folates, as well as their use for nucleotide synthesis [130–132]. Thus, an abundant supply of folate might be expected to optimize the proliferative capabilities of neoplastic cells.

Enhancement of tumorigenesis by the administration of abundant quantities of folic acid has been observed in several rodent models of colon cancer if the folate is administered after foci of neoplasia are already established or in settings in which an extraordinarily strong predisposition toward carcinogenesis is present [8,9,133]. Similarly, small clinical trials conducted in individuals with cancer in the 1940s resulted in precisely these unintended results [134,135]. Conversely, restriction of folate availability in those with established foci of neoplasia would be expected to attenuate tumorigenesis. Data from both animal [136–138] and some human studies [11,139,140] are consistent with this concept. Thus, folate is thought to exert a paradoxical tumor-enhancing effect in settings in which it is administered to individuals who harbor neoplastic cells because it provides additional substrate for cellular pathways that are needed for the rapid proliferation of these cells.

A discussion of the results of clinical trials that have examined adenoma recurrence as the primary endpoint is found in Chapter 9, but it is worth noting here that the results of the four placebo-controlled trials that have studied subjects with a history of adenomas have been rather inconsistent: Two demonstrate a protective effect of folate supplements [141,142], one demonstrates some indications of accelerated neoplasia [7], and in one the results are null [143]. Perhaps the lack of consensus among these studies reflects the delicate balance between the protective and promotional effects of folic acid supplements, the equilibrium of which is shifted by underlying factors such as age of the subjects, or the inadvertent presence of micro- or macroscopic foci of neoplasia at the onset of a trial. This diversity of outcomes underscores just how far we have yet to advance before our knowledge can successfully be translated into effective cancer prevention strategies.

VII. CONCLUSIONS

Our mechanistic understanding of the relationship between folate status and carcinogenesis has grown significantly but still falls short of having established the cellular pathway(s) through which the effect is mediated. Moreover, a new layer of complexity, manifested by a paradoxical promoting effect, is increasingly under investigation and appears to be a genuine phenomenon in select circumstances.

Preclinical studies, as well as a limited number of clinical observations, indicate that the central role of folate in nucleotide synthesis and biological methylation goes awry in states where there is folate inadequacy. Because aberrations in nucleotide synthesis and repair in addition to DNA methylation are among the most common pathways identified in carcinogenesis, these mechanistic avenues continue to be the most likely explanations for the protective effect of folate. Recent evidence supports the former mechanism as being the more important of the two.

Vigorous pursuit of the specific signaling pathway(s) through which folate exerts its effects needs to continue, in part because this field holds promise for the potential of translating our knowledge into various measures that will reduce the burden of cancer in our society. Further, issues pertinent to dose, timing, stage of life when the effects are exerted, and important genetic and exogenous codeterminants are also critical components of the puzzle. The complexity of the relationship between folate and tumorigenesis illustrates how important a thorough understanding of the underlying science is if programs to exploit these scientific principles for the benefit of public health are to be carried out in a safe and efficacious manner.

ACKNOWLEDGMENTS

This chapter was supported in part by National Institutes of Health K05 CA100048, U54 CA10097, and Agricultural Research Service 58-1950-7-707 (to JBM). Any opinions, findings, conclusions, or recommendations expressed herein are those of the authors and do not necessarily reflect the view of the US Department of Agriculture.

REFERENCES

1. Giovannucci E. Epidemiologic studies of folate and colorectal neoplasia: A review. *J Nutr* 2002; 132:2350S–55S.
2. Kim YI. Role of folate in colon cancer development and progression. *J Nutr* 2003; 133(Suppl 1):3731S–39S.
3. Beilby J, Ingram D, Hahnel R, Rossi E. Reduced breast cancer risk with increasing serum folate in a case-control study of the C677T genotype of the methylenetetra-hydrofolate reductase gene. *Eur J Cancer* 2004; 40:1250–54.
4. Ericson U, Sonestedt E, Gullberg B, Olsson H, Wirfält E. High folate intake is associated with lower breast cancer incidence in postmenopausal women in the Malmö Diet and Cancer cohort. *Am J Clin Nutr* 2007; 86:434–43.
5. Voorrips LE, Goldbohm RA, Brants HA, van Poppel GA, Sturmans F, Hermus RJ, van den Brandt PA. A prospective cohort study on antioxidant and folate intake and male lung cancer risk. *Cancer Epidemiol Biomarkers Prev* 2000; 9:357–65.
6. Larsson SC, Giovannucci E, Wolk A. Folate intake, MTHFR polymorphisms, and risk of esophageal, gastric, and pancreatic cancer: A meta-analysis. *Gastroenterology* 2006; 131:1271–83.
7. Cole BF, Baron JA, Sandler RS, Haile RW, Ahnen DJ, Bresalier RS, McKeown-Eyssen G, et al. Folic acid for the prevention of colorectal adenomas: A randomized clinical trial. *JAMA* 2007; 297:2351–59.
8. Song J, Sohn KJ, Medline A, Ash C, Gallinger S, Kim YI. Chemopreventive effects of dietary folate on intestinal polyps in *Apc+/– Msh2–/–* mice. *Cancer Res* 2000; 60:3191–99.
9. Song J, Medline A, Mason JB, Gallinger S, Kim YI. Effects of dietary folate on intestinal tumorigenesis in the *Apc*Min mouse. *Cancer Res* 2000; 60:5434–40.
10. Mason JB, Dickstein A, Jacques PF, Haggarty P, Selhub J, Dallal G, Rosenberg IH. A temporal association between folic acid fortification and an increase in colorectal cancer rates may be illuminating important biological principles: A hypothesis. *Cancer Epidemiol Biomarkers Prev* 2007; 16:1325–29.

11. Stolzenberg-Solomon RZ, Chang SC, Leitzmann MF, Johnson KA, Johnson C, Buys SS, Hoover RN, Ziegler RG. Folate intake, alcohol use, and postmenopausal breast cancer risk in the Prostate, Lung, Colorectal, and Ovarian Cancer Screening Trial. *Am J Clin Nutr* 2006; 83:895–904.

12. Grønbaek K, Hother C, Jones PA. Epigenetic changes in cancer. *APMIS* 2007; 115:1039–59.

13. Tudek B. Base excision repair modulation as a risk factor for human cancers. *Mol Aspects Med* 2007; 28:258–75.

14. Shpitz B, Bomstein Y, Mekori Y, Cohen R, Kaufman Z, Grankin M, Bernheim J.. Proliferating cell nuclear antigen as a marker of cell kinetics in aberrant crypt foci, hyperplastic polyps, adenomas, and adenocarcinomas of the human colon. *Am J Surg* 1997; 174:425–30.

15. Henderson L, Irving K, Gregory J. *National Diet and Nutrition Survey: Adults Aged 19–64. Vol. 4.* London: Her Majesty's Stationery Office, 2004. Available at www.food. gov.uk/science/dietarysurveys/ndnsdocuments/ndns4.

16. Lindenbaum J, Rosenberg IH, Wilson PW, Stabler SP, Allen RH. Prevalence of cobalamin deficiency in the Framingham elderly population. *Am J Clin Nutr* 1994; 60:2–11.

17. Planells E, Sanchez C, Montellano MA, Mataix J, Llopis J. Vitamins B6 and B12 and folate status in an adult Mediterranean population. *Eur J Clin Nutr* 2003; 57:777–85.

18. Theodoratou E, Farrington SM, Tenesa A, McNeill G, Cetnarskyj R, Barnetson RA, Porteous ME, Dunlop MG, Campbell H. Dietary vitamin B6 intake and the risk of colorectal cancer. *Cancer Epidemiol Biomarkers Prev* 2008; 17:171–82.

19. Wu K, Helzlsouer K, Comstock G, Hoffman SC, Nadeau MR, Selhub J. A prospective study on folate, B12, and PLP and breast cancer. *Cancer Epidemiol Biomarkers Prev* 1999; 8:209–17.

20. James SJ, Basnakian AG, Miller BJ. In vitro folate deficiency induces deoxynucleotide pool imbalance, apoptosis, and mutagenesis in Chinese hamster ovary cells. *Cancer Res* 1994; 54:5075–80.

21. Blount BC, Mack MM, Wehr CM, MacGregor JT, Hiatt RA, Wang G, Wickramasinghe SN, Everson RB, Ames BN. Folate deficiency causes uracil misincorporation into human DNA and chromosome breakage: Implications for cancer and neuronal damage. *Proc Natl Acad Sci USA* 1997; 94:3290–95.

22. Choi SW, Friso S, Dolnikowski GG, Bagley PJ, Edmondson AN, Smith DE, Mason JB. Biochemical and molecular aberrations in the rat colon due to folate depletion are age-specific. *J Nutr* 2003; 133:1206–12.

23. Duthie SJ, Hawdon A. DNA instability (strand breakage, uracil misincorporation, and defective repair) is increased by folic acid depletion in human lymphocytes in vitro. *FASEB J* 1997; 12:1491–97.

24. Duthie SJ, Hawdon A. DNA instability (strand breakage, uracil misincorporation, and defective repair) is increased by folic acid depletion in human lymphocytes in vitro. *FASEB J* 1998; 12:1491–97.

25. Duthie SJ, Grant G, Narayanan S. Increased uracil misincorporation in lymphocytes from folate-deficient rats. *Br J Cancer* 2000; 83:1532–37.

26. Duthie SJ, Narayanan S, Blum S, Pirie L, Brand GM. Folate deficiency in vitro induces uracil misincorporation and DNA hypomethylation and inhibits DNA excision repair in immortalized normal human colon epithelial cells. *Nutr Cancer* 2000; 37:245–51.

27. Crott JW, Mashiyama ST, Ames BN, Fenech MF. Methylenetetrahydrofolate reductase C677T polymorphism does not alter folic acid deficiency-induced uracil incorporation into primary human lymphocyte DNA in vitro. *Carcinogenesis* 2001; 22:1019–25.

28. Choi SW, Friso S, Ghandour H, Bagley PJ, Selhub J, Mason JB. Vitamin B_{12} deficiency induces anomalies of base substitution and methylation in the DNA of rat colonic epithelium. *J Nutr* 2004; 134:750–55.

29. Kapiszewska M, Kalemba M, Wojciech U, Milewicz T. Uracil misincorporation into DNA of leukocytes of young women with positive folate balance depends on plasma B12 concentrations and methylenetetrahydrofolate reductase polymorphisms. A pilot study. *J Nutr Biochem* 2005; 16:467–78.

30. Liu Z, Choi SW, Crott JW, Keyes MK, Jang H, Smith DE, Kim M, Laird PW, Bronson R, Mason JB. Mild depletion of dietary folate combined with other B vitamins alters multiple components of the Wnt pathway in mouse colon. *J Nutr* 2007; 137:2701–08.

31. Barnes DE, Lindahl T. Repair and genetic consequences of endogenous DNA base damage in mammalian cells. *Annu Rev Genet* 2004; 38:445–76.

32. Dianov GL, Timchenko TV, Sinitsina OI, Kuzminov AV, Medvedev OA, Salganik RI. Repair of uracil residues closely spaces on the opposite strands of plasmid DNA results in double-strand break and deletion formation. *Mol Gen Genet* 1991; 225:448–52.

33. Moynahan ME, Jasin M. Loss of heterozygosity induced by a chromosomal double-strand break. *Proc Natl Acad Sci USA* 1997; 94:8988–93.

34. Crott JW, Mashiyama ST, Ames BN, Fenech M. The effect of folic acid deficiency and MTHFR C677T polymorphism on chromosome damage in human lymphocytes in vitro. *Cancer Epidemiol Biomarkers Prev* 2001; 10:1089–96.

35. Elliott B, Jasin M. Double-strand breaks and translocations in cancer. *Cell Mol Life Sci* 2002; 59:373–85.

36. Jackson SP. Sensing and repairing DNA double strand breaks. *Carcinogenesis* 2002; 23:687–96.

37. Brison O. Gene amplification and tumor progression. *Biochim Biophys Acta* 1993; 1155:25–41.

38. Seeger RC, Brodeur GM, Sather H, Dalton A, Siegel SE, Wong KY, Hammond D. Association of multiple copies of the N-myc oncogene with rapid progression of neuroblastomas. *N Engl J Med* 1985; 313:1111–16.

39. Garinis GA, Mitchell JR, Moorhouse MJ, Hanada K, de Waard H, Vandeputte D, Jans J, et al. Transcriptome analysis reveals cyclobutane pyrimidine dimers as a major source of UV-induced DNA breaks. *EMBO J* 2005; 24:3952–62.

40. Kathe SD, Shen GP, Wallace SS. Single-stranded breaks in DNA but not oxidative DNA base damages block transcriptional elongation by RNA polymerase II in HeLa cell nuclear extracts. *J Biol Chem* 2004; 279:18511–20.

41. Kim YI, Shirwadkar S, Choi SW, Puchyr M, Wang Y, Mason JB. Effects of dietary folate on DNA strand breaks within mutation-prone exons of the p53 gene in rat colon. *Gastroenterology* 2000; 119:151–61.

42. Liu Z, Choi S-W, Crott J, Smith D, Mason JB. Multiple B-vitamin inadequacy amplifies alterations induced by isolated folate depletion in p53 expression and its downstream effector, MDM2. *Int J Cancer* 2008; 123:519–23.

43. Crott JW, Liu Z, Choi SW, Mason JB. Folate depletion in human lymphocytes up-regulates p53 expression despite marked induction of strand breaks in exons 5-8 of the gene. *Mutat Res* 2007; 626:171–79.

44. Pogribny IP, Basnakian AG, Miller BJ, Lopatina NG, Poirier LA, James SJ. Breaks in genomic DNA and within the p53 gene are associated with hypomethylation in livers of folate/methyl-deficient rats. *Cancer Res* 1995; 55:1894–901.

45. Kim YI, Pogribny IP, Basnakian AG, Miller JW, Selhub J, James SJ, Mason JB. Folate deficiency in rats induces DNA strand breaks and hypomethylation within the p53 tumor suppressor gene. *Am J Clin Nutr* 1997; 65:46–52.

46. Krokan HE, Drabløs F, Slupphaug G. Uracil in DNA—Occurrence, consequences and repair. *Oncogene* 2002; 21:8935–48.

47. Choi SW, Kim YI, Weitzel JN, Mason JB. Folate depletion impairs DNA excision repair in the colon of the rat. *Gut* 1998; 43:93–99.

48. Knock E, Deng L, Wu Q, Lawrance AK, Wang XL, Rozen R. Strain differences in mice highlight the role of DNA damage in neoplasia induced by low dietary folate. *J Nutr* 2008; 138:653–58.

49. Herbig K, Chiang EP, Lee LR, Hills J, Shane B, Stover PJ. Cytoplasmic serine hydroxymethyltransferase mediates competition between folate-dependent deoxyribonucleotide and S-adenosylmethionine biosyntheses. *J Biol Chem* 2002; 277:38381–89.

50. MacFarlane AJ, Liu X, Perry CA, Flodby P, Allen RH, Stabler SP, Stover PJ. Cytoplasmic serine hydroxymethyltransferase regulates the metabolic portioning of methylenetetrahydrofolate but is not essential in mice. *J Biol Chem* 2008; 283:25846–53. Remainder unpublished, presented at *Diet, Epigenetic Events, and Cancer Prevention* NIH Symposium, September 26–27, 2007.

51. Hayashi I, Sohn K-J, Stempak JM, Croxford R, Kim Y-I. Folate deficiency induces cell-specific changes in the steady-state transcript levels of genes involved in folate metabolism and 1-carbon transfer reactions in human colonic epithelial cells. *J Nutr* 2007; 137:607–13.

52. Fenech M. The in vitro micronucleus technique. *Mutat Res* 2000; 455:81–95.

53. Basten GP, Duthie SJ, Pirie L, Vaughan N, Hill MH, Powers HJ. Sensitivity of markers of DNA stability and DNA repair activity to folate supplementation in healthy volunteers. *Br J Cancer* 2006; 94:1942–47.

54. Fenech M, Aitken C, Rinaldi J. Folate, vitamin B12, homocysteine status and DNA damage in young Australian adults. *Carcinogenesis* 1998; 19:1163–71.

55. van den Donk M, Pellis L, Crott JW, van Engeland M, Friederich P, Nagengast FM, van Bergeijk JD, et al. Folic acid and vitamin B-12 supplementation does not favorably influence uracil incorporation and promoter methylation in rectal mucosa DNA of subjects with previous colorectal adenomas. *J Nutr* 2007; 137:2114–20.

56. Wagner C. Biochemical role of folate in cellular metabolism. In: Bailey LB, ed., *Folate in Health and Disease.* New York: Marcel Dekker, 1995: 23–42.

57. Hoffman DR, Cornatzer WE, Duerre JA. Relationship between tissue levels of S-adenosylmethionine, S-adenosylhomocysteine, and transmethylation reactions. *Can J Biochem* 1979; 57:56–65.

58. Akesson B, Fehling C, Jagerstad M, Stenram U. Effect of experimental folate deficiency on lipid metabolism in liver and brain. *Br J Nutr* 1982; 47:505–20.

59. Wainfan E, Moller ML, Maschio FA, Balis ME. Methionine induced changes in rat liver transfer RNA methylation. *Cancer Res* 1975; 35:2830–35.

60. Balaghi M, Wagner C. DNA methylation in folate deficiency: Use of CpG methylase. *Biochem Biophys Res Commun* 1993; 193:1184–90.

61. Jacob RA, Gretz DM, Taylor PC, James SJ, Pogribny IP, Miller BJ, Henning SM, Swendseid ME. Moderate folate depletion increases plasma homocysteine and decreases lymphocyte DNA methylation in postmenopausal women. *J Nutr* 1998; 128:1204–12.

62. Ghandour H, Lin BF, Choi SW, Mason JB, Selhub J. Folate status and age affect the accumulation of L-isoaspartyl residues in rat liver proteins. *J Nutr* 2002; 132:1357–60.

63. Ehrlich M, Gama-Sosa MA, Huang LH, Midgett RM, Kuo KC, McCune RA, Gehrke C. Amount and distribution of 5-methylcytosine in human DNA from different types of tissues of cells. *Nucleic Acids Res* 1982; 10:2709–21.

64. Rai K, Chidester S, Zavala CV, Manos EJ, James SR, Karpf AR, Jones DA, Cairns BR. Dnmt2 functions in the cytoplasm to promote liver, brain, and retina development in zebrafish. *Genes Dev* 2007; 21:261–66.

65. Denissenko MF, Chen JX, Tang MS, Pfeifer GP. Cytosine methylation determines hot spots of DNA damage in the human P53 gene. *Proc Natl Acad Sci USA* 1997; 94:3893–98.

66. Jones PA, Baylin SB. The epigenomics of cancer. *Cell* 2007; 128:683–92.

67. Kim YI, Giuliano A, Hatch KD, Schneider A, Nour MA, Dallal GE, Selhub J, Mason JB. Global DNA hypomethylation increases progressively in cervical dysplasia and carcinoma. *Cancer* 1994; 74:893–99.
68. Issa JP, Ottaviano YL, Celano P, Hamilton SR, Davidson NE, Baylin SB. Methylation of the oesterogen receptor CpG island links ageing and neoplasia in human colon. *Nat Genet* 1994; 7:536–40.
69. Agrawal A, Murphy RF, Agrawal DK. DNA methylation in breast and colorectal cancers. *Mod Pathol* 2007; 20:711–21.
70. Sakatani T, Kaneda A, Iacobuzio-Donahue CA, Carter MG, de Boom WS, Okano H, Ko MS, Ohlsson R, Longo DL, Feinberg AP. Loss of imprinting of Igf2 alters intestinal maturation and tumorigenesis in mice. *Science* 2005; 307:1976–78.
71. Chen RZ, Pettersson U, Beard C, Jackson-Grusby L, Jaenisch R. DNA hypomethylation leads to elevated mutation rates. *Nature* 1998; 395:89–93.
72. Hoffman M, Schulz W. Causes and consequences of DNA hypomethylation in human cancer. *Biochem Cell Biol* 2005; 83:296–321.
73. Wasson GR, McGlynn AP, McNulty H, O'Reilly SL, McKelvey-Martin VJ, McKerr G, Strain JJ, Scott J, Downes CS. Global DNA and p53 region-specific hypomethylation in human colonic cells is induced by folate depletion and reversed by folate supplementation. *J Nutr* 2006; 136:2748–53.
74. Rampersaud GC, Kauwell GPA, Hutson AD, Cerda JJ, Bailey LB. Genomic DNA methylation decreases in response to moderate folate depletion in elderly women. *Am J Clin Nutr* 2000; 72:998–1003.
75. Pogribny IP, Miller BJ, James SJ. Alterations in hepatic p53 gene methylation patterns during tumor progression with folate/methyl deficiency in the rat. *Cancer Lett* 1997; 115:31–38.
76. Sohn KJ, Stempack JM, Reid S, Shirwadkar S, Mason JB, Kim YI. The effect of dietary folate on genomic and p53-specific DNA methylation in rat colon. *Carcinogenesis* 2003; 24:81–90.
77. Lu SC, Alvarez L, Huang ZZ, Chen L, An W, Corrales F, Avila M, Kanel G, and Mato JM. Methionine adenosyltransferase 1A knockout mice are predisposed to liver injury and exhibit increased expression of genes involved in proliferation. *Proc Natl Acad Sci USA* 2001; 98:5560–65.
78. Yi J, Melnyk S, Pogribna M, Pogribny I, Hine RJ, James SJ. Increase in plasma homocysteine associated with parallel increases in plasma S-adenosylhomocysteine and lymphocyte DNA hypomethylation. *J Biol Chem* 2000; 275:29318–23.
79. James SJ, Melnyk S, Pogribna M, Pogribny IP, Caudill MA. Elevation in S-adenosylhomocysteine and DNA hypomethylation: Potential epigenetic mechanism for homocysteine-related pathology. *J Nutr* 2002; 132(Suppl):2361S–66S.
80. Jhaveri M, Wagner C, Trepel J. Impact of extracellular folate levels on global gene expression. *Mol Pharmacol* 2001; 60:1288–95.
81. Kim YI, Christman JK, Fleet JC, Cravo ML, Salomon RN, Smith D, Ordovas J, Selhub J, Mason JB. Moderate folate deficiency does not cause global hypomethylation of hepatic and colonic DNA or c-myc-specific hypomethylation of colonic DNA in rats. *Am J Clin Nutr* 1995; 61:1083–90.
82. Issa JP. Aging, DNA methylation and cancer. *Crit Rev Oncol Hematol* 1999; 32:31–43.
83. Keyes MK, Jang H, Mason JB, Liu Z, Crott JW, Smith DE, Friso S, Choi SW. Older age and dietary folate are determinants of genomic and p16-specific DNA methylation in mouse colon. *J Nutr* 2007; 137:1713–17.
84. Stern LL, Mason JB, Selhub J, Choi SW. Genomic DNA hypomethylation, a characteristic of most cancers, is present in peripheral leukocytes of individuals who are homozygous for the C677T polymorphism in the methylenetetrahydrofolate reductase gene. *Cancer Epidemiol Biomarkers Prev* 2000; 9:849–53.

85. Friso S, Choi SW, Girelli D, Mason JB, Dolnikowski GG, Bagley PJ, Olivieri O, et al. A common mutation in the 5,10-methylenetetrahydrofolate reductase gene affects genomic DNA methylation through an interaction with folate status. *Proc Natl Acad Sci USA* 2002; 99:5606–11.
86. Pufulete M, Al-Ghnaniem R, Rennie JA, Appleby P, Harris N, Gout S, Emery PW, Sanders TA. Influence of folate status on genomic DNA methylation in colonic mucosa of subjects without colorectal adenoma or cancer. *Br J Cancer* 2005; 92:838–42.
87. Cravo M, Fidalgo P, Pereira AD, Gouveia-Oliveira A, Chaves P, Selhub J, Mason JB, Mira FC, Leitao CN. DNA methylation as an intermediate biomarker in colorectal cancer: Modulation by folic acid supplementation. *Eur J Cancer Prev* 1994; 3:473–79.
88. Cravo ML, Pinto AG, Chaves P, Cruz JA, Lage P, Nobre-Leitao C, Costa Mira F. Effect of folate supplementation on DNA methylation of rectal mucosa in patients with colonic adenomas: Correlation with nutrient intake. *Clin Nutr* 1998; 17:45–49.
89. Kim YI, Baik HW, Fawaz K, Knox T, Mee Lee Y, Norton R, Libby E, Mason JB. Effects of folate supplementation on two provisional molecular markers of colon cancer: A prospective, randomized trial. *Am J Gastroenterol* 2001; 96:184–95.
90. Pufulete M, Al-Ghaniem R, Khushal A, Appleby P, Harris N, Gout S, Emery PW, Sanders TAB. Effect of folic acid supplementation on genomic DNA methylation in patients with colorectal adenoma. *Gut* 2005; 54:648–53.
91. Ghoshal K, Li X, Datta J, Bai S, Pogribny I, Pogribny M, Huang Y, Young D, Jacob ST. A folate- and methyl-deficient diet alters the expression of DNA methyltransferases and methyl CpG binding proteins involved in epigenetic gene silencing in livers of F344 rats. *J Nutr* 2006; 136:1522–27.
92. Kraunz K, Hsiung D, McClean M, Liu M, Osanyingbemi J, Nelson H, Kelsey K. Dietary folate is associated with p16INK4A methylation in head and neck squamous cell carcinoma. *Int J Cancer* 2006; 119:1553–57.
93. van den Donk M, van Engeland M, Pellis L, Witteman BJ, Kok FJ, Keijer J, Kampman E. Dietary folate intake in combination with MTHFR C677T genotype and promoter methylation of tumor suppressor and DNA repair genes in sporadic colorectal adenomas. *Cancer Epidemiol Biomarkers Prev* 2007; 16:327–33.
94. Holt PR, Higgins PJ, Atillasoy E, Davis PJ, Lipkin M. Abnormal cell proliferation and p52/p35-CSK expression in the colons of aging rats. *Exp Gerontol* 1995; 30:495–503.
95. Paganelli M, Santucci R, Biasco G, Miglioli M, Barbara L. Effect of sex and age on rectal cell renewal in humans. *Cancer Lett* 1990; 53:117–21.
96. Nishida N, Nagasaka T, Nishimura T, Ikai I, Boland C, Goel A. Aberrant methylation of multiple tumor suppressor genes in aging liver, chronic hepatitis, and hepatocellular carcinoma. *Hepatology* 2008; 47:908–18.
97. Youssef EM, Estecio MR, Issa JP. Methylation and regulation of expression of different retinoic acid receptor beta isoforms in human colon cancer. *Cancer Biol Ther* 2004; 3:82–86.
98. Crott JW, Choi SW, Ordovas JM, Ditelberg JS, Mason JB. Effects of dietary folate and aging on gene expression in the colonic mucosa of rats: Implications for carcinogenesis. *Carcinogenesis* 2004; 25:69–76.
99. Novakovic P, Stempak JM, Sohn KJ, Kim YI. Effects of folate deficiency on gene expression in the apoptosis and cancer pathways in colon cancer cells. *Carcinogenesis* 2006; 27:916–24.
100. Crott JW, Liu Z, Keyes MK, Choi SW, Jang H, Moyer MP, Mason JB. Moderate folate depletion modulates the expression of selected genes in the cell cycle, intracellular signaling and folate uptake in human colonic epithelial cell lines. *J Nutr Biochem* 2008; 19:328–35.
101. Sohn KJ, Puchyr M, Salomon RN, Graeme-Cook F, Fung L, Choi SW, Mason JB, Medline A, Kim YI. The effect of dietary folate on Apc and p53 mutations in the dimethylhydrazine rat model of colorectal cancer. *Carcinogenesis* 1999; 20:2345–50.

102. Bianchi NO, Bianchi MS, Richard SM. Mitochondrial genome instability in human cancer. *Mutat Res* 2001; 488:9–23.

103. Crott JW, Choi SW, Branda RF, Mason JB. Accumulation of DNA deletions is age, tissue, and folate-dependent in rats. *Mutat Res* 2005; 570:63–70.

104. Su F, Overholtzer M, Besser D, Levine AJ. WISP-1 attenuates p53-mediated apoptosis in response to DNA damage through activation of the Akt kinase. *Genes Dev* 2002; 16:46–57.

105. Cagatay T, Ozturk M. P53 mutation as a source of aberrant beta-catenin accumulation in cancer cells. *Oncogene* 2002; 21:7971–80.

106. Rocco JW, Sidransky D. p16(MTS-1/CDKN2/INK4a) in cancer progression. *Exp Cell Res* 2001; 264:42–55.

107. Pogribny IP, James SJ. De novo methylation of the p16INK4A gene in early preneoplastic liver and tumors induced by folate/methyl deficiency in rats. *Cancer Lett* 2002; 187:69–75.

108. Oyama K, Kawakami K, Maeda K, Ishiguro K, Watanabe G. The association between methylenetetrahydrofolate reductase polymorphism and promoter methylation in proximal colon cancer. *Anticancer Res* 2004; 24:649–54.

109. Krishnamurthy J, Torrice C, Ramsey MR, Kovalev GI, Al-Regaiey K, Su L, Sharpless NE. Ink4a/Arf expression is a biomarker of aging. *J Clin Invest* 2004; 114:1299–307.

110. Krishnamurthy J, Ramsey MR, Ligon KL, Torrice C, Koh A, Bonner-Weir S, Sharpless NE. p16INK4a induces an age dependant decline in islet regenerative potential. *Nature* 2006; 443:453–57.

111. Martinez ME, Maltzman T, Marshall JR, Einspahr J, Reid ME, Sampliner R, Ahnen DJ, Hamilton S, Alberts D. Risk factors for Ki-ras protooncogene mutation in sporadic colorectal adenomas. *Cancer Res* 1999; 59:5181–85.

112. Brink M, Weijenberg M, de Goeij A, Roemen GM, Lentjes MH, de Bruïne AP, van Engeland M, Goldbohm RA, van den Brandt PA. Dietary folate and k-ras mutations in sporadic colon and rectal cancer in the Netherlands Cohort Study. *Int J Cancer* 2005; 114:824–30.

113. Rideout WM 3rd, Coetzee GA, Olumi AF, Jones PA. 5-Methylcytosine as an endogenous mutagen in the human LDL receptor and p53 genes. *Science* 1990; 249:1288–90.

114. Shen JC, Rideout WM 3rd, Jones PA. High frequency mutagenesis by a DNA methyltransferase. *Cell* 1992; 71:1073–80.

115. Chen J, Giovannucci E, Kelsey K, Rimm EB, Stampfer MJ, Colditz GA, Spiegelman D, Willett WC, Hunter DJ. A methylenetetrahydrofolate reductase polymorphism and the risk of colorectal cancer. *Cancer Res* 1996; 56:4862–64.

116. Ma J, Stampfer MJ, Giovannucci E, Arigas C, Hunter DJ, Fuchs C, Willett WC, Selhub J, Henekens CH, Rozen R. Methylenetetrahydrofolate reductase polymorphism, dietary interactions, and risk of colorectal cancer. *Cancer Res* 1997; 57:1098–102.

117. Crott J, Mason JB. MTHFR polymorphisms and colorectal neoplasia. In: *MTHFR Polymorphisms and Disease*. Ueland P, Rozen R, eds., Georgetown, TX: Landes Bioscience, 2005:179–96.

118. Hubner R, Houlston R. MTHFR C677T and colorectal cancer risk: A meta-analysis of 25 populations. *Int J Cancer* 2007; 120:1027–35.

119. Huang Y, Han S, Liu Y, Mao Y, Xie Y. Different roles of MTHFR C677T and A1298C polymorphisms in colorectal adenoma and colorectal cancer: A meta-analysis. *J Hum Genet* 2007; 52:73–85.

120. Levine AJ, Siegmund KD, Ervin CM, Diep A, Lee ER, Frankl HD, Haile RW. The methylenetetrahydrofolate reductase 677C->T polymorphism and distal colorectal adenoma risk. *Cancer Epidemiol Biomark Prev* 2000; 9:657–63.

121. Li D, Ahmed M, Li Y, Jiao L, Chou TH, Wolff RA, Lenzi R, et al. 5,10-Methylenetetrahydrofolate reductase polymorphisms and the risk of pancreatic cancer. *Cancer Epidemiol Biomarkers Prev* 2005; 14:1470–76.

122. Green JM, MacKenzie RE, Matthews RG. Substrate flux through methylenetetrahy-drofolate dehydrogenase: Predicted effects of the concentration of methylenetetra-hydrofolate on its partitioning into pathways leading to nucleotide biosynthesis or methionine regeneration. *Biochemistry* 1988; 27:8014–22.

123. Quinlivan EP, Davis SR, Shelnutt KP, Henderson GN, Ghandour H, Shane B, Selhub J, Bailey LB, Stacpoole PW, Gregory JF 3rd. Methylenetetrahydrofolate reductase 677C->T polymorphism and folate status affect one-carbon incorporation into human DNA deoxynucleosides. *J Nutr* 2005; 135:389–96.

124. Davis SR, Quinlivan EP, Shelnutt KP, Maneval DR, Ghandour H, Capdevila A, Coats BS, et al. The methylenetetrahydrofolate reductase 677C->T polymorphism and dietary folate restriction affect plasma one-carbon metabolites and red blood cell folate concen-trations and distribution in women. *J Nutr* 2005; 135:1040–44.

125. Reed MC, Nijhout HF, Neuhouser ML, Gregory JF 3rd, Shane B, James SJ, Boynton A, Ulrich CM. A mathematical model gives insights into nutritional and genetic aspects of folate-mediated one-carbon metabolism. *J Nutr* 2006; 136:2653–61.

126. DeVos L, Chanson A, Liu Z, Ciappio ED, Parnell LD, Mason JB, Tucker KL, Crott JW. Associations between single nucleotide polymorphisms in folate uptake and metaboliz-ing genes with blood folate, homocysteine and DNA uracil levels. *Am J Clin Nutr* 2008; 88:1149–58.

127. Narayanan S, McConnell J, Little J, Sharp L, Piyathilake CJ, Powers H, Basten G, Duthie SJ. Association between two common variants C677T and A1298C in the methylenetetrahydrofolate reductase gene and measures of folate metabolism and DNA stability (strand breaks, misincorporated uracil, and DNA methylation status) in human lymphocytes in vivo. *Cancer Epidemiol Biomarkers Prev* 2004; 13:1436–43.

128. Halsted C, Villanueva J, Devlin A, Niemela O, Parkkila S, Garrow T, Wallock L, Shigenaga M, Melnyk S, James SJ. Folate deficiency disturbs hepatic methionine metabolism and promotes liver injury in the ethanol-fed micropig. *Proc Natl Acad Sci USA* 2002; 99:10072–77.

129. Mason JB, Choi S-W. Effects of alcohol on folate metabolism: Implications for carcinogenesis. *Alcohol* 2005; 35:235–41.

130. Egan MG, Sirlin S, Rumberger BG, Garrow TA, Shane B, Sirotnak FM. Rapid decline in folylpolyglutamate synthetase activity and gene expression during maturation of HL-60 cells. Nature of the effect, impact on folate compound polyglutamate pools, and evidence for programmed down-regulation during maturation. *J Biol Chem* 1995; 270:5462–68.

131. Kelemen LE. The role of folate receptor a in cancer development, progression and treatment: Cause, consequence or innocent bystander? *Int J Cancer* 2006; 119:243–50.

132. Voeller D, Rahman L, Zajac-Kaye M. Elevated levels of thymidylate synthase linked to neoplastic transformation of mammalian cells. *Cell Cycle* 2004; 3:1005–07.

133. Kim YI, Salomon RN, Graeme-Cook F, Choi SW, Smith DE, Dallal GE, Mason JB. Dietary folate protects against the development of macroscopic colonic neoplasia in a dose responsive manner in rats. *Gut* 1996; 39:732–40.

134. Farber S. Some observations on the effect of folic acid antagonists on acute leukemia and other forms of incurable cancer. *Blood* 1949; 4:160–67.

135. Heinle RW, Welch AD. Experiments with pteroylglutamic acid and pteroylglutamic acid deficiency in human leukemia. Abstract. *J Clin Invest* 1948; 27:539.

136. Kotsopoulos J, Sohn KJ, Martin R, Choi M, Renlund R, Mckerlie C, Hwang SW, Medline A, Kim YI. Dietary folate deficiency suppresses N-methyl-N-nitrosourea induced mam-mary tumorigenesis in rats. *Carcinogenesis* 2003; 24:937–44.

137. Kotsopoulos J, Medline A, Renlund R, Sohn KJ, Martin R, Hwang SW, Lu S, Archer MC, Kim YI. Effects of dietary folate on the development and progression of mammary tumors in rats. *Carcinogenesis* 2005; 26:1603–12.

138. Le Leu RK, Young GP, McIntosh GH. Folate deficiency reduces the development of colorectal cancer in rats. *Carcinogenesis* 2000; 21:2261–65.
139. Van Guelpen B, Hultdin J, Johansson I, Hallmans G, Stenling R, Riboli E, Winkvist A, Palmqvist R. Low folate levels may protect against colorectal cancer. *Gut* 2006; 55:1461–66.
140. Hultdin J, Van Guelpen B, Bergh A, Hallmans G, Stattin P. Plasma folate, vitamin B12, and homocysteine and prostate cancer risk: A prospective study. *Int J Cancer* 2005; 113:819–24.
141. Paspatis GA, Karamanolis DG. Folate supplementation and adenomatous colonic polyps. *Dis Colon Rectum* 1994; 37:1340–41.
142. Jaszewski R, Misra S, Tobi M, Ullah N, Naumoff JA, Kucuk O, Levi E, Axelrod BN, Patel BB, Majumdar AP. Folic acid supplementation inhibits recurrence of colorectal adenomas: A randomized chemoprevention trial. *World J Gastroenterol* 2008; 14:4492–98.
143. Logan RF, Grainge MJ, Shepherd VC, Armitage NC, Muir KR. ukCAP Trial Group. Aspirin and folic acid for the prevention of recurrent colorectal adenomas. *Gastroenterology* 2008; 134:29–38.
144. Popescu N, Dipaolo J, Amsbaugh D. Integration site of human papillomavirus-18 DNA sequences of HeLa cell chromosomes. *Cytogenet Cell Genet* 1987; 44:58–62.
145. Everson R, Wehr C, Erexson G, MacGregor J. Association of marginal folate depletion with increased human chromosomal damage in vivo: Demonstration by analysis of micronucleated erythrocytes. *J Natl Cancer Inst* 1988; 80:525–29.
146. Green R, Phillips D, Chen A, Reidy J, Ragab A. Effects of folate in culture medium on common fragile sites in lymphocyte chromosomes from normal and leukemic children. *Hum Genet* 1998: 91:9–12.
147. Williams E, Gross R, Newberne P. Effect of folate deficiency on the cell-mediated immune response in rats. *Nutr Reports Int* 1975; 12:137–48.
148. Kim YI, Hayek M, Mason JB, Meydani SN. Severe folate deficiency impairs natural killer cell-mediated cytotoxicity in rats. *J Nutr* 2002; 132:1361–67.
149. da Costa K, Cochary E, Blusztajn J, Garner S, Zeisel S. Accumulation of 1,2-sn-dua-cylglycerol with increased membrane-associated protein kinase C may be the mechanism for spontaneous hepatocarcinogenesis in choline deficient rats. *J Biol Chem* 1993; 268:2100–05.
150. Kim YI, Miller JW, da Costa KA, Nadeau M, Smith D, Selhub J, Zeisel SH, Mason JB. Severe folate deficiency causes secondary depletion of choline and phosphocholine in rat liver. *J Nutr* 1994; 124:2197–203.

11 Folate and Vascular Disease
Epidemiological Perspective

Sari R. Kalin and Eric B. Rimm

CONTENTS

I. INTRODUCTION

Epidemiological investigations of folate and vascular disease can trace their roots to a provocative article published by McCully nearly 40 years ago [1]. The article described the cases of two children who suffered from rare inborn enzymatic defects that led to extremely high blood levels of the amino acid homocysteine (Hcy) and, ultimately, to their deaths. Although these homocystinuria cases stemmed from distinctly different metabolic causes—one from a defect of methionine synthase [2], the other from a deficiency of cystathionine-β-synthase—autopsies revealed that the children had similarly widespread arteriosclerotic plaques and vascular damage. From these and other observations, McCully raised a question that has spurred decades of scientific work: Could elevated Hcy play a role in the pathogenesis of arteriosclerosis, even at only moderately elevated levels and when not accompanied by frank enzymatic defects?

Since then, population-based studies of Hcy and cardiovascular disease (CVD) have offered some support for the so-called Hcy hypothesis, although the relationship may be stronger for stroke than for heart disease—and may not be as strong as once thought [3–5]. Hcy is a byproduct of methionine metabolism, and several biological mechanisms have been proposed for its vascular toxicity [6]. Folate and vitamin B12 are required for the normal functioning of the Hcy-methionine cycle, whereas vitamin B6 is required for the cystathionine-β-synthase–mediated conversion of Hcy to cysteine. Furthermore, individuals with deficiencies in these vitamins tend to have higher blood levels of Hcy, and taking supplements of these vitamins can lower Hcy concentrations, with evidence that folic acid supplements have the greatest Hcy-lowering effect [7]. Thus, interest in the Hcy hypothesis has driven more than two decades worth of research to answer the question of whether folate might play a role in vascular disease prevention via its influence on Hcy levels or other mechanisms.

An influential meta-analysis by Boushey et al. [3] in 1995 quantitatively reviewed the association between Hcy, heart disease, and the possible benefit of folic acid supplementation. At the time, no observational study or randomized clinical trial had directly explored the effect of increasing folic acid intake on lower risk of heart disease. However, the Food and Drug Administration was considering mandatory fortification of flour and cereal products with folic acid, at the rate of 140 or 350 µg/100 g flour, to reduce the incidence of neural tube defects (NTDs) [8]. Amid the controversy over whether to embark on such a sweeping program to benefit a relatively small subgroup of the population, the public health community was keenly interested in whether folic acid fortification could reduce the incidence of heart disease as well. Boushey et al. estimated that fortifying grain products with 350 µg of folic acid/100 g of flour could reduce Hcy concentrations in the United States by an average of 5 µmol/L and prevent nearly 50,000 coronary artery disease deaths a year; the estimate was based on analyses showing a 60% to 80% increased odds of vascular disease for a 5 µmol/L increase in Hcy, as well as corresponding reductions in Hcy levels from modest amounts of folic acid supplementation (200 µg/day). Prospective observational studies followed, providing considerable [9–24], albeit not unanimous [25–32], evidence for an inverse relationship between folate status, coronary heart disease (CHD), and stroke, leading to calls for large-scale randomized trials to answer the question of folate's role in vascular disease prevention [6,33]. To date, results from seven major randomized controlled trials of high-dose folic acid, vitamin B6, and vitamin B12 supplementation for secondary prevention of CVD have been reported [34–40], as have findings from several smaller trials [41–44]. Although these have largely failed to find any benefit for folic acid supplementation, the interpretation of some of these studies has been complicated by the advent of mandatory folic acid fortification in the United States and Canada in 1998, at the level of 140 µg of folic acid/100 g of refined flour in the United States [45] (150 µg of folic acid/100 g of refined flour in Canada [46]), a level designed to increase average folic acid intake by approximately 100 µg/day [47]. The most recent data suggest that postfortification, average Hcy concentrations in the United States decreased by about 10% [48], enough to potentially obscure any benefit of additional folic acid supplementation.

Further complicating interpretation of these studies is the fact that the relationship between Hcy and heart disease appears to be somewhat less strong than once thought [4,49]. After controlling for blood pressure and other CVD risk factors, a 2002 meta-analysis found that decreasing Hcy concentration by about 3 µmol/L was associated with 11% lower odds of ischemic heart disease (odds ratio [OR] = 0.89; 95% confidence interval [CI], 0.83–0.96) and 19% lower odds of stroke (OR = 0.81; 95% CI, 0.69–0.95) [4]. Given that the randomized trials of folic acid supplementation were designed based on earlier estimates of a stronger relationship between Hcy concentrations and CVD risk, they may be underpowered to detect a modest benefit of supplementation [49]. Several major trials have, as of this writing, yet to report results [50–54], and a planned meta-analysis of all major trials, once completed, may have enough power to demonstrate a protective effect if one exists [49].

In this chapter, we review the major population-based studies on folate and CHD, stroke, and other vascular diseases. We explore the conflicting findings between the prospective observational studies and the randomized controlled trials as well as speculate as to whether it will be possible to demonstrate a benefit of folic acid supplementation in heavily fortified populations.

II. FOLATE AND CORONARY HEART DISEASE

A. PROSPECTIVE OBSERVATIONAL STUDIES

Investigators have studied the relationship between folate status and CHD development in several large prospective cohorts with mixed results. Some have found an inverse relationship between folate status and CHD in subjects who were healthy at baseline [10–14,17,18,22,26], whereas others have failed to show any significant relationship [24–29,31,32] (see Table 11.1 for a summary of studies). Of the latter group, however, some studies hint at folate's potential protective effect. In the Physicians' Health Study, although the finding failed to reach significance, men in the lowest 20th percentile of plasma folate had a 40% higher risk of myocardial infarction (MI) compared with men in the upper 80th percentile (multivariate adjusted relative risk [RR] = 1.4; 95% CI, 0.9–2.3) [25]. In the First National Health and Nutrition Examination Survey (NAHANES) Epidemiologic Follow-up Study, although low serum folate concentrations were not associated with CHD in the entire study population, they were inversely associated with disease risk in younger subjects (ages 35–54). Individuals in the lowest quartile of serum folate (≤9.9 nmol/L) had 2.4 times the risk of CHD as those in the highest quartile (≥21.8 nmol/L) (95% CI, 1.1–5.2) [28]. More recently, in the Japan Public Health Center-Based Prospective Study Cohort I, dietary folate intake was inversely associated with MI in smokers who did not take vitamin supplements. Smokers in the highest quintile of folate intake had a 72% lower risk of MI than smokers in the lowest quintile of intake (RR = 0.28; 95% CI, 0.09–0.88), but there was no significant relationship between folate and MI in nonsmokers (RR = 0.87; 95% CI, 0.43–1.76) [24]; these findings echo those of the Nurses' Health Study, where the inverse association between folate intake and CHD was stronger among smokers (RR = 0.55; 95% CI, 0.39–0.77) than among nonsmokers (RR = 0.87; 95% CI, 0.64–1.20) [12].

Studies that have measured dietary folate intake [10–12,14,15,22,24,31] have been more consistent in their findings of an inverse relationship between folate status and CHD, whereas studies that have measured folate biomarkers [10,18,25–29,32] have been more equivocal. In the dietary studies, investigators have assessed folate intake

TABLE 11.1

Summary of Prospective Observational Studies of Folate Status and Coronary Heart Disease

Authors (Publication Year)	Country (Cohort Name)	Gender	Age (y)	Number of Individuals	Number of Cases	Follow-up Period (y)	Primary Outcome	Folate Status	Multivariate Adjusted RR[a] (95% CI)
Chasan-Taber et al. (1996) [25]	United States (Physicians' Health Study)	M	40–84	14,916	333	7.5	Acute MI or death as a result of coronary disease	Plasma folate (ng/mL) ≤2.0 ng/mL ≥2.0 ng/mL	1.4 (0.9–2.3) 1.0 (Referent)
Morrison et al. (1996) [10]	Canada (Nutrition Canada Survey)	M/F	39–79	5,056	165	15	CHD mortality	Serum folate (nmol/L) <6.8 nmol/L [3 ng/mL] >13.6 nmol/L [6 ng/mL]	1.69 (1.10–2.61) 1.0 (Referent)
Zeitlin et al. (1997) [26]	United States (The Bronx Aging Study)	M/F	75–85	488	440	10	Total all-cause mortality, stroke, MI, CHD, and CVD	Serum folate mean (SD), (ng/mL), P = .89 No CVD events: 11.0 (8) CVD events: 10.8 (6.8)	

Reference	Study	Sex	Age	N	FU (yrs)	Outcome	Exposure	Category	Men	Women
Folsom et al. (1998) [27]	United States (Atherosclerosis Risk in Communities Study)	M/F	45–64	15,792	3.3	CHD	Plasma folate means (nmol/L) per tHcy Quintiles / Quintiles of tHcy	8.5 — 3.46–6.28	1.0 Ref	1.0 Ref
								8.7 — 6.29–7.83	0.61 (0.3–1.30)	0.81 (0.3–2.0)
								5.6 — 7.84–9.24	0.68 (0.3–1.4)	0.88 (0.3–2.2)
								4.9 — 9.25–11.49	0.87 (0.4–1.8)	0.34 (0.1–0.97)
								4.0 — 11.50–33.51	1.01 (0.5–2.2)	0.39 (0.1–1.06)
Giles et al. (1998) [28]	United States (NHANES I Epidemiologic Follow-Up Study)	M/F	35–74	1,921	20	CHD	Serum folate (nmol/L)	≤9.9	0.8 (0.6–1.1)	
								10.0–14.2	0.9 (0.6–1.3)	
								14.3–21.7	1.1 (0.8–1.5)	
								≥21.8	1.0 (Referent)	
Rimm et al. (1998) [12]	United States (The Nurses' Health Study)	F	30–55	80,082	14	Nonfatal MI and fatal CHD	Folate intake µg/day	<190	1.0 (Referent)	
								190–244	0.86 (0.71–1.05)	
								245–318	0.86 (0.7–1.06)	
								319–544	0.78 (0.63–0.98)	
								≥545	0.69 (0.55–0.87)	
Voutilainen et al. (2000) [13]	Finland (Kuopio Ischaemic Heart Disease Risk Factor [KIHD] Study)	M	46–64	2,682	5	Acute coronary events	Serum folate (nmol/L)	≤11.3	1.0 (Referent)	
								>11.3	0.3 (0.1–0.84)	

continued

TABLE 11.1 (continued)
Summary of Prospective Observational Studies of Folate Status and Coronary Heart Disease

Authors (Publication Year)	Country (Cohort Name)	Gender	Age (y)	Number of Individuals	Number of Cases	Follow-up Period (y)	Primary Outcome	Folate Status		Multivariate Adjusted RR[a] (95% CI)	
Voutilainen et al. (2001) [14]	Finland (KIHD Study)	M	42–60	1,980	199	10	Acute coronary events	Dietary folate (µg/d)	<211	1.0 (Referent)	
									211–236	0.76 (no CI)	
									237–261	0.64 (no CI)	
									262–297	0.53 (0.33–0.87)	
									>297	0.45 (0.25–0.81)	
de Bree et al. (2003) [17]	Netherlands (Monitoring Project on CVD Risk Factors)	M/F	20–59	36,000[b]	199	10.3	CHD	Plasma folate means (nmol/L) per tHcy tertiles	Tertiles of tHcy	Men	Women
								7.1	6.4–12.6	1.0 Ref	1.0 Ref
								6.3	12.7–15.3	1.15 (0.5–2.62)	0.45 (0.45–1.45)
								5.1	15.4–53.9	2.00 (0.82–4.87)	0.22 (0.06–0.87)
Hung et al. (2003) [29]	Australia (Busselton Health Survey)	M/F	20–90	2,950	1,016	29	Fatal CHD and CVD	Serum folate (ng/ml) men and women		Men	Women
								0–2.99		1.07 (0.8–1.43)	1.19 (0.88–1.61)
								3.0–4.49		1.13 (0.93–1.38)	1.15 (0.93–1.43)
								4.5–5.99		0.95 (0.78–1.17)	1.07 (0.84–1.35)
								≥6.0		1.0 Ref	1.0 Ref
Voutilainen et al. (2004) [18]	Finland (KIHD Study)	M	46–64	810	61	7.7	Acute coronary events	Serum folate (nmol/L)	<8.4	1.0 Referent	
									8.4–11.3	0.78 (0.44–1.38)	

Study	Country (Study)	Sex	Age	N	Cases	Outcome	Exposure	Rate ratio
Drogan et al. (2006) [22]	Germany (European Prospective Investigation into Cancer and Nutrition (EPIC)–Potsdam study)	M/F	35–64	22,245	129	MI	Dietary folate (μg/d) <103 >103	1.0 (Referent) 0.52 (0.33–0.81)
Dalmeijer et al. (2007) [31]	Netherlands (PROSPECT-EPIC)	F	49–70	16,165	717	CVD	Dietary folate (μg/d) ≤169 169–191 191–215 ≥215	1.0 (Referent) 0.86 (0.64–1.15) 1.05 (0.74–1.49) 1.23 (0.75–2.01)
Vanuzzo et al. (2007) [32]	Italy (The Martignacco Project)	M/F	40–59	218	109	CHD	Serum folate (nmol/L) 3.25–5.83 (controls) Median = 4.27 2.85–6.16 (cases) Median 4.33	0.93 (0.63–1.37)
Ishihara et al. (2008) [24]	Japan (The Japan Public Health Center-Based Prospective Study Cohort I)	M/F	40–59	40,803	251	CHD and definite MI	Dietary folate (μg/d), means of low, medium, and high quintiles 290 372 436	1.0 (Referent) 0.80 (0.54–1.18) 0.80 (0.52–1.21)

a For those studies for which direct rate ratios could not be calculated, odds ratios as estimates of rate ratios are presented.

b For the Debree et al. study [17], the base population was 36,000 participants, but the analysis was conducted as a case–cohort study, and only 630 participants were randomly selected from the base population for folate analysis.

via food frequency questionnaire (FFQ) [11,12,22,24,31], multiday diet record [14], or single 24-hour recall [10,15]. Whereas each of these dietary measures has potential for error and misclassification, FFQs and multiday diet records are better able to identify individual differences in nutrient intake than a single 24-hour recall [55], and five of the six studies that have used FFQs or multiday measurements of dietary folate intake have found an inverse association between folate and CHD in at least one of the study subgroups [11,12,14,22,24].

Dietary studies that have explored the relationship between folate intake, drinking patterns, and CHD provide further evidence that poor folate status increases CHD risk. Alcohol consumption is known to impair folate absorption and utilization [56–58], yet there is strong evidence that moderate alcohol consumption reduces the risk of CHD, possibly through its beneficial effects on HDL, insulin sensitivity, and clotting factors [59,60]; thus, individuals who consume alcohol may have a greater need for folate, and the beneficial effects of moderate drinking may be obscured in individuals who have poor folate status. The Nurses' Health Study [12,61] and the European Prospective Investigation into Cancer and Nutrition—Potsdam [22] cohorts have both found that the inverse relationship between folate and CHD was stronger in individuals who had higher alcohol intakes. In the Nurses' Health Study, moderate drinking combined with high folate intake conferred the greatest reduction in CHD risk [12]. Women who consumed at least one drink a day ($\geq$15 g of ethanol/day) and were in the highest quintile of folate consumption ($\geq$545 µg/day) had a 78% lower risk of CHD compared with women who abstained from alcohol and were in the lowest quintile of folate intake (<190 µg/day) (RR = 0.22; 95% CI, 0.11–0.44) (Figure 11.1). A subsequent study with further follow-up on the same cohort found that there was no significant relationship between folate status and CVD in women who abstained from alcohol or were light or moderate drinkers, but that folate status is inversely associated with CVD risk in the heaviest drinkers (>30 g of ethanol/day) [61]. In this group of heaviest alcohol consumers, women with adequate folate intake (400–599 µg/day) had a 40% lower risk of CVD mortality compared with women with similar alcohol intake but with an estimated folate intake of less than 180 µg/day. However, not all cohort studies have found stronger effects in individuals who have higher alcohol intakes [14,62]. The Kuopio Ischemic Heart Disease Risk Factor (KIHD) Study, for example, found that among light drinkers (<30 g/week of ethanol, mean 8 g/week), those in the highest folate quintile had a 73% lower RR of acute coronary events than those in the lowest quintile (RR = 0.27; 95% CI, 0.12–0.65), but in heavier drinkers (>30 g/week of ethanol, mean 132 g/week), there was no significant inverse relationship (for the highest vs. lowest quintiles of folate, RR = 0.72; 95% CI, 0.30–1.72) [14]. Folate intakes in the Kuopio cohort were relatively low (mean ~260 µg/day), however, and it is possible that in heavier drinkers, folate intakes were simply not high enough to offset alcohol's detrimental effects on folate metabolism.

Red blood cell folate is considered to be a relatively long-term indicator of folate status [63], but only one prospective study to date has measured its relationship to CHD [29]; the study, in an Australian cohort, failed to find an association between folate and CHD. Most prospective cohort studies have measured serum or plasma folate concentration at baseline [10,17,18,25–28,32], and most of those have failed to find a significant relationship between folate status and CHD [25–27,32]. However,

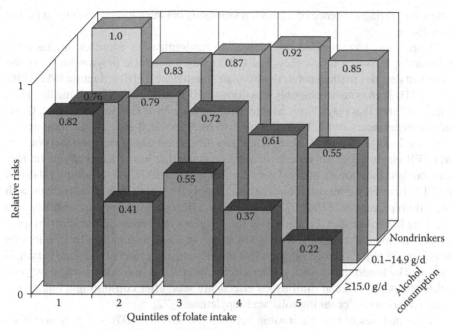

FIGURE 11.1 Relative risk of CHD (nonfatal MI and fatal CHD) by quintiles of energy-adjusted folate across levels of alcohol consumption among 80,082 women in the Nurses' Health Study. Women in the lowest quintile of folate who did not drink alcohol were the reference category. (Reprinted from Rimm EB, Willett WC, Hu FB, Sampson L, Colditz GA, Manson JE, Hennekens C, Stampfer MJ, *JAMA* 1998; 279:359–64. With permission.)

low serum or plasma concentrations can reflect—and fail to distinguish between—recent or long-term inadequacies in folate intake [63]; therefore, there is potential for misclassification that would bias findings toward the null.

B. Genetic Studies

Gene–disease association studies can be used to shed light on the relationship between environment and disease if the genetic polymorphism in question mimics the effect of an environmental exposure [64]. Under what is typically called Mendelian randomization, a genetic polymorphism serves as a proxy for the environmental exposure. Because most polymorphisms are distributed by the principles of Mendelian inheritance and would therefore not be associated with other lifestyle choices or characteristics later in life, an association between a polymorphism and a chronic disease outcome is not affected by confounding, reverse causation, or selection bias that may accompany observational studies of environment and disease [65]. The comparison of gene–disease and environment–disease relationships is central to this approach. If the gene–disease relationship is similar in strength and direction to what one would expect from an environmental exposure of the same magnitude, it offers supporting evidence of a causal relationship between environmental exposure and disease.

Researchers have applied the Mendelian randomization approach to study the relationship between folate, Hcy, and CHD using a common polymorphism of the gene that encodes methylenetetrahydrofolate (methylene-THF) reductase (MTHFR). The MTHFR enzyme irreversibly transforms 5,10-methylene-THF to 5-methyl-THF, a methyl donor that plays a crucial role in the conversion of Hcy to methionine. Gross inborn deficiencies in MTHFR lead to extremely elevated Hcy concentrations and vascular damage as well as other pathologies [66]. A variant of the gene that encodes MTHFR yields a thermolabile form of the enzyme that has reduced effects on Hcy metabolism. Individuals homozygous for the *MTHFR* 677C→T genotype (*MTHFR* 677 TT) have Hcy concentrations that are roughly 25% higher than individuals with the wild-type gene (*MTHFR* 677 CC) [67]—in effect, mimicking the conditions of a life-long low folate diet. Frequency of the TT genotype varies dramatically by geographic region and ethnicity, from a low of 1% in some populations to 15% to 35% in others [68,69]. Evidence suggests that the Hcy-raising effect of the gene variant is modified by folate status, with greater effects observed in individuals who have poor folate status [70,71], and diminished effects are seen after consuming a folate- and folic acid–rich diet or taking folic acid supplements [72].

Meta-analyses of the relationship between the *MTHFR* 677C→T polymorphism and the risk of CHD have had mixed results [5,73,74], perhaps reflecting limitations of the Mendelian randomization approach, chief among them the need for very large sample sizes to detect associations when the genotype influence on phenotype is small and when the association of the phenotype to outcome (in this example, the association of Hcy to CHD) is modest [65,74]. In 2002, a meta-analysis by Klerk et al. [73] of 40 studies (roughly 11,162 cases) found that, compared with individuals with the CC genotype, individuals with the TT genotype had 16% higher odds of CHD (95% CI, 1.05–1.28), an effect that was primarily seen in the setting of low folate status. The authors found significant heterogeneity between the studies, however. Stratification by country of origin reduced heterogeneity and revealed that the increased risk associated with the TT genotype was largely confined to European studies (comparing TT with CC, OR = 1.14; 95% CI, 1.01–1.28) but absent in North American studies (OR = 0.87; 95% CI, 0.73–1.05). The authors hypothesized that the continent-of-origin differences could be the result of effect modification by folate status, given that vitamin use and breakfast cereal fortification were more common in North America than in Europe.

That same year, Wald et al. [5] combined data from 46 studies (12,193 cases) on the *MTHFR* polymorphism and CHD and compared the strength of the association and the differences in Hcy concentrations with that of a combined analysis of 15 prospective studies (3,144 events) of Hcy and CHD. They found that having the TT genotype was associated with 21% higher odds of CHD compared with having the CC genotype (OR = 1.21; 95% CI, 1.06–1.39); they also noted significant heterogeneity between studies. Extrapolating from the genetic studies that had information on subjects' Hcy concentrations, they calculated that a 5-μmol/L increase in Hcy was associated with similarly higher risk of CHD in both the prospective studies (OR = 1.32; 95% CI, 1.19–1.45) and in the genetic studies

TABLE 11.2

Odds Ratio for Coronary Heart Disease Comparing *MTHFR* 677TT with *MTHFR* 677CC Genotypes

Region	Odds Ratio (95% CI)	Number of Cases: Controls	Number of Studies
Europe	1.08 (0.99–1.18)	17,275:313	41
North America	0.93 (0.80–1.10)	3,714:3,969	15
Middle East	2.61 (1.81–3.75)	971:1,316	5
Asia	1.23 (0.94–1.62)	2,755:4,735	16
Australia	1.04 (0.73–1.49)	1,285:480	3
Overall	1.14 (1.05–1.24)	26,000:31,813	80

Source: Lewis SJ, Ebrahim S, Davey Smith G, *BMJ* 2005; 331:1053. With permission.

(OR = 1.42; 95% CI, 1.11–1.84)—evidence, according to the authors, for a causal link between Hcy and CHD.

A more recent meta-analysis of the *MTHFR* 677C→T polymorphism by Lewis et al. [74], however, calls into question these earlier findings. Lewis et al.'s analysis, which included twice as many studies (81) and cases (26,000) as the earlier reports, found that the TT genotype was associated overall with 14% higher odds of CHD compared with the CC genotype (95% CI, 1.05–1.24), but after stratification by region, heterogeneity was reduced, and increased odds of CHD were found only in the Middle East and Asia (Table 11.2).

In conclusion, it is difficult to use the results from genetic associations alone in an argument for or against a causal association between folate and CHD. However, the evidence is at least supportive of a modest association between low folate status and increased disease risk.

III. FOLATE, STROKE, AND OTHER VASCULAR DISEASE ENDPOINTS

A. Prospective Observational Studies

Most [15,16,19–21,23,75], but not all [9,26,30], prospective cohort studies have found a significant inverse relationship between folate status and stroke or other cerebro-vascular outcomes in both North American and European cohorts (see Table 11.3 for a summary of studies). Data for these studies were largely collected before the start of mandatory folic acid fortification of cereal grains in the United States and Canada in 1998. However, fortification has provided intriguing ecological evidence consistent with an inverse relationship between folate status and stroke: A recent study compared national stroke mortality trends before and after the fortification mandate in the United States and Canada with trends in the United Kingdom, which does not mandate fortification [76]. Although all three countries showed a

TABLE 11.3

Summary of Prospective Observational Studies of Folate Status and Stroke

Authors (Publication Year)	Country (Cohort Name)	Gender	Age	Number of Individuals	Number of Cases	Follow-up Years	Primary Outcome	Folate Status	Multivariate Adjusted RR[a] (95% CI)	
Giles et al. (1995) [9]	United States (First National Health & Examination Survey (NHANES) Epidemiologic Follow-up Study)	M/F	35–74	2,006	98	13	Ischemic strokes	Serum folate (nmol/L)		
								≤9.2	1.37 (0.82–2.29)	
								>9.2	1.0 Referent	
Bazzano et al. (2002) [15]	United States (NHANES I Epidemiologic Follow-Up Study)	M/F	25–74	9,764	926 = incident stroke cases 3,758 = incident CVD cases	19	Stroke and CVD	Dietary folate (µg/d)	Stroke	CVD
								<136.0	1.0 Ref	1.0 Ref
								136.0–203.7	0.93 (0.74–1.16)	0.98 (0.89–1.07)
								203.7–300.6	0.85 (0.71–0.99)	0.88 (0.79–0.97)
								>300.6	0.8 (0.64–0.99)	0.87 (0.79–0.96)
Maxwell et al. (2002) [16]	Canada (Canadian Study of Health & Aging)	M/F	65+	10,263	369	5	Adverse cerebrovascular event (vascular dementia, vascular cognitive impairment, fatal stroke)	Serum folate (nmol/L)[c]		
								5–12	2.22 (1.0–4.93)	
								14–36	1.0 Referent	

Study	Country (cohort)	Sex	Age	N	Number of strokes	—	Outcome	Exposure	Ischemic stroke	Hemorrhagic stroke
He et al. (2004) [19]	United States (Health Professionals Follow-up Study)	M	40–75	43,732	725 incident stroke (455 = ischemic stroke, 125 = hemorrhagic, 145 = unknown)	14	Ischemic and hemorrhagic stroke	Median intake of dietary folate (µg/d)	Ischemic stroke	Hemorrhagic stroke
								262	1.0 Ref	1.0 Ref
								336	1.0 (0.74–1.36)	1.28 (0.71–2.32)
								413	0.75 (0.53–1.06)	1.49 (0.79–2.83)
								547	0.96 (0.68–1.35)	1.31 (0.67–2.55)
								821	0.66 (0.45–0.98)	0.86 (0.40–1.88)
Al-Delaimy et al. (2004) [30]	United States (Nurses' Health Study)	F	34–59	83,272	1,140	18	Total stroke (ischemic, thrombotic, embolic, subarachnoid hemorrhage, intraparenchymal hemorrhage)	Dietary folate (µg/d)		
								30–210	1.00 Referent	
								211–271	0.99 (0.82–1.20)	
								272–354	1.09 (0.89–1.33)	
								355–526	1.01 (0.81–1.25)	
								>526	0.99 (0.78–1.25)	
Van Guelpen et al. (2005) [20]	Sweden (Northern Swedish Health & Disease Cohort)	M/F	25–74	74,000[b]	334 ischemic strokes & 62 hemorrhagic strokes	21	Ischemic and hemorrhagic stroke	Plasma folate (nmol/L)	Referents (n) median plasma folate (25th–75th percentile)	Cases (n) median plasma folate (25th–75th percentile)
								Ischemic stroke (P = .872)	(593) 7.2 (5.0–9.9)	(295) 6.9 (4.9–10.1)
								Hemorrhagic stroke (P = .015)	(110) 7.1 (5.2–10.7)	(57) 6.3 (4.4–8.1)

continued

TABLE 11.3 (continued)
Summary of Prospective Observational Studies of Folate Status and Stroke

Authors (Publication Year)	Country (Cohort Name)	Gender	Age	Number of Individuals	Number of Cases	Follow-up Years	Primary Outcome	Folate Status	Multivariate Adjusted RR[a] (95% CI)	
									Any stroke	Ischemic stroke
Virtanen et al. (2005) [21]	Finland (KIHD Study)	M	46–64	1,015	49 (34 ischemic strokes)	9.6	Any stroke and ischemic stroke	Serum tHcy (mean)		
								Highest third	2.77 (1.23–6.24)	2.61 (1.02–6.71)
								Lowest third	1.0 (Referent)	1.0 (Referent)
								Serum folate (mean)		
								Highest third	0.35 (0.14–0.87)	0.40 (0.15–1.09)
								Lowest third	1.0 (Referent)	1.0 (Referent)
Weikert et al. (2007) [23]	Europe (European Prospective Investigation into Cancer & Nutrition –Potsdam Study)	M/F	35–65	967	188	6	Ischemic stroke or TIA	Plasma folate (nmol/L)		
								15.0 (13.6–16.5)	0.91 (0.58–1.42)	
								20.3 (19.3–22.2)	0.91 (0.58–1.45)	
								29.7 (26.3–35.3)	1.0 Referent	

a For those studies for which direct rate ratios could not be calculated, odds ratios as estimates of rate ratios are presented.

b For the Van Guelpen et al. study [20], the base population was derived from two large studies with 74,000 participants, but the analysis was conducted as nested case-referent study on 396 cases (352 of which had values for plasma folate) and matched double referents.

c For the Maxwell et al. study [16], each of the 15 study centers had its own lab; they differed in the normal range for serum folate values, so individuals were categorized into quartiles based on study center. The lowest quartile maximum values ranged from 5 to 12 nmol/L, and the highest quartile minimum values ranged from 14 to 36 nmol/L.

decrease in stroke mortality from 1990 to 2002, mortality rates in the United States and Canada decreased more rapidly after the start of mandatory folic acid fortification in 1998, whereas rates did not change consistently in the United Kingdom after 1998. Analysis of NHANES data pre- and postfortification showed that mean serum folate concentrations increased significantly in adults in the United States, whereas mean Hcy concentrations decreased. In this study, the sensitivity analysis conducted by Yang et al. [76] suggests that in the United States, changes in other stroke risk factors, such as smoking, hypertension, diabetes, and high cholesterol, were not responsible for the improved mortality rates during this period. These investigators note that, although the evidence is limited, there was no corresponding decrease in stroke incidence postfortification; thus, the decrease in mortality is likely the result of a decrease in the case-fatality rate.

There is more limited prospective observational evidence on the relationship between folate and other vascular outcomes. In the Health Professionals Follow-up Study, Merchant et al. [77] reported an inverse relationship between total folate intake (from food and supplements) and risk of peripheral arterial disease (PAD). After 12 years of follow-up, men in the top quintile of folate intake (mean, 840 μg/day) had roughly a 30% lower risk of developing the disease than men in the bottom quintile of intake (mean, 244 μg/day; RR = 0.67; 95% CI, 0.47–0.96). This effect was weakened and no longer significant after adjustment for vitamins E, B6, and B12. Further analysis revealed that the inverse relationship between folate and PAD was confined to men who obtained folate from supplements, not foods, raising the possibility that other components of multivitamins could be responsible for the observed effect.

Results for the Nurses' Health Study I and II suggest a significant inverse relationship between total folate intake and hypertension that was stronger in younger women than in older women [78]. Comparing the highest (≥1,000 μg/day) with the lowest (<200 μg/day) categories of folate intake, after 8 years of follow-up, the multivariate adjusted RR of hypertension in women aged 27 to 44 at baseline was 0.54 (95% CI, 0.45–0.66), whereas in women aged 43 to 70 at baseline, it was 0.82 (95% CI, 0.69–0.97). Among nonusers of supplements, the association between food folate and hypertension was not significant; the authors speculate that the lack of significance could be because of the relatively narrow range of food folate intakes or the higher bioavailability of folic acid from supplements.

B. Genetic Studies

Several meta-analyses have used the *MTHFR* 677C→T polymorphism (as described above) to shed light on whether the relationship between elevated Hcy concentrations and stroke is causal [5,79–81]. A paucity of data on the folate status of participants in the genome–stroke studies has limited analyses of effect modification by folate status, although some investigators have used continent of origin as a proxy for this well-documented gene–environment interaction.

Casas et al.'s [81] meta-analysis used the Mendelian randomization approach. First, they calculated an expected OR for stroke, based on Wald et al.'s [5] previous meta-analysis of prospective studies of Hcy and stroke, as well as their own meta-analysis of the differences in Hcy concentration associated with the TT versus CC genotype in healthy individuals (n = 15,635). They then conducted a meta-analysis of 30 studies (n cases = 6,324; n controls = 7,604) to calculate the OR of stroke associated with the TT versus CC genotype. Finally, they compared the OR with the estimate. They found that individuals with the TT genotype had 26% higher odds of stroke than individuals with the CC genotype (95% CI, 1.14–1.40), an effect comparable to the expected OR (OR = 1.20; 95% CI, 1.10–1.31) based on the elevation of Hcy associated with the TT genotype. This lends further evidence to support a causal relationship between Hcy and stroke. In the Hcy meta-analysis [81], when studies were stratified by continent of origin, the authors observed that mean Hcy concentration differences between TT and CC genotypes were higher in Europe and other continents than in North America; mean serum folate concentration were lower in Europe and other continents than in North America, perhaps reflecting differences in folate intake that modified the effect of the TT genotype on Hcy concentrations. However, the genome–stroke meta-analysis did not find any differences in OR when analyses were restricted by geographic region or ethnicity. A more recent meta-analysis by Ariyaratnam et al. [82] of 10 Asian studies (7 in China, 3 in Korea) found that, compared with the C allele genotype (CC+CT), the TT genotype was associated with a similarly increased risk of stroke (OR = 1.22; 95% CI, 0.98–1.52) to that found in a meta-analysis of European populations (OR = 1.24; 95% CI, 1.08–1.42) [83].

Meanwhile, a meta-analysis by Cronin et al. [80] found that the risk of stroke or transient ischemic attack (TIA) increased according to the dose of the T allele. The analysis combined data from 32 studies, with 6,110 cases and 8,760 controls. Compared with individuals with the CC genotype, the OR for stroke in individuals who had at least one T allele (CT or TT) was 1.17 (95% CI, 1.09–1.26); individuals with the TT genotype had an OR of 1.37 (95% CI, 1.15–1.64). Stratifying the data by continent of origin, the investigators found that the risk associated with the TT genotype was greater in Asia (OR = 1.37; 95% CI, 0.79–1.89; P = .02) than in Europe (OR = 1.17; 95% CI, 1.02–1.34; P = .03); the trend in North America had a similar magnitude of effect but failed to reach significance, possibly because of the small number studies included (OR = 1.58; 95% CI, 0.9–2.75; P = .1).

IV. RANDOMIZED CONTROLLED TRIALS

In general, from the results of the observational studies summarized above provide modest evidence for an inverse association between folate intake and CVD. Results from studies of the *MTHFR* polymorphism (as a proxy for Hcy and folate status) provide further supportive evidence. What have been missing are confirmatory results from randomized placebo-controlled intervention studies. The early observational studies of Hcy and CVD risk and studies of CVD benefit from folate led to several large randomized placebo-controlled intervention studies to test the hypothesis that folate alone or in combination with other B vitamins could prevent CVD. To improve power and to reduce the length of follow-up necessary to document hard clinical endpoints, the completed trials thus far have all been secondary prevention. We summarize the completed published trials in Table 11.4 and other ongoing trials in Table 11.5.

TABLE 11.4

Completed Major Randomized Controlled Trials of B Vitamin Supplementation and Vascular Disease

Authors (Publication Year)	Country (Cohort Name)	Fortification	Gender	Age (y)	Disease History at Baseline	Number Randomized: Number Events	Treatment Regimen (mg/day)	Length of Treatment (Mean)	Primary Endpoint	Multivariate Adjusted RR (95% CI), Treatment vs. Placebo
Baker et al. (2002) [34]	CHAOS-2	No	a	a	CHD	1,882:187	5 folic acid	1.7[b] year	Composite of nonfatal MI, cardiovascular death, or unplanned revascularization	0.97 (0.72–1.29)
Toole et al. (2004) [35]	United States, Canada, and Scotland (VISP)	Yes	M/F	35–75+	Acute ischemic stroke ≤120 days before randomization	3,680:300	25.0 B6 0.8 folic acid	2 year	Ischemic stroke recurrence	1.1 (0.8–1.3)
Bønaa et al. (2006) [36]	Norway (NORVIT)	No	M/F	30–85	Acute MI 7 days before randomization	3,749:716	40.0 B6 0.4 B12 0.8 folic acid	3.3 year	Composite of fatal and nonfatal MI and stroke, and sudden death attributed to CHD	1.22 (1.0–1.5)
Lonn et al. (2006) [37]	Canada, United States, Brazil, Western Europe, and Slovakia (HOPE-2)	Yes and no[c]	M/F	55+	Vascular disease or diabetes	5,522:1,066	50.0 B6 1.0 B12 2.5 folic acid	5 year	Composite of deaths from cardiovascular causes, MI, or stroke	0.95 (0.84–1.07)

continued

TABLE 11.4 (continued)
Completed Major Randomized Controlled Trials of B Vitamin Supplementation and Vascular Disease

Authors (Publication Year)	Country (Cohort Name)	Fortification	Gender	Age (y)	Disease History at Baseline	Number Randomized: Number Events	Treatment Regimen (mg/day)	Length of Treatment (Mean)	Primary Endpoint	Multivariate Adjusted RR (95% CI), Treatment vs. Placebo
Albert et al. (2008) [38]	United States (WAFACS)	Yes	F	42+	History of CVD or three cardiovascular risk factors	5,442:796	50.0 B6 1.0 B12 2.5 folic acid	7.3 y	Composite of morbidity/mortality from incident MI, stroke, CABG, PTCA, and cardiovascular mortality	1.03 (0.9–1.19)
Jamison et al. (2007) [39]	United States (HOST)	Yes	M/F	21+	End-stage renal disease	2,056:884	100.0 B6 2.0 B12 40.0 folic acid	3.2 y	All-cause mortality	1.04 (0.91–1.18)
Ebbing et al. (2008) [40]	Norway (WENBIT)	No	M/F	18+	Undergoing angiography for stable angina pectoris, an acute coronary syndrome or aortic valve stenosis	3,096:422	40.0 B6 0.4 B12 0.8 folic acid	38 mo	All cause death, acute MI, unstable angina pectoris, or thromboembolic stroke	No significant differences between treatment and control groups

a For the Baker et al. study [34], the study results were presented in abstract form, and information was not provided regarding the gender and age of participants.
b Median years.
c The Lonn et al. study [37] (HOPE-2) was conducted in 13 countries, only some of which had mandatory folic acid fortification.

TABLE 11.5

In-Progress Randomized Controlled Trials of B Vitamin Supplementation and Vascular Disease

Authors (Publication Year)	Country (Cohort Name)	Fortification	Gender	Age (y)	Disease History at Baseline	Expected Number Randomized	Treatment Regimen (mg/day)	Expected Length of Treatment (Mean Years)	Primary Endpoint
Galan et al. (2008) [50]	France (SU.FOL.OM3)	No	M/F	45–80	History of MI, unstable angina pectoris, or ischemic stroke in past year	2,501	3.0 B6 0.56 folic acid 0.02 B12 600 n-3 fatty acids	5	Combination of MI, ischemic stroke, and cardiovascular death
SEARCH Study Collaborative Group (2007) [51]	United Kingdom (SEARCH)	No	M/F	18–80	MI	12,064	80.0 simvastatin 0.8 B12 2.0 folic acid	7	Major vascular events
Bostom et al. (2006) [52]	United States (FAVORIT)	Yes	M/F	35–75	Renal transplant	4,000	5.0 folic acid 50.0 B6 1.0 B12	5	Composite of incident or recurrent CVD outcomes
VITATOPS (2002) [54]	20 countries/5 continents (VITATOPS)	No	M/F	—	Recent stroke/ TIA	8,000	2.0 folic acid 25.0 B6 0.5 B12	2	TIA, unstable angina, revascularization procedures, dementia, depression

Concurrent with the early development and initiation of clinical trials, folic acid fortification was mandated in many countries worldwide to reduce NTDs in the offspring of mothers. The mandated fortification of flour in enriched cereal grain products in 1998 in North America increased folic acid intake by an estimated 100 to 200 μg/day on a population level and significantly reduced the prevalence of low folate and high plasma Hcy concentrations in middle-aged individuals [47]. In addition to the effect this has had on decreasing NTDs, the most immediate consequence was that it became difficult to identify high-risk patients with elevated Hcy (or deficient folate status) for secondary prevention trials. For example, in the Vitamin Intervention for Stroke Prevention (VISP) study [35], a secondary prevention trial of 3,680 stroke patients from North America to keep enrollment numbers sufficiently high, the threshold for "elevated Hcy" used as the inclusion criteria was decreased twice because the recruitment time frame paralleled mandated folate fortification. The difference in Hcy concentrations between the arm randomized to high-dose and the arm randomized to low-dose B vitamins was narrower at the end of the trial compared with the beginning, suggesting that folic acid fortification of the food supply diluted the effective difference between treatment arms. Furthermore, both arms had lower Hcy by the end of the trial as a result of an overall substantial decrease in Hcy in the whole "at-risk" population. In general, this reduces the difference in exposure between the intervention and placebo arm and biases the results toward the null. After 2 years of follow-up in the VISP study, the RR of ischemic stroke was 1.0 (95% CI, 0.8–1.3), with virtually identical Kaplan-Meier survival curves between patients randomized to high-dose versus low-dose B vitamins.

In Heart Outcomes Prevention Evaluation-2 (HOPE-2), also a large-scale secondary prevention trial, 5,522 patients 55 years of age or older who had vascular disease or diabetes were randomly assigned to daily treatment either with the combination of 2.5 mg of folic acid, 50 mg of vitamin B6, and 1 mg of vitamin B12 or with placebo and were followed for an average of 5 years [37]. The authors reported no benefit in the primary outcomes of death from CVD. They did report significantly lower risk of stroke (mostly because of ischemic stroke) but adverse risk of angina. Interestingly, as with VISP, background fortification may have biased results toward the null because approximately 72% of the patients were in countries with folic acid fortification. As listed in Table 11.4, several other large, international, carefully conducted secondary prevention trials have now been published with similar null results with respect to most CVD outcomes. For example, in the Norwegian Vitamin Trial (NORVIT), 3,749 patients post-MI were randomized to 800 μg of folate and other B vitamins and followed for more than 3 years. No benefit for folic acid supplementation was found, and, if anything, a modest 22% increase in recurrent CHD, stroke, or sudden death was found [36]. In the Women's Antioxidant and Folic Acid Cardiovascular Study (WAFACS) trial, which followed 5,442 high-risk women in the United States for more than 7 years, those randomized to high-dose B supplements (2.5 mg of folic acid) had no difference in subsequent CVD (RR = 1.03; 95% CI, 0.90, 1.19) [36,38]. In these intervention studies and others, the arm randomized to the folic acid supplement typically had 20% to 25% lower Hcy on treatment and estimated compliance rates of 60% to 90%.

As discussed previously [84], the development of atherosclerosis and CVD is a multifaceted progression of biological processes that likely includes hyperlipidemia, endothelial dysfunction, oxidation, inflammation, coagulation, and other pathophysiological phenomena. It seems biologically implausible that a single vitamin should be instrumental across all etiological pathways from early fatty streak production to the ultimate clinical event sometimes 60 to 80 years later. Furthermore, it may be that any modest benefit for folate, at a magnitude similar to that documented in the observational studies above, would be dwarfed by the benefit achieved from careful clinical management of patients with statins, antihypertensives, aspirin, and nutritional counseling. For example, in the HOPE-2 trial mentioned above, baseline use of aspirin or an antiplatelet agent was reported by 78% of the treatment group, β-blockers by 46%, and angiotensin-converting enzyme (ACE) inhibitors by 65.9%. In the NORVIT study, baseline use of statins, antihypertensives, and aspirin ranged from 80 to 92% of participants. It is also possible that vitamins are beneficial in these selective "high-risk" patient populations, but when given at such high doses, the benefits of supplements may be offset by a modest adverse interaction with medications. We also do not know for sure whether the beneficial effects of folate on Hcy may affect redundant biological pathways to those impacted by these same medications. Thus, the results from trials of medically managed patients are still valid but may not be generalizable to the primary prevention setting for CVD. This makes the interpretation of the existing intervention studies more challenging because all were among individuals who had documented existing illnesses and presumably careful clinical management. Seven of the trials included patients with previous CHD; three included patients with previous stroke; and two included patients with previous renal disease.

In a recent meta-analysis on the efficacy of folic acid supplementation specifically for stroke prevention [85], the authors highlighted populations in whom greatest benefit could be achieved. In the eight randomized trials summarized, folic acid intervention significantly reduced risk of stroke by 18% (95% CI, 0%–32%). The risk reduction (percent reduction) was only in strata defined by supplementation longer than 3 years (29%), effective Hcy decreasing by 20% or more (23%), in countries without grain fortification (25%), and in patients without previous stroke (25%). In a similar style post hoc efficacy analysis of VISP, Spence [86] reported a significant reduction in stroke risk with B vitamin supplementation. He argued that the high-dose B vitamins would only be effective among those without renal failure and among those without extreme levels of baseline B12 (because in the study those with low levels of B12 at baseline were given B12 injections). Among the remaining 2,155 patients, the higher-dose vitamin B intervention did significantly decrease risk of CVD death by approximately 20%.

One final concern that has arisen with the interpretation of intervention studies is the wide range of dosages of B vitamins. These have ranged from 0.5–40.0 mg/day for folic acid, 0.02–1.0 mg/day for vitamin B12, and 3–100 mg/day for vitamin B6. For folate, this is up to 250 times the Recommended Dietary Allowance of 400 μg/day dietary folate equivalents, and in many cases above the folic acid Tolerable Upper Intake Level (1 mg/day) recommended by the Institute of Medicine [63]. Excess folic acid may lead to circulation of unmetabolized folic acid in plasma, which has been shown to potentially be associated with reduced immune function [87]. The effects on coronary disease progression are unknown. Further complicating the effects of excess folic acid supplementation is the metabolic interaction folate may have with alcohol consumption [12,61,88]. Future primary and secondary prevention studies of folate should consider the effects of folate stratified by alcohol consumption.

We did not include as a true randomized trial in Tables 11.4 and 11.5 the quasi-experimental intervention of folate fortification in North America. However, in some ways this may be the most important documentation of the health effects of folate because it encompasses all types of populations across the primary and secondary prevention spectrum. As discussed above, in an analysis of stroke mortality rates from 1990–2002, Yang et al. [76] compared rates before and after fortification in the United States and Canada with trends in rates for the United Kingdom. The slowly decreasing trend in stroke mortality rates observed after 1990 in the United States and Canada accelerated significantly after 1998, when mandatory folic acid fortification was implemented. Interestingly, this improvement in stroke mortality paralleled the anticipated reduction in rates for NTDs. In contrast, no improvement in the decrease of stroke mortality or in the occurrence of NTDs was seen in England and Wales, where folic acid fortification was not mandatory. This is not a true randomized study across worldwide populations because secular changes in other factors, such as diagnostic patterns, drug use, and dietary changes, may also have occurred concurrently and differentially across populations and could explain some of the benefit attributed to folic acid fortification, but these results are additional evidence that contribute to the hypothesis that better folate status does decrease risk of CVD across the general population.

V.   CURRENT CONTROVERSIES AND UNANSWERED QUESTIONS

After summarizing results from all the available epidemiological data, the most important unanswered question still remains: "Does improved folate status decrease the risk of CVD among otherwise healthy individuals?" To answer this question, evidence from primary prevention trials may be necessary, but these are unlikely to be conducted because of the prohibitive costs of following a sufficiently large population for decades. Additional support for the folate hypothesis may be forthcoming with the sophisticated network analyses from genome-wide association studies that will reveal the most important biological pathways in the etiology of CVD—and whether these pathways are folate dependent. Even if evidence does emerge that a folate-specific pathway is partly responsible for disease occurrence, the public health prevention (or intervention) message will still be controversial. The initial impetus behind the fortification of the flour supply with folic acid was based on the potential to reduce NTDs in susceptible populations and not on the unproven benefit on CVD. The major concern was that excessive folic acid would mask symptoms related to pernicious anemia from vitamin B12 deficiency. In a recent analysis of a representative sample of elderly participants from NHANES, high blood folate concentrations were associated with poor cognitive outcomes in men and women with low vitamin B12 concentrations. Interestingly, the opposite was true for folate and cognitive function for those with sufficient vitamin B12 concentrations [89]. Thus, this should continue to be an active area for research as markers for vitamin deficiency and cognitive function become better defined and the diagnostic technology improves. A recent cost-effective analysis of the folic acid fortification program in the United States suggested that health and economic gains of folic acid fortification far outweigh the losses and that increasing the level of fortification warrants further consideration [90].

VI. CONCLUSION

In summary, if there is benefit from greater folate intake or for folic acid supplementation on CHD or stroke, the overall benefit is likely to be modest and may only be in populations without previous CVD (or not medically managed for complications leading to CVD) or with baseline intake well below the estimated average requirement of 320 µg/day. There is now overwhelming evidence that folic acid alone or in combination with other B vitamins is not efficacious in the secondary prevention of CVD. However, the existing evidence, with support from observational and randomized interventions and with further support generated from genetic analyses, suggests that folate status may be inversely associated with CVD with the greatest reduction in risk specifically for stroke.

ACKNOWLEDGMENTS

We thank Christine Iannaccone for assistance with partial preparation of the manuscript.

REFERENCES

1. McCully KS. Vascular pathology of homocysteinemia: Implications for the pathogenesis of arteriosclerosis. *Am J Pathol* 1969; 56:111–28.
2. McCully KS. Homocysteine, vitamins, and vascular disease prevention. *Am J Clin Nutr* 2007; 86:1563S–68.
3. Boushey CJ, Beresford SA, Omenn GS, Motulsky AG. A quantitative assessment of plasma homocysteine as a risk factor for vascular disease. Probable benefits of increasing folic acid intakes. *JAMA* 1995; 274:1049–57.
4. Homocysteine Studies Collaboration. Homocysteine and risk of ischemic heart disease and stroke: A meta-analysis. *JAMA* 2002; 288:2015–22.
5. Wald DS, Law M, Morris JK. Homocysteine and cardiovascular disease: Evidence on causality from a meta-analysis. *BMJ* 2002; 325:1202.
6. Splaver A, Lamas GA, Hennekens CH. Homocysteine and cardiovascular disease: Biological mechanisms, observational epidemiology, and the need for randomized trials. *Am Heart J* 2004; 148:34–40.
7. Homocysteine Lowering Trialists' Collaboration. Dose-dependent effects of folic acid on blood concentrations of homocysteine: A meta-analysis of the randomized trials. *Am J Clin Nutr* 2005; 82:806–12.
8. FDA. Food labeling: Health claims and label statement: Folic acid and neural tube defects. *Fed Reg* 1993; 58:53254–97, 55305–17.
9. Giles WH, Kittner SJ, Anda RF, Croft JB, Casper ML. Serum folate and risk for ischemic stroke. First National Health and Nutrition Examination Survey epidemiologic follow-up study. *Stroke* 1995; 26:1166–70.
10. Morrison HI, Schaubel D, Desmeules M, Wigle DT. Serum folate and risk of fatal coronary heart disease. *JAMA* 1996; 275:1893–96.

11. Rimm EB, Stampfer MJ, Ascherio A, Giovannucci E, Willett WC. Dietary folate, vitamin B6, vitamin B12 intake and risk of CHD among a large population of men. Abstract. *Circulation* 1996; 93:625.

12. Rimm EB, Willett WC, Hu FB, Sampson L, Colditz GA, Manson JE, Hennekens C, Stampfer MJ. Folate and vitamin B6 from diet and supplements in relation to risk of coronary heart disease among women. *JAMA* 1998; 279:359–64.

13. Voutilainen S, Lakka TA. Low serum folate concentrations are associated with an excess incidence of acute coronary events: The Kuopio Ischaemic Heart Disease Risk Factor Study. *Eur J Clin Nutr* 2000; 54:424.

14. Voutilainen S, Rissanen TH, Virtanen J, Lakka TA, Salonen JT, Kuopio Ischemic Heart Disease Risk Factor Study. Low dietary folate intake is associated with an excess incidence of acute coronary events: The Kuopio Ischemic Heart Disease Risk Factor Study. *Circulation* 2001; 103:2674–80.

15. Bazzano LA, He J, Ogden LG, Loria C, Vupputuri S, Myers L, Whelton PK. Dietary intake of folate and risk of stroke in US men and women: NHANES I Epidemiologic Follow-up Study. National Health and Nutrition Examination Survey. *Stroke* 2002; 33:1183–88.

16. Maxwell CJ, Hogan DB, Ebly EM. Serum folate levels and subsequent adverse cerebrovascular outcomes in elderly persons. *Dement Geriatr Cogn Disord* 2002; 13:225–34.

17. de Bree A, Verschuren WM, Blom HJ, Nadeau M, Trijbels FJ, Kromhout D. Coronary heart disease mortality, plasma homocysteine, and B-vitamins: A prospective study. *Atherosclerosis* 2003; 166:369–77.

18. Voutilainen S, Virtanen JK, Rissanen TH, Alfthan G, Laukkanen J, Nyyssönen K, Mursu J, et al. Serum folate and homocysteine and the incidence of acute coronary events: The Kuopio Ischaemic Heart Disease Risk Factor Study. *Am J Clin Nutr* 2004; 80:317–23.

19. He K, Merchant A, Rimm EB, Rosner BA, Stampfer MJ, Willett WC, Ascherio A. Folate, vitamin B6, and B12 intakes in relation to risk of stroke among men. *Stroke* 2004; 35:169–74.

20. Van Guelpen B, Hultdin J, Johansson I, Stegmayr B, Hallmans G, Nilsson TK, Weinehall L, Witthöft C, Palmqvist R, Winkvist A. Folate, vitamin B12, and risk of ischemic and hemorrhagic stroke: A prospective, nested case-referent study of plasma concentrations and dietary intake. *Stroke* 2005; 36:1426–31.

21. Virtanen JK, Voutilainen S, Happonen P, Alfthan G, Kaikkonen J, Mursu J, Rissanen TH, et al. Serum homocysteine, folate and risk of stroke: Kuopio Ischaemic Heart Disease Risk Factor (KIHD) Study. *Eur J Cardiovasc Prev Rehabil* 2005; 12:369–75.

22. Drogan D, Klipstein-Grobusch K, Dierkes J, Weikert C, Boeing H. Dietary intake of folate equivalents and risk of myocardial infarction in the European Prospective Investigation into Cancer and Nutrition (EPIC)--Potsdam study. *Public Health Nutr* 2006; 9:465–71.

23. Weikert C, Dierkes J, Hoffmann K, Berger K, Drogan D, Klipstein-Grobusch K, Spranger J, Möhlig M, Luley C, Boeing H. B vitamin plasma levels and the risk of ischemic stroke and transient ischemic attack in a German cohort. *Stroke* 2007; 38:2912–18.

24. Ishihara J, Iso H, Inoue M, Iwasaki M, Okada K, Kita Y, Kokubo Y, Okayama A, Tsugane S, JPHC Study Group. Intake of folate, vitamin B6 and vitamin B12 and the risk of CHD: The Japan Public Health Center-Based Prospective Study Cohort I. *J Am Coll Nutr* 2008; 27:127–36.

25. Chasan-Taber L, Selhub J, Rosenberg IH, Malinow MR, Terry P, Tishler PV, Willett W, Hennekens CH, Stampfer MJ. A prospective study of folate and vitamin B6 and risk of myocardial infarction in US physicians. *J Am Coll Nutr* 1996; 15:136–43.

26. Zeitlin A, Frishman WH, Chang CJ. The association of vitamin B 12 and folate blood levels with mortality and cardiovascular morbidity incidence in the old old: The Bronx aging study. *Am J Ther* 1997; 4:275–81.

27. Folsom AR, Nieto FJ, McGovern PG, Tsai MY, Malinow MR, Eckfeldt JH, Hess DL, Davis CE. Prospective study of coronary heart disease incidence in relation to fasting total homocysteine, related genetic polymorphisms, and B vitamins: The Atherosclerosis Risk in Communities (ARIC) study. *Circulation* 1998; 98:204–10.

28. Giles WH, Kittner SJ, Croft JB, Anda RF, Casper ML, Ford ES. Serum folate and risk for coronary heart disease: Results from a cohort of US adults. *Ann Epidemiol* 1998; 8:490–96.

29. Hung J, Beilby JP, Knuiman MW, Divitini M. Folate and vitamin B-12 and risk of fatal cardiovascular disease: Cohort study from Busselton, Western Australia. *BMJ* 2003; 326:131.

30. Al-Delaimy WK, Rexrode KM, Hu FB, Albert CM, Stampfer MJ, Willett WC, Manson JE. Folate intake and risk of stroke among women. *Stroke* 2004; 35:1259–63.

31. Dalmeijer GW, Olthof MR, Verhoef P, Bots ML, van der Schouw YT. Prospective study on dietary intakes of folate, betaine, and choline and cardiovascular disease risk in women. *Eur J Clin Nutr* 2008; 62(3):386–94.

32. Vanuzzo D, Pilotto L, Lombardi R, Lazzerini G, Carluccio M, Diviacco S, Quadrifoglio F, et al. Both vitamin B6 and total homocysteine plasma levels predict long-term athero-thrombotic events in healthy subjects. *Eur Heart J* 2007; 28:484–91.

33. Stampfer MJ, Rimm EB. Folate and cardiovascular disease. Why we need a trial now. *JAMA* 1996; 275:1929–30.

34. Baker F, Picton D, Blackwood S, Hunt J, Eskine M, Oyas M, Ashby M, Anjana S, Brown MJ, et al. Blinded comparison of folic acid and placebo in patients with ischemic heart disease: An outcome trial. Abstract. *Circulation* 2002; 106:3642.

35. Toole JF, Malinow MR, Chambless LE, Spence JD, Pettigrew LC, Howard VJ, Sides EG, Wang CH, Stampfer M. Lowering homocysteine in patients with ischemic stroke to prevent recurrent stroke, myocardial infarction, and death: The Vitamin Intervention for Stroke Prevention (VISP) randomized controlled trial. *JAMA* 2004; 291:565–75.

36. Bønaa KH, Njølstad I, Ueland PM, Schirmer H, Tverdal A, Steigen T, Wang H, Nordrehaug JE, Arnesen E, Rasmussen K, NORVIT Trial Investigators. Homocysteine lowering and cardiovascular events after acute myocardial infarction. *N Engl J Med* 2006; 354:1578–88.

37. Lonn E, Yusuf S, Arnold MJ, Sheridan P, Pogue J, Micks M, McQueen MJ, et al. Homocysteine lowering with folic acid and B vitamins in vascular disease. *N Engl J Med* 2006; 354:1567–77.

38. Albert CM, Cook NR, Gaziano JM, Zaharris E, MacFadyen J, Danielson E, Buring JE, Manson JE. Effect of folic acid and B vitamins on risk of cardiovascular events and total mortality among women at high risk for cardiovascular disease: A randomized trial. *JAMA* 2008; 299:2027–36.

39. Jamison RL, Hartigan P, Kaufman JS, Goldfarb DS, Warren SR, Guarino PD, Gaziano JM, Veterans Affairs Site Investigators. Effect of homocysteine lowering on mortality and vascular disease in advanced chronic kidney disease and end-stage renal disease: A randomized controlled trial. *JAMA* 2007; 298:1163–70.

40. Ebbing M, Bleie Ø, Ueland PM, Nordrehaug JE, Nilsen DW, Vollset SE, Refsum H, Pedersen EK, Nygård O. Mortality and cardiovascular events in patients treated with homocysteine-lowering B vitamins after coronary angiography: A randomized controlled trial. *JAMA* 2008; 300:795–804.

41. Wrone EM, Hornberger JM, Zehnder JL, McCann LM, Coplon NS, Fortmann SP. Randomized trial of folic acid for prevention of cardiovascular events in end-stage renal disease. *J Am Soc Nephrol* 2004; 15:420–26.

42. Schnyder G, Roffi M, Flammer Y, Pin R, Hess OM. Effect of homocysteine-lowering therapy with folic acid, vitamin B12, and vitamin B6 on clinical outcome after

percutaneous coronary intervention: The Swiss Heart study: A randomized controlled trial. *JAMA* 2002; 288:973–79.

43. Liem A, Reynierse-Buitenwerf GH, Zwinderman AH, Jukema JW, van Veldhuisen DJ. Secondary prevention with folic acid: Results of the Goes extension study. *Heart* 2005; 91:1213–14.

44. Zoungas S, McGrath BP, Branley P, Kerr PG, Muske C, Wolfe R, Atkins RC, et al. Cardiovascular morbidity and mortality in the Atherosclerosis and Folic Acid Supplementation Trial (ASFAST) in chronic renal failure: A multicenter, randomized, controlled trial. *J Am Coll Cardiol* 2006; 47:1108–16.

45. Food and Drug Administration. Food additives permitted for direct addition to food for human consumption: Folic acid (folacin), final rule. *Fed Reg* 1996; 8797–807.

46. Health Canada. Regulations amending the food and drug regulations: Schedule No. 1066 (flour fortification). *Canada Gazette Part II* 1998; 132.

47. Jacques PF, Selhub J, Bostom AG, Wilson PW, Rosenberg IH. The effect of folic acid fortification on plasma folate and total homocysteine concentrations. *N Engl J Med* 1999; 340:1449–54.

48. Pfeiffer CM, Osterloh JD, Kennedy-Stephenson J, Picciano MF, Yetley EA, Rader JI, Johnson CL. Trends in circulating concentrations of total homocysteine among US adolescents and adults: Findings from the 1991-1994 and 1999-2004 National Health and Nutrition Examination Surveys. *Clin Chem* 2008; 54:801–13.

49. B-Vitamin Treatment Trialists' Collaboration. Homocysteine-lowering trials for prevention of cardiovascular events: A review of the design and power of the large randomized trials. *Am Heart J* 2006; 151:282–87.

50. Galan P, Briancon S, Blacher J, Czernichow S, Hercberg S. The SU.FOL.OM3 Study: A secondary prevention trial testing the impact of supplementation with folate and B-vitamins and/or Omega-3 PUFA on fatal and non fatal cardiovascular events, design, methods and participants characteristics. *Trials* 2008; 9:35.

51. SEARCH Study Collaborative Group, Bowman L, Armitage J, Bulbulia R, Parish S, Collins R. Study of the effectiveness of additional reductions in cholesterol and homocysteine (SEARCH): Characteristics of a randomized trial among 12064 myocardial infarction survivors. *Am Heart J* 2007; 154:815–23.e6.

52. Bostom AG, Carpenter MA, Kusek JW, Hunsicker LG, Pfeffer MA, Levey AS, Jacques PF, McKenney J, FAVORIT Investigators. Rationale and design of the Folic Acid for Vascular Outcome Reduction In Transplantation (FAVORIT) trial. *Am Heart J* 2006; 152:448 e1–7.

53. Dusitanond P, Eikelboom JW, Hankey GJ, Thom J, Gilmore G, Loh K, Yi Q, Klijn CJ, Langton P, van Bockxmeer FM, Baker R, Jamrozik K. Homocysteine-lowering treatment with folic acid, cobalamin, and pyridoxine does not reduce blood markers of inflammation, endothelial dysfunction, or hypercoagulability in patients with previous transient ischemic attack or stroke: A randomized substudy of the VITATOPS trial. *Stroke* 2005; 36:144–46.

54. The VITATOPS Trial Study Group. The VITATOPS (Vitamins to Prevent Stroke) trial: Rationale and design of an international, large, simple, randomised trial of homocysteine-lowering multivitamin therapy in patients with recent transient ischaemic attack or stroke. *Cerebrovasc Dis* 2002; 13:120–26.

55. Willett W. *Nutritional Epidemiology*, 2nd ed. New York: Oxford University Press, 1998.

56. Barak AJ, Beckenhauer HC, Hidiroglou N, Camilo ME, Selhub J, Tuma DJ. The relationship of ethanol feeding to the methyl folate trap. *Alcohol* 1993; 10:495–97.

57. Shaw S, Jayatilleke E, Herbert V, Colman N. Cleavage of folates during ethanol metabolism. Role of acetaldehyde/xanthine oxidase-generated superoxide. *Biochem J* 1989; 257:277–80.

58. Hidiroglou N, Camilo ME, Beckenhauer HC, Tuma DJ, Barak AJ, Nixon PF, Selhub J. Effect of chronic alcohol ingestion on hepatic folate distribution in the rat. *Biochem Pharmacol* 1994; 47:1561–66.

59. Rimm EB, Klatsky A, Grobbee D, Stampfer MJ. Review of moderate alcohol consumption and reduced risk of coronary heart disease: Is the effect due to beer, wine, or spirits. *BMJ* 1996; 312:731–36.

60. Mukamal KJ, Jensen MK, Grønbaek M, Stampfer MJ, Manson JE, Pischon T, Rimm EB. Drinking frequency, mediating biomarkers, and risk of myocardial infarction in women and men. *Circulation* 2005; 112:1406–13.

61. Jiang R, Hu FB, Giovannucci EL, Rimm EB, Stampfer MJ, Spiegelman D, Rosner BA, Willett WC. Joint association of alcohol and folate intake with risk of major chronic disease in women. *Am J Epidemiol* 2003; 158:760–71.

62. Morrison HI, Ellison LF, Schaubel D, Wigle DT. Relationship of dietary folate and vitamin B6 with coronary heart disease in women. *JAMA* 1998; 280:417–18; author reply 418–19.

63. Food and Nutrition Board and Institute of Medicine. *Dietary Reference Intakes for Thiamin, Riboflavin, Niacin, Vitamin B6, Folate, Vitamin B12, Pantothenic Acid, Biotin, and Choline—A Report of the Standing Committee on the Scientific Evaluation of Dietary Reference Intakes and Its Panel on Folate, Other B Vitamins, and Choline and Subcommittee on Upper Reference Levels of Nutrients.* Washington, DC: The National Academies Press, 2000.

64. Davey Smith G, Ebrahim S. "Mendelian randomization": Can genetic epidemiology contribute to understanding environmental determinants of disease? *Int J Epidemiol* 2003; 32:1–22.

65. Ebrahim S, Davey Smith G. Mendelian randomization: Can genetic epidemiology help redress the failures of observational epidemiology? *Hum Genet* 2008; 123:15–33.

66. Kanwar YS, Manaligod JR, Wong PW. Morphologic studies in a patient with homocystinuria due to 5, 10-methylenetetrahydrofolate reductase deficiency. *Pediatr Res* 1976; 10:598–609.

67. Brattstrom L, Wilcken DE, Ohrvik J, Brudin L. Common methylenetetrahydrofolate reductase gene mutation leads to hyperhomocysteinemia but not to vascular disease: The result of a meta-analysis. *Circulation* 1998; 98: 2520–26.

68. Botto LD, Yang Q. 5,10-Methylenetetrahydrofolate reductase gene variants and congenital anomalies: A HuGE review. *Am J Epidemiol* 2000; 151:862–77.

69. Guéant-Rodriguez RM, Guéant JL, Debard R, Thirion S, Hong LX, Bronowicki JP, Namour F, et al. Prevalence of methylenetetrahydrofolate reductase 677T and 1298C alleles and folate status: A comparative study in Mexican, West African, and European populations. *Am J Clin Nutr* 2006; 83:701–07.

70. Jacques PF, Bostom AG, Williams RR, Ellison RC, Eckfeldt JH, Rosenberg IH, Selhub J, Rozen R. Relation between folate status, a common mutation in methylenetetrahydrofolate reductase, and plasma homocysteine concentrations. *Circulation* 1996; 93:7–9.

71. de Bree A, Verschuren WM, Bjørke-Monsen AL, van der Put NM, Heil SG, Trijbels FJ, Blom HJ. Effect of the methylenetetrahydrofolate reductase 677C→T mutation on the relations among folate intake and plasma folate and homocysteine concentrations in a general population sample. *Am J Clin Nutr* 2003; 77:687–93.

72. Ashfield-Watt PA, Pullin CH, Whiting JM, Clark ZE, Moat SJ, Newcombe RG, Burr ML, Lewis MJ, Powers HJ, McDowell IF. Methylenetetrahydrofolate reductase 677C->T genotype modulates homocysteine responses to a folate-rich diet or a low-dose folic acid supplement: a randomized controlled trial. *Am J Clin Nutr* 2002; 76:180–86.

73. Klerk M, Verhoef P, Clarke R, Blom HJ, Kok FJ, Schouten EG; MTHFR Studies Collaboration Group. MTHFR 677C→T polymorphism and risk of coronary heart disease: A meta-analysis. *JAMA* 2002; 288:2023–31.

74. Lewis SJ, Ebrahim S, Davey Smith G. Meta-analysis of MTHFR 677C→T polymorphism and coronary heart disease: Does totality of evidence support causal role for homocysteine and preventive potential of folate? *BMJ* 2005; 331:1053.
75. Larsson SC, Männistö S, Virtanen MJ, Kontto J, Albanes D, Virtamo J. Folate, vitamin B6, vitamin B12, and methionine intakes and risk of stroke subtypes in male smokers. *Am J Epidemiol* 2008; 167:954–61.
76. Yang Q, Botto LD, Erickson JD, Berry RJ, Sambell C, Johansen H, Friedman JM Improvement in stroke mortality in Canada and the United States, 1990 to 2002. *Circulation* 2006; 113:1335–43.
77. Merchant AT, Hu FB, Spiegelman D, Willett WC, Rimm EB, Ascherio A. The use of B vitamin supplements and peripheral arterial disease risk in men are inversely related. *J Nutr* 2003; 133:2863–67.
78. Forman JP, Rimm EB, Stampfer MJ, Curhan GC. Folate intake and the risk of incident hypertension among US women. *JAMA* 2005; 293:320–29.
79. Kelly PJ, Rosand J, Kistler JP, Shih VE, Silveira S, Plomaritoglou A, Furie KL. Homocysteine, MTHFR 677C→T polymorphism, and risk of ischemic stroke: Results of a meta-analysis. *Neurology* 2002; 59:529–36.
80. Cronin S, Furie KL, Kelly PJ. Dose-related association of MTHFR 677T allele with risk of ischemic stroke: Evidence from a cumulative meta-analysis. *Stroke* 2005; 36:1581–87.
81. Casas JP, Bautista LE, Smeeth L, Sharma P, Hingorani AD. Homocysteine and stroke: Evidence on a causal link from mendelian randomisation. *Lancet* 2005; 365:224–32.
82. Ariyaratnam R, Casas JP, Whittaker J, Smeeth L, Hingorani AD, Sharma P. Genetics of ischaemic stroke among persons of non-European descent: A meta-analysis of eight genes involving approximately 32,500 individuals. *PLoS Med* 2007; 4:e131.
83. Casas JP, Hingorani AD, Bautista LE, Sharma P. Meta-analysis of genetic studies in ischemic stroke: Thirty-two genes involving approximately 18 000 cases and 58 000 controls. *Arch Neurol* 2004; 61:1652–61.
84. Moats C, Rimm EB. Vitamin intake and risk of coronary disease: Observation versus intervention. *Curr Atheroscler Rep* 2007; 9:508–14.
85. Wang X, Qin X, Demirtas H, Li J, Mao G, Huo Y, Sun N, Liu L, Xu X. Efficacy of folic acid supplementation in stroke prevention: A meta-analysis. *Lancet* 2007; 369:1876–82.
86. Spence JD. Perspective on the efficacy analysis of the Vitamin Intervention for Stroke Prevention trial. *Clin Chem Lab Med* 2007; 45:1582–85.
87. Troen AM, Mitchell B, Sorensen B, Wener MH, Johnston A, Wood B, Selhub J, et al. Unmetabolized folic acid in plasma is associated with reduced natural killer cell cytotoxicity among postmenopausal women. *J Nutr* 2006; 136:189–94.
88. Chiuve SE, Giovannucci EL, Hankinson SE, Hunter DJ, Stampfer MJ, Willett WC, Rimm EB. Alcohol intake and methylenetetrahydrofolate reductase polymorphism modify the relation of folate intake to plasma homocysteine. *Am J Clin Nutr* 2005; 82:155–62.
89. Morris MS, Jacques PF, Rosenberg IH, Selhub J. Folate and vitamin B-12 status in relation to anemia, macrocytosis, and cognitive impairment in older Americans in the age of folic acid fortification. *Am J Clin Nutr* 2007; 85:193–200.
90. Bentley TG, Weinstein MC, Willett WC, Kuntz KM. A cost-effectiveness analysis of folic acid fortification policy in the United States. *Public Health Nutr* 2008; 1–13.

12 Folate and Vascular Disease
Basic Mechanisms

*Luciana Hannibal, Alla V. Glushchenko,
and Donald W. Jacobsen*

CONTENTS

I. INTRODUCTION

Cardiovascular health depends on an adequate supply of folate in our diets. Suboptimal nutritional status with respect to folate places an individual at increased risk for the development of cardiovascular disease (CVD) [1–3]. Cardiovascular

291

cells and tissues, like all cells and tissues in the body, require folates for the maintenance of one-carbon metabolism. The myriad functions performed by folate substrates in intermediary metabolism include but are not limited to de novo synthesis of purines, biosynthesis of thymidylate, movement of reduced and oxidized one-carbon units throughout the cell, and maintenance of the methylation potential of the cell by providing an adequate supply of methyl groups for the synthesis of S-adenosylmethionine (AdoMet). In addition, 5-methyltetrahydrofolate (5-methyl-THF) serves as a substrate for the B12-dependent methylation of homocysteine (Hcy) back to methionine in the methionine cycle. Deficiency of either B12 or folate leads to hyperhomocysteinemia, an independent risk factor for CVD. As shown in Figure 12.1, the transsulfuration pathway and betaine-dependent remethylation pathway are not active in cardiovascular cells and tissues of adults, thus limiting the metabolism of Hcy to B12-dependent remethylation in the methionine cycle [4]. Therefore, cardiovascular cells and tissues may be particularly vulnerable to elevations in serum Hcy. Although hyperhomocysteinemia per se was thought to promote endothelial dysfunction, more recent evidence suggests that other factors are involved, as described in this chapter. It is now widely recognized that endothelial dysfunction is a mediator and contributes to the progression of CVD. The mechanisms that are responsible for the development of endothelial dysfunction include hyperhomocysteinemia, oxidative stress, and limited bioavailability of nitric oxide (NO). Remarkably, folic acid, 5-methyl-THF, and tetrahydrobiopterin (H_4B) can dramatically improve functional aspects of the vascular endothelium by mechanisms that only now are beginning to be understood. Recent evidence suggests that folates,

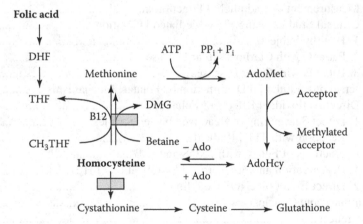

FIGURE 12.1 Homocysteine metabolism in cardiovascular cells and tissues. Homocysteine is an intermediary metabolite in the methionine cycle. Methionine is converted to S-adenosylmethionine (AdoMet), which then serves as a methyl group donor for methyltransferases. S-Adenosylhomocysteine (AdoHcy) is hydrolyzed to adenosine and homocysteine. The latter is remethylated back to methionine by B12-dependent methionine synthase using 5-methyl-THF (CH_3THF) as the methyl group donor. The transsulfuration and betaine remethylation pathways are inoperative in cardiovascular cells and tissues because of lack of expression of cystathionine-β-synthase and betaine-homocysteine methyltransferase, respectively [4].

operating either directly or indirectly on the vascular endothelium, promote coupling of NO production by endothelial NO synthase (eNOS). However, folates are also essential for AdoMet-dependent biological methylation reactions that are catalyzed by more than 100 methyltransferase enzymes. Thus, a decrease in methylation potential as a result of folate deficiency may also contribute to endothelial dysfunction. The biochemistry of cellular folates, the regulation of folate pathways, and the role of folates in DNA synthesis and cell division are described in Chapters 1 and 3, which should be consulted for more detailed information in these areas.

The term "vascular disease" encompasses a vast arena of pathological conditions—more than could possibly be covered in a single chapter. This chapter focuses on atherosclerosis, which is the leading cause of mortality and morbidity in developed and developing countries around the world. The role of folates in atherogenesis and progression of atherosclerosis will be examined with special emphasis on the vascular endothelium and how endothelial dysfunction contributes to the risk of CVD. The mechanisms underpinning folate-mediated improvement of endothelial function will then be addressed. It is entirely possible that during the next decade new therapeutic modalities using THFs and H_4Bs will be introduced to treat atherosclerosis and other forms of CVD.

II. LOW FOLATE STATUS AND RISK OF CARDIOVASCULAR DISEASE

In North America and several other countries with folic acid fortification programs, folate deficiency in the general population is seldom reported [5,6]. In 1996, the Food and Drug Administration mandated that folic acid be added to enriched cereal grain products, including flour, at the level of 140 µg/100 g, which was fully implemented by January 1998 [7]. However, before the folic acid fortification program in North America and in countries that do not fortify with folic acid, several reports suggested that low folate status was a risk factor for CVD. Pancharuniti et al. [8], studying 101 white men with angiographically defined coronary artery disease (CAD) and 108 aged-matched control subjects, found that low folate status was associated with increased risk of disease. In an evaluation of 5,056 participants from the Nutrition Canada Survey in a retrospective cohort study, Morrison et al. [1] found a progressive increased relative risk (RR) of mortality resulting from CAD in subjects with low folate status. For subjects with serum folate less than 6.8 nmol/L the RR was 1.69 (95% confidence interval [CI], 1.10–2.61). In a prospective cohort study involving 80,082 subjects from the Nurses' Health Study and controlling for common cardiovascular risk factors, Rimm et al. [9] found that those in the top quintile for dietary folate intake compared with those in the bottom quintile had a reduced RR of 0.69 (95% CI, 0.55–0.85) for nonfatal myocardial infarction (MI) or fatal CAD. In the same study, multiple vitamin users also had reduced RR. Additional studies have confirmed the observation that low folate status increases the RR of increased acute coronary events [2,3,10–12]. However, other studies reported no association between low folate status and increased risk of CVD [13–15].

There are also data suggesting that folate status may have a bearing on the incidence of stroke. Giles et al. [16], using data from the First National Health and Examination Survey Epidemiological Follow-up Study, found that low folate status

(≤9.2 nmol/L) was a risk factor for ischemic stroke, with the RR being much stronger in African Americans (3.60; 95% CI, 1.02–12.71) than in whites (1.18; 95% CI, 0.67–2.08). There has been an ongoing decrease in stroke mortality between 1990 and 1997 in the United States (−0.3%; 95% CI, −0.7 to 0.08) and Canada (−1.0%; 95% CI, −1.4 to −0.6). However, the decrease in stroke mortality accelerated significantly between 1998 and 2002 in the United States (−2.9%; 95% CI, −3.5 to −2.3) and Canada (−5.4%; 95% CI, −6.0 to −4.7) after the introduction of folic acid fortification as reported by Yang et al. [17]. In England and Wales, where food fortification with folic acid does not occur, the decrease in stroke mortality did not change appreciably between 1990 and 2002. Is food fortification with folic acid and the resulting improvement in folate nutritional status in the general population of North America responsible for the decrease in stroke mortality? If so, what might be the mechanisms behind the accelerated decrease in stroke mortality?

III. METABOLIC CONSEQUENCES OF LOW FOLATE STATUS IN CARDIOVASCULAR DISEASE

Although there is evidence for an association between low folate status and risk of CVD, mechanisms to explain this association have yet to be defined and in some cases have become controversial. This is particularly true for the "homocysteine theory of arteriosclerosis" coined by McCully and Wilson in 1975 [18]. Hyperhomocysteinemia, decreased methylation potential, and misincorporation of uracil into DNA leading to DNA fragility are important metabolic consequences of low folate status that may yield mechanistic understanding as to the role of folates in atherogenesis and the progression of CVD.

A. HYPERHOMOCYSTEINEMIA

Hcy is a naturally occurring sulfur-containing amino acid generated in the methionine cycle (Figure 12.1) by the hydrolysis of S-adenosylhomocysteine. The methionine cycle is operative in most, if not all, cells in the body and has three important functions: (1) dietary methionine is converted to S-adenosylmethionine (AdoMet in Figure 12.1), which serves as the methyl group donor substrate for more than 100 methyltransferase enzymes [19]; (2) 5-methyl-THF (CH_3THF in Figure 12.1) serves as the cosubstrate in the remethylation of Hcy back to methionine by cobalamin (B12)-dependent methionine synthase and in the process is converted to THF, the active substrate form of folate in cells [20]; and (3) Hcy, a branch-point metabolite, is converted to cysteine in the transsulfuration pathway [21]. The transsulfuration pathway is found in liver and kidney but not in other tissue and organ systems [22]. In adult cardiovascular cells and tissues, the first enzyme of the transsulfuration pathway, cystathionine-β-synthase, is not expressed, rendering the pathway inactive [4]. Because cardiovascular cells and tissues are incapable of converting Hcy to cysteine, they must capture cysteine from the circulation to supply their needs if cysteine from protein degradation is inadequate. Because adult cardiovascular cells and tissues do not express betaine/Hcy methyltransferase activity (Figure 12.1) [4], the only active pathway for removal of Hcy, which is cytotoxic at higher levels, is the remethylation pathway catalyzed by B12-dependent methionine synthase. Thus, optimal levels of both folate and B12 are required to drive this remethylation reaction at full capacity (Figure 12.1).

B. HYPOMETHYLATION

Methyl groups are essential for the regulation of gene expression, chromatin structure, and epigenetic phenomenon [23]. Human diseases, including vascular disease, are either caused or impacted by abnormal methylation [24]. Specifically, the impact of DNA methylation is associated with transcription silencing changes in gene expression: Loss of methylation activates gene expression [25]. Experimental studies have confirmed that a failure to establish the correct DNA methylation pattern during early embryogenesis can lead to apoptosis, embryonic lethality, or multiple developmental malformations [26–29]. As mentioned earlier, Hcy can promote arteriosclerotic development. One of the mechanisms to explain the vascular pathology of elevated Hcy is hypomethylation caused by excessive levels of S-adenosylhomocysteine (AdoHcy in Figure 12.1), which is an end-product inhibitor of AdoMet-dependent methyltransferases [30]. Wang et al. [31,32] showed that Hcy (20–50 μM) and homo-cystine inhibit [^{3}H]thymidine incorporation, an indicator of DNA synthesis, and cell proliferation specifically in human umbilical vein endothelial cells and porcine aortic endothelial cells. The same group has recently demonstrated that endothelial growth suppression by Hcy involves DNA hypomethylation of a CpG site in the promoter of the *cyclin A* gene [33]. Hcy did not inhibit DNA synthesis in aortic smooth muscle cells or fibroblasts. In fact, Hcy appears to be mitogenic to aortic smooth muscle cells [34]. The growth inhibition of endothelial cells may be one of the mechanisms for Hcy-induced arteriosclerosis [35]. Diet-related changes in DNA methylation can also contribute to carcinogenesis that occurs in livers of methyl-deficient rats and mice [36].

Hcy may also be involved in the regulation of expression of DNA epigenetic phenotype modifications [37–41]. Genomic hypomethylation occurs in lesions of apolipoprotein E (apoE) knockout mice and in the neointima of balloon-denuded New Zealand white rabbit aortas [42]. Hypomethylation is present in specific genes such as the *15-lipoxygenase* gene, *estrogen receptor-α gene*, and *extracellular superoxide dismutase* gene—all important in atherogenesis and progression of atherosclerosis [43,44]. Increased *estrogen receptor-α* gene methylation was observed in multiple tissue specimens collected from patients undergoing coronary artery bypass surgery and in atherosclerotic plaques collected from patients undergoing directional coronary atherectomy or carotid endarterectomy [45].

The diversity of phenotypes in differentiated organs is not because of genetic alterations but rather epigenetic changes: The genome is hypomethylated, but selected CpG-rich islands in the 5′-flanking regions of genes become densely hypermethylated [46]. Studies have shown that DNA methylation of CpG islands can be an important mechanism controlling gene expression in CVD [24]. Lund et al. [47] analyzed apoE-null mice and control wild-type mice in early stages of atherosclerosis (at 4 weeks of age with hyperlipidemia but with no histological signs of aortic lesions) and with advanced fibrocellular lesions (at 6 months of age). They found evidence of DNA hypo- and hypermethylation in both age groups, but significant excess hypomethylation in peripheral blood cells was observed only in older mice. Zaina et al. [48] concluded that atherogenic lipoprotein profiles promote DNA hypermethylation in cultured human macrophages. DNA hypomethylation may reflect hyperproliferation of cell types involved in immune or inflammatory responses during atherosclerosis [49,50].

C. DNA Synthesis and Repair

Folates are absolutely essential for DNA replication and repair processes. The de novo synthesis of purine deoxyribonucleotides depends on 10-formyl-THF, and thymidylate biosynthesis depends on 5,10-methylene-THF, as described in Chapter 3. The clinical hallmark of acute folate deficiency is megaloblastic anemia, which graphically illustrates impairment of DNA replication. When cellular levels of 5,10-methylene-THF are limited as a result of folate deficiency, uracil is misincorporated into DNA [51]. This causes chromosomal fragile sites, chromosome breakage, and micronucleus formation (reviewed by Fenech [52]). Although adult cardiovascular cells and tissues have low mitotic indices, there is turnover of cells, particularly in the vascular endothelium. Low folate status could impair regeneration of vascular endothelial cells in regions where the endothelium has been injured.

IV. THE VASCULAR ENDOTHELIUM AND CARDIOVASCULAR HEALTH

The cardiovascular system, consisting of the heart, arteries, capillaries, and veins, is lined with a continuous monolayer of endothelial cells that for decades was believed to act merely as a barrier for blood cells and large proteins and as a passive filter for small molecules. The mass of endothelial cells in the cardiovascular system, approximately 1.5 kg in the average adult, is now thought to have organ-like properties and is an active source of factors that elicit both local and systemic effects (reviewed in Le Brocq et al. [53]). Endothelial cells produce NO, endothelin, prostacyclin, and angiotensinogen among other important substances. These factors play a critical role in modulating vasodilatation and vasoconstriction and hence blood flow, shear stress, and blood pressure. Under normal conditions, the luminal surface of the vascular endothelium has an antithrombotic phenotype. Atherosclerosis is a systemic arterial disease initiated by areas of injured endothelium that become vulnerable to infiltration of inflammatory cells, lipid deposition, smooth muscle cell proliferation, and fibrosis. NO produced by the healthy endothelium is a key antiatherogenic molecule whose protective effects are lost if the tissue is damaged. Thus, assessment of the endothelial function is a useful marker for cardiovascular risk.

A. Endothelial Cell Dysfunction and Risk of Cardiovascular Disease

During the 1990s, several studies clearly demonstrated that loss of function of vascular endothelial cells was prognostic for atherogenesis and development of atherosclerosis [54–56]. Vita et al. [54] infused acetylcholine into the left anterior descending or circumflex coronary artery in 34 patients with angiographically smooth coronary arteries and assessed diameter changes with quantitative angiography. At peak acetylcholine dose, the response ranged from +37% (dilation) to −53% (constriction). Using multiple regression analysis, male gender ($P < .001$), total number of risk factors ($P < .001$), serum cholesterol ($P < .01$), family history ($P < .05$), and age ($P < .05$) were independently associated with the acetylcholine response, suggesting that coronary risk factors are associated with loss of endothelium-dependent vasodilation. They concluded that "the development of vasoconstriction is likely to be an abnormal endothelial function that precedes atherosclerosis or an early marker of atherosclerosis not detectable by angiography." Zeiher et al. [55] found evidence for progressive endothelial dysfunction in patients with different early stages of coronary atherosclerosis. In a prospective study involving 147 patients followed for 7.7 years, Schächinger et al. [56] determined that atherosclerotic disease progression and cardiovascular event rates can be predicted by coronary endothelial vasodilator dysfunction. Other studies have made similar observations and support the position that assessment of coronary endothelial vasoreactivity has both diagnostic and prognostic value in patients at risk for CAD [57–59].

B. Measurement of Endothelial Function

There are both in vitro and in vivo techniques to measure functionality of the vascular endothelium (for a recent review, see Le Brocq et al. [53]). Flow-mediated dilatation (FMD) of the brachial artery is widely used to measure endothelial function and assess risk of CVD [60–62]. FMD is an indicator of the functional integrity of the endothelium using high-resolution ultrasound and wall tracking. It represents the ability of the brachial artery to dilate in response to ischemia-induced hyperemia in the forearm and reflects the bioavailability of endogenous NO [63]. Brachial artery FMD correlates well with coronary endothelial function and carotid intimal medial thickness [64]. This is a sensitive and specific screening test to predict CAD. This method can assess the reversibility of endothelial dysfunction among asymptomatic subjects at high risk of arterial disease [65]. However, a caveat should be mentioned. Bots et al. [66] found considerable variation in mean FMD values across studies. For healthy subjects, mean FMD varied from 0.20% to 19.2%. For patients with CAD, FMD varied from −1.30% to 14.0%, and for subjects with diabetes mellitus, FMD varied from 0.75% to 12.0%. Thus, there is great overlap between healthy and patient populations, which has been attributed to technical aspects of the procedure.

C. Clinical Studies Using Flow-Mediated Dilatation

1. Healthy Subjects

Although endothelial dysfunction contributes to the genesis and development of CVD, a mechanistic understanding to explain the pathological changes in the vasculature remains incomplete. Endothelial cell injury by chemical insult (e.g., elevated Hcy), pathogens, and mechanical stress may be initiating events in atherogenesis [67,68]. Early studies have shown a strong clinical association between total plasma Hcy (tHcy) and CVD risk [69–71]. However, the mechanism(s) of Hcy-induced endothelial dysfunction remains elusive. Endothelial dysfunction has been observed in the subjects with minor elevation of tHcy [72,73]. In other studies, correlations between endothelial dysfunction and tHcy in both healthy subjects and patients with CAD were not observed [74,75]. Other studies were unable to show an effect of folic acid on FMD in healthy individuals (Table 12.1). However, two of nine studies in healthy volunteers [73,76] reported that FMD was improved on long-term supplementation with folic acid. Usui et al. [77] and Doshi et al. [74,78] suggest that improvement in FMD is the result of a rapid and acute effect of folic acid and not of Hcy decrease.

De Bree at al. [63] did a meta-analysis of randomized, double-blind, and placebo-controlled folic acid trials evaluating the effect of folic acid on endothelial function. Fourteen trials were identified through MEDLINE based on inclusion criteria where 732 persons were treated with folic acid (with or without vitamin B6 or vitamin B12 or both) or placebo for a median of 8 weeks. Six of these trials used a cross-over design, and eight trials used a parallel design. The net change in FMD was evaluated to assess the effect of treatment on endothelial function. Folic acid improved FMD by 1.08% (95% CI, 0.57, 1.59; $P = 0.0005$) when compared with placebo groups. Importantly, the subjects at greater risk of CVD had a better improvement in FMD. The dose of folic acid also was very important. Treatment with a lower dose of folic acid (<5 mg/day) did not have a beneficial effect on FMD (−0.07% FMD; 95% CI, −0.37, 0.22% FMD). The studies with a higher dose (≥5 mg/day) did show improved FMD (1.42% FMD; 95% CI, 1.25, 1.58% FMD) (Figure 12.2) [63].

Oral methionine loading (0.1 mg/kg) has been used to increase tHcy and to assess the efficiency of the transsulfuration pathway [75]. tHcy was increased threefold with peak concentration occurring at 4 to 8 hours after receiving the oral methionine load (Figure 12.3). This acute increase in tHcy resulted in endothelial cell dysfunction and an abnormal FMD. Others have made similar observations with methionine loading [77,79]. In a second study of methionine loading in healthy elderly volunteers, tHcy increased from 9.4 μmol/L at baseline to 26.6 μmol/L after 6 hours. However, in this study, methionine-induced hyperhomocysteinemia did not impair FMD [80]. In contrast, the reduction in the increase in plasma tHcy concentrations by folic acid (10 mg/day), betaine (3 g/day), or serine (5 g/day) together with an oral methionine load, did not affect FMD. Other studies have shown that supplementation with folic acid together with a methionine load [77], folic acid alone [78], or 5-methyl-THF alone [74,81,82] can improve vascular function. This suggests that Hcy impairs vascular function in patients with CVD or patients at high risk for CVD.

2. Patients with Cardiovascular Disease

Hyperhomocysteinemia is a biomarker of inflammatory disease, including atherosclerosis [83]. Chemotactic cytokines (chemokines) are a family of inflammatory cytokines that are characterized by their ability to cause migration of leukocytes into inflamed tissue [84]. In patients with atherosclerosis, increased levels of chemokines like interleukin 8 (IL-8) and monocyte chemoattractant peptide 1 (MCP-1) were found in the plasma and within the atherosclerotic vessel [85–89]. Holven et al., [90] investigating 26 adults with hyperhomocysteinemia (fasting plasma tHcy >15 μmol/L), have shown that folic acid normalized the Hcy concentrations. This

TABLE 12.1
Overview of Placebo-Controlled Studies into the Effect of Folic Acid Supplementation on Vascular Function Measured by FMD

Reference	Participants	Participant Characteristics	Study Design	Findings
Bellamy et al. [76]	Healthy volunteers	18 participants; tHcy > 13 µmol/L at entry (age not reported)	Randomized, double-blind, placebo-controlled, cross-over study Oral folic acid (5 mg/d) and placebo for 6 wk each (6-wk washout)	tHcy 28% lower after folic acid (8.7 ± 2.5 µmol/L) than after placebo (12.1 ± 3.6 µmol/L; $P = .003$) Folic acid improved FMD vs. placebo (2.5% ± 0.4% vs. 1.1% ± 0.3%; $P = .02$)
Woo et al. [73]	Healthy volunteers	17 participants (mean age, 54 ± 10 y; 15 males)	Randomized, double-blind, placebo-controlled, cross-over study Oral folic acid (10 mg/d) and placebo for 8 wk (4-wk washout)	tHcy was lower after folic acid (8.1 ± 3.1 µmol/L) than after placebo (9.5 ± 2.5 µmol/L; $P = .03$) Folic acid improved FMD vs. placebo (8.2% ± 1.6% vs. 6.0% ± 1.3%; $P = .001$)
Wilmink et al. [147]	Healthy volunteers	20 participants (mean age, 23 ± 3.4 y; 10 males)	Randomized, double-blind, placebo-controlled, cross-over study Oral folic acid (10 mg/d) and placebo for 2 wk (8-wk washout)	Fasting Hcy was 2.2 µmol/L lower after folic acid (5.0 ± 0.7 µmol/L) than after placebo (7.2 ± 2.1 µmol/L; $P = .05$) Folic acid did not affect FMD
van Dijk et al. [148]	Healthy volunteers	130 participants (mean age 45 y; siblings of patients with atherothrombotic disease)	Randomized, double-blind, placebo-controlled, parallel study Treatment for 1–2 y: (1) 5 mg/d folic acid + 250 mg/d vitamin B6 ($n = 63$; age 45 ± 7 y; 37 males) (2) Placebo ($n = 67$; age 46 ± 8 y; 29 males)	Fasting Hcy decreased by 40% in B vitamin group relative to the placebo group ($P = .001$) No effect of B vitamin treatment on FMD

continued

TABLE 12.1 (continued)
Overview of Placebo-Controlled Studies into the Effect of Folic Acid Supplementation on Vascular Function Measured by FMD

Reference	Participants	Participant Characteristics	Study Design	Findings
Pullin et al. [100]	Healthy volunteers	126 participants (42 of each MTHFR genotype; mean age, 39 ± 12 y; 53 males)	Randomized, placebo-controlled, crossover study Treatments, 4 mo: (1) Placebo (dietary folate intake, ~200 μg/d) (2) 400 μg/d dietary folate (total folate intake, ~600 μg/d) (3) 400 μg of folic acid (total folate intake, ~600 μg/d)	tHcy decreased by 14% and 16% after dietary folate and folic acid supplementation, respectively No effect of treatment on FMD irrespective of the MTHFR genotype
Hirsch et al. [149]	Healthy volunteers	20 participants and 20 age-matched patients with hyperhomocysteinemia (mean age, 30 ± 6 y)	Randomized, double-blind, placebo-controlled, parallel study Folic acid (0.6 mg/d), vitamin B12 (0.8 mg/d), vitamin B6 (2 mg/d) (9 pairs, $n = 18$), or placebo for 8 wk (11 pairs, $n = 22$)	tHcy decreased as a result of vitamin treatment in normohomocysteinemic and in hyperhomocysteinemic participants ($P < .0001$) No effect of vitamin treatment on FMD
Woodman et al. [150]	Healthy volunteers	26 participants (mean age, 49 ± 2 y) with high Hcy at baseline (15.6 ± 1.5 μmol/L)	Randomized, double-blind, placebo-controlled, crossover study Oral folic acid (5 mg/d) and placebo for 8 wk (4-wk washout)	Folic acid decreased Hcy by 34% Folic acid treatment did not affect FMD
Carlsson et al. [151]	Healthy volunteers	20 participants (mean age, 78 ± 1 y), mean Hcy concentration 12.8 ± 0.5 (SEM) μmol/L	Single-blind intervention study Treatments, each for 10 wk: (1) Placebo (2) Multivitamins: folic acid (0.4 mg), vitamin B12 (0.025 mg), vitamin B6 (6 mg) daily (3) Placebo (4) Multivitamins: folic acid (0.4 mg), vitamin B12 (0.025 mg), vitamin B6	Multivitamin intake decreased Hcy concentrations by 6% ($P = .06$), and multivitamin + 1 mg folic acid intake did not further lower Hcy; during the 40-wk study, tHcy was decreased by 11% (P trend = .03) FMD did not improve after either of those treatments relative to the preceding placebo period

Olthof et al. [152]	Healthy volunteers	39 participants (mean age, 59 ± 5 y), mean tHcy concentration 12.0 ± 2.0 μM	Randomized, double-blind, placebo-controlled, cross-over study. Folic acid (0.8 mg/d), betaine (6 g/d), and placebo for 6 wk each (6-wk washout)	Fasting Hcy was lower after folic acid by 20%, after betaine by 12% relative to placebo. Treatment did not affect FMD
Title et al. [96]	Patients with CAD	75 patients (age, 59 ± 10 y)	Randomized, double-blind, placebo-controlled, parallel study. Intervention for 4 mo with: (1) Placebo ($n = 25$) (2) Folic acid (5 mg/d) ($n = 25$) (3) Folic acid (5 mg/d) + antioxidant vitamin C (2 g/d), and vitamin E (800 IU/d) ($n = 25$)	Folic acid reduced tHcy by 11% ($P = .23$) relative to placebo. Folic acid improved FMD from 3.2% ± 3.6% at baseline to 5.2% ± 3.9% after treatment ($P = .04$ folic acid vs. placebo). The improvement in FMD correlated with the reduction in Hcy ($r = 0.5$; $P = .01$). Folic acid + antioxidants reduced tHcy by 9% ($P = .56$) relative to placebo. Folic acid + antioxidants did not improve FMD (2.6% ± 2.4% at baseline; 4.0% ± 3.7% after treatment, $P = .45$, folic acid + antioxidants vs. placebo) relative to placebo
Chambers et al. [98]	Patients with CHD	89 male patients (mean age, 56 y; range, 39–67 y)	Randomized, double-blind, placebo-controlled, parallel study. Intervention for 8 wk with: (1) Folic acid (5 mg/d) + vitamin B12 (1 mg/d) ($n = 59$) (2) Placebo ($n = 30$)	B vitamins reduced tHcy by –30% ($P = .001$) relative to placebo. FMD is improved in B vitamin group (+1.5% ± 3.5% change from baseline) relative to placebo (−0.3% ± 2.5%) ($P = .008$). There was an independent relationship between FMD and free, but not protein-bound, Hcy
Thambyrajah et al. [153]	Patients with CAD	86 patients (mean age, 63 y; range, 46–79 y; 79 males), tHcy > 11 μmol/L	Randomized, double-blind, placebo-controlled, parallel study. Intervention for 12 wk with: (1) Folic acid (5 mg/d) ($n = 43$) (2) Placebo ($n = 43$)	Folic acid reduced tHcy by 24% ($P = .001$) relative to placebo. No significant difference in FMD between folic acid and placebo group, but the improvement in FMD was larger in the folic acid group (+1.2%; 95% CI, 0.7%–1.8%) than in the placebo group (+0.4%; −0.3% to 1.1%) ($P = .07$)

continued

TABLE 12.1 (continued)
Overview of Placebo-Controlled Studies into the Effect of Folic Acid Supplementation on Vascular Function Measured by FMD

Reference	Participants	Participant Characteristics	Study Design	Findings
Doshi et al. [74]	Patients with CAD	52 patients (mean age, 57 ± 8 y)	Randomized, double-blind, placebo-controlled, cross-over study. Folic acid (5 mg/d) and placebo for 6 wk (4-mo washout)	Folic acid decreased tHcy by ~14% (10.8 μmol/L after placebo; 9.3 μmol/L after folic acid). Folic acid improved FMD vs. placebo (P <.001). Decreases in tHcy were not correlated with improvement in FMD
Doshi et al. [78]	Patients with CAD	33 patients (mean age, 55 ± 7 y)	Randomized, double-blind, placebo-controlled, parallel study. Intervention for 6 wk with: (1) Folic acid (5 mg/d) (n = 16) (2) Placebo (n = 17). FMD measured before and 2 and 4 h after first dose of folic acid, and after 6 wk of treatment	tHcy was lower (~20%) in the folic group relative to the placebo (P <.001). No difference in tHcy between the intervention groups during initial 4 h after intake of supplements on the first day. FMD improved within 2–4 h after first dose of folic acid, which persisted after 6 wk of folic acid intake. No correlation between FMD improvement and reduction in tHcy or changes in serum folate
Moat et al. [99]	Patients with CAD	84 patients (mean age, 60 ± 7 y; 74 males)	Randomized, placebo-controlled, parallel. Intervention for 6 wk with: (1) High dose of folic acid (5 mg/d) (2) Low dose of folic acid (0.4 mg/d) (3) Placebo	High-dose, but not low-dose, folic acid treatment improved FMD, despite a significant reduction in tHcy concentrations in both folic acid treatment groups relative to placebo

Study	Patients	Study design and intervention	Results
Sydow et al. [154]	27 patients with peripheral arterial occlusive disease	Randomized, placebo-controlled, parallel study Intervention for 8 wk with: (1) Folic acid (10 mg/d), vitamin B6 (20 mg/d), vitamin B12 (0.2 mg/d) (n = 9; 69 ± 4 y) (2) Arginine (24 g/d) (n = 9; 64 ± 4 y) (3) Placebo (n = 9; 69 ± 4 y)	Mean tHcy at baseline was 15.0 μmol/L; after 8-wk treatment with B vitamins, tHcy was decreased to 8.7 μmol/L; neither arginine nor placebo treatment affected tHcy. Neither B vitamin treatment nor placebo affected FMD; arginine enhanced FMD from 7.2 FMD% at baseline to 10.2 FMD% after 8 wk
Lekakis et al. [155]	34 patients with hypercholesterolemia receiving statins	Randomized, placebo-controlled, parallel study Intervention for 4 wk with: (1) Folic acid (5 mg/d) (n = 17) (2) Placebo (n = 17)	Hcy concentrations were not reported. Within the folic acid treatment group, FMD improved after treatment (4.7% ± 3.2% to 7.1% ± 3.1%; P = .02), whereas there was no improvement after placebo (5.7% ± 3.8% to 5.6% ± 2.2%; NS). Final FMD between the folic acid–treated group and the placebo group were not significantly different
Thambyrajah et al. [156]	100 patients with chronic renal failure (mean age, 62 y; range, 22–84 y)	Randomized, double-blind, placebo-controlled, parallel study Intervention for 12 wk with: (1) Folic acid (5 mg/d) (n = 50) (2) Placebo (n = 50)	Hcy concentrations were 25% lower in the folic acid group relative to placebo. Folic acid supplementation did not affect FMD
Bennet-Richards et al. [157]	25 normotensive children with chronic renal failure (mean age, 12 ± 3 y)	Randomized, double-blind, placebo-controlled, cross-over study Folic acid (5 mg/d) and placebo for 8 wk (8-wk washout)	tHcy decreased during folic acid treatment (from 10.3 ± 4.2 to 8.6 ± 2.3 μmol/L; P = .03) but not during placebo (from 9.0 ± 2.2 to 9.8 ± 2.7 μmol/L; P = .3). Final FMD after the folic acid and after placebo period were not significantly different
Pena et al. [158]	36 patients with type 1 diabetes (mean age, 13.6 ± 2.5y)	Randomized, double-blind, placebo-controlled, cross-over study Folic acid (5 mg/d) and placebo for 8 wk (8-wk washout)	tHcy did not change significantly but were already low at baseline (~5 μmol/L). Folic acid improved FMD relative to placebo (P < .001)

Source: Modified from Olthof MR, Bots ML, Katan MB, Verhoef P, *PLoS Clin Trials* 2006; 1:e4. With permission.

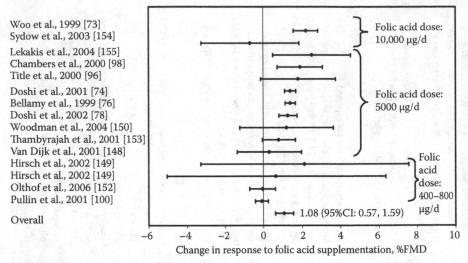

FIGURE 12.2 Change (and 95% CI) in the percentage of flow-mediated dilatation (%FMD) resulting from folic acid supplementation per included intervention group and the overall estimated change (and 95% CI). Half of the participants in the study by Hirsch et al. had high concentrations of homocysteine. (Reprinted from de Bree A, van Mierlo LA, Draijer R, *Am J Clin Nutr* 2007; 86:610–17. With permission.)

was accompanied by a reduction in oxidized low-density lipoprotein–stimulated release of CXC chemokines (IL-8) and CC chemokines (MCP-1) from peripheral blood mononuclear cells. In another prospective, randomized, double-blind, placebo-controlled, cross-over study, the effects of 5 mg of oral folic acid supplementation on 20 patients with familial hypercholesterolemia were investigated. This treatment restored the impaired endothelium-dependent vasodilation. Lipid profiles were not different between the placebo- and the folic acid–treated groups. Oral folic acid supplementation significantly increased both serum and red cell folate and decreased tHcy concentrations [91]. Patients with familial hypercholesterolemia have impaired endothelium-dependent FMD. These changes reversed after treatment coinfusion of 5-methyl-THF. This effect appeared to be the result of greater bioavailability of NO [81]. Also, 5-methyl-THF improved NO-mediated endothelium-dependent vasomotor responses and reduced vascular superoxide after incubating vessels with 5-methyl-THF (1–100 μmol/L) (ex vivo) and after intravenous infusion of 5-methyl-THF (in vivo) using saphenous veins and internal mammary arteries from 117 patients undergoing coronary artery bypass grafting [92].

Recent observations from clinical intervention studies indicate that low-dose folic acid supplementation can lower tHcy with no measurable reduction in cardiovascular risk, and high-dose folic acid can improve endothelial function before any change in plasma tHcy level [93]. A low (400 μg/day) and a high (5 mg/day) dose of folic acid can reduce the concentration of plasma tHcy by 15% to 25% [94]. Folic acid has a maximal effect on lowering plasma tHcy at daily doses of 400 μg [95]. Endothelial function was improved using high-dose folic acid between 6 weeks and 1 year (Table 12.1)

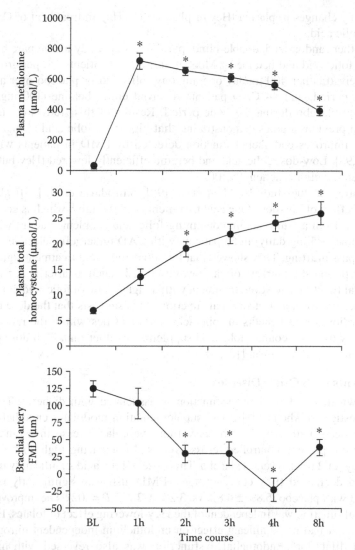

FIGURE 12.3 Time course of endothelial function (flow-mediated dilatation; FMD) induced by methionine loading. Methionine (100 mg/kg body weight) was administered to 10 healthy subjects. Plasma methionine, homocysteine, and FMD of the brachial artery were measured from 0 to 8 h following the methionine load. Values are mean ± SEM; *P < .001, comparing change with baseline. (Reprinted from Ashfield-Watt PA, Moat SJ, Doshi SN, McDowell IF, *Biomed Pharmacother* 2001; 55:425–33. With permission.)

[74,96,97]. In some studies, improvement in endothelial function was observed before decrease of Hcy [96,98]. There is a high possibility that folic acid may influence endothelial function through mechanisms other than decrease of tHcy. Doshi et al. [78] reported an acute improvement in endothelial function within 2 hours without any changes in plasma tHcy or plasma-free Hcy in treatment of CAD with 5 mg of folic acid.

In another randomized, double-blind, parallel group study to compare high- and low-dose folic acid and betaine by Moat et al. [99], 90 patients (30 per group) with CAD received either 400 μg/day or 5 mg/day folic acid or placebo over a 6-week treatment period, and 44 CAD patients received either betaine (100 mg/kg/day) or matched placebo during the same period. Results of this study were in agreement with previous studies demonstrating that high-dose folic acid (5 mg/day) significantly improves endothelial function detected by FMD in patients with CAD [74,78,96,98]. Low-dose folic acid and betaine efficiently lowered tHcy but did not improve endothelial function [99,100].

In contrast to the study by Moat et al. [99], Shirodaria et al. [101] also compared the effect of low-dose folic acid treatment (400 μg daily, which is comparable with intake from a multivitamin containing folic acid supplementation) with high-dose folic acid (5 mg daily) in 56 patients with CAD undergoing elective coronary artery bypass grafting. They showed that low-dose folic acid treatment significantly improved prognostic markers of cardiovascular risk, such as arterial stiffness and endothelial function. However, treatment with a higher dose of folic acid did not have any further improvement in vascular function. This suggests that the dose response of the cardiovascular benefits of folic acid treatment lies within the range of that provided by over-the-counter folic acid supplements rather than high-dose pharmacological folic acid treatment [101].

3. Patients with Other Diseases

It is known that endothelium dysfunction is associated with diabetes. Title et al. [102] investigated whether folic acid supplementation modulates endothelial function in patients with type 2 diabetes without vascular disease in a randomized, double-blind, placebo-controlled, cross-over trial comparing high-dose folic acid (10 mg/day for 2 weeks) versus placebo. This dose of folic acid significantly increased folate and decreased tHcy concentrations. FMD also was significantly improved compared with placebo (5.8% ± 4.8% vs. 3.2% ± 2.7%; $P = .02$). The improvement in endothelial function was independent of the Hcy-lowering effect of folates. However, this treatment had no significant effect on endothelium-independent nitroglycerin-mediated dilatation. Endothelial dysfunction was also reversed with high-dose folic acid in patients with diabetes [82]. Using venous plethysmography, Mangoni et al. [103] observed improvement in endothelium-dependent acetylcholine-induced forcarm blood flow after 4 weeks of treatment with folic acid (5 mg/day). In the same study, endothelium-independent vasodilation was not changed in 26 patients with type 2 diabetes without vascular disease. In another interesting study, MacKenzie et al. [104] showed that high-dose folic acid (5 mg/day) and vitamin B6 (100 mg/day) rapidly normalized endothelial dysfunction assessed by FMD in 124 children with type 1 diabetes. Although these children had severe endothelial dysfunction, FMD improved with folic acid treatment from 2.6% ± 4.3% to 9.7% ± 6.0%, with vitamin B6 from 3.5% ± 4.0% to 8.3% ± 4.2%, and with combination folic acid and vitamin B6 from 2.8% ± 3.5% to 10.5% ± 4.4% within 8 weeks. FMD improved within 2 hours and persisted for the 8-week treatment period. Glyceryl trinitrate-induced vasodilation (endothelium-independent vasodilation) did not change under these treatment protocols, indicating little or no direct effect on smooth muscle function.

Hyperhomocysteinemia also is an important risk factor for end-stage renal disease patients, where hemodialysis patients have an increased risk of cardiovascular morbidity and mortality [105,106]. Cianciolo et al. [107] have shown that intravenous 5-methyl-THF treatment improved survival in hemodialysis patients and reduced inflammation in end-stage renal disease patients independent of Hcy lowering when compared with oral folic acid treatment. The form of folic acid may be important in terms of endothelial function. The same beneficial effect of the metabolically active form of folic acid (5-methyl-THF) in improving endothelial-dependent vasodilatation was found in hemodialysis patients [108] and in peritoneal dialysis patients [109].

Understanding how "folates" improve endothelial function in CAD via mechanisms, independent of Hcy lowering, is addressed in the next section. In summary, folates are effective agents for improving endothelial function in a number of different pathological conditions.

V. REVERSAL OF ENDOTHELIAL DYSFUNCTION BY FOLATES: MECHANISMS

The mechanisms underlying the protective effects of folate on endothelial dysfunction, which is widely believed to be an initiating factor in atherogenesis, are only partially understood. At the biochemical level, 5-methyl-THF is required to support the activity of the enzyme methionine synthase, which catalyzes the methylation of Hcy to form methionine. Methionine synthase is inactivated by reactive oxygen species (ROS) and reactive nitrogen species (RNS) both in vivo and in vitro [110,111]. As a consequence, pathophysiological conditions of oxidative stress lead to partial or total inactivation of the enzyme with the concomitant accumulation of its substrate, Hcy. The action of folate in lowering Hcy has been well documented [73,96,98,112,113].

Interestingly, more recent studies indicate that folic acid and 5-methyl-THF can also exert protective effects by mechanisms independent of Hcy lowering [74,78,91,92,114–124]. For example, Title et al. [102] have recently shown that brachial artery FMD significantly increased following 2 weeks of folic acid supplementation compared with placebo in patients with type 2 diabetes (Figure 12.4). However, no significant correlation between levels of FMD and changes in tHcy or serum folate concentrations were observed in this study. Mechanisms of folate action leading to improved vascular function but independent of Hcy lowering include (1) direct antioxidant effects of folate, and (2) interactions of folate with eNOS and/or its cofactor H_4B.

A. DIRECT ANTIOXIDANT EFFECTS OF FOLATE

Oxidative stress, defined as a status where free radical production exceeds the antioxidant capacity of cells, is associated with endothelial dysfunction, decreased bioavailability of ˙NO, and atherothrombotic vascular disease [125]. Nitric oxide (˙NO), superoxide ($O_2^{˙-}$), peroxynitrite ($ONOO^-$), and hydroxyl radical (˙OH) are forms of ROS and RNS involved in the development of oxidative and nitrosative stress-related pathologies.

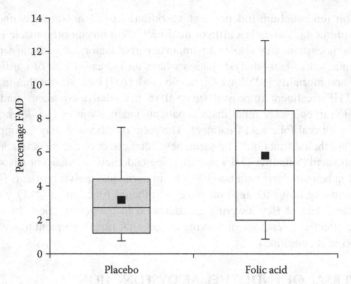

FIGURE 12.4 Brachial artery flow-mediated dilatation (FMD) after placebo and folic acid treatment in patients with type 2 diabetes. The box represents the interquartile range (between 25th and 75th percentiles). Mean values for FMD are shown as the small black squares within each box (3.2% ± 2.7% vs. 5.8% ± 4.8%; $P = .02$ by one-way ANOVA, $n = 19$). (From Title LM, Ur E, Giddens K, McQueen MJ, Nassar BA, *Vasc Med* 2006; 11:101–09. With permission.)

The fact that high concentrations of 5-methyl-THF (100–500 µM) may have direct antioxidant properties has attracted much interest in the literature recently [74,81,92]. Model studies indicate that the observed direct antioxidant effects of folate in biological systems involve (1) direct scavenging of free radicals, and (2) repair of thiyl radicals [126].

1. Direct Scavenging of Reactive Oxygen Species

Joshi et al. [126] have investigated the direct reaction of folic acid with oxidant species such as $CCl_3O_2^{\cdot}$ (a model of peroxyl radical) and $O_2^{\cdot-}$ and $^{\cdot}OH$. The reaction of folic acid with $CCl_3O_2^{\cdot}$, $O_2^{\cdot-}$, and $^{\cdot}OH$ is rapid. The bimolecular rate constants were found to be 4.10×10^7 $L \cdot mol^{-1} \cdot s^{-1}$ for $CCl_3O_2^{\cdot}$ and 1.13×10^{10} $L \cdot mol^{-1} \cdot s^{-1}$ for $^{\cdot}OH$, at pH 6.8. The reaction of folic acid with $O_2^{\cdot}-$ was investigated at pH 12.8, and the bimolecular rate constant was found to be 2.8×10^9 $L \cdot mol^{-1} \cdot s^{-1}$ [126]. The superoxide-scavenging capacity of 5-methyl-THF has been also documented by direct electron paramagnetic resonance measurements using the spin trap 5-(diethoxyphosphoryl)-5-methyl-L-pyrroline-*N*-oxide [127]. The authors observed that the scavenging potency of 5-methyl-THF is about 20-fold lower than that of ascorbic acid, a well-known antioxidant vitamin. In agreement with these findings, Verhaar et al. [128] reported a dose-dependent reduction of superoxide produced by xanthine oxidase and eNOS by 5-methyl-THF. Again, it is important to note that the concentrations of 5-methyl-THF used in this study are well beyond physiological or even therapeutic dosages.

Interestingly, Antoniades et al. [92] showed that superoxide production in intact human vessel segments decreased significantly ($P < .01$) after 45 minutes of intravenous infusion of 5-methyl-THF (Figure 12.5). In agreement with previous findings [81], they found that the effect of 5-methyl-THF as a scavenger of super-oxide generated from the xanthine/xanthine oxidase system is significant only at concentrations greater than 10 μM. In contrast, 5-methyl-THF had a strong direct peroxynitrite ($ONOO^-$) scavenging effect at concentrations as low as 1 μM, i.e., comparable to that of equal concentrations of uric acid, a known scavenger of peroxynitrite [92].

In summary, the in vitro and in vivo studies on the reactivity of 5-methyl-THF toward ROS indicate that (1) 5-methyl-THF has a significant peroxynitrite but not superoxide scavenging effect; and (2) the poor direct superoxide scavenging capacity of 5-methyl-THF does not account for the observed reduction in vascular superoxide production. For example, it was observed that low concentrations of 5-methyl-THF (1 μM) caused a significant decrease in vascular superoxide production both ex vivo and in vivo, with no evidence of direct superoxide scavenging [92]. An alternative explanation for the observed 5-methyl-THF–lowering effect of vascular superoxide production will be considered later in this chapter.

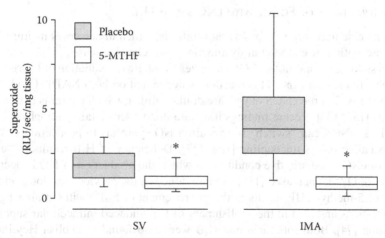

FIGURE 12.5 Superoxide production from intact vessels segments after about 45 minutes of intravenous infusion of 5-methyl-THF (5-MTHF) (0.13 mg/kg body weight). Placebo: $n = 25$; treated patients: $n = 15$. Measurements were performed in paired samples of both SV (saphenous vein) and IMA (internal mammary artery) from the same patients using 5 mM lucigenin-enhanced chemiluminescence. *$P < .01$ versus placebo. RLU/s/mg indicates relative light units per second per milligram. (Reprinted from Antoniades C, Shirodaria C, Warrick N, Cai S, de Bono J, Lee J, Leeson P, et al., *Circulation* 2006; 114:1193–201. With permission.)

2. Reaction with Thiyl Radical

In addition to participating in redox processes, thiols take part in scavenging of free radicals (reactions A and B, respectively).

$$RSH \rightarrow RS^{\bullet} + e^- + H^+ \hspace{3cm} \text{Reaction A}$$

$$R_1CH_2^{\bullet} + RSH \rightarrow R_1CH_3 + RS^{\bullet} \hspace{2cm} \text{Reaction B}$$

Both reactions involve formation of thiyl radicals ($RS^{\bullet}$). Thiyl radicals are oxidants that can initiate lipid peroxidation reactions by hydrogen abstraction from polyunsaturated fatty acids. In addition, thiyl radicals can induce *cis/trans*-isomerization of mono-and polyunsaturated fatty acids by addition to the double bond. Thus, repair of the thiyl radicals is important for both the maintenance of the antioxidant function of thiols and to prevent lipid damage [129].

Model studies suggested that folic acid not only scavenges thiyl radical but also repairs it back to its reduced form (RSH) at physiological pH [126]. The bimolecular rate constant for the reaction of folic acid with thiyl radical was found to be 6×10^8 $L \cdot mol^{-1} \cdot s^{-1}$ at pH 6. In support of this finding, it was found that folic acid inhibits microsomal lipid peroxidation in a dose-dependent fashion, with 37% protection at a concentration of folic acid of 500 μM [126]. The limited solubility of folic acid in the lipid phase could account for the high concentration required to achieve significant levels of protection.

B. INTERACTIONS OF FOLATE WITH eNOS AND H₄B

H₄B is an essential cofactor for NO biosynthesis, which underscores its importance in the prevention of endothelial dysfunction and related diseases [121]. Under normal physiological conditions eNOS catalyzes the stepwise oxidation of L-arginine to form NO and L-citrulline. This reaction is dependent on both NADPH and O_2 and takes place within the eNOS oxygenase domain dimer, which contains bound heme and H₄B [130–133]. Recent findings illustrate that under certain pathophysiological conditions, eNOS can "switch" from mainly NO synthesis to production of $O_2^{\bullet-}$, a process called eNOS uncoupling [134–137]. Deficiency of H₄B results in "uncoupling" of eNOS, a disruptive condition in which the production of NO is decreased and that of $O_2^{\bullet-}$ is increased [138]. As mentioned in the previous sections, administration of 5-methyl-THF results in the improvement of FMD without altering tHcy concentrations and also in the abolishment of Hcy-induced intracellular superoxide generation [74]. Both folic acid and H₄B were also found to abolish Hcy-induced superoxide production in cell culture [74]. This suggests that folic acid, 5-methyl-THF, and H₄B restore endothelial function by suppressing superoxide production and enhancing NO generation and/or increasing its half-life. In fact, it was noted that 5-methyl-THF has no effect on in vitro NO production by eNOS but induced a dose-dependent reduction in eNOS and xanthine oxidase–induced superoxide generation and reversed impaired endothelium-dependent vasodilation in patients with familial hypercholesterolemia [81]. The mechanism of this effect was attributed to the ability of 5-methyl-THF to reduce superoxide and enhance NO production [127].

Although incompletely understood, some of the actions of 5-methyl-THF and H_4B on the endothelium display a certain degree of specificity. Griffith et al. [119] have demonstrated that 5-methyl-THF and H_4B, but not folic acid or dihydrobiopterin, can modulate arterial function through effects on gap junctional communication and electrotonic signaling. Hyndman et al. [139] have shown that 5-methyl-THF binds to one of the active sites of eNOS and mimics the orientation of H_4B. Remarkably, the relative binding energy for 5-methyl-THF and H_4B were −16.92 and −13.96, respectively. The same group also reported that 5-methyl-THF attenuates superoxide production (induced by inhibition of H_4B synthesis) by eNOS and improves endothelial function in aortas isolated from H_4B-deficient rats. More specifically, a dose of 100 μM of either 5-methyl-THF or H_4B improved acetylcholine-mediated vasorelaxation of rat aorta rings to a similar degree [139].

Although our understanding of the interactions between folate, eNOS, and H_4B is incomplete, two potential mechanisms for the beneficial effects of folate on eNOS can be pictured in light of the recent in vitro and in vivo evidence [120].

1. Regeneration and/or Chemical Stabilization of H_4B

The structural similarity of 5-methyl-THF and H_4B makes it feasible for these cofactors to be interreplaceable as far as steric hindrance considerations go. Very interestingly, Mayer et al. [140] reported the presence of a pteridine-binding domain in NO synthase with similarities to the folate-binding site of dihydrofolate reductase. It was found that a synthetic peptide whose sequence mimics the putative dihydrofolate reductase domain of eNOS caused a concentration-dependent inhibition of enzyme activity. The inhibition appeared to be caused by interference with the enzymatic one-electron reduction of molecular oxygen. It has been speculated that this dihydrofolate reductase domain may act as a locus through which 5-methyl-THF can facilitate electron transfer by H_4B from the reductase domain of eNOS to heme [140]. Alternatively, 5-methyl-THF may enhance the binding of H_4B to eNOS or increase H_4B availability by chemical stabilization as it was described for ascorbic acid [141]. In addition, it has been suggested that folates can stimulate the regeneration of H_4B from the inactive oxidized $q-H_2B$ [142]. In support of these ideas, it has been confirmed that high-dose folate supplementation (as folinic acid) produced clinical improvement in children with H_4B deficiency [143].

2. Direct Effect on eNOS Coupling

Recent findings show that under certain pathophysiological conditions, eNOS can "switch" from mainly NO synthesis to production of $O_2^{\cdot-}$, a process called eNOS uncoupling [134–137]. Addition of H_4B results in a substantial reduction of superoxide production by eNOS in vitro [135,144] and in an improvement of NO availability in vivo [145,146]. This suggests that H_4B restores eNOS uncoupling. In a series of in vitro experiments, Stroes et al. [127] obtained strong evidence that 5-methyl-THF can also influence the enzymatic activity of uncoupled eNOS: 5-methyl-THF reduces superoxide generation and increases NO synthesis. Interestingly, the authors observed that in pterin-free eNOS, addition of 25 μM 5-methyl-THF did not cause significant changes in superoxide formation (Figure 12.6). However, addition of 5-methyl-THF to partially replete eNOS (still H_4B deficient) causes a substantial

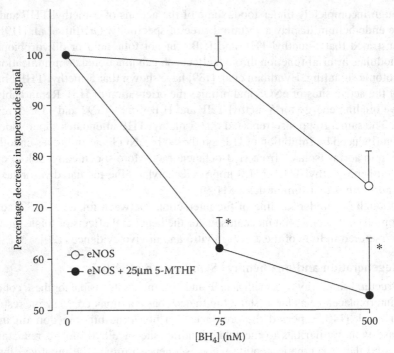

FIGURE 12.6 Effect of H_4B on superoxide production by eNOS in the presence and absence of 5-methyl-THF (5-MTHF). $P < .05$. The detection was performed by competitive superoxide trapping (CST) using 5-diethoxyphosphoryl-5-methyl-1-pyrroline-N-oxide (DEPMPO) as the spin trap. (From Stroes ES, van Faassen EE, Yo M, Martasek P, Boer P, Govers R, Rabelink TJ, *Circ Res* 2000; 86:1129–34. With permission.)

reduction in the amount of superoxide formed. Furthermore, the authors also found that preincubation of endothelial cells in culture with 1 to 10 μM 5-methyl-THF or 100 μM sepiapterin significantly enhances acetylcholine-induced nitrite production, an indirect measurement of NO production (Figure 12.7) [127]. In support of direct effects of 5-methyl-THF on eNOS, Antoniades et al. [92] found that short-term incubation of internal mammary artery with 1 μM 5-methyl-THF resulted in a significant increase in the eNOS dimer/monomer ratio, indicative of improvement in eNOS protein dimerization (Figure 12.8).

Finally, a comprehensive study performed in rats showed that high-dose folic acid pretreatment blunts cardiac dysfunction during ischemia [115]. The authors proposed that the observed effect involves preservation of high-energy phosphates, reduction of ROS generation, eNOS uncoupling, and myocardial necrosis. A rather dramatic result was observed on the protective effect of folic acid pretreatment against coronary flow decrease resulting from ischemia-reperfusion events. As expected, bradykinin administered to hearts in vitro before versus after ischemia-reperfusion showed a marked decrease in endothelium-dependent flow response. This was restored to a normal response by pretreatment with folic acid (Figure 12.9) [115].

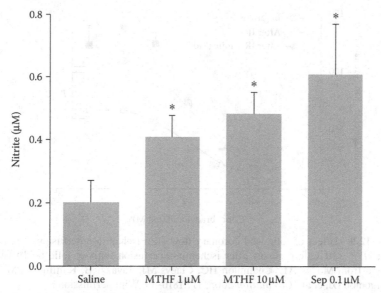

FIGURE 12.7   Effect of 5-methyl-THF (5-MTHF) and sepiapterin on NO production by endothelial cells in culture. $P < .05$ vs. saline. (From Stroes ES, van Faassen EE, Yo M, Martasek P, Boer P, Govers R, Rabelink TJ,. *Circ Res* 2000; 86:1129–34. With permission.)

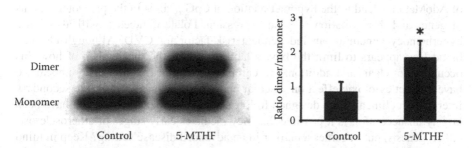

FIGURE 12.8   Ex vivo incubation of internal mammary artery with 1 mM 5-methyl-THF (5-MTHF) on eNOS dimerization. Dimer/monomer ratio was evaluated by immunoblotting after quantification of eNOS band intensity. $*P < .05$ vs. control. (Reprinted from Antoniades C, Shirodaria C, Warrick N, Cai S, de Bono J, Lee J, Leeson P, et al., *Circulation* 2006; 114:1193–201. With permission.)

VI.   SUMMARY AND CONCLUSIONS

To function properly, the cardiovascular system requires folate, an essential micronutrient that drives one-carbon metabolism. Thus, folate substrates are used for de novo purine biosynthesis, thymidylate synthesis, Hcy remethylation, and AdoMet

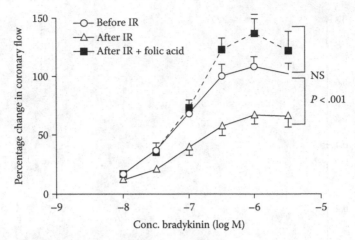

FIGURE 12.9 Effect of folic acid coronary flow after ischemia-reperfusion. NS, not significant; *P < .001 before versus after ischemia-reperfusion without folic acid treatment. (Reprinted from Moens AL, Champion HC, Claeys MJ, Tavazzi B, Kaminski PM, Wolin MS, Borgonjon DJ, et al., *Circulation* 2008; 117:1810–19. With permission.)

production. Folate deficiency can affect the cardiovascular system in a variety of ways. Impaired DNA replication may prevent the regeneration of endothelial stem cells that are needed to repair damaged endothelium. A decrease in the production of AdoMet may lead to the hypomethylation of CpG islands in the promoter regions of genes and dysregulation of gene expression. Folate deficiency will also cause hyperhomocysteinemia—an independent risk factor for CVD. Although elevated blood Hcy appears to limit the bioavailability of NO, the mechanism of how this occurs is not clear, and additional research is needed in this area. Hcy appears to have a direct cytotoxic effect on vascular endothelial cells. However, the secondary intervention clinical trials designed to lower tHcy in patients with CVD have been largely unsuccessful. Is it possible that Hcy mediates early stages of atherosclerosis (atherogenesis) but becomes a marker in an advanced disease setting? Keep in mind that all the secondary intervention trials enlist cohorts with advanced atherosclerosis, i.e., patients who have suffered an MI or stroke. The "mediator to marker hypothesis" could explain why the recent secondary intervention clinical trials have been, for the most part, negative.

On a more positive note, folic acid, 5-methyl-THF, and H_4B improve vascular endothelial cell function by mechanisms that only now are being worked out. This is an exciting area of research that could possibly lead to novel treatment modalities in the future.

REFERENCES

1. Morrison HI, Schaubel D, Desmeules M, Wigle DT. Serum folate and risk of fatal coronary heart disease. *JAMA* 1996; 275:1893–96.

2. Robinson K, Arheart K, Refsum H, Brattström L, Boers G, Ueland P, Rubba P, et al. Low circulating folate and vitamin B_6 concentrations—Risk factors for stroke, peripheral vascular disease, and coronary artery disease. *Circulation* 1998; 97:437–43.

3. Voutilainen S, Rissanen TH, Virtanen J, Lakka TA, Salonen JT. Low dietary folate intake is associated with an excess incidence of acute coronary events: The Kuopio Ischemic Heart Disease Risk Factor Study. *Circulation* 2001; 103:2674–80.

4. Chen P, Poddar R, Tipa EV, DiBello PM, Moravec CD, Robinson K, Green R, Kruger WD, Garrow TA, Jacobsen DW. Homocysteine metabolism in cardiovascular cells and tissues: Implications for hyperhomocysteinemia and cardiovascular disease. *Adv Enzyme Regul* 1999; 39:93–109.

5. Jacques PF, Selhub J, Bostom AG, Wilson PWF, Rosenberg IH. The effect of folic acid fortification on plasma folate and total homocysteine concentrations. *N Engl J Med* 1999; 340:1449–54.

6. Pfeiffer CM, Caudill SP, Gunter EW, Osterloh J, Sampson EJ. Biochemical indicators of B vitamin status in the US population after folic acid fortification: Results from the National Health and Nutrition Examination Survey 1999–2000. *Am J Clin Nutr* 2005; 82:442–50.

7. Anonymous. Food standards: Amendment of standards of identity for enriched grain products to require addition of folic acid. Final rule. *Fed Reg* 1996; 61:8781–97.

8. Pancharuniti N, Lewis CA, Sauberlich HE, Perkins LL, Go RCP, Alvarez JO, Macaluso M, et al. Plasma homocyst(e)ine, folate, and vitamin B_{12} concentrations and risk for early onset coronary artery disease. *Am J Clin Nutr* 1994; 59:940–48.

9. Rimm EB, Willett WC, Hu FB, Sampson L, Colditz GA, Manson JE, Hennekens C, Stampfer MJ. Folate and vitamin B_6 from diet and supplements in relation to risk of coronary heart disease among women. *JAMA* 1998; 279:359–64.

10. Verhoef P, Stampfer MJ, Buring JE, Gaziano JM, Allen RH, Stabler SP, Reynolds RD, Kok FJ, Hennekens CH, Willett WC. Homocysteine metabolism and risk of myocardial infarction: Relation with vitamins B_6, B_{12}, and folate. *Am J Epidemiol* 1996; 143:845–59.

11. Ford ES, Byers TE, Giles WH. Serum folate and chronic disease risk: Findings from a cohort of United States adults. *Int J Epidemiol* 1998; 27:592–98.

12. Loria CM, Ingram DD, Feldman JJ, Wright JD, Madans JH. Serum folate and cardiovascular disease mortality among US men and women. *Arch Intern Med* 2000; 160:3258–62.

13. Chasan-Taber L, Selhub J, Rosenberg IH, Malinow MR, Terry P, Tishler PV, Willett W, Hennekens CH, Stampfer MJ. A prospective study of folate and vitamin B_6 and risk of myocardial infarction in US physicians. *J Am Coll Nutr* 1996; 15:136–43.

14. Folsom AR, Nieto FJ, McGovern PG, Tsai MY, Malinow MR, Eckfeldt JH, Hess DL, Davis CE. Prospective study of coronary heart disease incidence in relation to fasting total homocysteine, related genetic polymorphisms, and B vitamins. The Atherosclerosis Risk in Communities (ARIC) study. *Circulation* 1998; 98:204–10.

15. Siri PW, Verhoef P, Kok FJ. Vitamins B_6, B_{12}, and folate: Association with plasma total homocysteine and risk of coronary atherosclerosis. *J Am Coll Nutr* 1998; 17:435–41.

16. Giles WH, Kittner SJ, Anda RF, Croft JB, Casper ML. Serum folate and risk for ischemic stroke: First National Health and Nutrition Examination Survey Epidemiologic Follow-up Study. *Stroke* 1995; 26:1166–70.

17. Yang Q, Botto LD, Erickson JD, Berry RJ, Sambell C, Johansen H, Friedman JM. Improvement in stroke mortality in Canada and the United States, 1990 to 2002. *Circulation* 2006; 113:1335–43.

18. McCully KS, Wilson RB. Homocysteine theory of arteriosclerosis. *Atherosclerosis* 1975; 22:215–27.

19. Clarke S, Banfield K. S-Adenosylmethionine-dependent methyltransferases. In: Carmel R, Jacobsen DW, eds., *Homocysteine in Health and Disease*. Cambridge, UK: Cambridge University Press, 2001:63–78.

20. Olteanu H, Banerjee R. Cobalamin-dependent remethylation. In: Carmel R, Jacobsen DW, eds., *Homocysteine in Health and Disease*. Cambridge, UK: Cambridge University Press, 2001:135–44.

21. Kruger WD. The transsulfuration pathway. In: Carmel R, Jacobsen DW, eds., *Homocysteine in Health and Disease*. Cambridge, UK: Cambridge University Press, 2001:153–61.

22. Finkelstein JD. Methionine metabolism in mammals. *J Nutr Biochem* 1990; 1:228–37.

23. Stover PJ, Garza C. Bringing individuality to public health recommendations. *J Nutr* 2002; 132:2476S–80S.

24. Dong C, Yoon W, Goldschmidt-Clermont PJ. DNA methylation and atherosclerosis. *J Nutr* 2002; 132:2406S–09S.

25. Jaenisch R, Bird A. Epigenetic regulation of gene expression: How the genome integrates intrinsic and environmental signals. *Nat Genet* 2003; 33(Suppl):245–54.

26. Zagris N, Podimatas T. 5-Azacytidine changes gene expression and causes developmental arrest of early chick embryo. *Int J Dev Biol* 1994; 38:741–44.

27. Kakutani T, Jeddeloh JA, Flowers SK, Munakata K, Richards EJ. Developmental abnormalities and epimutations associated with DNA hypomethylation mutations. *Proc Natl Acad Sci USA* 1996; 93:12406–11.

28. Alonso-Aperte E, Ubeda N, Achon M, Perez-Miguelsanz J, Varela-Moreiras G. Impaired methionine synthesis and hypomethylation in rats exposed to valproate during gestation. *Neurology* 1999; 52:750–56.

29. Finnell RH, Spiegelstein O, Wlodarczyk B, Triplett A, Pogribny IP, Melnyk S, James JS. DNA methylation in Folbp1 knockout mice supplemented with folic acid during gestation. *J Nutr* 2002; 132:2457S–61S.

30. Lee ME, Wang H. Homocysteine and hypomethylation. A novel link to vascular disease. *Trends Cardiovasc Med* 1999; 9:49–54.

31. Wang H, Yoshizumi M, Lai K, Tsai J-C, Perrella MA, Haber E, Lee M-E. Inhibition of growth and p21^{ras} methylation in vascular endothelial cells by homocysteine but not cysteine. *J Biol Chem* 1997; 272:25380–85.

32. Wang H, Jiang X, Yang F, Chapman GB, Durante W, Sibinga NE, Schafer AI. Cyclin A transcriptional suppression is the major mechanism mediating homocysteine-induced endothelial cell growth inhibition. *Blood* 2002; 99:939–45.

33. Yamada K, Gravel RA, Toraya T, Matthews RG. Human methionine synthase reductase is a molecular chaperone for human methionine synthase. *Proc Natl Acad Sci USA* 2006; 103:9476–81.

34. Tsai J-C, Perrella MA, Yoshizumi M, Hsieh C-M, Haber E, Schlegel R, Lee M-E. Promotion of vascular smooth muscle growth by homocysteine: A link to atherosclerosis. *Proc Natl Acad Sci USA* 1994; 91:6369–73.

35. Yang F, Tan HM, Wang H. Hyperhomocysteinemia and atherosclerosis. *Sheng Li Xue Bao* 2005; 57:103–14.

36. Baylin SB, Herman JG, Graff JR, Vertino PM, Issa JP. Alterations in DNA methylation: A fundamental aspect of neoplasia. *Adv Cancer Res* 1998; 72:141–96.

37. Yi P, Melnyk S, Pogribna M, Pogribny IP, Hine RJ, James SJ. Increase in plasma homocysteine associated with parallel increases in plasma S-adenosylhomocysteine and lymphocyte DNA hypomethylation. *J Biol Chem* 2000; 275:29318–23.

38. Friso S, Choi SW, Girelli D, Mason JB, Dolnikowski GG, Bagley PJ, Olivieri O, et al. A common mutation in the 5,10-methylenetetrahydrofolate reductase gene affects genomic DNA methylation through an interaction with folate status. *Proc Natl Acad Sci U S A* 2002; 99:5606–11.

39. Hiltunen MO, Turunen MP, Hakkinen TP, Rutanen J, Hedman M, Makinen K, Turunen AM, Aalto-Setala K, Yla-Herttuala S. DNA hypomethylation and methyltransferase expression in atherosclerotic lesions. *Vasc Med* 2002; 7:5–11.

40. Hiltunen MO, Yla-Herttuala S. DNA methylation, smooth muscle cells, and atherogenesis. *Arterioscler Thromb Vasc Biol* 2003; 23:1750–53.
41. Devlin AM, Bottiglieri T, Domann FE, Lentz SR. Tissue-specific changes in H19 methylation and expression in mice with hyperhomocysteinemia. *J Biol Chem* 2005; 280:25506–11.
42. Weiner AM. SINEs and LINEs: The art of biting the hand that feeds you. *Curr Opin Cell Biol* 2002; 14:343–50.
43. Prak ET, Kazazian HH Jr. Mobile elements and the human genome. *Nat Rev Genet* 2000; 1:134–44.
44. Deininger PL, Moran JV, Batzer MA, Kazazian HH Jr. Mobile elements and mammalian genome evolution. *Curr Opin Genet Dev* 2003; 13:651–58.
45. Post WS, Goldschmidt-Clermont PJ, Wilhide CC, Heldman AW, Sussman MS, Ouyang P, Milliken EE, Issa JP. Methylation of the estrogen receptor gene is associated with aging and atherosclerosis in the cardiovascular system. *Cardiovasc Res* 1999; 43:985–91.
46. Feinberg AP, Tycko B. The history of cancer epigenetics. *Nat Rev Cancer* 2004; 4:143–53.
47. Lund G, Andersson L, Lauria M, Lindholm M, Fraga MF, Villar-Garea A, Ballestar E, Esteller M, Zaina S. DNA methylation polymorphisms precede any histological sign of atherosclerosis in mice lacking apolipoprotein E. *J Biol Chem* 2004; 279:29147–54.
48. Zaina S, Lindholm MW, Lund G. Nutrition and aberrant DNA methylation patterns in atherosclerosis: More than just hyperhomocysteinemia? *J Nutr* 2005; 135:5–8.
49. Ross R. Atherosclerosis—An inflammatory disease. *N Engl J Med* 1999; 340:115–26.
50. Hansson GK, Libby P, Schonbeck U, Yan ZQ. Innate and adaptive immunity in the pathogenesis of atherosclerosis. *Circ Res* 2002; 91:281–91.
51. Blount BC, Mack MM, Wehr CM, MacGregor JT, Hiatt RA, Wang G, Wickramasinghe SN, Everson RB, Ames BN. Folate deficiency causes uracil misincorporation into human DNA and chromosome breakage: Implications for cancer and neuronal damage. *Proc Natl Acad Sci USA* 1997; 94:3290–95.
52. Fenech M. The role of folic acid and vitamin B12 in genomic stability of human cells. *Mutat Res* 2001; 475:57–67.
53. Le Brocq M, Leslie SJ, Milliken P, Megson IL. Endothelial dysfunction: From molecular mechanisms to measurement, clinical implications, and therapeutic opportunities. *Antioxid Redox Signal* 2008; 10:1631–74.
54. Vita JA, Treasure CB, Nabel EG, McLenachan JM, Fish RD, Yeung AC, Vekshtein VI, Selwyn AP, Ganz P. Coronary vasomotor response to acetylcholine relates to risk factors for coronary artery disease. *Circulation* 1990; 81:491–97.
55. Zeiher AM, Drexler H, Wollschlager H, Just H. Modulation of coronary vasomotor tone in humans. Progressive endothelial dysfunction with different early stages of coronary atherosclerosis. *Circulation* 1991; 83:391–401.
56. Schächinger V, Britten MB, Zeiher AM. Prognostic impact of coronary vasodilator dysfunction on adverse long-term outcome of coronary heart disease. *Circulation* 2000; 101:1899–906.
57. Zeiher AM, Krause T, Schachinger V, Minners J, Moser E. Impaired endothelium-dependent vasodilation of coronary resistance vessels is associated with exercise-induced myocardial ischemia. *Circulation* 1995; 91:2345–52.
58. Hasdai D, Gibbons RJ, Holmes DR Jr, Higano ST, Lerman A. Coronary endothelial dysfunction in humans is associated with myocardial perfusion defects. *Circulation* 1997; 96:3390–95.
59. Suwaidi JA, Hamasaki S, Higano ST, Nishimura RA, Holmes DR Jr, Lerman A. Long-term follow-up of patients with mild coronary artery disease and endothelial dysfunction. *Circulation* 2000; 101:948–54.

60. Celermajer DS, Sorensen KE, Gooch VM, Spiegelhalter DJ, Miller OI, Sullivan ID, Lloyd JK, Deanfield JE. Non-invasive detection of endothelial dysfunction in children and adults at risk of atherosclerosis. *Lancet* 1992; 340:1111–15.

61. Anderson TJ, Uehata A, Gerhard MD, Meredith IT, Knab S, Delagrange D, Lieberman EH, et al. Close relation of endothelial function in the human coronary and peripheral circulations. *J Am Coll Cardiol* 1995; 26:1235–41.

62. Takase B, Uehata A, Akima T, Nagai T, Nishioka T, Hamabe A, Satomura K, Ohsuzu F, Kurita A. Endothelium-dependent flow-mediated vasodilation in coronary and brachial arteries in suspected coronary artery disease. *Am J Cardiol* 1998; 82:1535–39, A7–8.

63. de Bree A, van Mierlo LA, Draijer R. Folic acid improves vascular reactivity in humans: A meta-analysis of randomized controlled trials. *Am J Clin Nutr* 2007; 86:610–17.

64. Ravikumar R, Deepa R, Shanthirani C, Mohan V. Comparison of carotid intima-media thickness, arterial stiffness, and brachial artery flow mediated dilatation in diabetic and nondiabetic subjects (The Chennai Urban Population Study [CUPS-9]). *Am J Cardiol* 2002; 90:702–07.

65. Schroeder S, Enderle MD, Ossen R, Meisner C, Baumbach A, Pfohl M, Herdeg C, Oberhoff M, Haering HU, Karsch KR. Noninvasive determination of endothelium–mediated vasodilation as a screening test for coronary artery disease: Pilot study to assess the predictive value in comparison with angina pectoris, exercise electrocardiography, and myocardial perfusion imaging. *Am Heart J* 1999; 138:731–39.

66. Bots ML, Westerink J, Rabelink TJ, de Koning EJ. Assessment of flow-mediated vasodilatation (FMD) of the brachial artery: Effects of technical aspects of the FMD measurement on the FMD response. *Eur Heart J* 2005; 26:363–68.

67. Ross R, Glomset JA. The pathogenesis of atherosclerosis (Part 1). *N Engl J Med* 1976; 295:369–77.

68. Ross R, Glomset JA. The pathogenesis of atherosclerosis (Part 2). *N Engl J Med* 1976; 295:420–25.

69. Boushey CJ, Beresford SA, Omenn GS, Motulsky AG. A quantitative assessment of plasma homocysteine as a risk factor for vascular disease. Probable benefits of increasing folic acid intakes. *JAMA* 1995; 274:1049–57.

70. Danesh J, Lewington S. Plasma homocysteine and coronary heart disease: Systematic review of published epidemiological studies. *J Cardiovasc Risk* 1998; 5:229–32.

71. Christen WG, Ridker PM. Blood levels of homocysteine and atherosclerotic vascular disease. *Curr Atheroscler Rep* 2000; 2:194–99.

72. Tawakol A, Omland T, Gerhard M, Wu JT, Creager MA. Hyperhomocyst(e)inemia is associated with impaired endothelium-dependent vasodilation in humans. *Circulation* 1997; 95:1119–21.

73. Woo KS, Chook P, Lolin YI, Sanderson JE, Metreweli C, Celermajer DS. Folic acid improves arterial endothelial function in adults with hyperhomocysteinemia. *J Am Coll Cardiol* 1999; 34:2002–06.

74. Doshi SN, McDowell IF, Moat SJ, Lang D, Newcombe RG, Kredan MB, Lewis MJ, Goodfellow J. Folate improves endothelial function in coronary artery disease: An effect mediated by reduction of intracellular superoxide? *Arterioscler Thromb Vasc Biol* 2001; 21:1196–202.

75. Ashfield-Watt PA, Moat SJ, Doshi SN, McDowell IF. Folate, homocysteine, endothelial function and cardiovascular disease. What is the link? *Biomed Pharmacother* 2001; 55:425–33.

76. Bellamy MF, McDowell IF, Ramsey MW, Brownlee M, Newcombe RG, Lewis MJ. Oral folate enhances endothelial function in hyperhomocysteinaemic subjects. *Eur J Clin Invest* 1999; 29:659–62.

77. Usui M, Matsuoka H, Miyazaki H, Ueda S, Okuda S, Imaizumi T. Endothelial dysfunction by acute hyperhomocyst(e)inaemia: Restoration by folic acid. *Clin Sci (Lond)* 1999; 96:235–39.

78. Doshi SN, McDowell IF, Moat SJ, Payne N, Durrant HJ, Lewis MJ, Goodfellow J. Folic acid improves endothelial function in coronary artery disease via mechanisms largely independent of homocysteine lowering. *Circulation* 2002; 105:22–26.

79. Bellamy MF, McDowell IF, Ramsey MW, Brownlee M, Bones C, Newcombe RG, Lewis MJ. Hyperhomocysteinemia after an oral methionine load acutely impairs endothelial function in healthy adults. *Circulation* 1998; 98:1848–52.

80. Olthof MR, Bots ML, Katan MB, Verhoef P. Acute effect of folic acid, betaine, and serine supplements on flow-mediated dilation after methionine loading: A randomized trial. *PLoS Clin Trials* 2006; 1:e4.

81. Verhaar MC, Wever RM, Kastelein JJ, van Dam T, Koomans HA, Rabelink TJ. 5-Methyltetrahydrofolate, the active form of folic acid, restores endothelial function in familial hypercholesterolemia. *Circulation* 1998; 97:237–41.

82. van Etten RW, de Koning EJ, Verhaar MC, Gaillard CA, Rabelink TJ. Impaired NO-dependent vasodilation in patients with type II (non-insulin-dependent) diabetes mellitus is restored by acute administration of folate. *Diabetologia* 2002; 45:1004–10.

83. Ross R. The pathogenesis of atherosclerosis: A perspective for the 1990s. *Nature* 1993; 362:801–09.

84. Terkeltaub R, Boisvert WA, Curtiss LK. Chemokines and atherosclerosis. *Curr Opin Lipidol* 1998; 9:397–405.

85. Riesenberg K, Levy R, Katz A, Galkop S, Schlaeffer F. Neutrophil superoxide release and interleukin 8 in acute myocardial infarction: Distinction between complicated and uncomplicated states. *Eur J Clin Invest* 1997; 27:398–404.

86. Matsumori A, Furukawa Y, Hashimoto T, Yoshida A, Ono K, Shioi T, Okada M, et al. Plasma levels of the monocyte chemotactic and activating factor/monocyte chemoattractant protein-1 are elevated in patients with acute myocardial infarction. *J Mol Cell Cardiol* 1997; 29:419–23.

87. Aukrust P, Ueland T, Muller F, Andreassen AK, Nordoy I, Aas H, Kjekshus J, Simonsen S, Froland SS, Gullestad L. Elevated circulating levels of C-C chemokines in patients with congestive heart failure. *Circulation* 1998; 97:1136–43.

88. Damas JK, Gullestad L, Ueland T, Solum NO, Simonsen S, Froland SS, Aukrust P. CXC-chemokines, a new group of cytokines in congestive heart failure—Possible role of platelets and monocytes. *Cardiovasc Res* 2000; 45:428–36.

89. Aukrust P, Berge RK, Ueland T, Aaser E, Damas JK, Wikeby L, Brunsvig A, et al. Interaction between chemokines and oxidative stress: Possible pathogenic role in acute coronary syndromes. *J Am Coll Cardiol* 2001; 37:485–91.

90. Holven KB, Aukrust P, Holm T, Ose L, Nenseter MS. Folic acid treatment reduces chemokine release from peripheral blood mononuclear cells in hyperhomocysteinemic subjects. *Arterioscler Thromb Vasc Biol* 2002; 22:699–703.

91. Verhaar MC, Wever RM, Kastelein JJ, van Loon D, Milstien S, Koomans HA, Rabelink TJ. Effects of oral folic acid supplementation on endothelial function in familial hypercholesterolemia. A randomized placebo-controlled trial. *Circulation* 1999; 100:335–38.

92. Antoniades C, Shirodaria C, Warrick N, Cai S, de Bono J, Lee J, Leeson P, et al. 5-Methyltetrahydrofolate rapidly improves endothelial function and decreases superoxide production in human vessels: Effects on vascular tetrahydrobiopterin availability and endothelial nitric oxide synthase coupling. *Circulation* 2006; 114:1193–201.

93. Moat SJ, Doshi SN, Lang D, McDowell IF, Lewis MJ, Goodfellow J. Treatment of coronary heart disease with folic acid: Is there a future? *Am J Physiol Heart Circ Physiol* 2004; 287:H1–7.

94. Lobo A, Naso A, Arheart K, Kruger WD, Abou-Ghazala T, Alsous F, Nahlawi M, et al. Reduction of homocysteine levels in coronary artery disease by low-dose folic acid combined with vitamins B6 and B12. *Am J Cardiol* 1999; 83:821–25.

95. Lowering blood homocysteine with folic acid based supplements: Meta-analysis of randomised trials. Homocysteine Lowering Trialists' Collaboration. *BMJ* 1998; 316:894–98.

96. Title LM, Cummings PM, Giddens K, Genest JJ Jr, Nassar BA. Effect of folic acid and antioxidant vitamins on endothelial dysfunction in patients with coronary artery disease. *J Am Coll Cardiol* 2000; 36:758–65.

97. Woo KS, Chook P, Chan LL, Cheung AS, Fung WH, Qiao M, Lolin YI, et al. Long-term improvement in homocysteine levels and arterial endothelial function after 1-year folic acid supplementation. *Am J Med* 2002; 112:535–39.

98. Chambers JC, Ueland PM, Obeid OA, Wrigley J, Refsum H, Kooner JS. Improved vascular endothelial function after oral B vitamins: An effect mediated through reduced concentrations of free plasma homocysteine. *Circulation* 2000; 102:2479–83.

99. Moat SJ, Madhavan A, Taylor SY, Payne N, Allen RH, Stabler SP, Goodfellow J, McDowell IF, Lewis MJ, Lang D. High- but not low-dose folic acid improves endothelial function in coronary artery disease. *Eur J Clin Invest* 2006; 36:850–59.

100. Pullin CH, Ashfield-Watt PA, Burr ML, Clark ZE, Lewis MJ, Moat SJ, Newcombe RG, Powers HJ, Whiting JM, McDowell IF. Optimization of dietary folate or low-dose folic acid supplements lower homocysteine but do not enhance endothelial function in healthy adults, irrespective of the methylenetetrahydrofolate reductase (C677T) genotype. *J Am Coll Cardiol* 2001; 38:1799–805.

101. Shirodaria C, Antoniades C, Lee J, Jackson CE, Robson MD, Francis JM, Moat SJ, et al. Global improvement of vascular function and redox state with low-dose folic acid: Implications for folate therapy in patients with coronary artery disease. *Circulation* 2007; 115:2262–70.

102. Title LM, Ur E, Giddens K, McQueen MJ, Nassar BA. Folic acid improves endothelial dysfunction in type 2 diabetes—An effect independent of homocysteine-lowering. *Vasc Med* 2006; 11:101–09.

103. Mangoni AA, Sherwood RA, Asonganyi B, Swift CG, Thomas S, Jackson SH. Short-term oral folic acid supplementation enhances endothelial function in patients with type 2 diabetes. *Am J Hypertens* 2005; 18:220–26.

104. MacKenzie KE, Wiltshire EJ, Gent R, Hirte C, Piotto L, Couper JJ. Folate and vitamin B6 rapidly normalize endothelial dysfunction in children with type 1 diabetes mellitus. *Pediatrics* 2006; 118:242–53.

105. Buccianti G, Baragetti I, Bamonti F, Furiani S, Dorighet V, Patrosso C. Plasma homocysteine levels and cardiovascular mortality in patients with end-stage renal disease. *J Nephrol* 2004; 17:405–10.

106. Mallamaci F, Bonanno G, Seminara G, Rapisarda F, Fatuzzo P, Candela V, Scudo P, et al. Hyperhomocysteinemia and arteriovenous fistula thrombosis in hemodialysis patients. *Am J Kidney Dis* 2005; 45:702–07.

107. Cianciolo G, La Manna G, Coli L, Donati G, D'Addio F, Persici E, Comai G, et al. 5-Methyltetrahydrofolate administration is associated with prolonged survival and reduced inflammation in ESRD patients. *Am J Nephrol* 2008; 28:941–48.

108. Buccianti G, Raselli S, Baragetti I, Bamonti F, Corghi E, Novembrino C, Patrosso C, Maggi FM, Catapano AL. 5-Methyltetrahydrofolate restores endothelial function in uraemic patients on convective haemodialysis. *Nephrol Dial Transplant* 2002; 17:857–64.

109. Baragetti I, Raselli S, Stucchi A, Terraneo V, Furiani S, Buzzi L, Garlaschelli K, Alberghini E, Catapano AL, Buccianti G. Improvement of endothelial function in uraemic patients on peritoneal dialysis: A possible role for 5-MTHF administration. *Nephrol Dial Transplant* 2007; 22:3292–97.

110. Danishpajooh IO, Gudi T, Chen Y, Kharitonov VG, Sharma VS, Boss GR. Nitric oxide inhibits methionine synthase activity in vivo and disrupts carbon flow through the folate pathway. *J Biol Chem* 2001; 276:27296–303.

111. Nicolaou A, Waterfield CJ, Kenyon SH, Gibbons WA. The inactivation of methionine synthase in isolated rat hepatocytes by sodium nitroprusside. *Eur J Biochem* 1997; 244:876–82.

112. Symons JD, Mullick AE, Ensunsa JL, Ma AA, Rutledge JC. Hyperhomocysteinemia evoked by folate depletion: Effects on coronary and carotid arterial function. *Arterioscler Thromb Vasc Biol* 2002; 22:772–80.

113. Zhang X, Chen S, Li L, Wang Q, Le W. Folic acid protects motor neurons against the increased homocysteine, inflammation and apoptosis in SOD1(G93A) transgenic mice. *Neuropharmacology* 2008; 54:1112–19.

114. Moens AL, Vrints CJ, Claeys MJ, Timmermans JP, Champion HC, Kass DA. Mechanisms and potential therapeutic targets for folic acid in cardiovascular disease. *Am J Physiol Heart Circ Physiol* 2008; 294:H1971–77.

115. Moens AL, Champion HC, Claeys MJ, Tavazzi B, Kaminski PM, Wolin MS, Borgonjon DJ, et al. High-dose folic acid pretreatment blunts cardiac dysfunction during ischemia coupled to maintenance of high-energy phosphates and reduces postreperfusion injury. *Circulation* 2008; 117:1810–19.

116. Tousoulis D, Antoniades C, Koumallos N, Marinou K, Stefanadi E, Latsios G, Stefanadis C. Novel therapies targeting vascular endothelium. *Endothelium* 2006; 13:411–21.

117. Leopold JA, Loscalzo J. Organic nitrate tolerance and endothelial dysfunction: Role of folate therapy. *Minerva Cardioangiol* 2003; 51:349–59.

118. Stanger O. Physiology of folic acid in health and disease. *Curr Drug Metab* 2002; 3:211–23.

119. Griffith TM, Chaytor AT, Bakker LM, Edwards DH. 5-Methyltetrahydrofolate and tetra-hydrobiopterin can modulate electrotonically mediated endothelium-dependent vascular relaxation. *Proc Natl Acad Sci USA* 2005; 102:7008–13.

120. Verhaar MC, Stroes E, Rabelink TJ. Folates and cardiovascular disease. *Arterioscler Thromb Vasc Biol* 2002; 22:6–13.

121. Das UN. Folic acid says NO to vascular diseases. *Nutrition* 2003; 19:686–92.

122. Huang RF, Yaong HC, Chen SC, Lu YF. In vitro folate supplementation alleviates oxidative stress, mitochondria-associated death signaling and apoptosis induced by 7-ketoc-holesterol. *Br J Nutr* 2004; 92:887–94.

123. Zabihi S, Eriksson UJ, Wentzel P. Folic acid supplementation affects ROS scavenging enzymes, enhances Vegf-A, and diminishes apoptotic state in yolk sacs of embryos of diabetic rats. *Reprod Toxicol* 2007; 23:486–98.

124. Schulz E, Jansen T, Wenzel P, Daiber A, Munzel T. Nitric oxide, tetrahydrobiopterin, oxidative stress, and endothelial dysfunction in hypertension. *Antioxid Redox Signal* 2008; 10:1115–26.

125. Munzel T, Sinning C, Post F, Warnholtz A, Schulz E. Pathophysiology, diagnosis and prognostic implications of endothelial dysfunction. *Ann Med* 2008; 40:180–96.

126. Joshi R, Adhikari S, Patro BS, Chattopadhyay S, Mukherjee T. Free radical scavenging behavior of folic acid: Evidence for possible antioxidant activity. *Free Radic Biol Med* 2001; 30:1390–99.

127. Stroes ES, van Faassen EE, Yo M, Martasek P, Boer P, Govers R, Rabelink TJ. Folic acid reverts dysfunction of endothelial nitric oxide synthase. *Circ Res* 2000; 86:1129–34.

128. Verhaar MC, Wever RMF, Kastelein JJP, Van Dam T, Koomans HA, Rabelink TJ. 5-Methyltetrahydrofolate, the active form of folic acid, restores endothelial function in familial hypercholesterolemia. *Circulation* 1998; 97:237–41.

129. Ferreri C, Kratzsch S, Landi L, Brede O. Thiyl radicals in biosystems: Effects on lipid structures and metabolisms. *Cell Mol Life Sci* 2005; 62:834–47.

130. Wei CC, Wang ZQ, Arvai AS, Hemann C, Hille R, Getzoff ED, Stuehr DJ. Structure of tetrahydrobiopterin tunes its electron transfer to the heme-dioxy intermediate in nitric oxide synthase. *Biochemistry* 2003; 42:1969–77.

131. Wei CC, Wang ZQ, Hemann C, Hille R, Stuehr DJ. A tetrahydrobiopterin radical forms and then becomes reduced during Nomega-hydroxyarginine oxidation by nitric-oxide synthase. *J Biol Chem* 2003; 278:46668–73.

132. Wei CC, Wang ZQ, Tejero J, Yang YP, Hemann C, Hille R, Stuehr DJ. Catalytic reduction of a tetrahydrobiopterin radical within nitric-oxide synthase. *J Biol Chem* 2008; 283:11734–42.

133. Wei CC, Wang ZQ, Wang Q, Meade AL, Hemann C, Hille R, Stuehr DJ. Rapid kinetic studies link tetrahydrobiopterin radical formation to heme-dioxy reduction and arginine hydroxylation in inducible nitric-oxide synthase. *J Biol Chem* 2001; 276:315–19.

134. Pritchard KA Jr, Groszek L, Smalley DM, Sessa WC, Wu M, Villalon P, Wolin MS, Stemerman MB. Native low-density lipoprotein increases endothelial cell nitric oxide synthase generation of superoxide anion. *Circ Res* 1995; 77:510–18.

135. Stroes E, Hijmering M, van Zandvoort M, Wever R, Rabelink TJ, van Faassen EE. Origin of superoxide production by endothelial nitric oxide synthase. *FEBS Lett* 1998; 438:161–64.

136. Xia Y, Roman LJ, Masters BS, Zweier JL. Inducible nitric-oxide synthase generates superoxide from the reductase domain. *J Biol Chem* 1998; 273:22635–39.

137. Xia Y, Tsai AL, Berka V, Zweier JL. Superoxide generation from endothelial nitric-oxide synthase. A Ca2+/calmodulin-dependent and tetrahydrobiopterin regulatory process. *J Biol Chem* 1998; 273:25804–08.

138. Ozkor MA, Quyyumi AA. Tetrahydrobiopterin. *Curr Hypertens Rep* 2008; 10:58–64.

139. Hyndman ME, Verma S, Rosenfeld RJ, Anderson TJ, Parsons HG. Interaction of 5-methyltetrahydrofolate and tetrahydrobiopterin on endothelial function. *Am J Physiol Heart Circ Physiol* 2002; 282:H2167–72.

140. Mayer B, Pitters E, Pfeiffer S, Kukovetz WR, Schmidt K. A synthetic peptide corresponding to the putative dihydrofolate reductase domain of nitric oxide synthase inhibits uncoupled NADPH oxidation. *Nitric Oxide* 1997; 1:50–55.

141. Heller R, Unbehaun A, Schellenberg B, Mayer B, Werner-Felmayer G, Werner ER. L-ascorbic acid potentiates endothelial nitric oxide synthesis via a chemical stabilization of tetrahydrobiopterin. *J Biol Chem* 2001; 276:40–47.

142. Kaufman S. Some metabolic relationships between biopterin and folate: Implications for the "methyl trap hypothesis." *Neurochem Res* 1991; 16:1031–36.

143. Smith I, Hyland K, Kendall B. Clinical role of pteridine therapy in tetrahydrobiopterin deficiency. *J Inherit Metab Dis* 1985; 8(Suppl 1):39–45.

144. Vasquez-Vivar J, Kalyanaraman B, Martasek P, Hogg N, Masters BS, Karoui H, Tordo P, Pritchard KA Jr. Superoxide generation by endothelial nitric oxide synthase: The influence of cofactors. *Proc Natl Acad Sci U S A* 1998; 95:9220–25.

145. Stroes E, Kastelein J, Cosentino F, Erkelens W, Wever R, Koomans H, Luscher T, Rabelink T. Tetrahydrobiopterin restores endothelial function in hypercholesterolemia. *J Clin Invest* 1997; 99:41–46.

146. Tiefenbacher CP, Chilian WM, Mitchell M, DeFily DV. Restoration of endothelium-dependent vasodilation after reperfusion injury by tetrahydrobiopterin. *Circulation* 1996; 94:1423–29.

147. Wilmink HW, Stroes ES, Erkelens WD, Gerritsen WB, Wever R, Banga JD, Rabelink TJ. Influence of folic acid on postprandial endothelial dysfunction. *Arterioscler Thromb Vasc Biol* 2000; 20:185–88.

148. van Dijk RA, Rauwerda JA, Steyn M, Twisk JW, Stehouwer CD. Long-term homocysteine-lowering treatment with folic acid plus pyridoxine is associated with decreased blood pressure but not with improved brachial artery endothelium-dependent vasodilation or carotid artery stiffness: A 2-year, randomized, placebo-controlled trial. *Arterioscler Thromb Vasc Biol* 2001; 21:2072–79.

149. Hirsch S, Pia De la Maza M, Yanez P, Glasinovic A, Petermann M, Barrera G, Gattas V, Escobar E, Bunout D. Hyperhomocysteinemia and endothelial function in young subjects: Effects of vitamin supplementation. *Clin Cardiol* 2002; 25:495–501.
150. Woodman RJ, Celermajer DE, Thompson PL, Hung J. Folic acid does not improve endothelial function in healthy hyperhomocysteinaemic subjects. *Clin Sci (Lond)* 2004; 106:353–58.
151. Carlsson CM, Pharo LM, Aeschlimann SE, Mitchell C, Underbakke G, Stein JH. Effects of multivitamins and low-dose folic acid supplements on flow-mediated vasodilation and plasma homocysteine levels in older adults. *Am Heart J* 2004; 148:E11.
152. Olthof MR, Bots ML, Katan MB, Verhoef P. Effect of folic acid and betaine supplementation on flow-mediated dilation: A randomized, controlled study in healthy volunteers. *PLoS Clin Trials* 2006; 1:e10.
153. Thambyrajah J, Landray MJ, Jones HJ, McGlynn FJ, Wheeler DC, Townend JN. A randomized double-blind placebo-controlled trial of the effect of homocysteine-lowering therapy with folic acid on endothelial function in patients with coronary artery disease. *J Am Coll Cardiol* 2001; 37:1858–63.
154. Sydow K, Schwedhelm E, Arakawa N, Bode-Boger SM, Tsikas D, Hornig B, Frolich JC, Boger RH. ADMA and oxidative stress are responsible for endothelial dysfunction in hyperhomocyst(e)inemia: Effects of L-arginine and B vitamins. *Cardiovasc Res* 2003; 57:244–52.
155. Lekakis JP, Papamichael CM, Papaioannou TG, Dagre AG, Stamatelopoulos KS, Tryfonopoulos D, Protogerou AD, Stamatelopoulos SF, Mavrikakis M. Oral folic acid enhances endothelial function in patients with hypercholesterolaemia receiving statins. *Eur J Cardiovasc Prev Rehabil* 2004; 11:416–20.
156. Thambyrajah J, Landray MJ, McGlynn FJ, Jones HJ, Wheeler DC, Townend JN. Does folic acid decrease plasma homocysteine and improve endothelial function in patients with predialysis renal failure? *Circulation* 2000; 102:871–75.
157. Bennett-Richards K, Kattenhorn M, Donald A, Oakley G, Varghese Z, Rees L, Deanfield JE. Does oral folic acid lower total homocysteine levels and improve endothelial function in children with chronic renal failure? *Circulation* 2002; 105:1810–15.
158. Pena AS, Wiltshire E, Gent R, Hirte C, Couper J. Folic acid improves endothelial function in children and adolescents with type 1 diabetes. *J Pediatr* 2004; 144:500–04.

13 Folate and Neurological Function

Epidemiological Perspective

Martha Savaria Morris and Paul F. Jacques

CONTENTS

I. INTRODUCTION

We have Victor Herbert's scientific zeal to thank for the inception of many of our current ideas about the functions of folate in the body and the consequences of folate deficiency. In 1961, Herbert made himself folate deficient over a period of months and documented psychiatric symptoms, including forgetfulness, irritability, and sleeplessness, which were cured by 2 days of folic acid treatment [1]. Although no general consensus exists today regarding the role that folate status plays in cognitive and affective disorders such as Alzheimer's disease (AD) and depression, many epidemiological studies conducted since the late 1990s have attempted to shed light on the subject. Reports of low circulating folate concentration in psychiatric patients [2] sparked some early case–control studies involving comparisons among different groups of psychiatric inpatients and between patients and nonpatients [3]. However, the main instigator of the flurry of epidemiological research activity that began at the end of the past century was the pressure to prove that elevated homocysteine (Hcy) concentrations contributed to the burden of cardiovascular disease, including stroke. Landmark studies published in the 1990s showed that AD and cerebrovascular disease were related [4] and that folate status was the principal determinant of circulating Hcy concentrations [5]. This latter finding came as a surprise because, although folate's role in Hcy remethylation was known, the variability of folate status in developed countries was thought insufficient to explain the variation in Hcy concentrations. The now-famous "nun" studies that established the link between brain infarcts and AD also showed that low serum folate was strongly related to neuropathological indicators of AD and to cognitive impairment when such pathology was present [6]. Together, these various discoveries raised the hope that the risk of stroke, vascular dementia, AD, and cognitive impairment in AD might be lowered by a simple dietary modification that was already virtually guaranteed in some countries by manda-tory folic acid fortification policies. Although microvascular disease, silent brain infarcts, or direct neurotoxic effects of Hcy or its metabolites could have contributed to Victor Herbert's symptoms and the nuns' brain lesions and cognitive impairment [7,8], modern epidemiological studies have identified Hcy-independent associations between folate status and cognition in the elderly population [9–11]. These findings are consistent with older ideas about how folate status influences central nervous system (CNS) function, namely, through effects on biogenic amine metabolism [12] and/or via folate's role in the synthesis of S-adenosylmethionine (SAM), the principal methyl group donor for the CNS [13]. Despite the long-held view that folate status, through its role in methylation reactions in the brain, is involved in mood regulation [14] and the touting of SAM supplements as mood enhancers [15], epidemiological studies evaluating the contribution of low folate status to the burden of depression in populations have appeared in the literature only very recently. In this chapter, the large and growing body of epidemiological literature examining associations between folate status indicators and age-related cognitive impairment and depression is reviewed. The findings of key studies are put into perspective with a focus on methodological details.

II. HCY, FOLATE, AND COGNITIVE FUNCTION IN OLDER ADULTS

A. METHODOLOGICAL CONSIDERATIONS

1. Study Design

Early epidemiological studies linking hyperhomocysteinemia or low folate status to a higher prevalence of cognitive impairment or AD had limited ability to revolution-ize thinking because of very small sample sizes, selected populations, and biases inher-ent in case–control designs [16–18]. By the end of 2005, however, findings had been published from several studies with more subjects and stronger designs, including a number of prospective investigations.

An important source of confusion has been the contribution of stroke to associa-tions between circulating Hcy concentration and cognitive impairment. Studies have established hyperhomocysteinemia as an independent risk factor for stroke [19,20], and stroke is one of the two main causes of dementia [21]. Consequently, studies that do not take stroke into account by excluding prospective subjects with stroke history, controlling for such history analytically, or considering stroke and AD as separate outcomes cannot distinguish between direct effects of folate or Hcy on brain function and the already elucidated connection between hyperhomocysteinemia and stroke. Another important consideration is the influence on results of temporal changes in folate intake caused by the increased health consciousness that comes with aging, the institution of folic acid fortification policies, and illness. If folate status is causally related to cognition and the induction time is long, people who have changed to high-folate diets may be misclassified in cross-sectional studies because their folate status was lower during the relevant period. Furthermore, prospective studies that follow subjects over the long term, but only assess diet at a single time point, may misclassify subjects if the induction time is short.

Confounding can also plague observational studies. For example, diabetes needs to be controlled for because it is a common illness that can simultaneously affect cognitive function [22], dietary habits, and circulating Hcy concentrations [23]. Some authors have mutually controlled data analyses for Hcy and folate in an attempt to shed light on the question of whether folate might have any effect on neurological function that is independent of Hcy. Results of such analyses are difficult to interpret, however. Specifically, confounding by folate (i.e., a direct effect of folate and no direct effect of Hcy) and mediation by Hcy in the causal pathway between low folate status and neurological function would both be reflected by attenuation of the Hcy association by controlling for folate status. Furthermore, although an association between folate status and neurological function that remains after control for Hcy could reflect effects of folate that are independent of the pathway mediated by Hcy, they could also merely reflect measurement error (i.e., a residual effect of Hcy caused by incomplete control).

Finally, in Hcy-lowering trials and in observational studies carried out where the food supply is fortified with folic acid, it is important to consider any potential inter-action between extremely high folic acid intake and vitamin B12 status. Consistent with the idea that neurocognitive consequences of vitamin B12 deficiency may be exacerbated by high folic acid intake [24], cognitive impairment was observed significantly more frequently among senior participants in the National Health and Nutrition Examination Survey (NHANES) with low vitamin B12 status and high circulating folate concentrations than it was among those with other combinations of the two factors [25].

2. Assessment of Cognitive Function

The diverse outcomes considered in studies evaluating a possible connection between nutrition and cognitive function reflect subtle differences in the hypotheses being addressed. Several studies have considered AD as an outcome, and a few have subcategorized patients with dementia as having vascular dementia or AD. Because AD cannot be definitively diagnosed in life [26], AD diagnosis in these studies was based on the natural history of dementia. Some recent research suggests that cognitive impairment in the elderly population generally constitutes some stage of AD [27] and that preclinical AD is not necessarily associated with any cognitive impairment [28]. Consequently, the application of strict AD criteria may result in misclassification as a result of contamination of the comparison group with subjects in an early stage of AD. Other studies have focused on cognitive impairment or cognitive decline, either because distinguishing subtypes of cognitive impairment was not feasible or because the authors were specifically interested in identifying factors that protect against the earliest age-related cognitive changes. However, if cognitive impairment can, as many suspect, indicate different disease processes or even normal cognitive aging [29], use of a nonspecific outcome such as poor cognitive test performance might contribute to negative study results when a true causal relation exists between folate status and some, but not all, forms of age-related cognitive impairment. It is also worth pointing out that, unless a permanent change in cognitive function is demonstrated, studies that reveal associations between dietary factors and cognitive test scores may be demonstrating short-term performance-enhancing effects that apply to generally healthy people and have nothing to do with the prevention of age-related cognitive decline. After all, it was just such a short-term phenomenon that Victor Herbert demonstrated in his famous experiment.

Many studies assessed cognitive function using the Mini-Mental State Examination (MMSE) developed by Folstein et al. in 1975 [30]. The test is in wide usage in clinical settings to quickly determine whether geriatric patients have dementia by assessing awareness of the time and place of testing, basic motor skills, language use and comprehension, and the ability to repeat lists of words. Use of the MMSE in epidemiological studies is somewhat problematic, however. Specifically, people with memory impairment but relative preservation of other cognitive domains, a group very likely to progress to dementia within 6 years [26], may perform relatively well on the MMSE. Consequently, despite the MMSE's utility at identifying people who may already have dementia, it may not be appropriate for identifying an at-risk population. Furthermore, rather than remaining stable or steadily declining with age, MMSE scores may increase over the short term [31]. Perhaps most importantly, low folate status or hyperhomocysteinemia may be associated with specific cognitive functions, whereas MMSE scores may be low only for people with multiple cognitive deficits, which is consistent with AD diagnostic criteria [32].

The problem for some large epidemiological studies is the goal of assessing many exposures and health outcomes simultaneously, such that a single test may be considered the only practical option. The choice of test(s) in some investigations has been made in the interest of replicating results of previous studies. For example, the only cognitive problem found to be associated with low folate status and hyperhomocysteinemia in a landmark study conducted by Riggs et al. [33] was impairment in visuoconstruction ability, which along with memory and language deficits is a prominent neuropsychological deficit of AD [34]. Visuoconstruction ability is variously assessed, but commonly used tests require subjects to arrange items in a pattern, copy a complex drawing, or create a freehand drawing of a familiar figure, such as a clock face. Tests of executive function, or the ability to connect past experience with present action, are commonly used, probably because dementia is defined as severe impairment of memory and executive function [35]. The transition from normal cognitive aging to early AD is marked by atrophy of the hippocampus [36], a brain area that appears crucial for episodic memory [37]. Consequently, a test of episodic memory was chosen as the cognitive function test administered to senior participants in the third NHANES (NHANES III). However, the idea that episodic memory has a unique status in distinguishing people who will and will not progress to AD has been challenged [38]. Furthermore, different forms of mild cognitive impairment (MCI) are now recognized [26], and a memory test may misclassify as normal subjects with nonamnestic MCI. Although some clinical MCI subtypes may not progress to AD, it is believed that most not only affect everyday functioning but will also evolve into recognized clinical entities, such as frontotemporal dementia, Lewy body dementia, Parkinson's disease with dementia, or progressive supranuclear palsy [39]. Therefore, the goal of characterizing the cognitive effects of low or high folate status, regardless of how they may relate to AD, seems worthwhile. Possibly because one theory of cognitive aging explains the decline as a decrease in the speed with which many processing operations can be executed [40], recent NHANES data collection cycles used the Digit Symbol Substitution Test (DSST) of attention and information processing speed. The DSST, which is more sensitive than the MMSE to changes in higher-level cognitive functioning [41], has also been included in many comprehensive test batteries.

Reporting results from individual cognitive function tests from a comprehensive battery increases the possibility of overinterpreting associations that have arisen merely by chance. However, properly cautious interpretation of epidemiological data implies recognition of the limitations of any single study. The motivation behind reporting a single composite score from a neuropsychological test battery is similar to that behind use of the MMSE. Because a clinical AD diagnosis requires multiple cognitive deficits, the calculation of a composite score from the individual test results makes sense. On the other hand, use of composite scores of global cognitive function might miss associations between folate status and/or hyperhomocysteinemia and cognitive impairment if these factors affect certain cognitive domains but not others. Creating composite scores for a defined cognitive domain also makes sense, in that a given test usually requires the application of a number of cognitive abilities, although even such combination of test results can mask effects. For example, recent research suggests that impairments in psychomotor speed and speed of information processing reflect dysfunction of two different domains [42].

B. Landmark Studies

After development of the serum folate assay in 1960, reports began to surface from Great Britain of low folate status in institutionalized dementia patients [43]. If those associations reflected causal relations, the direction was suspect because of likely deterioration of nutritional status brought about by mental illness or institutionalization. Inspired by these reports and by the general lack of data on effects of vitamin deficiencies in the elderly population, Goodwin et al. [44] conducted the landmark cross-sectional study relating intakes and circulating concentrations of micronutrients to cognitive test results in 1983. The authors focused on 300 normal, community-dwelling older people and found that those with low B vitamin status performed worse than other subjects on tests of delayed story recall and abstract thinking and problem solving. In 1997, results of analyses relating test performance in 1986 to concurrent and past nutritional status were described for 137 surviving cohort members [45]. Current folate intake and circulating and red blood cell (RBC) folate concentrations were once again related to results of a test of abstract thinking, whereas plasma and RBC folate concentrations measured in 1980 did not predict 1986 cognitive test performance. Furthermore, no association was found between folate status assessed in 1986 and results of memory tests administered concurrently.

In 1996, Riggs et al. [33] reported on 70 male veterans being followed in the Boston-based Normative Aging Study. Cross-sectional analyses carried out with data collected in 1993 revealed associations between both low plasma folate and higher plasma Hcy and poor performance on a visuoconstruction test but not on tests of language, perceptual speed and attention, memory, or spatial reasoning. Results of multivariate analyses mutually controlled for plasma folate and Hcy suggested that the association between folate status and figure copying ability was attributable to hyperhomocysteinemia. Several years later, Tucker et al. [11] reported on the baseline folate and Hcy concentrations of more than 300 of the veterans as predictors of decline in the various cognitive abilities over 1 to 4 years of follow-up. Consistent with the earlier cross-sectional study, results revealed associations between low folate status and high circulating Hcy concentrations and decline in figure copying ability that were not entirely independent of each other. However, in the multivariate analysis mutually controlled for folate and Hcy, only low folate status remained significantly associated with decline in this cognitive function. On the other hand, high plasma Hcy at baseline was related to decline in recall ability, but low B vitamin status was not. Consequently, the prospective data gave the impression that folate and Hcy affected different cognitive domains. Another possibility is that hyperhomocysteinemia at baseline indicated prodromal AD or microvascular disease predisposing the subjects to accelerated memory loss.

C. FOLATE, HCY, AND ALZHEIMER'S DISEASE

Results of formal tests of the hypothesis that low folate status or high circulating Hcy concentration is related to dementia or AD have been presented in 13 published articles in addition to Snowdon's above-mentioned report on the Sisters of Notre Dame (Table 13.1) [6,46–58]. All the investigators applied dementia diagnostic criteria specified in the *Diagnostic and Statistical Manual of Mental Disorders* (DSM) and/or by the National Institute for Neurological Disorders and Stroke Association–Alzheimer Disease and Related Disorders Association (NINDS-ADRDA), and most who reported on AD either required that cases meet criteria for probable AD or considered the effect on results of excluding possible AD cases. The earliest reports came from case-control studies. However, by February 2008, eight prospective studies, with follow-up time ranging from 2.4 to 8 years had been published [46–52], along with three cross-sectional analyses [48,53,54]. Potentially confounding factors accounted for in the studies varied but always included age and sex, and in all but one case [55], education. Ten studies specifically considered folate status in relation to AD or any dementia [10,47,49–54,56,57], and six linked low folate status to a higher

TABLE 13.1

Studies Investigating the Relationship between Folate or Homocysteine (Hcy) Status and Dementia

First Author	Design	n	Age Range	Outcomes	Significant Findings Hcy	Significant Findings Folate
McCaddon [55]	Case–control	60	Median = 79 y	AD	√	NA
Clarke [56]	Case–control	272	≥55 y	AD	√	√
Wang [46]	3-y follow-up	370	≥75 y	AD, dementia	NA	–
McIlroy [63]	Case–control	232	Mean = 74.3 y	AD, VAD	√, √	NA
Seshadri [47]	8-y follow-up	1,092	Mean ≅ 77 y	AD, dementia	√, √	–
Quadri [57]	Cross-sectional	232	≥60 y	AD/VAD, MCI	√, —	√, √
Luchsinger [48]	Cross-sectional	909	>65 y	AD	—	NA
Luchsinger [48]	4-y follow-up	679	>65 y	AD	—	NA
Ramos [54]	Cross-sectional	1,721	≥60 y	AD	—	√
Ravaglia [49]	4-y follow-up	816	>65 y	AD, dementia	√, √	√, √
Luchsinger [53]	6-y follow-up	965	>65 y	AD	—	√
Morris [50]	4-y follow-up	1,041	≥65 y	AD	NA	—
Haan [52]	4.5-y follow-up	1,405	≥60 y	AD/CIND	√[a]	—
Kim [51]	2.4-y follow-up	518	≥65 y	Dementia	√[b]	√

[a] The relationship between Hcy and AD/CIND was no longer significant when stroke was controlled for.
[b] Change in Hcy over the follow-up period was associated with AD; Hcy at baseline was not.

AD prevalence [54,56,57] or incidence [49,51,53]. An analysis of data collected in the prospective Framingham Study was among the four investigations that failed to link low folate status to AD. Importantly, however, hyperhomocysteinemia at baseline was significantly associated with a subsequent AD diagnosis [47], and the folate results were complicated by the institution of government-mandated folic acid fortification of foods during the 8-year follow-up period. At first glance, the prospective results from the postfortification Sacramento Area Latino Study on Aging (SALSA) [52] appear similar. However, the association between hyperhomocysteinemia and dementia/cognitive impairment in the SALSA was reduced and became nonsignificant when results were adjusted for incident stroke. The SALSA's findings may have been affected by the combination of AD and cognitive impairment without dementia (CIND) into a single outcome category. To elaborate, CIND cases are heterogeneous, and some may improve to an unimpaired state within 3 years [31,58]. Moreover, previously conducted cross-sectional analyses involving baseline (1998) data revealed an association between lower RBC folate concentrations and dementia [54,59] but not CIND [59].

The Chicago Health and Aging Project (CHAP) failed to find an association between baseline folate intake and subsequent AD. Furthermore, CHAP authors had concluded from a previous analysis that, in contrast to both expectation and results of cross-sectional analyses of baseline data, the rate of cognitive decline among cohort members increased significantly with increasing folate intake at baseline. Users of supplements providing 401 to 1,200 µg/day folic acid also declined significantly more rapidly over a median 5.5 years of follow-up than nonsupplement users [60]. The authors suspected that high folic acid intake might have exacerbated neurological syndromes associated with vitamin B12 deficiency. Indeed, postfortification NHANES data suggested that high folate status was associated with poor cognitive function in subjects with low vitamin B12 status [25]. However, higher folate status was associated with better cognitive function in all seniors combined. The CHAP was another prospective American study whose follow-up period encompassed the year 1998, when mandatory folic acid fortification went into effect. If folate intake during follow-up was relevant to diagnosis, it follows from evidence of marked increases in folate intake [61] and status [62] effected by fortification that relevant intake was underestimated by baseline data. CHAP authors reported that almost all the final cognitive assessments occurred after government-mandated folic acid fortification was instituted, whereas nutritional assessments mainly occurred before fortification. Thus, the appearance of relative protection from cognitive decline by low baseline folate status might have reflected unequal distribution of the cognitive benefits of fortification (i.e., fortification may have effected stabilization or improvement of cognition among folate-deficient subjects alone).

A final report with no significant association between baseline folate status and AD incidence was based on data collected in the Swedish Kungsholmen Project [46]. Two unique aspects of this investigation were the relatively advanced age of the subjects and oversampling from among those whose MMSE scores at age 75 years were below the typically applied cut-off point for suspicion of AD. Because of these design features, the study's negative findings may argue against any benefits of increased folate status on progression from prodromal to clinically evident AD.

Except under conditions of food folic acid fortification, circulating Hcy concentrations mainly reflect folate status [5]. Consequently, studies that reported on Hcy, but not folate, as main effects are also relevant to the hypothesis that higher folate status protects against AD [48,55,63]. Using a case–control design, McIlroy et al. [63] found that patients diagnosed with AD, patients diagnosed with vascular dementia (VAD), and stroke patients without dementia were all significantly more likely than controls to have plasma Hcy concentrations of 13.3 µmol/L or greater. Consistent with that report, McCaddon et al. [55] found a large difference in Hcy concentration between AD patients and high-functioning controls. In contrast to these case–control studies, the Washington Heights-Inwood Columbia Aging Project (WHICAP) revealed no associations between circulating Hcy concentrations and AD risk or prevalence after controlling for age and other covariates [48], although a connection between higher folate intake and protection from AD was later found in the same cohort [53]. As the preliminary analyses demonstrated, the prevalence of diabetes in the cohort was high, and the diabetic subjects had significantly lower circulating Hcy concentrations than the nondiabetic subjects, possibly accounting for the lack of association between Hcy and AD.

A few investigators who linked both folate status and Hcy concentrations to AD or dementia attempted to determine whether folate bore any relation to the outcome that was independent of folate's connection to Hcy. Multivariate adjustment for Hcy had virtually no effect on odds ratios (ORs) relating low folate status to AD, VAD, or any dementia in Quadri et al.'s [57] Italian cross-sectional study. Furthermore, significant associations were found between low folate status and dementia after analyses conducted by Ramos et al. [54] and Ravaglia et al. [49] were controlled for Hcy. Also, although Clarke et al. [56] reported that observed associations between folate status and AD operated through folate's connection with Hcy, Kim et al. [51] found that an association between Hcy increase and dementia incidence in a Korean population was largely explained by change in folate status.

D. FOLATE, HCY, AND COGNITIVE TEST PERFORMANCE

A strong research focus on AD is not surprising considering that adults over age 55 years fear AD more than any other health problem [64]. However, when Goodwin et al. [44] embarked on their landmark study of vitamin status and cognitive test performance, they were interested in subtle aberrations in cognitive function, perhaps because it seemed unlikely that the commonly encountered subclinical malnutrition that concerned them could cause such a devastating outcome as AD. Today, MCI is considered an important public health problem because it either is AD or predisposes to it. In fact, cognitive function tests administered to elderly NHANES participants were selected because they were believed to be more sensitive to dementia than the MMSE [65]. However, Goodwin et al. [44] pointed out that subtle cognitive deficits are important in their own right because of strong associations with mortality. Moreover, the World Health Organization, in its charter, affirmed the right of every human to enjoy the highest attainable standard of health, defined as a state of complete physical, mental, and social well-being and not merely the absence of disease or infirmity [66]. Analytic epidemiological studies that focus on cognitive test performance address the combined purpose of preventing life-threatening disease, including AD, and optimizing the mental health of elderly people who are experiencing so-called "normal" aging.

Cross-sectional analyses relating Hcy concentration and/or folate status to MMSE scores or modified MMSE scores have been described in 11 articles (Table 13.2), 8 of which reported significant [54,67–72] or marginally significant [73] associations. Most of the studies reported exclusively on Hcy, and only three of the nine cross-sectional studies that considered associations between Hcy concentrations and MMSE failed to demonstrate them. Two of the exceptions were based on Rotterdam data [74,75], and the third was the small Oxford Project to Investigate Memory and Aging (OPTIMA) [76]. The most likely explanation for the failure of the Rotterdam Scan Study and the OPTIMA to link Hcy concentrations to MMSE scores was the requirement for participants to not have dementia or have MMSE scores above a certain cut-off point. Feng et al. [73] also studied subjects without dementia, and they demonstrated only marginally significant associations between Hcy and folate concentrations and MMSE scores. The status of the MMSE as a dementia-screening tool bears emphasis here. Hyperhomocysteinemia may also be related to more subtle cognitive deficits. However, such effects may not be demonstrable using the MMSE. In fact, both studies that failed to find cross-sectional associations between Hcy concentrations and MMSE scores, and also used other cognitive function tests, linked high Hcy concentrations to low scores on some other tests [75,76]. The negative

TABLE 13.2

Studies Investigating the Relationship between Folate or Homocysteine (Hcy) Status and Mini-Mental State Examination (MMSE) Scores

First Author	Design	n	Age Range	Exclusions for Dementia	Significant Findings Hcy	Folate
Kalmijn [74]	Cross-sectional	630	≥55 y	None	—	NA
Kalmijn [74]	Nested case–control	702	≥55 y	None	—	NA
Lindeman [68]	Cross-sectional	793	≥65 y	None	NA	√
Prins [75]	Cross-sectional	1,027	≥60 y	MMSE < 26	—	NA
Seshadri [47]	8-y follow-up	1,092	Mean ≅ 77 y	Demented	√	NA
Duthie [69]	Cross-sectional	186	79 y	None	√	√
Duthie [69]	Cross-sectional	148	64 y	None	—	—
Budge [76]	Cross-sectional	158	60–91 y	None	—	NA
Dufouil [67]	Cross-sectional	1,241	Mean = 67 y	None	√	NA
Dufouil [67]	4-y follow-up	1,241	Mean = 67 y	None	$P = .05$	NA
Ravaglia [71]	Cross-sectional	650	≥65 y	MMSE < 24	√	—
Miller[a] [70]	Cross-sectional	1,789	≥60 y	None	√	NA
Wright [72]	Cross-sectional	2,871	>65 y	None	√	NA
Wright [72]	Cross-sectional	1,049	40–65 y	None	—	NA
Ramos[a] [54]	Cross-sectional	1,356	≥60 y	None	NA	√
Tucker [11]	3-y follow-up	321	Mean = 67 y	None	—	—
Feng [73]	Cross-sectional	451	Mean = 64.2 y	MMSE < 24	$P = .07$	$P = .06$
Kang[b] [78]	10-y follow-up	635	≥70 y	None	NA	—

[a] The Sacramento Area Latino Study on Aging used the 3MSE, which is a modified MMSE on a 100-point scale.

[b] The Nurses' Health Study used a version of the MMSE adapted for telephone interviews.

results for younger subgroups of participants in studies set in Aberdeen, Scotland [69] and northern Manhattan [72] may also be explained by the insensitivity of the MMSE to subtle cognitive impairment, which would be the main type of cognitive impairment affecting nonelderly adults. Indeed, the mean MMSE score for members of the 64-year-old Aberdeen cohort was 28.9 [69], indicating a lack of dementia but not necessarily near-perfect cognitive function, as the MMSE score might seem to suggest.

Seven cross-sectional studies considered folate status as a main effect [54,68,69,71–73,77]. No association was reported in the 64-year-old Aberdeen cohort only [69] or for participants in the Italian Conselice Study of Brain Aging (CABS) [71]. The CABS was another study involving only people without dementia. However, its authors reported an association between MMSE scores and circulating concentrations of Hcy but not folate. Unique attributes of that study's subjects were low educational achievement and low folate status. Specifically, only 20% of the subjects had more than 5 years of formal education, and the mean plasma folate concentration of less than 12 nmol/L characterized only a minority of subjects in other studies. The

MMSE may be able to detect subtle defects in cognitive function in poorly educated populations, in which the chance of encountering mainly perfect scores would be low. However, the CABS population may have presented an analogous impediment to the detection of an association, namely, a lack of high folate concentrations.

Few investigators have considered prospective associations between Hcy and/or folate concentrations and either MMSE scores or MMSE score decline, and only one study found a statistically significant association. It is instructive, however, to consider the results in relation to follow-up time. In two negative studies focusing on Hcy, subjects without dementia were followed for 2 to 3 years [11,74]. On the other hand, a marginally significant association between baseline Hcy concentrations and subsequent MMSE performance was found in a study that assessed cognitive function 4 years after baseline [67]. Finally, Seshadri et al. [47] reported that a significant association between baseline Hcy concentration and MMSE scores was detectable in Framingham cohort members only after 4 years of follow-up. Together with the results of cross-sectional studies, results of the prospective studies add support to the idea that some negative findings reflect the insensitivity of the MMSE to minor cognitive changes. Specifically, MMSE scores may remain high for a long period in people who are progressing toward dementia.

Only two studies evaluated the prospective association between folate status and MMSE scores. Tucker et al. [11] found no association despite linking folate status to scores on a visuoconstruction task. A sample of Nurses' Health Study (NHS) participants were administered a version of the MMSE adapted for use in telephone interviews, and the investigators found no association between folate status in 1989 and 1990 and either scores obtained approximately 10 years later or a 4-year decrease in scores after the baseline cognitive assessments [78]. Two additional findings from that study are worth noting. First, women who were in the second quartile category for plasma folate had nonsignificantly higher scores on the Telephone Interview for Cognitive Status (TICS) than women in the first quartile category, whereas women with higher plasma folate performed very slightly worse than women in the referent category. Second, the authors noted an interaction between multivitamin use and vitamin B12 status, suggesting that whether multivitamin use was beneficial or detrimental to cognition depended on vitamin B12 status. To elaborate, women whose vitamin B12 status remained low despite multivitamin use had the lowest cognitive scores, and women who used multivitamins and had high vitamin B12 status had the highest cognitive scores. Because 67% of the women in the highest quartile category for plasma folate were multivitamin users, these results may be consistent with findings from a postfortification NHANES cycle suggesting that whether high folate status was beneficial or detrimental to cognition depended on vitamin B12 status [25].

Associations between folate status and/or Hcy concentrations and performance on cognitive tests other than the MMSE have been reported in 22 articles (Table 13.3). Included among the studies were nine prospective analyses with follow-up times ranging from 2.3 to 10 years. Sample sizes ranged from less than 200 to almost 4,000 subjects, and 11 studies involved more than 1,000 people. Only the previously mentioned NHS and CHAP investigations, both of which focused on folate status alone, reported null or negative results. Findings of the positive studies

TABLE 13.3

Studies Investigating the Relationship between Folate or Homocysteine (Hcy) Status and Neuropsychological Test Performance

First Author	Design	n	Age Range	Test Used	Significant Findings Hcy	Significant Findings Folate
Lindeman [68]	Cross-sectional	793	≥65 y	Several	NA	$\sqrt{}$[a,b]
Morris [10]	Cross-sectional	1,270	≥60 y	Story recall	$\sqrt{}$[a]	$\sqrt{}$[a]
Prins [75]	Cross-sectional	1,027	≥60 y	Several	$\sqrt{}$[b,c]	NA
Duthie [69]	Cross-sectional	186	79 y	Several	$\sqrt{}$[c,d]	$\sqrt{}$
Duthie [69]	Cross-sectional	148	64 y	Several	—	$\sqrt{}$[d]
Budge [76]	Cross-sectional	158	60–91 y	CAMCOG[e]	$\sqrt{}$[a]	NA
Dufouil [67]	Cross-sectional	1,241	Mean = 67 y	Several	$\sqrt{}$[b (P = .06),c]	NA
Dufouil [67]	4-y follow-up	1,241	Mean = 67 y	Several	$\sqrt{}$[b (P = .08),c]	NA
Miller [70]	Cross-sectional	1,789	≥60 y	Several	$\sqrt{}$	NA
Garcia [82]	2.4-y follow-up	180	≥65 y	Stroop test	$\sqrt{}$[b]	NA
Ramos [54]	Cross-sectional	1,356	≥60 y	Several	NA	$\sqrt{}$[a]
Nurk [79]	6-y follow-up	2,189	65–68 y	KOLT[f]	$\sqrt{}$[a]	—
Tucker [11]	3-y follow-up	321	Mean = 67 y	Several	$\sqrt{}$[a,d]	$\sqrt{}$[d]
Morris [60]	5.5-y follow-up	3,718	Mean = 74 y	Global ability	NA	Negative
Kado [134]	Cross-sectional	370	70–79 y	Global ability	$\sqrt{}$	—
Kado [134]	7-y follow-up	370	70–79 y	Global ability	—	$\sqrt{}$
Shafer [83]	Cross-sectional	1,140	50–70 y	Several	$\sqrt{}$[a,b,c,d]	NA
Durga [9]	Cross-sectional	819	50–70 y	Several	NA	$\sqrt{}$[a,c]
Clark [135]	Cross-sectional	200	56–67 y	Several	$\sqrt{}$[a]	NA
Elias [80]	7.6-y follow-up	659	40–49 y	Global ability	—	NA
Elias [80]	7.6-y follow-up	732	50–59 y	Global ability	—	NA
Elias [80]	7.6-y follow-up	705	60–82 y	Global ability	$\sqrt{}$	NA
Feng [73]	Cross-sectional	451	≥55 y	Several	$\sqrt{}$[b,c,d]	$\sqrt{}$[a,b]
Kang [78]	10-y follow-up	635	≥70 y	None	NA	—
Morris [25]	Cross-sectional	1,302	≥60 y	DSST[g]	$\sqrt{}$[c]	$\sqrt{}$[c]
Elias [136]	Cross-sectional	812	Mean = 62 y	Several	$\sqrt{}$[a,b]	$\sqrt{}$[b]
de Lau [137]	Cross-sectional	1,033	≥60 y	Several	NA	$\sqrt{}$[c]

[a] A significant association was found for a test of recall or memory.
[b] A significant association was found for a test of executive function.
[c] A significant association was found for a test of speed.
[d] A significant association was found for a test of visuospatial ability.
[e] CAMCOG = Cambridge Cognitive Examination.
[f] KOLT = Kendrick Object Learning Test.
[g] DSST = Digit-Symbol Substitution Test.

are not easily summarized because of variation in the test batteries used and the cognitive domains assessed. Memory function was specifically related to Hcy concentration in eight studies [10,11,76,79–83], three of which were prospective [11,79,80]. In fact, after following Framingham Offspring Cohort members for

7.6 years, Elias et al. [80] reported that in cohort members aged 60 to 82 years, higher Hcy concentrations were associated with poorer performance on a wide variety of tests, including tests of abstract thinking and verbal learning and memory. An important feature of that study was stratification of the analyses by age group, which, consistent with results obtained by Duthie et al. [69] and Wright et al. [72] using MMSE scores, revealed no associations between Hcy status and cognitive function in subjects who were younger than 60 years of age. This finding probably reflects the generally high cognitive function of younger adults, regardless of their exposures. On the other hand, Duthie et al. [69] linked poor visuoconstruction ability, but no other cognitive impairment, to low folate status in their younger cohort. Although this finding could have been the result of chance, it may also highlight an early cognitive effect of low folate status. This idea is reinforced by results obtained for veterans participating in the Normative Aging Study [11]. Although the men were followed for only 3 years, those with low folate status at baseline were significantly more impaired in visuoconstruction ability than those with higher folate status at baseline, although no other cognitive differences were observed. Another interesting finding regarding visuoconstruction obtained by Duthie et al. was a significant association with Hcy concentration, but not folate status, for a 79-year-old cohort.

Considering the possibility that cognitive speed is a heterogeneous concept and slow information processing is pathognomonic for cognitive decline, the several studies that reported results from a letter/symbol-digit substitution-type test are of interest. Most of these studies evaluated the association between Hcy concentration and test performance, and all that did found a significant association [25,67,69,73,75], including both cross-sectional and prospective analyses of data collected in the Epidemiology of Vascular Aging study. Three studies that considered folate status in relation to letter/symbol-digit substitution performance found no association [9,69,73]. On the other hand, the analysis of postfortification NHANES data revealed that, in subjects with normal vitamin B12 status, high folate status was associated with protection from poor test performance even when a term for hyperhomocysteinemia was in the multivariate model [25]. Consequently, although no conclusion can be reached regarding a specific link between folate status and information processing speed, there seems to be relatively strong support for an association between slow information processing and higher Hcy concentrations. It is important to note that slow cerebration is a particular hallmark of vitamin B12 deficiency [81]. However, associations between slow information processing and Hcy concentration were revealed by Dufouil et al. [67] from both cross-sectional and prospective analyses after controlling for vitamin B12 status.

One of the early reports from an epidemiological study of a link between hyperhomocysteinemia and cognitive impairment was based on results of the Stroop test [82], which supposedly evaluates executive function, a reputation shared with verbal fluency, Trails B, Purdue Pegboard Assembly, and tests of nonverbal fluency and abstract thinking. Ten authors reported on results of such tests [9,11,54,67,68,70,73,75,82,83], but only five of them considered folate [9,11,54,68,73]. One report of significant relationships came from the Singapore Longitudinal Aging Study, in which a cross-sectional association was observed between folate status and verbal fluency but not design fluency. Results from that study were similarly mixed but reversed for Hcy, in that higher Hcy was related to poor performance on design fluency but not verbal fluency. These results were not entirely consistent with those of other studies that reported on verbal fluency, however. Specifically, although Hcy concentration was also unrelated to verbal fluency in the Normative Aging Study [11], it was related to both verbal fluency and Stroop scores in the Rotterdam Scan Study [75]. Furthermore, neither Tucker et al. [11] nor Durga et al. [9] linked folate status to verbal fluency. Results for Trails B were similarly mixed, with one study finding a significant association with folate status [68], two studies finding no association with Hcy concentration [73,83], and one study finding marginally significant associations with Hcy concentration both cross-sectionally and prospectively [67]. In the Baltimore Memory Study, Hcy concentration was related to poor performance on the Purdue Pegboard Assembly Test and a test of abstract thinking, but not the Stroop test [83]. The SALSA found no association between either folate status [54] or Hcy concentration [70] and performance on a test of abstract thinking.

Few authors have reported on the effect of mutually controlling for Hcy and folate on results of analyses relating folate and/or Hcy to performance on specific neuropsychological tests, and even fewer have considered the possibility of interactions. Although an analysis of NHANES III data revealed cross-sectional associations between both folate status and circulating Hcy concentrations and delayed recall ability, results of a test of interaction suggested that this ability was preserved in senior survey participants with higher folate status, regardless of their Hcy concentrations. This finding suggests that, despite the significant associations found between Hcy concentration and memory function in several studies, there are circumstances under which memory function is relatively preserved in seniors with hyperhomocysteinemia, and the condition of higher folate status may be among them. Such a finding could suggest Hcy-independent effects of folate, at least on verbal memory function. Results from the Singapore Longitudinal Study of Aging seem to support this idea. In that study, circulating concentrations of Hcy and folate were related to results of completely different tests. Specifically, Hcy was related to tests of nonverbal fluency, speed of information processing, and visuoconstruction ability, whereas folate was related to verbal fluency, immediate and delayed recall ability, and verbal learning.

E. FOLIC ACID TREATMENT AND COGNITIVE FUNCTION

A small number of randomized clinical trials have assessed the effect of treatment with folic acid supplements, or combined B vitamin supplements, on neuropsychological test performance (Table 13.4). The focus here is on those trials that were carried out neither in populations with dementia nor in subjects deficient in some specific nutrient other than folate. Except for the Folic Acid and Carotid Intima Thickness (FACIT) trial [84], the studies have generally been small and of short duration, with more than half revealing no benefits of folic acid treatment [85–87]. One small study that reported several treatment effects after only 2 months involved folate-deficient, cognitively impaired subjects [88], which likely explains its success. Specifically,

TABLE 13.4
Randomized Placebo-Controlled Trials Investigating the Effect of Supplements Containing Folic Acid on Cognition

First Author	Subject Characteristics	n	Treatment	Duration	Significant Benefits
Fioravanti [88]	Folate deficient, mild/moderate cognitive impairment	30	15 mg folic acid	60 d	√[a]
Bryan[b] [89]	Stratified random sample of women in three age ranges from electoral rolls, aged 20–30 y, 45–55 y, and 65–92 y	221	750 μg folic acid, 15 μg B12, 75 mg B6	5 wk	√[c]
Pathansali [87]	Healthy volunteers with MMSE[d] > 27 who were not B vitamin deficient, aged ≥65 y	24	5 mg folic acid	4 wk	—
Lewerin[e] [86]	Community members, median age of 76 y	126	800 μg folic acid, 500 μg B12, 3 mg B6	4 mo	—
Stott [138]	Ischemic vascular disease patients, aged ≥65 y	47	2.5 mg folic acid, 500 μg B12	12 wk	—
McMahon[f] [85]	Service club members, aged ≥65 y, homocysteine >13 μmol/L	276	1,000 μg methylfolate, 500 μg B12, 10 mg B6	2 y	—
Durga [84]	Community members, aged 50–70 y, homocysteine 13–25 μmol/L, plasma B12 > 200 pmol/L	818	800 μg folic acid	3 y	√[a,c,g]

[a] The treatment group outperformed the placebo group on a test of recall or memory.
[b] $P = .06$ for immediate recall, youngest group.
[c] The treatment group outperformed the placebo group on a test of executive function.
[d] MMSE = Mini-Mental State Examination.
[e] $P = .093$ for the Digit-Symbol Substitution Test of information processing speed. However, $P = .039$, favoring the placebo group, was found for a test of perceptual speed.
[f] $P = .05$, favoring the placebo group, was found for the combined score from eight tests, results of all but one of which favored the placebo group. However, the only significant finding was for a test of executive function ($P = .007$, favoring the placebo group).
[g] The treatment group outperformed the placebo group on a test of speed. Furthermore, $P < .05$ was calculated for a global score generated by averaging five composite scores variously created from results of five cognitive function tests.

the treatment provided a nutrient the subjects lacked, and the benefits of replacement were detectable because the subjects were declining. A very brief trial also demonstrated some cognitive benefits of daily treatment with 750 μg of folic acid combined with 15 μg of vitamin B12 and 75 mg of vitamin B6 [89]. In contrast to these two trials, a 2-year study of cognitively healthy subjects with hyperhomocysteinemia conducted in New Zealand by McMahon et al. [85] failed to demonstrate any cognitive benefits despite Hcy normalization. That the treated group performed somewhat worse than the placebo group on nearly all of the eight tests in the battery was reflected in the marginally significant P value ($P = .05$) for the composite score. Furthermore, treated subjects performed significantly worse than members of the placebo group on Trails B. This may have been associated with the high folic acid intake (1000 µg) the supplement provided in the treated group, which was equivalent to the Tolerable Upper Intake Level [90]. Also, considering that the mean age of the subjects was 73 years and that an elevated Hcy concentration was an entrance requirement for the study, some low vitamin B12 status (which might not be detectable with the serum vitamin B12 assay [91]) would be expected. Although the supplement delivered a very high dose of vitamin B12, and mean plasma vitamin B12 was high as a result, total vitamin B12 intake might not have been sufficient to normalize vitamin B12 function in subjects who were vitamin B12 deficient [92].

The 3-year Dutch FACIT trial, the longest and largest of the published trials, reported treatment benefits for global cognitive function and the specific domains of memory and speed of information processing [84]. The cognitive function tests used in the Dutch and New Zealand trials differed, but both assessed multiple cognitive functions. The folic acid dose used in the FACIT trial was lower, and prospective subjects with deficient concentrations of circulating vitamin B12 were excluded. Although FACIT subjects were not supplemented with vitamin B12, they were younger than the participants in the New Zealand trial, such that the circulating vitamin B12 concentration may not have misclassified as many subjects as it might have with an older group, and the prevalence of deficiency should also have been lower [93,94].

III.   HCY, FOLATE, AND DEPRESSION

A.   BACKGROUND AND METHODOLOGICAL CONSIDERATIONS

In 1978, Carney and Sheffield [95] reported on the folate and vitamin B12 status of 272 psychiatric hospital admissions and documented the link between low folate status and the diagnosis of depression. This relationship continues to be demonstrated and extended [96,97]. For example, in a case review similar to that of Carney and Sheffields, Lerner et al. [98] recently found low folate status to be 3.5 times as common in depressed patients as it was in those diagnosed with mania. Low folate status is also related to the severity of depression among depressed patients [99], and higher folate status has been shown to accelerate recovery [97] and enhance the effects of conventional antidepressants [100,101]. These observations, along with knowledge of the high concentration of folates in the cerebrospinal fluid [102] and their importance to brain function, generate the hypothesis that folate status plays a role in the incidence of depression in populations. However, few relevant epidemiological investigations have been published, and standardization of methods has not occurred.

One published study classified subjects based on self-report of past depressive episodes and use of antidepressants [103]. However, assessing depression, rather than asking about previous diagnosis and treatment, is considered important because most depression goes undiagnosed [104], although overdiagnosis is also a problem [105–107]. On the other hand, subjects frequently underreport symptoms in surveys [108], and a lay-administered interview may identify transient phenomena rather than clinical disorders [109].

For the same reason that the MMSE has been used in epidemiological studies of age-related cognitive impairment, depressive symptom scales designed as quick screening tools have been used almost exclusively for depression classification in epidemiological studies of depression. However, no single scale has been used consistently. This makes some sense because the populations studied have varied among adult municipal employees [110], elderly disabled women [111], new mothers [112], young adults [113], middle-aged men [114–116], and unselected elderly people [68,103,116–119]. A previous study using NHANES III data [113] was the only one to use the National Institutes of Mental Health Diagnostic Interview Schedule (NIMH-DIS), which was developed specifically to assess whether participants in epidemiological studies meet DSM-III criteria for major depression and dysthymia [120]. This instrument might not be suitable for some populations, however. For example, studies have shown that for the elderly population a brief symptom inventory is preferable to an intensive interview [121] or a Likert response format, such as that used by the Center for Epidemiologic Studies Depression (CES-D) Scale [122]. One Korean study [51] used the Geriatric Mental State (GMS) schedule, which is a structured diagnostic interview designed for use in elderly populations that has been adapted for epidemiological research [123]. Unlike the NIMH-DIS, it does not allow distinction between major depression and dysthymia [51], but rather the GMS scores subjects on how well their responses correspond to eight different possible psychiatric syndromes. It is also possible that even when elderly people meet criteria for depressive diagnoses, they experience a different phenomenon than that experienced by younger people receiving the same diagnosis [124].

In clinical settings, a high depression scale score is supposed to be followed by a clinical interview to distinguish mere symptoms from a depression disorder [125]. This is because any checklist, and particularly the abbreviated ones recommended for the elderly population, miss some requirements for a depressive diagnosis, specifically those related to age of onset, the length of time symptoms have persisted, the clustering of other symptoms with dysphoria, and the exclusion of symptoms clearly resulting from a general medical condition [126]. Where use of a symptom scale may lead to overascertainment, a DIS or semistructured clinical interview may underascertain depression in the elderly population. That is, although elderly people frequently experience depressive symptoms [127], they seem to meet criteria for depression diagnoses less frequently than do younger people [128]. One reason for this is that elderly people, and particularly those who are cognitively impaired, may deny feelings of sadness [126]. The Geriatric Depression Scale (GDS) was specifically designed to characterize the "geriatric depression construct" [122]. However, there is controversy over whether the elements are appropriately labeled depression, or whether they simply characterize "old age" and thus poorly discriminate between depressed and nondepressed seniors [122]. Even if the so-called "subsyndromal" depression commonly observed in elderly persons is clinically significant, using a nonstandard definition of depression for a particular age group may make results of analytic epidemiological studies difficult to interpret because the causes of this special "geriatric" depression may differ from those of depressive syndromes that occur throughout the lifespan.

Studies of a possible link between nutritional status and depression are particularly susceptible to reverse causation and confounding. For example, depression classification is based on symptoms, with appetite disturbance being one of them. Furthermore, low nutritional status is strongly related to factors that seem capable of causing depression, such as poverty and serious illness. Some studies comparing depressed patients with other psychiatric patients and healthy controls [99,129], as well as some cross-sectional community studies [113,115], have provided evidence against appetite disturbance or weight change as the sole cause of the connection between folate status and depression. Nevertheless, reverse causation is still possible, in that depression might lower folate status by nondietary means, such as an effect on oxidative stress [17]. Of course, low folate status could be both a cause and effect of depression, with any lowering of folate status caused by depression posing a threat to recovery.

B. Epidemiological Studies of Folate Status in Relation to Depression

The first population-based observational study of a possible connection between folate status and depression was published in 2000 [118]. Results of 13 such investigations, including one short-term [51] and one long-term [114] follow-up study, have now been published (Table 13.5). Six of the studies [103,111,113,114,116,118] were included in a meta-analysis published in early 2008 [130], and the pooled, multivariate-adjusted OR (95% confidence interval) relating low folate status to depression was 1.42 (1.10–1.83).

Some of the investigations detailed in Table 13.5 focused exclusively on women [111,112] or men [114,115,117]. Six of the 13 evaluated the association between Hcy concentration and depression [113,116–119], and all considered associations between circulating folate concentrations [68,103,111,113,116,119], RBC folate concentrations [113], or folate intake [110,114,115,117] and depression. Despite wide variation in folate status, depression assessment methodology, and proportion of subjects classified as depressed, all the studies of young or middle-aged people [10,110,114–116,119], except a study of postpartum depression [112], found some evidence of an association between low folate status and depression after multivariate adjustment for important potentially confounding factors. A study of Japanese office workers linked lower energy-adjusted folate intakes to depression only among the men [110]. However, a sex-by-folate interaction was not formally tested, and men and women may have responded differently to the brief food frequency questionnaire that had been adapted from a longer, validated version.

Half of the studies of elderly people did not find associations between folate status and depression [68,103,111]. The exceptions were a study of 60 to 64-year-olds [119], an age range that is sometimes referred to as "young-old," an analysis of postfortification SALSA data that revealed a relationship for women only [118], and the Korean study that used the structured interview schedule [51]. Because comorbidity

TABLE 13.5
Studies Investigating the Relationship between Folate or Homocysteine (Hcy) Status and Depression

First Author	Design	n	Age Range	Depression Assessment[a]	Significant Findings Hcy	Significant Findings Folate
Penninx [111]	Cross-sectional	700[b]	≥65 y	GDS	NA	—
Lindeman [68]	Cross-sectional	883	≥65 y	GDS	NA	—
Tiemeier [139]	Nested case–control	419	≥55 y	CES-D/work-up	—	—
Morris [113]	Cross-sectional	2,948	15–39 y	NIH-DIS	—	√
Bjelland [116]	Cross-sectional	2,291	46–49 y	HADS-D	√	√[c]
Bjelland [116]	Cross-sectional	2,558	70–74 y	HADS-D	√	—
Tolmunen [115]	Cross-sectional	2,442	42–60 y	HPLDS	NA	√
Tolmunen [114]	13-y follow-up	2,600	42–60 y	Hospitalization	NA	√
Ramos [118]	Cross-sectional	1,510	>60 y	CES-D	—	√[d]
Sachdev [119]	Cross-sectional	412	60–64 y	PRIME-MD	√	√
Miyake [112]	2–9-mo follow-up	865[b]	Pregnant	EPDS	NA	—
Kamphuis [117]	Cross-sectional	332[e]	Mean = 75 y	Zung	—	—
Murakami [110]	Cross-sectional	309[e]	Mean = 45 y	CES-D	NA	√
Murakami [110]	Cross-sectional	208[b]	Mean = 41 y	CES-D	NA	—
Kim [51]	Cross-sectional	732	Mean = 73 y	GMS-DIS	√	—
Kim [51]	2.4-y follow-up	521	Mean = 73 y	GMS-DIS	√	√

[a] GDS, Geriatric Depression Scale; CES-D, Center for Epidemiology Studies Depression Scale; NIH-DIS, National Institutes of Health Diagnostic Interview Schedule; HADS-D, Hospital Anxiety and Depression Scale; HPLDS, Human Population Depression Scale; PRIME-MD, Primary Care Evaluation of Mental Disorders; EPDS, Edinburgh Postnatal Depression Scale; Zung, Zung Self-Rating Depression Scale; GMS-DIS, Geriatric Mental State Diagnostic Interview Schedule.

[b] Study or analysis involved women only.

[c] Subgroup analysis revealed a significant association for men only.

[d] Subgroup analysis revealed a significant association for women only.

[e] Study or analysis involved men only.

and bereavement increase with age, the study of 60 to 64-year-olds may have been able to detect an association where studies of older seniors were not, as a result of the greater ease of diagnosing depression when there is less physical illness and fewer short-term reactions to emotionally stressful events to confuse the presentation. There is also evidence suggesting that depression occurring in later old age is a different disease from depression occurring at earlier ages [124,128]. Consistent with most of the other cross-sectional studies involving older seniors, the Korean investigation found no association between folate status and prevalent depression. However, a significant association was revealed between folate status and depression incidence after an average of 2.4 years of follow-up. The authors thought that the discrepant results of their two analyses might be explained by nonresponse bias or dietary improvement in those with pre-existing depression. However, it could also be that the long-standing cases, which were excluded from the follow-up analyses, were etiologically distinct from cases that arose during follow-up. Thus, it is noteworthy that the NHANES III data on younger people did not reveal any association between serum folate concentration and dysthymia, which, by definition, is a chronic form of depression [32]. Blazer [128] has pointed out that dysthymia rarely begins in late life but may persist from mid-life into late life.

The SALSA, which focused on an American Latino population in the era of food-folate fortification, was the only investigation of "old-old" subjects to find a cross-sectional association between folate status and depression [118]. The finding was restricted to women, for whom median plasma folate was 28.6 nmol/L. If the SALSA findings reflect a true association between folate status and depressive symptoms in the elderly population, they could mean that very high folate status is needed to prevent depressive symptoms in elderly persons. Alternatively, the high folate concentrations of the participants may merely have facilitated detection of an association, or residual confounding by some correlate of depression, such as acculturation, might explain the relationship.

The study of 60- to 64-year-olds [119], as well as another whose subjects fell into the narrow age ranges of 46 to 49 years and 70 to 74 years [116], found significant associations between high Hcy concentrations and depression. In the former study, Hcy remained significantly related to depression after controlling for folate status, whereas the association between folate status and depression decreased somewhat and became nonsignificant after controlling for Hcy. The NHANES III data revealed no associations between Hcy concentration and major depression or dysthymia [113], but the subjects who underwent depression assessment in that survey were very young, and their Hcy concentrations were low. Presumably as a result of food folic acid fortification, Hcy concentrations of the SALSA participants were also low [118], and that study did not link Hcy concentration to depression either.

Kim et al. [51] found a cross-sectional association between Hcy concentration and depression in the elderly Korean sample. Furthermore, in that study, both high Hcy concentration at baseline and an increase in circulating Hcy between baseline and follow-up were associated with higher depression incidence. All of these associations remained significant after multivariate control for important confounders, including a vascular risk score based on self-report of not only cardiovascular diseases but also a variety of vascular disease risk factors. Controlling for vascular risk had little effect on the ORs, but the association between Hcy and depression appeared to be largely explained by folate status. In contrast to Kim et al.'s findings from the Korean study, a significant association between hyperhomocysteinemia and depression found in the Rotterdam Study was greatly reduced by controlling for potential confounders that included cardiovascular risk factors, MMSE score, and functional disability [103]. Finally, in the Zutphen Elderly Study, no association was found between either Hcy concentration or folate status and depression, whether terms for cardiovascular risk factors were in the model or not [117]. It seems likely that the discrepancies among the studies of older people relate, in part, to variation among the depression assessment scales in their tendency to detect symptoms of somatic disease. When this tendency is high, true associations may be masked by misclassification and spurious associations may emerge.

A few small trials have evaluated the effect of folic acid supplementation on recovery from depression in patients with major depression. In one trial, subjects with borderline or frank folate deficiency were randomized to treatment with an antidepressant plus either 15 mg/day methylfolate or placebo for 6 months. The antidepressant varied among the patients, but clinical outcome assessments and rating scale scores of the 13 folate-treated patients showed significantly more improvement than those of the 11 patients who received no treatment for their folate deficiency [101]. In a larger trial that was similar, except that folate deficiency was not required, 127 depressed subjects were randomized to 20 mg/day fluoxetine plus either 500 µg/day folic acid or placebo for 10 weeks [131]. Hamilton Rating Scale scores of the folic acid–treated group decreased significantly more than those of the antidepressant plus placebo group, but the effect was restricted to the 82 female patients, who had been randomized separately from the 45 male patients. In a third trial, normo-folatemic elderly patients with both dementia and depression were randomized to 50 mg/day of methylfolate ($n = 47$) or 100 mg/day of trazodone ($n = 49$) for 8 weeks, and depression ratings improved significantly in both groups [132].

On the whole, the small but growing body of published community-based epidemiological studies on folate status and depression seems highly inconsistent. However, much of the inconsistency is likely because of the contribution of "aging" studies. Results from the Hordaland Homocysteine Studies, which included both young and elderly subjects, are telling in this regard. Although a strong association between Hcy concentration and depression was revealed in the full data set, an association between folate status and depression could only be detected in a young subgroup. The conclusion that higher folate status is associated with the prevention of depression in young but not elderly persons is contradicted by the only follow-up study thus far conducted in an elderly population. Results mirrored findings from cross-sectional [113,115,119] and follow-up [114] analyses of data collected on young [113], middle-aged [114,115], and "young-old" [119] samples in suggesting that lower folate status was a risk factor for depression. Precisely what depressive symptoms folate status relates to would be of interest in reconciling the different results for different age groups.

IV. SUMMARY

The low folate concentrations of psychiatric inpatients sparked epidemiological interest in relationships between folate status and dementia/AD and depression, but research exploded after studies linked hyperhomocysteinemia to vascular disease, and vascular disease to AD. Most epidemiological studies supported the idea that low folate status and/or hyperhomocysteinemia was an independent risk factor for AD, and results inconsistent with this conclusion appear explicable by selection factors, misclassification, and confounding.

Heterogeneity in the literature regarding possible links between folate status and cognitive test performance and depression illustrates a struggle with what Roberts and Vermon [133] termed "the central unresolved issue in psychiatric epidemiology," i.e., how to measure psychiatric impairment in community settings. Early experience with a dementia screening test widely used in clinical settings revealed its poor ability to discriminate between cognitively intact people and those with subtle cognitive deficits. Furthermore, although many studies linked low folate status and/or hyperhomocysteinemia to poor cognitive performance, different results obtained with tests reputed to tap the same cognitive domain highlighted the need for standard assessment methods. Unfortunately, results of the first two Hcy-lowering trials to consider cognition disagree, and effort must now be invested in defining circumstances under which folic acid is beneficial and in determining whether, when, and at what level it might cause harm.

Studies of young and middle-aged people support the idea that low folate status is a risk factor for depression. The association is more difficult to detect in the elderly population because of confusion between depressive symptoms and somatic complaints, and perhaps because low folate status makes a relatively small contribution to the burden of clinically significant depression in elderly persons. Attempts to capture the "geriatric depression construct" by designing special screening instruments help to ensure treatment for clinically depressed elderly people, but epidemiological studies that used such instruments may have generated false-negative results for that age group. Clinical trial data suggest that folic acid supplementation may benefit depressed patients, but the usefulness of folic acid supplementation in the primary prevention of depression has not been tested.

REFERENCES

1. Herbert V. Experimental nutritional folate deficiency in man. *Trans Assoc Am Physicians* 1962; 75:307–20.
2. Young SN, Ghadirian AM. Folic acid and psychopathology. *Prog Neuropsychopharmacol Biol Psychiatry* 1989; 13:841–63.
3. Muntjewerff JW, Blom HJ. Aberrant folate status in schizophrenic patients: What is the evidence? *Prog Neuropsychopharmacol Biol Psychiatry* 2005; 29:1133–39.
4. Snowdon DA, Greiner LH, Mortimer JA, Riley KP, Greiner PA, Markesbery WR. Brain infarction and the clinical expression of Alzheimer disease. The Nun Study. *JAMA* 1997; 277:813–17.
5. Selhub J, Jacques PF, Wilson PW, Rush D, Rosenberg IH. Vitamin status and intake as primary determinants of homocysteinemia in an elderly population. *JAMA* 1993; 270:2693–98.
6. Snowdon DA, Tully CL, Smith CD, Riley KP, Markesbery WR. Serum folate and the severity of atrophy of the neocortex in Alzheimer disease: Findings from the Nun study. *Am J Clin Nutr* 2000; 71:993–98.
7. Obeid R, Herrmann W. Mechanisms of homocysteine neurotoxicity in neurodegenerative diseases with special reference to dementia. *FEBS Lett* 2006; 580:2994–3005.
8. Seshadri S. Elevated plasma homocysteine levels: Risk factor or risk marker for the development of dementia and Alzheimer's disease? *J Alzheimers Dis* 2006; 9:393–98.
9. Durga J, van Boxtel MP, Schouten EG, Bots ML, Kok FJ, Verhoef P. Folate and the methylenetetrahydrofolate reductase 677C-->T mutation correlate with cognitive performance. *Neurobiol Aging* 2006; 27:334–43.
10. Morris, MS, Jacques PF, Rosenberg IH, Selhub J. Hyperhomocysteinemia associated with poor recall in the third National Health and Nutrition Examination Survey. *Am J Clin Nutr* 2001; 73:927–33.

11. Tucker KL, Qiao N, Scott T, Rosenberg I, Spiro A 3rd. High homocysteine and low B vitamins predict cognitive decline in aging men: The Veterans Affairs Normative Aging Study. *Am J Clin Nutr* 2005; 82:627–35.
12. Bottiglieri T. Homocysteine and folate metabolism in depression. *Prog Neuropsychopharmacol Biol Psychiatry* 2005; 29:1103–12.
13. Bottiglieri T, Hyland K, Reynolds EH. The clinical potential of ademetionine (S-adenosylmethionine) in neurological disorders. *Drugs* 1994; 48:137–52.
14. Reynolds EH, Carney MW, Toone BK. Methylation and mood. *Lancet* 1984; 2:196–98.
15. Shu L, Lee NP. SAMe targets consumers via the web. *West J Med* 2000; 173:229–30.
16. Bell IR, Edman JS, Selhub J, Morrow FD, Marby DW, Kayne HL, Cole JO. Plasma homocysteine in vascular disease and in nonvascular dementia of depressed elderly people. *Acta Psychiatr Scand* 1992; 86:386–90.
17. Leblhuber F, Walli J, Widner B, Artner-Dworzak E, Fuchs D, Vrecko K. Homocysteine and B vitamins in dementia. *Am J Clin Nutr* 2001; 73:127–28.
18. Joosten E, Lesaffre E, Riezler R, Ghekiere V, Dereymaeker L, Pelemans W, Dejaeger E. Is metabolic evidence for vitamin B-12 and folate deficiency more frequent in elderly patients with Alzheimer's disease? *J Gerontol A Biol Sci Med Sci* 1997; 52:M76–79.
19. Boushey CJ, Beresford SA, Omenn GS, Motulsky AG. A quantitative assessment of plasma homocysteine as a risk factor for vascular disease. Probable benefits of increasing folic acid intakes. *JAMA* 1995; 274:1049–57.
20. Refsum H, Ueland PM, Nygard O, Vollset SE. Homocysteine and cardiovascular disease. *Annu Rev Med* 1998; 49:31–62.
21. Lindeboom J, Weinstein H. Neuropsychology of cognitive ageing, minimal cognitive impairment, Alzheimer's disease, and vascular cognitive impairment. *Eur J Pharmacol* 2004; 490:83–86.
22. Strachan MW, Price JF, Frier BM. Diabetes, cognitive impairment, and dementia. *BMJ* 2008; 336:6.
23. Wijekoon EP, Brosnan ME, Brosnan JT. Homocysteine metabolism in diabetes. *Biochem Soc Trans* 2007; 35:1175–79.
24. Reynolds E. Vitamin B12, folic acid, and the nervous system. *Lancet Neurol* 2006; 5:949–60.
25. Morris MS, Jacques PF, Rosenberg I, Selhub J. Folate and vitamin B-12 status in relation to anemia, macrocytosis, and cognitive impairment in older Americans in the age of folic acid fortification. *Am J Clin Nutr* 2007; 85:193–200.
26. Petersen RC. Mild cognitive impairment as a diagnostic entity. *J Intern Med* 2004; 256:183–94.
27. Morris JC, Storandt M, Miller JP, McKeel DW, Price JL, Rubin EH, Berg L. Mild cognitive impairment represents early-stage Alzheimer disease. *Arch Neurol* 2001; 58: 397–405.
28. Goldman WP, Price JL, Storandt M, Grant EA, McKeel DW Jr, Rubin EH, Morris JC. Absence of cognitive impairment or decline in preclinical Alzheimer's disease. *Neurology* 2001; 56:361–67.
29. Andrews-Hanna JR, Snyder AZ, Vincent JL, Lustig C, Head D, Raichle ME, Buckner RL. Disruption of large-scale brain systems in advanced aging. *Neuron* 2007; 56:924–35.
30. Folstein MF, Folstein SE, McHugh PR. "Mini-mental state." A practical method for grading the cognitive state of patients for the clinician. *J Psychiatr Res* 1975; 12:189–98.
31. Palmer K, Wang HX, Backman L, Winblad B, Fratiglioni L. Differential evolution of cognitive impairment in nondemented older persons: Results from the Kungsholmen Project. *Am J Psychiatry* 2002; 159:436–42.
32. American Psychiatric Association. *Diagnostic and Statistical Manual of Mental Disorders*, 4th ed., Washington, DC: American Psychiatric Press Inc., 1994.

33. Riggs KM, Spiro A 3rd, Tucker K, Rush D. Relations of vitamin B-12, vitamin B-6, folate, and homocysteine to cognitive performance in the Normative Aging Study. *Am J Clin Nutr* 1996; 63:306–14.

34. Huff FJ, Corkin S. Recent advances in the neuropsychology of Alzheimer's disease. *Prog Neuropsychopharmacol Biol Psychiatry* 1984; 8:643–48.

35. Hinman JD, Abraham CR. What's behind the decline? The role of white matter in brain aging. *Neurochem Res* 2007; 32:2023–31.

36. de Leon MJ, DeSanti S, Zinkowski R, Mehta PD, Pratico D, Segal S, Clark C, et al. MRI and CSF studies in the early diagnosis of Alzheimer's disease. *J Intern Med* 2004; 256:205–23.

37. Bird CM, Burgess N. The hippocampus and memory: Insights from spatial processing. *Nat Rev Neurosci* 2008; 9:182–94.

38. Backman L, Jones S, Berger AK, Laukka EJ, Small BJ. Multiple cognitive deficits during the transition to Alzheimer's disease. *J Intern Med* 2004; 256:195–204.

39. Wadley VG, Crowe M, Marsiske M, Cook SE, Unverzagt FW, Rosenberg AL, Rexroth D. Changes in everyday function in individuals with psychometrically defined mild cognitive impairment in the Advanced Cognitive Training for Independent and Vital Elderly Study. *J Am Geriatr Soc* 2007; 55:1192–98.

40. Salthouse TA. The processing-speed theory of adult age differences in cognition. *Psychol Rev* 1996; 103:403–28.

41. Proust-Lima C, Amieva H, Dartigues JF, Jacqmin-Gadda H. Sensitivity of four psychometric tests to measure cognitive changes in brain aging-population-based studies. *Am J Epidemiol* 2007; 165:344–50.

42. Morrens M, Hulstijn W, Sabbe B. Psychomotor slowing in schizophrenia. *Schizophr Bull* 2007; 33:1038–53.

43. Strachan RW, Henderson JG. Dementia and folate deficiency. *Q J Med* 1967; 36:189–204.

44. Goodwin JS, Goodwin JM, Garry PJ. Association between nutritional status and cognitive functioning in a healthy elderly population. *JAMA* 1983; 249:2917–21.

45. La Rue A, Koehler KM, Wayne SJ, Chiulli SJ, Haaland KY, Garry PJ. Nutritional status and cognitive functioning in a normally aging sample: A 6-y reassessment. *Am J Clin Nutr* 1997; 65:20–29.

46. Wang HX, Wahlin A, Basun H, Fastbom J, Winblad B, Fratiglioni L. Vitamin B(12) and folate in relation to the development of Alzheimer's disease. *Neurology* 2001; 56:1188–94.

47. Seshadri S, Beiser A, Selhub J, Jacques PF, Rosenberg IH, D'Agostino RB, Wilson PW, Wolf PA. Plasma homocysteine as a risk factor for dementia and Alzheimer's disease. *N Engl J Med* 2002; 346:476–83.

48. Luchsinger JA, Tang MX, Shea S, Miller J, Green R, Mayeux R. Plasma homocysteine levels and risk of Alzheimer disease. *Neurology* 2004; 62:1972–76.

49. Ravaglia G, Forti P, Maioli F, Martelli M, Servadei L, Brunetti N, Porcellini E, Licastro F. Homocysteine and folate as risk factors for dementia and Alzheimer disease. *Am J Clin Nutr* 2005; 82:636–43.

50. Morris MC, Evans DA, Schneider JA, Tangney CC, Bienias JL, Aggarwal NT. Dietary folate and vitamins B-12 and B-6 not associated with incident Alzheimer's disease. *J Alzheimers Dis* 2006; 9:435–43.

51. Kim JM, Stewart R, Kim SW, Yang SJ, Shin HY, Shin IS, Yoon JS. Changes in folate, vitamin B12, and homocysteine associated with incident dementia. *J Neurol Neurosurg Psychiatry* 2008; 79:864–68.

52. Haan MN, Miller JW, Aiello AE, Whitmer RA, Jagust WJ, Mungas DM, Allen LH, Green R. Homocysteine, B vitamins, and the incidence of dementia and cognitive impairment: Results from the Sacramento Area Latino Study on Aging. *Am J Clin Nutr* 2007; 85:511–17.

53. Luchsinger JA, Tang MX, Miller J, Green R, Mayeux R. Relation of higher folate intake to lower risk of Alzheimer disease in the elderly. *Arch Neurol* 2007; 64:86–92.
54. Ramos MI, Allen LH, Mungas DM, Jagust WJ, Haan MN, Green R, Miller JW. Low folate status is associated with impaired cognitive function and dementia in the Sacramento Area Latino Study on Aging. *Am J Clin Nutr* 2005; 82:1346–52.
55. McCaddon A, Davies G, Hudson P, Tandy S, Cattell H. Total serum homocysteine in senile dementia of Alzheimer type. *Int J Geriatr Psychiatry* 1998; 13:235–39.
56. Clarke R, Smith AD, Jobst KA, Refsum H, Sutton L, Ueland, PM. Folate, vitamin B12, and serum total homocysteine levels in confirmed Alzheimer disease. *Arch Neurol* 1998; 55:1449–55.
57. Quadri P, Fragiacomo C, Pezzati R, Zanda E, Forloni G, Tettamanti M, Lucca U. Homocysteine, folate, and vitamin B-12 in mild cognitive impairment, Alzheimer disease, and vascular dementia. *Am J Clin Nutr* 2004; 80:114–22.
58. Monastero R, Palmer K, Qiu C, Winblad B, Fratiglioni L. Heterogeneity in risk factors for cognitive impairment, no dementia: Population-based longitudinal study from the Kungsholmen Project. *Am J Geriatr Psychiatry* 2007; 15:60–69.
59. Campbell AK, Jagust WJ, Mungas DM, Miller JW, Green R, Haan MN, Allen LH. Low erythrocyte folate, but not plasma vitamin B-12 or homocysteine, is associated with dementia in elderly Latinos. *J Nutr Health Aging* 2005; 9:39–43.
60. Morris MC, Evans DA, Bienias JL, Tangney CC, Hebert LE, Scherr PA, Schneider JA. Dietary folate and vitamin B12 intake and cognitive decline among community-dwelling older persons. *Arch Neurol* 2005; 62:641–45.
61. Choumenkovitch SF, Selhub J, Wilson PW, Rader JI, Rosenberg IH, Jacques PF. Folic acid intake from fortification in United States exceeds predictions. *J Nutr* 2002; 132:2792–98.
62. Choumenkovitch SF, Jacques PF, Nadeau MR, Wilson PW, Rosenberg IH, Selhub J. Folic acid fortification increases red blood cell folate concentrations in the Framingham study. *J Nutr* 2001; 131:3277–80.
63. McIlroy SP, Dynan KB, Lawson JT, Patterson CC, Passmore AP. Moderately elevated plasma homocysteine, methylenetetrahydrofolate reductase genotype, and risk for stroke, vascular dementia, and Alzheimer disease in Northern Ireland. *Stroke* 2002; 33:2351–56.
64. Harris Interactive. MetLife Foundation Alzheimer's Survey: What America Thinks. Metlife Foundation; 2006 [cited March 20, 2008]. Available from: http://www.metlife.com/WPSAssets/20538296421147208330V1FAlzheimersSurvey.pdf.
65. U.S. Department of Health and Human Services. National Health and Nutrition Examination Survey 1999–2000 [cited March 21, 2008]. National Center for Health Statistics. Available from: http://www.cdc.gov/nchs/data/nhanes/frequency/cfq_doc.pdf.
66. Constitution of the World Health Organization. *Am J Public Health Nations Health* 1946 Nov; 36(11):1315–23.
67. Dufouil C, Alperovitch A, Ducros V, Tzourio C. Homocysteine, white matter hyperintensities, and cognition in healthy elderly people. *Ann Neurol* 2003; 53:214–21.
68 Lindeman RD, Romero LJ, Koehler KM, Liang HC, LaRue A, Baumgartner RN, Garry PJ. Serum vitamin B12, C and folate concentrations in the New Mexico elder health survey: Correlations with cognitive and affective functions. *J Am Coll Nutr* 2000; 19:68–76.
69. Duthie SJ, Whalley LJ, Collins AR, Leaper S, Berger K, Deary IJ. Homocysteine, B vitamin status, and cognitive function in the elderly. *Am J Clin Nutr* 2002; 75:908–13.
70. Miller JW, Green R, Ramos MI, Allen LH, Mungas DM, Jagust WJ, Haan MN. Homocysteine and cognitive function in the Sacramento Area Latino Study on Aging. *Am J Clin Nutr* 2003; 78:441–47.

71. Ravaglia G, Forti P, Maioli F, Muscari A, Sacchetti L, Arnone G, Nativio V, Talerico T, Mariani E. Homocysteine and cognitive function in healthy elderly community dwellers in Italy. *Am J Clin Nutr* 2003; 77:668–73.

72. Wright CB, Lee HS, Paik MC, Stabler SP, Allen RH, Sacco RL. Total homocysteine and cognition in a tri-ethnic cohort: The Northern Manhattan Study. *Neurology* 2004; 63:254–60.

73. Feng L, Ng TP, Chuah L, Niti M, Kua EH. Homocysteine, folate, and vitamin B-12 and cognitive performance in older Chinese adults: Findings from the Singapore Longitudinal Ageing Study. *Am J Clin Nutr* 2006; 84:1506–12.

74. Kalmijn S, Launer LJ, Lindemans J, Bots ML, Hofman A, Breteler MM. Total homocysteine and cognitive decline in a community-based sample of elderly subjects: The Rotterdam Study. *Am J Epidemiol* 1999; 150:283–89.

75. Prins ND, Den Heijer T, Hofman A, Koudstaal PJ, Jolles J, Clarke R, Breteler MM. Homocysteine and cognitive function in the elderly: The Rotterdam Scan Study. *Neurology* 2002; 59:1375–80.

76. Budge MM, de Jager C, Hogervorst E, Smith AD. Total plasma homocysteine, age, systolic blood pressure, and cognitive performance in older people. *J Am Geriatr Soc* 2002; 50:2014–18.

77. Lindeman RD, Romero LJ, Schade DS, Wayne S, Baumgartner RN, Garry PJ. Impact of subclinical hypothyroidism on serum total homocysteine concentrations, the prevalence of coronary heart disease (CHD), and CHD risk factors in the New Mexico Elder Health Survey. *Thyroid* 2003; 13:595–600.

78. Kang JH, Irizarry MC, Grodstein F. Prospective study of plasma folate, vitamin B12, and cognitive function and decline. *Epidemiology* 2006; 17:650–57.

79. Nurk E, Refsum H, Tell GS, Engedal K, Vollset SE, Ueland PM, Nygaard HA, Smith AD. Plasma total homocysteine and memory in the elderly: The Hordaland Homocysteine Study. *Ann Neurol* 2005; 58:847–57.

80. Elias MF, Sullivan LM, D'Agostino RB, Elias PK, Jacques PF, Selhub J, Seshadri S, Au R, Beiser A, Wolf PA. Homocysteine and cognitive performance in the Framingham offspring study: Age is important. *Am J Epidemiol* 2005; 162:644–53.

81. Hector M, Burton JR. What are the psychiatric manifestations of vitamin B12 deficiency? *J Am Geriatr Soc* 1988; 36:1105–12.

82. Garcia A, Haron Y, Pulman K, Hua L, Freedman M. Increases in homocysteine are related to worsening of stroop scores in healthy elderly persons: A prospective follow-up study. *J Gerontol A Biol Sci Med Sci* 2004; 59:1323–27.

83. Schafer JH, Glass TA, Bolla KI., Mintz M, Jedlicka AE, Schwartz BS. Homocysteine and cognitive function in a population-based study of older adults. *J Am Geriatr Soc* 2005; 53:381–88.

84. Durga J, van Boxtel MP, Schouten EG, Kok FJ, Jolles J, Katan MB, Verhoef P. Effect of 3-year folic acid supplementation on cognitive function in older adults in the FACIT trial: A randomised, double blind, controlled trial. *Lancet* 2007; 369:208–16.

85. McMahon JA, Green TJ, Skeaff CM, Knight RG, Mann JI, Williams SM. A controlled trial of homocysteine lowering and cognitive performance. *N Engl J Med* 2006; 354:2764–72.

86. Lewerin C, Nilsson-Ehle H, Matousek M, Lindstedt G, Steen B. Reduction of plasma homocysteine and serum methylmalonate concentrations in apparently healthy elderly subjects after treatment with folic acid, vitamin B12 and vitamin B6: A randomised trial. *Eur J Clin Nutr* 2003; 57:1426–36.

87. Pathansali R, Mangoni AA, Creagh-Brown B, Lan ZC, Ngow GL, Yuan XF, Ouldred EL, Sherwood RA, Swift CG, Jackson SH. Effects of folic acid supplementation on psychomotor performance and hemorheology in healthy elderly subjects. *Arch Gerontol Geriatr* 2006; 43:127–37.

88. Fioravanti M, Frerrario E, Massaia M, Cappa G, Rivolta G, Grossi E, Buckley AE. Low folate levels in the cognitive decline of elderly patients and the efficacy of folate as a treatment for improving memory deficits. *Arch Gerontol Geriatr* 1997; 26:1–3.

89. Bryan J, Calvaresi E, Hughes D. Short-term folate, vitamin B-12 or vitamin B-6 supplementation slightly affects memory performance but not mood in women of various ages. *J Nutr* 2002; 132:1345–56.

90. Institute of Medicine. *Dietary reference intakes for thiamin, riboflavin, niacin, vitamin B6, folate, vitamin B12, pantothenic acid, biotin, and choline.* Washington, DC: National Academy Press, 1998.

91. Stabler SP, Lindenbaum J, Allen RH. The use of homocysteine and other metabolites in the specific diagnosis of vitamin B-12 deficiency. *J Nutr* 1996; 126:1266S–72S.

92. Rajan S, Wallace JI, Brodkin KI, Beresford SA, Allen RH, Stabler SP. Response of elevated methylmalonic acid to three dose levels of oral cobalamin in older adults. *J Am Geriatr Soc* 2002; 50:1789–95.

93. Lindenbaum J, Rosenberg IH, Wilson PW, Stabler SP, Allen RH. Prevalence of cobalamin deficiency in the Framingham elderly population. *Am J Clin Nutr* 1994; 60:2–11.

94. Morris MS, Jacques PF, Rosenberg IH, Selhub J. Elevated serum methylmalonic acid concentrations are common among elderly Americans. *J Nutr* 2002; 132:2799–803.

95. Carney MW, Sheffield BF. Serum folic acid and B12 in 272 psychiatric in-patients. *Psychol Med* 1978; 8:139–44.

96. Bottiglieri T, Crellin R, Reynolds EH. Folate and neuropsychiatry. In: Bailey LB, ed., *Folate in Health and Disease*, New York: Marcel Dekker, 1995:435–62.

97. Papakostas GI, Petersen T, Lebowitz BD, Mischoulon D, Ryan JL, Nierenberg AA, Bottiglieri T, Alpert JE, Rosenbaum JF, Fava M. The relationship between serum folate, vitamin B12, and homocysteine levels in major depressive disorder and the timing of improvement with fluoxetine. *Int J Neuropsychopharmacol* 2005; 8:523–28.

98. Lerner V, Kanevsky M, Dwolatzky T, Rouach T, Kamin R, Miodownik C. Vitamin B12 and folate serum levels in newly admitted psychiatric patients. *Clin Nutr* 2006; 25:60–67.

99. Abou-Saleh MT, Coppen A. Serum and red blood cell folate in depression. *Acta Psychiatr Scand* 1989; 80:78–82.

100. Coppen A, Chaudhry S, Swade C. Folic acid enhances lithium prophylaxis. *J Affect Disord* 1986; 10:9–13.

101. Godfrey PS, Toone BK, Carney MW, Flynn TG, Bottiglieri T, Laundy M, Chanarin I, Reynolds EH. Enhancement of recovery from psychiatric illness by methylfolate. *Lancet* 1990; 336:392–95.

102. Spector R, Lorenzo AV. Folate transport in the central nervous system. *Am J Physiol* 1975; 229:777–82.

103. Tiemeier H, van Tuijl HR, Hofman A, Meijer J, Kiliaan AJ, Breteler MM. Vitamin B12, folate, and homocysteine in depression: The Rotterdam Study. *Am J Psychiatry* 2002; 159:2099–101.

104. Nierenberg AA. Current perspectives on the diagnosis and treatment of major depressive disorder. *Am J Manag Care* 2001; 7:S353–66.

105. Aragones E, Pinol JL, Labad A. The overdiagnosis of depression in non-depressed patients in primary care. *Fam Pract* 2006; 23:363–68.

106. Boland RJ, Diaz S, Lamdan RM, Ramchandani D, McCartney JR. Overdiagnosis of depression in the general hospital. *Gen Hosp Psychiatry* 1996; 18:28–35.

107. Perry SW, Cella DF. Overdiagnosis of depression in the medically ill. *Am J Psychiatry* 1987; 144:125–26.

108. Eaton WW, Neufeld K, Chen LS, Cai G. A comparison of self-report and clinical diagnostic interviews for depression: Diagnostic interview schedule and schedules for clinical assessment in neuropsychiatry in the Baltimore epidemiologic catchment area follow-up. *Arch Gen Psychiatry* 2000; 57:217–22.

109. Murphy JM, Laird NM, Monson RR, Sobol AM, Leighton AH. A 40-year perspective on the prevalence of depression: The Stirling County Study. *Arch Gen Psychiatry* 2000; 57:209–15.

110. Murakami K, Mizoue T, Sasaki S, Ohta M, Sato M, Matsushita Y, Mishima N. Dietary intake of folate, other B vitamins, and omega-3 polyunsaturated fatty acids in relation to depressive symptoms in Japanese adults. *Nutrition* 2008; 24:140–47.

111. Penninx BW, Guralnik JM, Ferrucci L, Fried LP, Allen RH, Stabler SP. Vitamin B(12) deficiency and depression in physically disabled older women: Epidemiologic evidence from the Women's Health and Aging Study. *Am J Psychiatry* 2000; 157:715–21.

112. Miyake Y, Sasaki S, Tanaka K, Yokoyama T, Ohya Y, Fukushima W, Saito K, Ohfuji S, Kiyohara C, Hirota Y. Dietary folate and vitamins B12, B6, and B2 intake and the risk of postpartum depression in Japan: The Osaka Maternal and Child Health Study. *J Affect Disord* 2006; 96:133–38.

113. Morris MS, Fava M, Jacques PF, Selhub J, Rosenberg IH. Depression and folate status in the US population. *Psychother Psychosom* 2003; 72:80–87.

114. Tolmunen T, Hintikka J, Ruusunen A, Voutilainen S, Tanskanen A, Valkonen VP, Viinamaki H, Kaplan GA, Salonen JT. Dietary folate and the risk of depression in Finnish middle-aged men. A prospective follow-up study. *Psychother Psychosom* 2004; 73:334–39.

115. Tolmunen T, Voutilainen S, Hintikka J, Rissanen T, Tanskanen A, Viinamaki H, Kaplan GA, Salonen JT. Dietary folate and depressive symptoms are associated in middle-aged Finnish men. *J Nutr* 2003; 133:3233–36.

116. Bjelland I, Tell GS, Vollset SE, Refsum H, Ueland PM. Folate, vitamin B12, homocysteine, and the MTHFR 677C->T polymorphism in anxiety and depression: The Hordaland Homocysteine Study. *Arch Gen Psychiatry* 2003; 60:618–26.

117. Kamphuis MH, Geerlings MI, Grobbee DE, Kromhout D. Dietary intake of B(6-9-12) vitamins, serum homocysteine levels and their association with depressive symptoms: The Zutphen Elderly Study. *Eur J Clin Nutr* 2008; 62:939–45.

118. Ramos MI, Allen LH, Haan MN, Green R, Miller JW. Plasma folate concentrations are associated with depressive symptoms in elderly Latina women despite folic acid fortification. *Am J Clin Nutr* 2004; 80:1024–28.

119. Sachdev PS, Parslow RA, Lux O, Salonikas C, Wen W, Naidoo D, Christensen H, Jorm AF. Relationship of homocysteine, folic acid and vitamin B12 with depression in a middle-aged community sample. *Psychol Med* 2005; 35:529–38.

120. American Psychiatric Association. *Diagnostic and Statistical Manual of Mental Disorders*, 3rd ed. Washington, DC: American Psychiatric Association, 1980.

121. Tison P. [Structured interview guide for evaluating depression in elderly patients, adapted from DSM IV and the GDS, HDRS and MADRS scales]. *Encephale* 2000; 26:33–43.

122. Adams KB. Depressive symptoms, depletion, or developmental change? Withdrawal, apathy, and lack of vigor in the Geriatric Depression Scale. *Gerontologist* 2001; 41:768–77.

123. Copeland JR, Prince M, Wilson KC, Dewey ME, Payne J, Gurland B. The Geriatric Mental State Examination in the 21st century. *Int J Geriatr Psychiatry* 2002; 17:729–32.

124. Devanand DP, Adorno E, Cheng J, Burt T, Pelton GH, Roose SP, Sackeim HA. Late onset dysthymic disorder and major depression differ from early onset dysthymic disorder and major depression in elderly outpatients. *J Affect Disord* 2004; 78:259–67.

125. Scogin F, Rohen N, Bailey E. Geriatric Depression Scale. In: Maruish ME, ed., *Handbook of Psychological Assessment in Primary Care Settings*, Mahwah, NJ: Lawrence Erlbaum Associates, Inc, 2000:491–508.

126. Galloway M, Rushworth L. Red cell or serum folate? Results from the National Pathology Alliance benchmarking review. *J Clin Pathol* 2003; 56:924–26.

127. VanItallie TB. Subsyndromal depression in the elderly: Underdiagnosed and undertreated. *Metabolism* 2005; 54:39–44.
128. Blazer DG. Depression in late life: Review and commentary. *J Gerontol A Biol Sci Med Sci* 2003; 58:249–65.
129. Fava M, Borus JS, Alpert JE, Nierenberg AA, Rosenbaum JF, Bottiglieri T. Folate, vitamin B12, and homocysteine in major depressive disorder. *Am J Psychiatry* 1997; 154:426–28.
130. Gilbody S, Bower P, Torgerson D, Richards D. Cluster randomized trials produced similar results to individually randomized trials in a meta-analysis of enhanced care for depression. *J Clin Epidemiol* 2008; 61:160–68.
131. Coppen A, Bailey J. Enhancement of the antidepressant action of fluoxetine by folic acid: A randomised, placebo controlled trial. *J Affect Disord* 2000; 60:121–30.
132. Passeri M, Cucinotta D, Abate G, Senin U, Ventura A, Stramba Badiale M, Diana R, La Greca P, Le Grazie C. Oral 5'-methyltetrahydrofolic acid in senile organic mental disorders with depression: Results of a double-blind multicenter study. *Aging (Milano)* 1993; 5:63–71.
133. Roberts RE, Vernon SW. The Center for Epidemiologic Studies Depression Scale: Its use in a community sample. *Am J Psychiatry* 1983; 140:41–46.
134. Kado DM, Karlamangla AS, Huang MH, Troen A, Rowe JW, Selhub J, Seeman TE. Homocysteine versus the vitamins folate, B6, and B12 as predictors of cognitive function and decline in older high-functioning adults: MacArthur Studies of Successful Aging. *Am J Med* 2005; 118:161–67.
135. Clark MS, Guthrie JR, Dennerstein L. Hyperhomocysteinemia is associated with lower performance on memory tasks in post-menopausal women. *Dement Geriatr Cogn Disord* 2005; 20:57–62.
136. Elias MF, Robbins MA, Budge MM, Elias PK, Brennan SL, Johnston C, Nagy Z, Bates CJ. Homocysteine, folate, and vitamins B6 and B12 blood levels in relation to cognitive performance: The Maine-Syracuse study. *Psychosom Med* 2006; 68:547–54.
137. de Lau LM, Refsum H, Smith AD, Johnston C, Breteler MM. Plasma folate concentration and cognitive performance: Rotterdam Scan Study. *Am J Clin Nutr* 2007; 86:728–34.
138. Stott DJ, MacIntosh G, Lowe GD, Rumley A, McMahon AD, Langhorne P, Tait RC, et al. Randomized controlled trial of homocysteine-lowering vitamin treatment in elderly patients with vascular disease. *Am J Clin Nutr* 2005; 82:1320–26.
139. Tettamanti M, Garri MT, Nobili A, Riva E, Lucca U. Low folate and the risk of cognitive and functional deficits in the very old: The Monzino 80-plus study. *J Am Coll Nutr* 2006; 25:502–08.

14 Folate and Neurological Disease
Basic Mechanisms

Teodoro Bottiglieri and Edward Reynolds

CONTENTS

I. INTRODUCTION

Folate was first chemically synthesized in 1945, 3 years before the isolation of vitamin B12 [1]. In the past 30 years it has become well established that this vitamin plays an essential role in central nervous system (CNS) development and function. More recently there has been growing evidence that folates are of fundamental importance in brain growth, differentiation, development, repair, mood, cognition, and aging [2,3]. This is illustrated by the many cases of inborn errors of folate metabolism, which lead to profound deleterious effects in the CNS such as mental retardation, psychiatric disorders, seizures, and myelopathy [4–6], and also by the role of prophylactic folic acid in enhancing neurological recovery from spinal cord injury in animal models [7] and preventing neural tube defects (NTDs) [8]. The neuropsychiatric complications of folate deficiency from various causes are remarkably similar to those described for vitamin B12 deficiency [3,9], but the former is particularly associated with depression and dementia, especially in the elderly population [2,10–13].

The intimate metabolic relationship that exists between folate and vitamin B12 has focused attention on a number of different basic neurochemical mechanisms. The one central biochemical reaction that unifies folate and vitamin B12 metabolism involves the methylation of homocysteine (Hcy) to methionine, which is catalyzed by methionine synthase (MS). This reaction is a primary metabolic control point for the synthesis of S-adenosylmethionine (SAM), a key substrate involved in numerous methylation reactions affecting gene activity, the post-translational modification of proteins and lipids, neurotransmitter synthesis and inactivation, and the modification of many other crucial metabolic intermediates. Furthermore, reduced folates are required in the synthesis of purines and thymidylate, essential structural components of RNA and DNA. Hence folate deficiency invariably leads to impaired cellular proliferation. The plethora of folate-dependent metabolic processes has provided a fertile ground to investigate basic mechanisms associated with folate deficiency. The functional activity of folate-dependent pathways is essential to all the cells in the body, and consequently folate deficiency is associated with many different pathological states. This review is confined to the role of folate in the CNS and basic mechanisms associated with neurological disease.

II. TRANSPORT OF FOLATE IN THE CENTRAL NERVOUS SYSTEM

Because mammalian cells are unable to synthesize folates, de novo specific transport mechanisms have evolved to allow the absorption and transport of folate derivatives from food sources. Specialized carrier-mediated systems for the uptake of folates are also necessary because reduced and oxidized folate forms are hydrophilic molecules that do not traverse the lipid bilayer easily by diffusion [14]. There are three main types of carrier-mediated transport systems: the proton-coupled folate transporter (PCFT), the reduced folate carrier (RFC1), and the small family of folate receptors (FRs) that is encoded by three distinct genes known as $FR\alpha$, $FR\beta$, and $FR\gamma$. The PCFT is involved primarily in the transport of folates in the upper small intestine [15]. The RFC1 is expressed ubiquitously throughout the body and functions as an anion exchanger with a high affinity for reduced folates. It performs specialized transport in the intestinal tract [16], in proximal renal tubules [17], in the placenta [18], and at the blood-brain barrier [19]. The high-affinity folate receptors FRα and FRβ are glycosylphosphatidylinositol (GPI)-anchored receptors, which function via a classical mechanism of receptor-mediated endocytosis. FRα has a high affinity for 5-methyltetrahydrofolate (5-methyl-THF) but a lower affinity for other reduced folates [20,21].

The transport of folate into the CNS takes place across the choroid plexus located in the lateral ventricles that separates the blood compartment from the cerebrospinal fluid (CSF). Both FRα and the RFC1 are involved in this transport process (Figure 14.1). FRα is localized in the basal side of the choroid plexus epithelial cells, and uptake

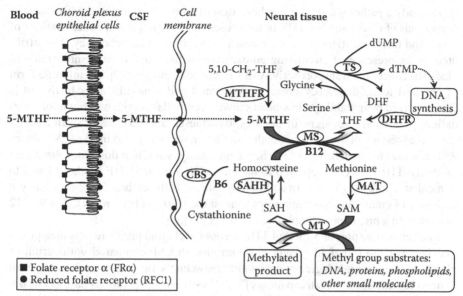

FIGURE 14.1 Blood-brain barrier transport of folate and metabolism. 5-MTHF, 5-methyltetrahydrofolate; 5,10-CH$_2$-THF, 5,10-methylenetetrahydrofolate, CBS, cystathione-β-synthetase; CSF, cerebrospinal fluid; DHF, dihydrofolate; dTMP, deoxythymidine monophosphate; dUMP, deoxyuridine monophosphate; MAT, methionine adenosyltransferase; MS, methionine synthase; MT, methyltransferase; SAH, S-adenosylhomocysteine; SAHH, SAH hydrolase; SAM, S-adenosylmethionine; THF, tetrahydrofolate; TS, thymidylate synthase.

of 5-methyl-THF occurs via receptor-mediated endocytosis. In the cytosol of the epithelial cells, 5-methyl-THF is transported out into CSF via the RFC1, which is localized in the apical membrane of the choroid plexus. Once in the CSF compartment, 5-methyl-THF is transported into neuronal cells via the RFC1. Studies in mice lacking the folic acid–binding protein (Folbp1; now termed Folr1, the murine homologue of human FRα) provided evidence that this receptor plays a critical role in folate homeostasis and is crucial to neural development and survival of the mouse embryo [22]. The uptake of folate has recently been studied in choroid plexus epithelial cells in vitro, providing evidence that two distinct processes are involved: in one FRα facilitates the transcellular movement of 5-methyl-THF, and in another PCFT is responsible for the export of metabolized folates from the endocytic compartment of epithelial cells [23]. Interestingly the high-affinity uptake of 5-methyl-THF by FRα was shown to be blocked by low levels of folic acid, which brings into question the correct form of folate that should be used to treat CNS disorders. These data suggest that low levels of folic acid in plasma may inhibit the transport of 5-methyl-THF across the blood-brain barrier via FRα. Transport of 5-methyl-THF into the CNS may also be inhibited by drugs such as corticosteroids, retinoids, and inhibitors of protein kinase C that disrupt the actin cytoskeleton and modulate FRα production [24,25]. Similarly, drugs that disrupt GPI-anchored proteins, such as sulfonylureas and antifungal agents, may also affect FRα recycling, and therefore transport of 5-methyl-THF into the CNS [26,27].

Recently a pathological state has been described that is associated with low concentrations of CSF 5-methyl-THF in the presence of normal blood concentrations of folate and total Hcy (tHcy) [28,29]. Known as cerebral folate deficiency, it is attributed to the presence of circulating autoantibodies that have been demonstrated to block the functional transport activity of FRα in cell cultures [30]. An infantile form of cerebral folate deficiency presents between 4 and 6 months after birth and is characterized by irritability, slow head growth, cerebellar ataxia, psychomotor retardation, pyramidal tract signs in the legs, dyskinesia, and seizures [28]. In another study, the presence of these autoantibodies to FRα in sera was found in 25 of 28 children with cerebral folate deficiency [31]. Supplementation with high doses of folinic acid (5-formyl-THF) has been reported to increase CSF 5-methyl-THF levels and lead to clinical amelioration [32,33]. In addition to patients with cerebral folate deficiency, a high titer of circulating autoantibodies against the FRα has been reported in 9 of 12 women with a pregnancy complicated by an NTD [30].

The active transport of 5-methyl-THF across the choroid plexus results in approximately a two- to threefold greater concentration in CSF compared with serum or plasma [34], and a high degree of correlation between the two has been shown to exist in neurological and psychiatric patients [35]. These early observations have been confirmed by further studies in pediatric and adult patients [36–42]. Surtees and Hyland [36] reported that there was no age-related change in CSF 5-methyl-THF concentration in 80 children and young adults with the reference range being 40 to 120 nmol/L. In a more recent study involving 63 pediatric controls (age range, 2 days–18 years), a negative correlation between CSF 5-methyl-THF and age was observed with higher levels in the first year of life (range, 63–129 nmol/L) compared with 2 to 3 years of age (range, 44–122 nmol/L) and 4 to 18 years of age (range, 42–81 nmol/L) [37]. A similar age-related effect has recently been reported in 89 pediatric patients [38]. Interestingly, studies in elderly subjects (range, 50–99 years old) showed that CSF 5-methyl-THF concentrations markedly decrease after 70 years of age [39]. In other studies, this age-related decrease in CSF 5-methyl-THF is associated with increased CSF tHcy [40,41], a sensitive marker of folate deficiency. It remains to be seen whether the age-related decrease in CSF 5-methyl-THF is caused by impaired transport at the choroid plexus, resulting from an increase in circulating autoantibodies to FRα. Transport of folate across the blood-brain barrier has been assessed indirectly by determination of the ratio of CSF/serum folate in 205 elderly subjects with suspected cognitive disorder [42]. The CSF/serum folate ratio was significantly lower in a dementia subgroup with vascular disease compared with a group without dementia, suggestive of a defect in the transport of folate across the blood-brain barrier.

III.   FOLATE METABOLISM IN THE CENTRAL NERVOUS SYSTEM

For an extensive review of folate metabolism, the reader is referred to Chapters 1 and 3. All the folate-dependent enzymes that are found in peripheral tissues are also present in neural tissues. Folate is present in every CNS region at a concentration range of 3% to 14% of that present in liver tissue [43]. Once 5-methyl-THF is transported across the blood-brain barrier and into neural tissues it participates in a reaction catalyzed by MS to transfer its methyl group to Hcy to produce methionine and THF (Figure 14.1). This de novo synthesis of methionine requires vitamin B12 as an additional cofactor. There is an essential and important difference between peripheral and CNS tissue in the metabolism of Hcy. An alternative pathway involving betaine/Hcy methyltransferase, which catalyzes the transfer of a methyl group from betaine to Hcy to form methionine, is present in peripheral tissues (i.e., hepatic and renal) but absent in CNS tissue [44]. Therefore, CNS tissue is solely dependent on the MS pathway and 5-methyl-THF to support the synthesis of methionine. Methionine is an essential amino acid that is required for the synthesis of SAM (or AdoMet), an important metabolite that functions as a methyl donor in numerous methylation reactions that are critical for normal cellular function (Figure 14.1). S-Adenosylhomocysteine (SAH) produced from methylation-dependent reactions is rapidly metabolized by SAH hydrolase (SAHH) to Hcy. The metabolic fate of Hcy is then determined by the activity of cystathionine-β-synthetase (CBS) and MS to produce cystathionine and methionine, respectively. However, if the metabolism of Hcy is restricted through either of these pathways, an alternative route is its conversion back to SAH by SAHH. There is no dietary source of Hcy, and as such its concentration in biological fluids and tissues is determined primarily by the functional activity of MS and CBS. This is an important metabolic consideration because the concentration of Hcy bound to protein in blood (tHcy) is a sensitive marker of folate and vitamin B12 deficiency [45,46], of which the major source is from peripheral tissues. Similarly, the concentration of tHcy in CSF, which is approximately 50-fold lower than in plasma, can be an indicator of the functional activity of the folate and vitamin B12–dependent MS enzyme in the CNS [47].

The folate/B12-dependent MS pathway produces THF, which enters the pool of reduced folates that are involved in the recycling of one-carbon units. These are supplied to the cycle in the form of serine and transferred to 5,10-methylene-THF, which plays an important role in the synthesis of deoxythymidine monophosphate (dTMP), which is incorporated into DNA (Figure 14.1). The folate cycle is completed with the conversion of 5,10-methylene-THF to 5-methyl-THF via 5,10-methylene-THF reductase (MTHFR). The homeostasis of folate metabolism in CNS tissue, as can also occur in peripheral tissues, may be altered by various factors, including nutritional deficiencies and the effects of drugs or genetic factors. In some instances the impact of these factors on folate metabolism can be compounded by nutrient–drug–genetic interactions.

IV. BASIC MECHANISMS OF FOLATE DEFICIENCY

The neurological features of inherited disorders of folate metabolism have been extensively reviewed [5,6]. These can vary with age of presentation but typically occur in the neonatal period, infancy, and childhood with clinical features such as lethargy, hyper- or hypotonia, behavioral disturbances, mental retardation, seizures, encephalopathy, neuropathy, and myelopathy. In adults the neuropsychiatric complications of acquired folate deficiency have been previously described in detail [3,9,10] and include depression, cognitive impairment, peripheral neuropathy, and myelopathy. Furthermore, the reported neuropsychiatric effects of folate deficiency are remarkably similar to those described for vitamin B12 deficiency. Deficiency of either vitamin may also lead to an indistinguishable megaloblastic anemia, which may or may not precede neurological complications [1,3,9,46]. There is evidence to

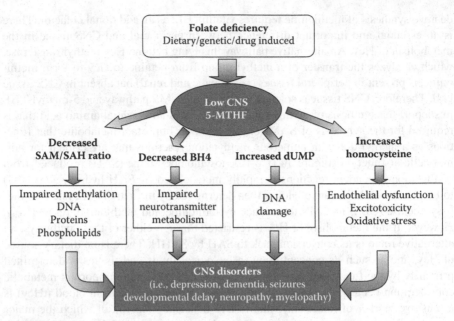

FIGURE 14.2 Mechanisms of folate-induced neurotoxicity. 5-MTHF, 5-methyltetra-hydrofolate; dUMP, deoxyuridine monophosphate; SAH, *S*-adenosylhomocysteine; SAM, *S*-adenosylmethionine; BH4, tetrahydrobiopterin.

show that impaired DNA synthesis as a result of altered one-carbon metabolism is the biochemical lesion responsible for the megaloblastic anemia of folate and vitamin B12 deficiency [47]. However, the biochemical mechanisms involved in the neuropsychiatric complications associated with a deficiency of these B vitamins have been more difficult to define.

Our current understanding of the biochemical mechanisms involved in folate deficiency–induced neurological dysfunction is based on associations between metabolic intermediates of the folate and methylation cycle with clinical syndromes as well as from studies of in vitro cell cultures and experimental animal models. These approaches have identified a number of probable mechanisms (summarized in Figure 14.2) that involve defects in many methylation-dependent pathways, DNA synthesis, direct and indirect effects of hyperhomocysteinemia, and decreased synthesis of monoamine neurotransmitters. It is likely that more than one mechanism may play a significant role as an underlying cause of neurological and psychiatric disorders. In other cases these mechanisms may accelerate disease progression or interfere with standard pharmacotherapy. Table 14.1 summarizes the clinical and biochemical associations that are described in more detail in the following sections.

A. IMPAIRED METHYLATION-DEPENDENT PATHWAYS IN THE CENTRAL NERVOUS SYSTEM

Substrate-specific methyltransferase enzymes are responsible for catalyzing the transfer of a methyl group to the carboxyl moiety of amino acids in proteins, cytosine

TABLE 14.1

Metabolic Mechanisms Associated with Folate Deficiency and Age-Related Central Nervous System Disorders

Age	CNS Disorder	Possible Metabolic Mechanisms
Embryo, fetus, infant, child	Disorders of CNS growth and development	Impaired DNA synthesis and transcription; impaired genomic methylation and epigenetic mechanisms
Adult	Myelopathy (SACD) or neuropathy	As above and impaired nongenomic methylation (e.g., myelin proteins, phospholipids)
	Depression or psychiatric disorders	Decreased synthesis of BH4 and reduced monoamine turnover; impaired genomic methylation (e.g., CpG sites in promoter region of COMT gene) and nongenomic methylation
Old age	Brain aging, cognitive decline, dementia	All the above including genomic and nongenomic methylation; decreased synthesis of membrane phospholipids, reduced choline, and ACH pools; misincorporation of dUMP into DNA
	Alzheimer's dementia and mixed dementias	All the above including impaired genomic methylation (e.g., CpG sites in promoter region of PSI gene), increased β-amyloid formation; impaired nongenomic methylation (e.g., reduced methylation of PP2A subunit C), increased phosphor-Tau formation; excitotoxicity and oxidative stress
	Cerebrovascular disease/stroke	Homocysteine-mediated vascular disease, oxidative stress

Source: Adapted from Reynolds E. *Lancet Neurol* 2006; 5:949–60. With permission.
ACH, acetylcholine; COMT, catecholamine-*O*-methyltransferase; dUMP, deoxyuridine monophosphate; PS1, presenilin-1; PP2A, protein phosphatase 2A; SACD, subacute combined; BH4, tetrahydrobiopterin.

residues of DNA, and to the amino moiety of phosphatidylethanolamine. In addition, numerous other small-molecular-weight compounds such as catecholamines and other biogenic amines are methylated. The activity of methyltransferase enzymes is subject to substrate availability and product inhibition. The universal methyl group donor for all the methylation reactions is SAM, and a common byproduct is SAH. Under normal physiological conditions SAH is hydrolyzed to Hcy. Experimental studies in animals have shown when Hcy metabolism is restricted, as can occur in folate and vitamin B12 deficiency, conversion back to SAH will occur and result in a marked increase in intracellular concentrations in peripheral and CNS tissue [49–51]. Increased SAH concentrations in the cell can lead to severe metabolic consequences as it has been shown to be a strong competitive inhibitor of methylation reactions [52,53]. The analysis of folate and metabolites related to the methylation cycle in CSF has been used to assess methylation status in the CNS. Considerable evidence points to a defect in methylation being involved in CNS disorders associated with folate and vitamin B12 deficiencies.

1. Studies on Cerebrospinal Fluid Folate and Methylation Metabolites

Increased tHcy and decreased SAM concentrations in CSF have been reported in patients diagnosed with subacute combined degeneration of the cord (SACD) resulting from either a folate or vitamin B12 deficiency [54–56]. Evidence to support a role for methylation in the maintenance of myelin has come mainly from studies on congenital defects of folate metabolism. Subnormal concentrations of 5-methyl-THF, SAM, and methionine in CSF have been reported in children with SACD, white matter disease, and cerebral atrophy resulting from severe MTHFR deficiency [37,57]. Treatment with betaine, which provides an alternative source of methyl groups, was associated with an increase in CSF SAM concentrations and in one case with magnetic resonance imaging (MRI) evidence of remyelination after 1 year of therapy [37]. More recently, Strauss et al. [48] studied five children with severe MTHFR deficiency and determined that high-dose betaine treatment led to an increase in plasma SAM, improved markers of methyltransferase activity, and a threefold increase of methionine uptake into the brain. Early intervention with betaine was associated with improved neurological outcome because one child treated from the newborn period had normal brain growth and development at 3 years of age. Two other children diagnosed during infancy showed improved neurological function, although still with developmental delay, and two older children had minimal neurological improvement [48]. It is likely that in these cases uptake of methionine into the brain supports the synthesis of SAM and promotes methylation that can protect the brain from neurological damage, which is most effective if this treatment occurs at an early stage. Confirmation that SAM is required for myelin synthesis has come from the study of a child with presumed methionine adenosyltransferase (MAT) deficiency, which catalyzes the conversion of methionine to SAM (Figure 14.1). At diagnosis, CSF methionine was grossly elevated; CSF SAM was greatly decreased; and there was MRI evidence of demyelination and basal ganglia calcification. Twelve months of therapy with oral SAM (400 mg twice daily) decreased CSF methionine and increased CSF SAM, and there was MRI evidence of remyelination [49]. In other studies, patients with acute lymphoblastic leukemia treated with the antifolate methotrexate (MTX) were found to have decreased concentrations of SAM and increased levels of SAH in CSF that were associated with leukoencephalopathy [58]. Progressive hypomethylation in the CNS was suggested to be responsible for the demyelination induced by MTX.

Analyses of CSF metabolites related to folate metabolism and the methylation cycle have also been studied in adult CNS disorders. Decreased concentrations of folate and SAM in CSF were reported in folate-deficient patients with depression and dementia, especially Alzheimer's disease (AD) [59,60], although changes in these CSF metabolites were not confirmed in another study in patients with dementia [61]. Other studies have demonstrated that there is an age-related increase in CSF tHcy [40] and decrease in CSF folate [39], which may play a role in age-related cognitive decline. Studies of the steady-state concentrations of folate and methylation metabolites in CSF, although useful in assessing global methylation status in the CNS, do not allow any measure of flux through the pathways or indicate specific methylation pathways that may be directly responsible for CNS disorders. Experimental studies in animal models have been useful in this regard as discussed in the following sections.

2. Protein Methylation in the Central Nervous System

Experimental studies have shown that inactivation of MS after exposure to nitrous oxide in the monkey [62], fruit bat [63], and pig [64] produces a myelopathy similar to that seen in SACD in humans. Supplementation with methionine in these models protected against the neurological damage. In the pig model, a decrease in the SAM/SAH ratio in neural tissues was shown to cause a generalized inhibition of "O" and "N" methyltransferase activity using an in vitro assay [65]. In another model, chickens injected with cycloleucine, an inhibitor of methionine adenosyltransferase and SAM synthesis, develop vacuolation of myelin similar to that seen in SACD [66]. Reduced incorporation of methyl groups into methyl-arginine 107 in myelin basic protein (MBP) was observed and proposed to be a major biochemical cause of demyelination. Carboxymethylation of arginine residues at position 107 in MBP is required to maintain compaction of the myelin sheath along the axon, which is essential for neurotransmission [67].

Carboxymethylation of amino acids is an important process in the post-translational modification of proteins that can alter the structure and function of enzymes. Recent studies have demonstrated a strong link between the methylation of protein phosphatase 2A (PP2A) and key CNS proteins involved in the pathogenesis of AD, such as phosphorylated Tau (p-Tau) and amyloid precursor protein (APP). PP2A is a heterotrimeric enzyme belonging to a class of serine (Ser) and threonine (Thr) phosphatases. It contains a 65-kDa scaffold A (also termed PR65 or PPP2R1) subunit, which binds a 36-kDa catalytic C (PPP2C) subunit and one of a variety of regulatory B subunits [68]. In neural tissue, Bα (also termed PPP2R2A, B55α, or PR55α) is the major regulatory subunit that increases the binding affinity of PP2A to Tau protein and markedly and specifically facilitates dephosphorylation of Tau by PP2A [69–71]. Several studies have shown that methylation of the conserved Leu-309 residue on the catalytic C subunit promotes the formation of Bα-containing PP2A holoenzymes [68] (Figure 14.3). This is catalyzed by a specific methyltransferase, leucine carboxyl methyltransferase-1 (LCMT-1; or PP2A methyltransferase-1) [72,73]. Demethylation of the catalytic C subunit by protein phosphatase methylesterase-1 may also occur [74]. In cultured cells, SAM-dependent, LCMT-1–mediated methylation of catalytic C subunit promotes the accumulation of Bα-containing PP2A holoenzymes and Tau dephosphorylation [75,76]. The role of PP2A in the CNS is recognized by studies demonstrating that LCMT-1 and methylation of PP2A subunit C are down-regulated in the cortex from AD brain, correlating with the severity of Tau pathology [77]. Studies in rat primary neuronal cell cultures have shown that MTX treatment increases levels of p-Tau which was associated with reduced PP2A methylation and reduced neuronal viability [78]. More interestingly, mice maintained on either a low folate or folate-deficient diet for 2 months had mild and severe hyperhomocysteinemia, respectively, and brain region–specific changes in SAM and SAH. This was associated with down-regulation of LCMT-1, methylated PP2A methylation, Bα expression, and enhanced Tau phosphorylation [76]. In this study, dietary modification of folate intake led to a significant decrease in SAM concentrations

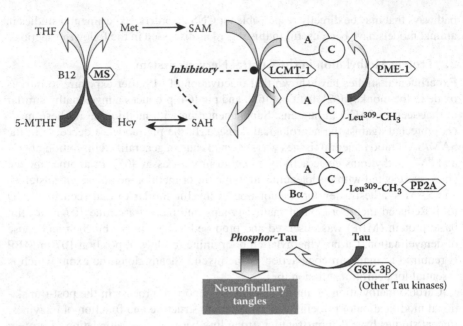

FIGURE 14.3 Relationship between 5-methyltetrahydrofolate, methylation of PP2A, and Tau phosphorylation. 5-MTHF, 5-methyltetrahydrofolate; GSK-3β, glycogen synthase kinase 3-beta; Hcy, homocysteine; LCMT, leucine carboxymethyltransferase-1; Met, methionine; MS, methionine synthase; PME-1, protein phosphatase methylesterase-1; PP2A, protein phosphatase 2A; SAH, *S*-adenosylhomocysteine; SAM, *S*-adenosylmethionine; THF, tetrahydrofolate.

in the striatum but not in other regions of the brain. Conversely, SAH concentrations were increased in all the brain regions except the striatum. These observations strongly suggest that SAH inhibition and/or down-regulation of LCMT-1 is primarily responsible for the effect of folate deficiency on PP2A substrate specificity and accumulation of p-Tau. Similar observations were reported in heterozygous mice for targeted deletion of the gene that expresses CBS [75]. In this study, regardless of the genotype (wild type or heterozygote), mice fed a high methionine and low folate diet had normal SAM but increased SAH concentrations in the brain, which was associated with decreased methylated PP2A and increased p-Tau and APP in brain tissue. The increase in phosphorylated APP is of significant interest because this has been linked to increased formation of amyloidogenic amyloid-β-peptide (Aβ) fragments [79,80]. These experimental studies provide novel mechanistic insights to the links between folate metabolism, methylation, and the pathogenesis of AD and other forms of dementia. It is important to note that studies in patients with neurological abnormalities showed that concentrations of CSF SAH and CSF folate correlated significantly with CSF p-Tau [41].

3. DNA Methylation and Transcription

Genomic DNA methylation plays a critical role in epigenetic mechanisms involving the regulation of gene expression and maintenance of gene integrity. DNA methyltransferases catalyze the transfer of a methyl group provided by SAM to cytosine residues located within CpG dinucleotide sequences. Folate provides one-carbon units to support the synthesis of SAM and thus appears to be a determinant of genomic DNA methylation and gene expression [81,82]. The promoters of housekeeping and tissue-specific genes contain CpG-rich segments. Methylation of CpG residues can directly interfere with transcription factor binding to DNA [83] or complex with methyl binding protein that affect the binding of transcriptional repressor proteins such as histone deacetylases, which results in silencing of genes [84]. Mutations in the gene encoding MeCP2, a methyl CpG binding protein linked to transcriptional repression, are associated with mental retardation. More specifically, several mutations have been identified in the *MeCP2* gene in patients with Rett syndrome, which is characterized by mental retardation, autistic behavior, severe dementia, and epilepsy. Reports of decreased concentrations of CSF 5-methyl-THF, as well as the presence of serum folate receptor autoantibodies [32,85] in patients with Rett syndrome, bring into question whether CNS folate deficiency contributes to the phenotype in this disorder. However, one study failed to confirm CNS folate deficiency in a large number of patients with Rett syndrome [86]. Geographical differences may be responsible for the discrepancy in these reports because the positive studies were performed in Europe and the negative study originated from food folate-fortified North America [32,85,86]. More recently, a European study reported low CSF folate concentrations in 8 of 25 patients with Rett syndrome, although the folate-deficient patients failed to show clinical improvement after treatment with folinic acid [87].

DNA methylation in the CNS has been linked with neural plasticity changes in response to neuronal activity and other stimuli such as learning and memory. Hypomethylation of CpG sites in the promoter region of brain-derived neurotrophic factor (*BDNF*) gene results in overexpression of BDNF in long-term cultures of cortical neurons under depolarizing conditions [88,89]. In resting nondepolarizing neurons the mouse *BDNF* promoter is hypermethylated and more tightly associated with MeCP2. In depolarizing conditions, MeCP2 associated with BDNF becomes phosphorylated, which leads to dissociation from the *BDNF* promoter and increased expression. BDNF plays an important role in neuronal survival and plasticity. More recently it has been shown that chronic overexpression of BDNF in mice causes learning deficits, as well as short-term memory impairments, both in spatial and instrumental learning tasks [90].

The transcriptional activities of several other neural-specific genes are regulated by methylated CpG residues in the promoter region. These include nicotinic receptors implicated in AD and other CNS disorders, reelin (an extracellular protein important for brain development), glial fibrillary acidic protein involved in neurogenesis and gliogenesis during CNS development, and synapsin I involved in the regulation of neurotransmitter release [91]. Recently studies have shown that membrane-bound catechol-*O*-methyltransferase (*COMT*) promoter DNA is frequently hypomethylated in frontal lobe brain tissue from schizophrenic and bipolar disorder patients [92]. The increase in transcriptional activity of *COMT* augments dopamine degradation. Interestingly, an interaction between the *MTHFR* 677C→T and *COMT* 1947G→A polymorphisms has been shown to increase the risk for reduced prefrontal activation and working memory impairment in schizophrenic subjects [93], which is associated with abnormal dopamine signaling.

DNA hypomethylation is linked to silencing of genes involved in APP processing and increased formation of amyloidogenic Aβ fragments. Aggregates of Aβ fragments occur as extracellular deposits in specific brain regions and lead to the formation of diffuse plaques that are characteristic of the neuropathology of AD. Known mutations of the *presenilin* and *APP* genes [94] result in increased activity of the γ-secretase (PS1) and β-secretase (BACE) that produce Aβ fragments. These mutations contribute to the familial form of AD, which comprises a small percentage of AD cases. The majority (90%–95%) of AD cases are sporadic in nature and occur from other underlying causes of unknown origin but also are characterized by deposition of amyloid plaques. The promoter region of the *APP* gene has CpG residues that regulate transcriptional activity. Hypomethylation of the *APP* gene promoter occurs with age in the cerebral cortex and is also observed in brain tissue from patients with AD [95,96]. In neuroblastoma SK-N-SH cells, treatment with SAM inhibits RNA expression of PS1 by methylation of its gene promoter and leads to down-regulation of Aβ peptide [97]. Medium deprived of folate and vitamin B12 decreased neuroblastoma intracellular SAM concentrations and induced PS1 and BACE promoter hypomethylation [98]. This was associated with increased PS1 and BACE protein expression and increased Aβ production, an effect that could be reversed by exogenous administration of SAM. These in vitro effects have been confirmed in a transgenic mouse model for AD (TgCRND8) in which dietary deficiency of folate, vitamin B12, and vitamin B6 induced PSI and BACE up-regulation and Aβ deposition [99]. Increased brain tissue SAH and decreased SAM/SAH ratio were proposed to cause inhibition of site-specific promoter DNA methylation. Interestingly, early cognitive impairment in a water maze task was evident in this model [99].

4. Methylation of Phospholipids

Phospholipid methylation is a reaction in which phosphatidylethanolamine (PE) is converted to phosphatidylcholine (PC). Two distinct phospholipid methyltransferase enzymes are involved with the addition of three methyl groups provided by SAM to the amino moiety of a PE molecule. The intermediate products of these enzymes are phosphatidyl-*N*-methyl ethanolamine (PME) and phosphatidyl-*N*-*N*-dimethyl ethanolamine (PDE). The sequential methylation of PE to PC involves the translocation of PE localized on the cytoplasmic side of the cell membrane to PC facing the external surface. This change in methylated phospholipid content increases the fluidity of the membrane and facilitates the lateral movement of proteins, such as receptors within the cell membrane lipid bilayer [100]. In the CNS β-adrenergic [101], muscarinic [102], and γ-aminobutyric acid receptor function [103] are influenced by phospholipid methylation.

Folate metabolism supports the synthesis of PC by providing methyl groups donated by SAM. Furthermore, membrane-bound PC is an endogenous source of choline that can be used in the synthesis of acetylcholine [104], a cholinergic neurotransmitter that plays an important role in memory function. Diminished PC concentrations are found in brain tissue from rats maintained on folate-deficient diets [105]. In a more recent study, mice maintained on a folate-deficient diet for 10 weeks were shown to have significantly depleted content of PC in brain tissue, which was associated with impaired spatial memory and learning [106]. The addition of methionine to the folate-deficient diet restored the PC content and reversed impaired memory function. Because the cognitive outcomes did not relate to hyperhomocysteinemia or reduced SAM/SAH ratios, changes in brain tissue PC content and choline availability were suggested to contribute to the manifestation of folate deficiency–related cognitive dysfunction. It is relevant to note that altered phospholipid content has been reported in postmortem brain tissue from AD patients, and significant changes in brain phospholipids that are dependent on SAM metabolism were detected in vivo with 31p magnetic resonance spectroscopy in the early stages of AD [107,108].

B. FOLATE AND MONOAMINERGIC NEUROTRANSMITTER METABOLISM

The neurotransmitter monoamines dopamine (DA), serotonin (5-hydroxytryptophan, 5HT), and norepinephrine (NE) have all been implicated in the etiology of a wide variety of neurological and psychiatric disorders. These monoamine neurotransmitters are the targets of many neuroleptic and psychopharmacotherapies directed toward correcting a CNS neurotransmitter imbalance. There is evidence to show that folate is involved in the regulation of monoamine neurotransmitters and that it is likely to play a role in depressive disorders and clinical response to antidepressant treatment. Low concentrations of CSF 5-hydroxyindole acetic acid (5-HIAA), a metabolite of 5HT that reflects global CNS tissue concentrations, have been reported in folate-deficient patients with various neuropsychiatric illnesses [109], epilepsy [110], and severe depression [111]. In a subgroup of depressed patients, CSF amine metabolites 5-HIAA, homovanillic acid (HVA, an indicator of dopamine turnover), and 3-methoxy-4-hydroxyphenylglycol (an indicator of noradrenaline turnover) were all significantly reduced in association with low red cell and CSF folate, low CSF SAM, and high CSF tHcy [39]. Experimental studies in folate-deficient mice have shown that the hypothalamic 5HIAA/5HT ratio and caudate DA and HVA concentrations were lower in deficient than control mice [112]. These neurochemical changes were associated with increased food spilling activity, a measure of motor function. Both clinical and experimental studies have confirmed that folic acid and SAM administration increase the turnover of these trimonoamines [2].

A putative mechanism linking folate deficiency and monoamine neurotransmitter function may involve tetrahydrobiopterin (BH4) metabolism, a cofactor required in the synthesis of monoamine neurotransmitters [113]. BH4 is formed by two routes: either a de novo pathway or a salvage pathway (Figure 14.4). In the de novo pathway, guanidine triphosphate (GTP) is converted to BH4 by GTP cyclohydrolase, 6-pyruvoltetrahydrobiopterin synthetase, and sepiaterin reductase (SR). In endothelial cells increasing Hcy concentrations is reported to reduce de novo synthesis of BH4 by inhibition of SR [114]. The salvage pathway of BH4 synthesis involves the conversion of quinoid-tetrahydrobiopterin by dihydropteridine reductase. There are structural similarities between folate and BH4, as both contain a pterin moiety. There is evidence to indicate that the folate enzymes MTHFR and dihydrofolate reductase (DHFR) are active in this salvage pathway (Figure 14.4). The synthesis of BH4 in the rat brain has been shown to be increased by 5-methyl-THF [115] and that DHFR can facilitate the synthesis of BH4 from BH2 [116]. More recently, studies in mice have shown that MTX, an inhibitor of DHFR, can impair the regeneration of BH4

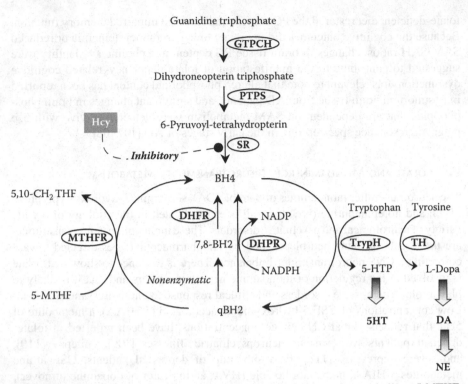

FIGURE 14.4 Relationship between folate and tetrahydrobiopterin metabolism, 5-MTHF, 5-methyltetrahydrofolate; 5-HT, serotonin; 5-HTP, 5-hydroxytryptophan; 5,10-CH$_2$THF, 5-10-methylene-tetrahydrofolate; 7,8-BH2, 7,8-dihydrobiopterin; DHFR, dihydrofolate reductase; DA, dopamine; DHPR, dihydropterin reductase; GTPCH, guanidine triphosphate cyclo-hydrolase; Hcy, homocysteine; L-dopa, 3,4-dihydroxy-L-phenylalanine; MTHFR, methylenetetrahydrofolate reductase; NE, norepinephrine; PTPS, 6-pyruvoyl-tetrahydrobiopterin synthetase; qBH2, quiniod-tetrahydrobiopterin; SR, sepiapterin reductase; TH, tyrosine hydroxylase; TrypH, tryptophan hydroxylase.

from BH2 [117]. Furthermore, in depressed patients there are significant correlations between red blood cell folate, CSF BH4, and CSF monoamine metabolites (5-HIAA and HVA) [111]. Reduced concentrations of CSF BH4 and monoamine metabolites have also been found in patients with MTHFR deficiency [116], consistent with a role for folate in BH4 synthesis and monoamine neurotransmitter metabolism.

There is a substantial body of literature to support a strong association between folate deficiency and depression [3,11,12]. It is of particular interest that a common polymorphism in the *MTHFR* gene (677C→T) is over-represented in patients with depression [118,119], providing further support for the link between folate and depression. In other studies it has been observed that folate-deficient depressed patients have a poorer clinical outcome in response to antidepressant treatment [11,120–122] and conversely that additional folate supplementation to antidepressant medication can improve clinical outcome [123,124]. Furthermore, folate deficiency can lower SAM concentrations in CSF [60], and a dietary supplement form of SAM has been shown to have an antidepressant effect. Based on these observations we have proposed that a vicious cycle of events can occur in which folate deficiency may lead to impaired methylation and neurotransmitter metabolism, increasing the risk for depression and a poor response to antidepressant therapy. This cycle may be broken with folic acid supplementation that restores methylation, improves neurotransmitter function, and enhances clinical outcome [11,125].

C. Folate Deficiency and Genomic Uracil Misincorporation

Folate is required for the synthesis of dTMP from deoxyuridine monophosphate (dUMP) (Figure 14.1). Thymidylate synthase catalyzes this reaction, which if blocked results in the accumulation of dUMP and deoxyuridine triphosphate (dUTP) and a concomitant decrease in dTMP. The consequence of increased dUTP is the misincorporation of uracil bases into DNA instead of thymidine, resulting in A/U mismatches in DNA strands, which can lead to genomic instability [126] and induce neuronal apoptosis [127]. dUMP is a normal intracellular metabolite, and small amounts of dUTP may be incorporated by DNA polymerase but is promptly removed by a base excision repair (BER) pathway involving uracil-DNA N-glycosylate (UNG). CNS tissue is particularly sensitive to DNA-damaging agents, and neurons are more vulnerable than astrocytes to DNA-damaging conditions [128]. Furthermore, the aging brain is likely to be more susceptible to DNA damage because in murine models the functional activity of the BER pathway peaks at middle age and significantly decreases in the elderly population [129].

Folate deficiency and inhibitors of folate metabolism such as MTX have been shown to induce cellular accumulation of dUTP that can lead to DNA damage [130,131,133]. Kruman et al. [133] investigated the effect of folate deficiency on Aβ-induced DNA damage in cultured hippocampal neurons. Folate deficiency resulted in increased neuronal cell death and promoted uracil misincorporation and impaired DNA repair. These effects were attenuated in the presence of Aβ, although Aβ alone did not induce these effects. In transgenic mice overexpressing APP, when maintained on a folate-deficient diet for 3 months there was a selective loss of CA3 pyramidal neurons of the hippocampus, a region sensitive to oxidative stress and DNA damage [133].

The effect of folate deficiency on uracil misincorporation into DNA has been studied in other mouse models. Mice lacking UNG maintained for 3 months on a folate-deficient diet were shown to have neurodegeneration of the CA3 hippocampal neurons, which was associated with a decrease in brain-derived nerve growth factor (BDNF) and decreased brain levels of the antioxidant glutathione [134]. BDNF is an important signaling molecule, whose synthesis and release is regulated by glutamate receptors. It is required in maintaining structural and functional changes at hippocampal synapses that underlie long-term potentiation and long-term memory [135,136]. In addition to the effects on brain BDNF, folate-deficient mice performed poorly in behavior tests for cognition, depression, and anxiety, an effect that was aggravated by the UNG$^{-/-}$ genotype. Changes in monoamines were also noted in folate-deficient mice with lower 5-HIAA/5HT ratios in the amygdala and striatum. However, this was not affected by UNG$^{-/-}$ genotype and appears therefore to be unrelated to the BER pathway [134].

D. Effect of Hyperhomocysteinemia in the Central Nervous System

1. Endothelial Dysfunction and Vascular Disease

There is a substantial amount of literature indicating Hcy is injurious to vascular endothelium and that hyperhomocysteinemia is a strong independent risk factor for cardiovascular, peripheral vascular, and cerebrovascular disease [137]. Various mechanisms have been implicated in Hcy-induced vascular dysfunction, including oxidative stress, inhibition of nitric oxide production, endoplasmic reticulum stress, and apoptotic cell death, which have been reviewed in detailed in Chapter 12 and elsewhere [138–140]. These mechanisms are particularly relevant in stroke, vascular dementia, and other cerebrovascular diseases in which hyperhomocysteinemia associated with folate deficiency is implicated. It is important to note that studies in murine models have shown that cerebral arterioles are more sensitive than the aorta to endothelial dysfunction caused by diet-induced hyperhomocysteinemia [141,142].

2. Excitotoxicity

Hyperhomocysteinemia may promote excitotoxicity and lead to increased neuronal injury and cell death. Excitotoxicity has been implicated in a wide variety of neurodegenerative and psychiatric disorders [143,144]. A pathway of oxidation of Hcy to Hcy sulfinic acid (HCSA) and homocysteic acid (HCA) has been proposed by analogy to the cysteine oxidation pathway, although enzymes catalyzing these reactions have not yet been described [143]. It has been shown by ^{35}S methionine and ^{35}S Hcy labeling studies that HCSA and HCA can be generated in brain tissue [145,146]. These compounds are putative neurotransmitters and endogenous agonists of the N-methyl-d-aspartate (NMDA) receptor. NMDA receptors are a subgroup of excitatory glutaminergic receptors involved in synaptic transmission and therefore important in excitotoxicity [143,144]. Activation of NMDA receptors results in an increase in intracellular Ca^{2+}, consequent release of cellular proteases, and eventual cell death.

In the brain, Hcy may either partially block the glycine site of the NMDA receptor complex or act as an agonist at the glutamate site of the same receptor [143]. Hcy may also be an agonist of group I metabotropic glutamate receptors [147,148]. Furthermore, Hcy has been shown to inhibit production of kynurenic acid, an endogenous antagonist of glutamate ionotropic receptors [149]. In vitro, SAH acted similar to but more potently than Hcy, suggesting that hyperhomocysteinemia-related disturbances of brain function are mediated partially by changes in brain kynurenic acid levels.

Elevated concentrations of tHcy in CSF have been reported in children with severe inborn errors affecting MTHFR [150], in folate-deficient patients with subacute combined degeneration of the cord [56], and in patients with acute lymphoblastic leukemia (ALL) treated with MTX [151,152]. In ALL patients the MTX-induced increase in CSF tHcy was associated with substantial increases in HCA and CSA. There was a definite threshold effect with increased HCA and CSA evident when CSF tHcy levels were more than 355 nmol/L. Moreover, ALL patients with neurological toxicity had many of the highest values of these sulfur-containing excitatory amino acids [151,152]. In other studies involving neuronal cell cultures, HCA has been shown to increase intracellular concentrations of the amyloidogenic fragment Aβ1-42, which was associated with cytotoxicity [153].

3. Oxidative Stress

Free radical–mediated oxidative stress is implicated as an underlying cause in a number of neurodegenerative and psychiatric diseases [154]. Several studies support the notion that Hcy neurotoxicity may be mediated through increased formation of reactive oxygen species (ROS). In cortical neuronal cell cultures, exogenous administration of Hcy was shown to interact with transition metals such as copper and attenuate the formation of hydrogen peroxide and Aβ, resulting in an increase in cell death [155]. Another study showed that cortical neuronal and neuroblastoma cell cultures grown in folate-free medium led to an increase in Hcy, ROS, and apoptosis [156]. The addition of 3-deazaadenosine, an inhibitor of Hcy formation, reduced the concentration Hcy and ROS and prevented neuronal cell death induced by folate deprivation. Folate deprivation was also associated with a decrease in cellular glutathione, a major cellular antioxidant [156]. Hyperhomocysteinemia induced in rats was shown to lead to the disruption of brain antioxidant defense, as assessed by measuring the total radical-trapping antioxidant potential [157], an effect that could be prevented by parenteral administration of folic acid [158]. In a mouse model of mild hyperhomocysteinemia, enhanced staining of superoxide radicals in peripheral vessels [141] and cerebral arterioles [142] has been demonstrated using dihydroethidium bromide, providing direct evidence of the presence of oxidative stress. Interestingly, cerebral arterioles are more sensitive to the formation of ROS than peripheral vessels, an effect that is consistent with the increased sensitivity of cerebral arterioles to Hcy-induced endothelial dysfunction [142].

The relationship between Hcy and oxidative stress has been studied in a small group of patients with AD. Increased concentrations of plasma and CSF 4-hydroxy-2-nonenol (4-HNE), a marker of lipid oxidation, have been reported in eight AD patients compared with six controls [159]. The AD patients had significantly lower levels of folate and vitamin B12 and increased plasma and CSF tHcy compared with the control group. Total Hcy and 4-HNE were significantly correlated in both plasma and CSF compartments.

V. SUMMARY

In the CNS, as in other tissues, maintaining an adequate supply of folate is essential to provide one-carbon units to support the synthesis of DNA and methionine, an essential amino acid required for the formation of SAM, which is vital for methylation-dependent pathways. In the CNS, as in other tissues, maintaining an adequate supply of folate is essential to provide one-carbon units to support the synthesis of methionine, an essential amino acid required for the formation of SAM, which is vital for methylation–dependent pathways. The aging brain may be at further risk of the effects of folate deficiency because evidence suggests that reduced transport of 5-methyl-THF across the blood-brain barrier occurs in the elderly population. This is particularly relevant for two major CNS disorders, dementia and depression, both of which are associated with folate deficiency and are prevalent in the aging population.

Our understanding of the role of folate in CNS function has increased considerably during the past decade. Several neurochemical mechanisms have been postulated to be involved in the etiology of different CNS disorders at various ages as a result of folate deficiency (Table 14.1). It is highly likely that the clinical neurological and psychiatric manifestations are the result of more than one mechanism and will also be dependent on the duration and severity of folate deficiency, as well as genetic susceptibility to CNS disorders. Additionally, a nutritional–drug–genetic interaction will play a significant role in the expression of clinical symptoms and the extent of CNS involvement.

There is increasing interest in the role of folate in AD and age-related cognitive decline. There are strong epidemiological associations linking folate deficiency and hyperhomocysteinemia with decreased cognitive function. Furthermore, positive preclinical studies have identified a central role of folate in the processing of amyloid and p-Tau protein that is linked to methylation-dependent pathways and mainstream theories related to the etiology of AD. These biochemical mechanisms that have been explored and proven in animal models and the clinical associations will provide the justification and impetus for conducting clinical trials of folate and other methyl group donors in patients with dementia and other CNS disorders.

REFERENCES

1. Reynolds EH. Folic acid, vitamin B12 and the nervous system: Historical aspects. In Botez MI, Reynolds EH, eds., *Folic Acid in Neurology, Psychiatry and Internal Medicine.* New York: Raven Press, 1979:1–5.
2. Bottiglieri T, Crellin R, Reynolds EH. Folates and neuropsychiatry. In Bailey L, ed., *Folate in Health and Disease*, 1st ed. New York: Marcel Dekker, 1995:435–62.
3. Reynolds E. Vitamin B12, folic acid, and the nervous system. *Lancet Neurol* 2006; 5:949–60.
4. Goyette P, Frosst P, Rosenblatt DS, Rozen R. Seven novel mutations in the methylenetetrahydrofolate reductase gene and genotype/phenotype correlations in severe methylenetetrahydrofolate reductase deficiency. *Am J Hum Genet* 1995; 56:1052–59.
5. Rosenblatt DS, Fenton WA. Inherited disorders of folate and cobalamin transport and metabolism. In Scriver CS, Beaudet AL, Sly WS, Calle D, eds., *The Metabolic Basis of Inherited Disease*, 8th ed. New York: McGraw-Hill, 2001:3897–933.
6. Whitehead VM. Acquired and inherited disorders of cobalamin and folate in children. *Br J Haematol* 2006; 134:125–36.
7. Iskandar BJ, Nelson A, Resnick D, Skene JH, Gao P, Johnson C, Cook TD, Hariharan N. Folic acid supplementation enhances repair of the adult central nervous system. *Ann Neurol* 2004; 56:221–27.
8. MRC Vitamin Study Research Group. Prevention of neural tube defects: Results of the Medical Research Council Vitamin Study. *Lancet* 1991; 338:131–37.
9. Shorvon SD, Carney MW, Chanarin I, Reynolds EH. The neuropsychiatry of megaloblastic anaemia. *BMJ* 1980; 281:1036–38.
10. Reynolds EH. Neurological aspects of folate and vitamin B12 metabolism. *Clin Haematol* 1976; 5:661–96.
11. Reynolds EH. Folic acid, ageing, depression, and dementia. *BMJ* 2002; 324:1512–15.
12. Morris MS. Folate, homocysteine, and neurological function. *Nutr Clin Care* 2002; 5:124–32.
13. D'Anci KE, Rosenberg IH. Folate and brain function in the elderly. *Curr Opin Clin Nutr Metab Care* 2004; 7:659–64.

14. Matherly LH, Godman ID. Membrane transport of folates. *Vitam Horm* 2003; 66:403–56.
15. Qiu A, Jansen M, Sakaris A, Min SH, Chattopadhyay S, Tsai E, Sandoval C, Zhao R, Akabas MH, Goldman ID. Identification of an intestinal folate transporter and the molecular basis for hereditary folate malabsorption. *Cell* 2006; 127:917–28.
16. Balamurugan K, Said HM. Role of reduced folate carrier in intestinal folate uptake. *Am J Physiol Cell Physiol* 2006; 291:C189–93.
17. Kneuer C, Honscha KU, Honscha W. Rat reduced-folate carrier-1 is localized basolaterally in MDCK kidney epithelial cells and contributes to the secretory transport of methotrexate and fluoresceinated methotrexate. *Cell Tissue Res* 2005; 320:517–24.
18. Sweiry JH, Yudilevich DL. Transport of folates at maternal and fetal sides of the placenta: Lack of inhibition by methotrexate. *Biochim Biophys Acta* 1985; 19;821:497–501.
19. Spector R, Johanson C. Micronutrient and urate transport in choroid plexus and kidney: Implications for drug therapy. *Pharm Res* 2006; 23:2515–24.
20. Antony AC. The biological chemistry of folate receptors. *Blood* 1992; 79:2807–20.
21. Westerhof GR, Schornagel JH, Kathmann I, Jackman AL, Rosowsky A, Forsch RA, Hynes JB, Boyle FT, Peters GJ, Pinedo HM. Carrier- and receptor-mediated transport of folate antagonists targeting folate-dependent enzymes: Correlates of molecular-structure and biological activity. *Mol Pharmacol* 1995; 48:459–71.
22. Piedrahita JA, Oetama B, Bennett GD, van Waes J, Kamen BA, Richardson J, Lacey SW, Anderson RG, Finnell RH. Mice lacking the folic acid-binding protein Folbp1 are defective in early embryonic development. *Nat Genet* 1999; 23:228–32.
23. Wollack JB, Makori B, Ahlawat S, Koneru R, Picinich SC, Smith A, Goldman ID, et al. Characterization of folate uptake by choroid plexus epithelial cells in a rat primary culture model. *J Neurochem* 2008; 104:1494–503.
24. Kamen BA, Smith AK. A review of folate receptor alpha cycling and 5-methyltetra-hydrofolate accumulation with an emphasis on cell models in vitro. *Adv Drug Deliv Rev* 2004; 56:1085–97.
25. Tran T, Shatnawi A, Zheng X, Kelley KM, Ratnam M. Enhancement of folate receptor alpha expression in tumor cells through the glucocorticoid receptor: A promising means to improved tumor detection and targeting. *Cancer Res* 2005; 65:4431–41.
26. Rothberg KG, Ying YS, Kamen BA, Anderson RG. Cholesterol controls the clustering of the glycophospholipid-anchored membrane receptor for 5-methyltetrahydrofolate. *J Cell Biol* 1990; 111:2931–38.
27. Müller G, Dearey EA, Pünter J. The sulphonylurea drug, glimepiride, stimulates release of glycosylphosphatidylinositol-anchored plasma-membrane proteins from 3T3 adipocytes. *Biochem J* 1993; 289:509–21.
28. Ramaekers VT, Häusler M, Opladen T, Heimann G, Blau N. Psychomotor retardation, spastic paraplegia, cerebellar ataxia and dyskinesia associated with low 5-methyltetrahydrofolate in cerebrospinal fluid: A novel neurometabolic condition responding to folinic acid substitution. *Neuropediatrics* 2002; 33:301–08.
29. Ramaekers VT, Blau N. Cerebral folate deficiency. *Dev Med Child Neurol* 2004; 46:843–51.
30. Rothenberg SP, da Costa MP, Sequeira JM, Cracco J, Roberts JL, Weedon J, Quadros EV. Autoantibodies against folate receptors in women with a pregnancy complicated by a neural-tube defect. *N Engl J Med* 2004; 350:134–42.
31. Ramaekers VT, Rothenberg SP, Sequeira JM, Opladen T, Blau N, Quadros EV, Selhub J. Autoantibodies to folate receptors in the cerebral folate deficiency syndrome. *N Engl J Med* 2005; 352:1985–91.
32. Ramaekers VT, Hansen SI, Holm J, Opladen T, Senderek J, Häusler M, Heimann G, Fowler B, Maiwald R, Blau N. Reduced folate transport to the CNS in female Rett patients. *Neurology* 2003; 61:506–15.

33. Moretti P, Sahoo T, Hyland K, Bottiglieri T, Peters S, del Gaudio D, Roa B, et al. Cerebral folate deficiency with developmental delay, autism, and response to folinic acid. *Neurology* 2005; 64:1088–90.

34. Spector R, Lorenzo AV. Folate transport in the central nervous system. *Am J Physiol* 1975; 229:777–82.

35. Reynolds EH, Gallagher BB, Mattson RH, Bowers M, Johnson AL. Relationship between serum and cerebrospinal fluid folate. *Nature* 1972; 240:155–57.

36. Surtees R, Hyland K. Cerebrospinal fluid concentrations of S-adenosylmethionine, methionine, and 5-methyltetrahydrofolate in a reference population: Cerebrospinal fluid S-adenosylmethionine declines with age in humans. *Biochem Med Metab Biol* 1990; 44:192–99.

37. Ormazabal A, García-Cazorla A, Pérez-Dueñas B, Gonzalez V, Fernández-Alvarez E, Pineda M, Campistol J, Artuch R. Determination of 5-methyltetrahydrofolate in cerebrospinal fluid of paediatric patients: Reference values for a paediatric population. *Clin Chim Acta* 2006; 371:159–62.

38. Verbeek MM, Blom AM, Wevers RA, Lagerwerf AJ, van de Geer J, Willemsen MA. Technical and biochemical factors affecting cerebrospinal fluid 5-MTHF, biopterin and neopterin concentrations. *Mol Genet Metab* 2008; 95:127–32.

39. Bottiglieri T, Reynolds EH, Laundy M. Folate in CSF and age. *J Neurol Neurosurg Psychiatry* 2000; 69:562.

40. Serot JM, Barbé F, Arning E, Bottiglieri T, Franck P, Montagne P, Nicolas JP. Homocysteine and methylmalonic acid concentrations in cerebrospinal fluid: Relation with age and Alzheimer's disease. *J Neurol Neurosurg Psychiatry* 2005; 76:1585–87.

41. Obeid R, Kostopoulos P, Knapp JP, Kasoha M, Becker G, Fassbender K, Herrmann W. Biomarkers of folate and vitamin B12 are related in blood and cerebrospinal fluid. *Clin Chem* 2007; 53:326–33.

42. Hagnelius NO, Wahlund LO, Nilsson TK. CSF/serum folate gradient: Physiology and determinants with special reference to dementia. *Dement Geriatr Cogn Disord* 2008; 25:516–23.

43. Neymeyer V, Tephly TR, Miller MW. Folate and 10-formyltetrahydrofolate dehydrogenase (FDH) expression in the central nervous system of the mature rat. *Brain Res* 1997; 766:195–204.

44. Sunden SL, Renduchintala MS, Park EI, Miklasz SD, Garrow TA. Betaine-homocysteine methyltransferase expression in porcine and human tissues and chromosomal localization of the human gene. *Arch Biochem Biophys* 1997; 345:171–74.

45. Stabler SP, Marcell PD, Podell ER, Allen RH, Savage DG, Lindenbaum J. Elevation of total homocysteine in the serum of patients with cobalamin or folate deficiency detected by capillary gas chromatography-mass spectrometry. *J Clin Invest* 1988; 81:466–74.

46. Lindenbaum J, Healton EB, Savage DG, Brust JC, Garrett TJ, Podell ER, Marcell PD, Stabler SP, Allen RH. Neuropsychiatric disorders caused by cobalamin deficiency in the absence of anemia or macrocytosis. *N Engl J Med* 1988; 318:1720–28.

47. Chanarin I, Deacon R, Lumb M, Perry J. Cobalamin and folate: Recent developments. *J Clin Pathol* 1992; 45:277–83.

48. Strauss KA, Morton DH, Puffenberger EG, Hendrickson C, Robinson DL, Wagner C, Stabler SP, et al. Prevention of brain disease from severe 5,10-methylenetetrahydrofolate reductase deficiency. *Mol Genet Metab* 2007; 91:165–75.

49. Bottiglieri T. Isocratic high performance liquid chromatographic analysis of S-adenosylmethionine and S-adenosylhomocysteine in animal tissues: The effect of exposure to nitrous oxide. *Biomed Chromatogr* 1990; 4:239–41.

49. Surtees R, Leonard J, Austin S. Association of demyelination with deficiency of cerebrospinal-fluid S-adenosylmethionine in inborn errors of methyl-transfer pathway. *Lancet* 1991; 338:1550–54.

50. Devlin AM, Arning E, Bottiglieri T, Faraci FM, Rozen R, Lentz SR. Effect of Mthfr genotype on diet-induced hyperhomocysteinemia and vascular function in mice. *Blood* 2004; 103:2624–29.
51. Dayal S, Devlin AM, McCaw RB, Liu ML, Arning E, Bottiglieri T, Shane B, Faraci FM, Lentz SR. Cerebral vascular dysfunction in methionine synthase-deficient mice. *Circulation* 2005; 112:737–44.
52. Cantoni GL. The role of S-adenosylhomocysteine in the biological utilization of S-adenosylmethionine. *Prog Clin Biol Res* 1985; 198:47–65.
53. Chiang PK. Biological effects of inhibitors of S-adenosylhomocysteine hydrolase. *Pharmacol Ther* 1998; 77:115–34.
54. Lever EG, Elwes RD, Williams A, Reynolds EH. Subacute combined degeneration of the cord due to folate deficiency: Response to methyl folate treatment. *J Neurol Neurosurg Psychiatry* 1986; 49:1203–07.
55. Reynolds EH, Bottiglieri T, Laundy M, Stern J, Payan J, Linnell J, Faludy J. Subacute combined degeneration with high serum vitamin B12 level and abnormal vitamin B12 binding protein. New cause of an old syndrome. *Arch Neurol* 1993; 50:739–42.
56. Bottiglieri T. Folate, vitamin B12, and neuropsychiatric disorders. *Nutr Rev* 1996; 54:382–90.
57. Hyland K, Smith I, Bottiglieri T, Perry J, Wendel U, Clayton PT, Leonard JV. Demyelination and decreased S-adenosylmethionine in 5,10-methylenetetrahydrofolate reductase deficiency. *Neurology* 1988; 38:459–62.
58. Kishi T, Tanaka Y, Ueda K. Evidence for hypomethylation in two children with acute lymphoblastic leukemia and leukoencephalopathy. *Cancer* 2000; 89:925–31.
59. Bottiglieri T, Godfrey P, Flynn T, Carney MW, Toone BK, Reynolds EH. Cerebrospinal fluid S-adenosylmethionine in depression and dementia: Effects of treatment with parenteral and oral S-adenosylmethionine. *J Neurol Neurosurg Psychiatry* 1990; 53:1096–98.
60. Bottiglieri T, Laundy M, Crellin R, Toone BK, Carney MW, Reynolds EH. Homocysteine, folate, methylation, and monoamine metabolism in depression. *J Neurol Neurosurg Psychiatry* 2000; 69:228–32.
61. Mulder C, Schoonenboom NS, Jansen EE, Verhoeven NM, van Kamp GJ, Jakobs C, Scheltens P. The transmethylation cycle in the brain of Alzheimer patients. *Neurosci Lett* 2005; 386:69–71.
62. Scott JM, Dinn JJ, Wilson P, Weir DG. Pathogenesis of subacute combined degeneration: A result of methyl group deficiency. *Lancet* 1981; 2:334–37.
63. Metz J. Cobalamin deficiency and the pathogenesis of nervous system disease. *Annu Rev Nutr* 1992; 12:59–79.
64. Weir DG, Molloy AM, Keating JN, Young PB, Kennedy S, Kennedy DG, Scott JM. Correlation of the ratio of S-adenosyl-L-methionine to S-adenosyl-L-homocysteine in the brain and cerebrospinal fluid of the pig: Implications for the determination of this methylation ratio in human brain. *Clin Sci (Lond)* 1992; 82:93–97.
65. McKeever M, Molloy A, Weir DG, Young PB, Kennedy DG, Kennedy S, Scott JM. An abnormal methylation ratio induces hypomethylation in vitro in the brain of pig and man, but not in rat. *Clin Sci (Lond)* 1995; 88:73–79.
66. Small DH, Carnegie PR. In vivo methylation of an arginine in chicken myelin basic protein. *J Neurochem* 1982; 38:184–90.
67. Kim S, Lim IK, Park GH, Paik WK. Biological methylation of myelin basic protein: Enzymology and biological significance. *Int J Biochem Cell Biol* 1997; 29:743–51.
68. Janssens V, Longin S, Goris J. PP2A holoenzyme assembly: In cauda venenum (the sting is in the tail). *Trends Biochem Sci* 2008; 33:113–21.
69. Sontag E, Nunbhakdi-Craig V, Lee G, Bloom GS, Mumby MC. Regulation of the phosphorylation state and microtubule-binding activity of Tau by protein phosphatase 2A. *Neuron* 1996; 17:1201–07.

70. Sontag E, Nunbhakdi-Craig V, Lee G, Brandt R, Kamibayashi C, Kuret J, White CL 3rd, Mumby MC, Bloom GS. Molecular interactions among protein phosphatase 2A, tau, and microtubules. Implications for the regulation of tau phosphorylation and the development of tauopathies. *J Biol Chem* 1999; 274:25490–98.

71. Xu Y, Chen Y, Zhang P, Jeffrey PD, Shi Y. Structure of a protein phosphatase 2A holoenzyme: Insights into B55-mediated Tau dephosphorylation. *Mol Cell* 2008; 31:873–85.

72. De Baere I, Derua R, Janssens V, Van Hoof C, Waelkens E, Merlevede W, Goris J. Purification of porcine brain protein phosphatase 2A leucine carboxyl methyltransferase and cloning of the human homologue. *Biochemistry* 1999; 38:16539–47.

73. Leulliot N, Quevillon-Cheruel S, Sorel I, de La Sierra-Gallay IL, Collinet B, Graille M, Blondeau K, et al. Structure of protein phosphatase methyltransferase 1 (PPM1), a leucine carboxyl methyltransferase involved in the regulation of protein phosphatase 2A activity. *J Biol Chem* 2004; 279:8351–58.

74. Ogris E, Du X, Nelson KC, Mak EK, Yu XX, Lane WS, Pallas DC. A protein phosphatase methylesterase (PME-1) is one of several novel proteins stably associating with two inactive mutants of protein phosphatase 2A. *J Biol Chem* 1999; 274:14382–91.

75. Sontag E, Nunbhakdi-Craig V, Sontag JM, Diaz-Arrastia R, Ogris E, Dayal S, Lentz SR, Arning E, Bottiglieri T. Protein phosphatase 2A methyltransferase links homocysteine metabolism with tau and amyloid precursor protein regulation. *J Neurosci* 2007; 27:2751–59.

76. Sontag JM, Nunbhakdi-Craig V, Montgomery L, Arning E, Bottiglieri T, Sontag E. Folate deficiency induces in vitro and mouse brain region-specific downregulation of leucine carboxyl methyltransferase-1 and protein phosphatase 2A B(alpha) subunit expression that correlate with enhanced tau phosphorylation. *J Neurosci* 2008; 28:11477–87.

77. Sontag E, Hladik C, Montgomery L, Luangpirom A, Mudrak I, Ogris E, White CL 3rd. Downregulation of protein phosphatase 2A carboxyl methylation and methyltransferase may contribute to Alzheimer disease pathogenesis. *J Neuropathol Exp Neurol* 2004; 63:1080–91.

78. Yoon SY, Choi HI, Choi JE, Sul CA, Choi JM, Kim DH. Methotrexate decreases PP2A methylation and increases tau phosphorylation in neuron. *Biochem Biophys Res Commun* 2007; 363:811–16.

79. Lee MS, Kao SC, Lemere CA, Xia W, Tseng HC, Zhou Y, Neve R, Ahlijanian MK, Tsai LH. APP processing is regulated by cytoplasmic phosphorylation. *J Cell Biol* 2003; 163:83–95.

80. Chang KA, Kim HS, Ha TY, Ha JW, Shin KY, Jeong YH, Lee JP, et al. Phosphorylation of amyloid precursor protein (APP) at Thr668 regulates the nuclear translocation of the APP intracellular domain and induces neurodegeneration. *Mol Cell Biol* 2006; 26:4327–38.

81. Jacob RA. Folate, DNA methylation, and gene expression: Factors of nature and nurture. *Am J Clin Nutr* 2000; 72:903–04.

82. Ulrey CL, Liu L, Andrews LG, Tollefsbol TO. The impact of metabolism on DNA methylation. *Hum Mol Genet* 2005; 14:139–47.

83. Watt F, Molloy PL. Cytosine methylation prevents binding to DNA of a HeLa cell transcription factor required for optimal expression of the adenovirus major late promoter. *Genes Dev* 1988; 2:1136–43.

84. Robertson KD, Wolffe AP. DNA methylation in health and disease. *Nat Rev Genet* 2000; 1:11–19.

85. Ramaekers VT, Sequeira JM, Artuch R, Blau N, Temudo T, Ormazabal A, Pineda M, et al. Folate receptor autoantibodies and spinal fluid 5-methyltetrahydrofolate deficiency in Rett syndrome. *Neuropediatrics* 2007; 38:179–83.

86. Neul JL, Maricich SM, Islam M, Barrish J, Smith EO, Bottiglieri T, Hyland K, Humphreys P, Percy A, Glaze D. Spinal fluid 5-methyltetrahydrofolate levels are normal in Rett syndrome. *Neurology* 2005; 64:2151–52.

87. Temudo T, Rios M, Prior C, Carrilho I, Santos M, Maciel P, Sequeiros J, et al. Evaluation of CSF neurotransmitters and folate in 25 patients with Rett disorder and effects of treatment. *Brain Dev* 2009; 31:46–51.

88. Martinowich K, Hattori D, Wu H, Fouse S, He F, Hu Y, Fan G, Sun YE. DNA methylation-related chromatin remodeling in activity-dependent BDNF gene regulation. *Science* 2003; 302:890–93.

89. Chen WG, Chang Q, Lin Y, Meissner A, West AE, Griffith EC, Jaenisch R, Greenberg ME. Derepression of BDNF transcription involves calcium-dependent phosphorylation of MeCP2. *Science* 2003; 302:885–89.

90. Cunha C, Angelucci A, D'Antoni A, Dobrossy MD, Dunnett SB, Berardi N, Brambilla R. Brain-derived neurotrophic factor (BDNF) overexpression in the forebrain results in learning and memory impairments. *Neurobiol Dis* 2009; 33:358–68.

91. Liu L, van Groen T, Kadish I, Tollefsbol TO. DNA methylation impacts on learning and memory in aging. *Neurobiol Aging* 2009; 30:549–60.

92. Abdolmaleky HM, Cheng KH, Faraone SV, Wilcox M, Glatt SJ, Gao F, Smith CL, et al. Hypomethylation of MB-COMT promoter is a major risk factor for schizophrenia and bipolar disorder. *Hum Mol Genet* 2006; 15:3132–45.

93. Roffman JL, Gollub RL, Calhoun VD, Wassink TH, Weiss AP, Ho BC, White T, et al. MTHFR 677C --> T genotype disrupts prefrontal function in schizophrenia through an interaction with COMT 158Val --> Met. *Proc Natl Acad Sci USA* 2008; 105:17573–78.

94. Lippa CF. Familial Alzheimer's disease: Genetic influences on the disease process. Review. *Int J Mol Med* 1999; 4:529–36.

95. Tohgi H, Utsugisawa K, Nagane Y, Yoshimura M, Genda Y, Ukitsu M. Reduction with age in methylcytosine in the promoter region -224 approximately -101 of the amyloid precursor protein gene in autopsy human cortex. *Brain Res Mol Brain Res* 1999; 70:288–92.

96. West RL, Lee JM, Maroun LE. Hypomethylation of the amyloid precursor protein gene in the brain of an Alzheimer's disease patient. *J Mol Neurosci* 1995; 6:141–46.

98. Fuso A, Seminara L, Cavallaro RA, D'Anselmi F, Scarpa S. S-adenosylmethionine/homocysteine cycle alterations modify DNA methylation status with consequent deregulation of PS1 and BACE and beta-amyloid production. *Mol Cell Neurosci* 2005; 28:195–204.

97. Scarpa S, Fuso A, D'Anselmi F, Cavallaro RA. Presenilin 1 gene silencing by S-adenosylmethionine: A treatment for Alzheimer disease? *FEBS Lett* 2003; 541: 145–48.

99. Fuso A, Nicolia V, Cavallaro RA, Ricceri L, D'Anselmi F, Coluccia P, Calamandrei G, Scarpa S. B-vitamin deprivation induces hyperhomocysteinemia and brain S-adenosylhomocysteine, depletes brain S-adenosylmethionine, and enhances PS1 and BACE expression and amyloid-beta deposition in mice. *Mol Cell Neurosci* 2008; 37:731–46.

100. Crews FT. Effects of membrane fluidity on secretion and receptor stimulation. *Psychopharmacol Bull* 1982; 18:135–43.

101. Hirata F, Strittmatter WJ, Axelrod J. beta-Adrenergic receptor agonists increase phospholipid methylation, membrane fluidity, and beta-adrenergic receptor-adenylate cyclase coupling. *Proc Natl Acad Sci USA* 1979; 76:368–72.

102. Muccioli G, Scordamaglia A, Bertacco S, Di Carlo R. Effect of S-adenosyl-L-methionine on brain muscarinic receptors of aged rats. *Eur J Pharmacol* 1992; 227:293–99.

103. Di Perri B, Calderini G, Battistella A, Raciti R, Toffano G. Phospholipid methylation increases [3H]diazepam and [3H]GABA binding in membrane preparations of rat cerebellum. *J Neurochem* 1983; 41:302–08.

104. Blusztajn JK, Liscovitch M, Richardson UI. Synthesis of acetylcholine from choline derived from phosphatidylcholine in a human neuronal cell line. *Proc Natl Acad Sci USA* 1987; 84:5474–77.

105. Akesson B, Fehling C, Jägerstad M, Stenram U. Effect of experimental folate deficiency on lipid metabolism in liver and brain. *Br J Nutr* 1982; 47:505–20.

106. Troen AM, Chao WH, Crivello NA, D'Anci KE, Shukitt-Hale B, Smith DE, Selhub J, Rosenberg IH. Cognitive impairment in folate-deficient rats corresponds to depleted brain phosphatidylcholine and is prevented by dietary methionine without lowering plasma homocysteine. *J Nutr* 2008; 138:2502–09.

107. Pettegrew JW, Kopp SJ, Minshew NJ, Glonek T, Feliksik JM, Tow JP, Cohen MM. 31P nuclear magnetic resonance studies of phosphoglyceride metabolism in developing and degenerating brain: Preliminary observations. *J Neuropathol Exp Neurol* 1987; 46:419–30.

108. Forlenza OV, Wacker P, Nunes PV, Yacubian J, Castro CC, Otaduy MC, Gattaz WF. Reduced phospholipid breakdown in Alzheimer's brains: A 31P spectroscopy study. *Psychopharmacology (Berl)* 2005; 180:359–65.

109. Botez MI, Young SN, Bachevalier J, Gauthier S. Folate deficiency and decreased brain 5-hydroxytryptamine synthesis in man and rat. *Nature* 1979; 278:182–83.

110. Botez MI, Young SN. Effects of anticonvulsant treatment and low levels of folate and thiamine on amine metabolites in cerebrospinal fluid. *Brain* 1991; 114:333–48.

111. Bottiglieri T, Hyland K, Laundy M, Godfrey P, Carney MW, Toone BK, Reynolds EH. Folate deficiency, biopterin and monoamine metabolism in depression. *Psychol Med* 1992; 22:871–76.

112. Gospe SM Jr, Gietzen DW, Summers PJ, Lunetta JM, Miller JW, Selhub J, Ellis WG, Clifford AJ. Behavioral and neurochemical changes in folate-deficient mice. *Physiol Behav* 1995; 58:935–41.

113. Kaufman S. Regulatory properties of pterin-dependent hydroxylases: Variations on a theme. In Usdin E, Weiner N, Youdim MBH, eds., *Function and Regulation of Monoamine Enzymes*. New York: Macmillian, 1981:165–73.

114. Topal G, Brunet A, Millanvoye E, Boucher JL, Rendu F, Devynck MA, David-Dufilho M. Homocysteine induces oxidative stress by uncoupling of NO synthase activity through reduction of tetrahydrobiopterin. *Free Radic Biol Med* 2004; 36:1532–41.

115. Hamon CBG, Blair JA, Barford PA. The effect of methyltetrahydrofolate on tetrahydrobiopterin metabolism. *J Mental Def Res* 1986; 30:170–83.

116. Kaufman S. Some metabolic relationships between biopterin and folate: Implications for the methyl trap hypothesis. *Neurochem Res* 1991; 16:1031–36.

117. Sawabe K, Wakasuqi K, Haseqwa H. Tetrahydrobiopterin uptake in supplemental administration: Elevation of tissue tetrahydrobiopterin in mice following uptake of the exogenously oxidized product 7,8-dihydrobiopterin and subsequent reduction by an anti-folate-sensitive process. *J Pharmacol Sci* 2004; 96:124–33.

118. Gilbody S, Lewis S, Lightfoot T. Methylenetetrahydrofolate reductase (MTHFR) genetic polymorphisms and psychiatric disorders: A HuGE review. *Am J Epidemiol* 2007; 165:1–13.

119. Kelly CB, McDonnell AP, Johnston TG, Mulholland C, Cooper SJ, McMaster D, Evans A, Whitehead AS. The MTHFR C677T polymorphism is associated with depressive episodes in patients from Northern Ireland. *J Psychopharmacol* 2004; 18:567–71.

120. Wesson VA, Levitt AJ, Joffe RT. Change in folate status with antidepressant treatment. *Psychiatry Res* 1994; 53:313–22.

121. Fava M, Borus JS, Alpert JE, Nierenberg AA, Rosenbaum JF, Bottiglieri T. Folate, vitamin B12, and homocysteine in major depressive disorder. *Am J Psychiatry* 1997; 154:426–28.

122. Coppen A, Abou-Saleh MT. Plasma folate and affective morbidity during long-term lithium therapy. *Br J Psychiatry* 1982; 141:87–89.

123. Godfrey PS, Toone BK, Carney MW, Flynn TG, Bottiglieri T, Laundy M, Chanarin I, Reynolds EH. Enhancement of recovery from psychiatric illness by methylfolate. *Lancet* 1990; 336:392–95.

124. Coppen A, Bailey J. Enhancement of the antidepressant action of fluoxetine by folic acid: A randomised, placebo controlled trial. *J Affect Disord* 2000; 60:121–30.

125. Bottiglieri T. Homocysteine and folate metabolism in depression. *Prog Neuropsychopharmacol Biol Psychiatry* 2005; 29:1103–12.

126. Beetstra S, Thomas P, Salisbury C, Turner J, Fenech M. Folic acid deficiency increases chromosomal instability, chromosome 21 aneuploidy and sensitivity to radiation-induced micronuclei. *Mutat Res* 2005; 578:317–26.

127. Kruman II, Schwartz E, Kruman Y, Cutler RG, Zhu X, Greig NH, Mattson MP. Suppression of uracil-DNA glycosylase induces neuronal apoptosis. *J Biol Chem* 2004; 279:43952–60.

128. Gobbel GT, Bellinzona M, Vogt AR, Gupta N, Fike JR, Chan PH. Response of post-mitotic neurons to X-irradiation: Implications for the role of DNA damage in neuronal apoptosis. *J Neurosci* 1998; 18:147–55.

129. Weissman L, de Souza-Pinto NC, Stevnsner T, Bohr VA. DNA repair, mitochondria, and neurodegeneration. *Neuroscience* 2007; 145(4):1318–29.

130. Goulian M, Bleile B, Tseng BY. The effect of methotrexate on levels of dUTP in animal cells. *J Biol Chem* 1980; 255:10630–37.

131. Goulian M, Bleile B, Tseng BY. Methotrexate-induced misincorporation of uracil into DNA. *Proc Natl Acad Sci USA* 1980; 7:1956–60.

132. Bertino JR, Mini E, Fernandes DJ. Sequential methotrexate and 5-fluorouracil: Mechanisms of synergy. *Semin Oncol* 1983; 10(Suppl 2):2–5.

133. Kruman II, Kumaravel TS, Lohani A, Pedersen WA, Cutler RG, Kruman Y, Haughey N, Lee J, Evans M, Mattson MP. Folic acid deficiency and homocysteine impair DNA repair in hippocampal neurons and sensitize them to amyloid toxicity in experimental models of Alzheimer's disease. *J Neurosci* 2002; 22:1752–62.

134. Kronenberg G, Harms C, Sobol RW, Cardozo-Pelaez F, Linhart H, Winter B, Balkaya M, et al. Folate deficiency induces neurodegeneration and brain dysfunction in mice lacking uracil DNA glycosylase. *J Neurosci* 2008; 28:7219–30.

135. Lu Y, Christian K, Lu B. BDNF: A key regulator for protein synthesis-dependent LTP and long-term memory? *Neurobiol Learn Mem* 2008; 89:312–23.

136. Hu Y, Russek SJ. BDNF and the diseased nervous system: A delicate balance between adaptive and pathological processes of gene regulation. *J Neurochem* 2008; 105:1–17.

137. McCully KS. Homocysteine, vitamins, and vascular disease prevention. *Am J Clin Nutr* 2007; 86:1563S–68S.

138. Wilson KM, Lentz SR. Mechanisms of the atherogenic effects of elevated homocysteine in experimental models. *Semin Vasc Med* 2005; 5:163–71.

139. Lentz SR. Mechanisms of homocysteine-induced atherothrombosis. *J Thromb Haemost* 2005; 3:1646–54.

140. Cook JW, Taylor LM, Orloff SL, Landry GJ, Moneta GL, Porter JM. Homocysteine and arterial disease. Experimental mechanisms. *Vascul Pharmacol* 2002; 38:293–300.

141. Dayal S, Arning E, Bottiglieri T, Böger RH, Sigmund CD, Faraci FM, Lentz SR. Cerebral vascular dysfunction mediated by superoxide in hyperhomocysteinemic mice. *Stroke* 2004; 35:1957–62.

142. Dayal S, Bottiglieri T, Arning E, Maeda N, Malinow MR, Sigmund CD, Heistad DD, Faraci FM, Lentz SR. Endothelial dysfunction and elevation of S-adenosylhomocysteine in cystathionine beta-synthase-deficient mice. *Circ Res* 2001; 88:1203–09.

143. Lipton SA, Kim WK, Choi YB, Kumar S, D'Emilia DM, Rayudu PV, Arnelle DR, Stamler JS. Neurotoxicity associated with dual actions of homocysteine at the N-methyl-D-aspartate receptor. *Proc Natl Acad Sci USA* 1997; 94:5923–28.

144. Olney JW. Excitatory amino acids and neuropsychiatric disorders. *Biol Psychiatry* 1989; 26:505–25.

145. Do KQ, Benz B, Binns KE, Eaton SA, Salt TE. Release of homocysteic acid from rat thalamus following stimulation of somatosensory afferents in vivo: Feasibility of glial participation in synaptic transmission. *Neuroscience* 2004; 124:387–93.

146. Cuenod M, Grandes P, Zangerle L, Streit P, Do KQ. Sulphur-containing excitatory amino acids in intercellular communication. *Biochem Soc Trans* 1993; 21:72–77.

147. Lazarewicz J, Urbanska EM. Dual effect of DL-homocysteine and S-adenosylhomo-cysteine on brain synthesis of the glutamate receptor antagonist, kynurenic acid. *J Neurosci Res* 2005; 79:375–82.

148. Zieminska E, Stafiej A, Lazarewicz JW. Role of group I metabotropic glutamate receptors and NMDA receptors in homocysteine-evoked acute neurodegeneration of cultured cerebellar granule neurones. *Neurochem Int* 2003; 43:481–92.

149. Luchowska E, Luchowski P, Paczek R, Ziembowicz A, Kocki T, Turski WA, Wielosz M, Azarewicz J, Urbanska EM. Dual effect of DL-homocysteine and S-adenosylhomo-cysteine on brain synthesis of the glutamate receptor antagonist, kynurenic acid. *J Neurosci Res* 2005; 79:375–82.

150. Surtees R, Bowron A, Leonard J. Cerebrospinal fluid and plasma total homocysteine and related metabolites in children with cystathionine beta-synthase deficiency: The effect of treatment. *Pediatr Res* 1997; 42:577–82.

151. Quinn CT, Griener JC, Bottiglieri T, Hyland K, Farrow A, Kamen BA. Elevation of homocysteine and excitatory amino acid neurotransmitters in the CSF of children who receive methotrexate for the treatment of cancer. *J Clin Oncol* 1997; 15:2800–06.

152. Quinn CT, Griener JC, Bottiglieri T, Arning E, Winick NJ. Effects of intraventricular methotrexate on folate, adenosine, and homocysteine metabolism in cerebrospinal fluid. *J Pediatr Hematol Oncol* 2004; 26:386–88.

153. Hasegawa T, Ukai W, Jo DG, Xu X, Mattson MP, Nakagawa M, Araki W, Saito T, Yamada T. Homocysteic acid induces intraneuronal accumulation of neurotoxic Abeta42: Implications for the pathogenesis of Alzheimer's disease. *J Neurosci Res* 2005; 80:869–76.

154. Bains JS, Shaw CA. Neurodegenerative disorders in humans: The role of glutathione in oxidative stress-mediated neuronal death. *Brain Res Brain Res Rev* 1997; 25:335–58.

155. White AR, Huang X, Jobling MF, Barrow CJ, Beyreuther K, Masters CL, Bush AI, Cappai R. Homocysteine potentiates copper- and amyloid beta peptide-mediated toxicity in primary neuronal cultures: Possible risk factors in the Alzheimer's-type neurodegen-erative pathways. *J Neurochem* 2001; 76:1509–20.

156. Ho PI, Ashline D, Dhitavat S, Ortiz D, Collins SC, Shea TB, Rogers E. Folate deprivation induces neurodegeneration: Roles of oxidative stress and increased homocysteine. *Neurobiol Dis* 2003; 14:32–42.

157. Wyse AT, Zugno AI, Streck EL, Matté C, Calcagnotto T, Wannmacher CM, Wajner M. Inhibition of Na(+),K(+)-ATPase activity in hippocampus of rats subjected to acute administration of homocysteine is prevented by vitamins E and C treatment. *Neurochem Res* 2002; 27:1685–89.

158. Matté C, Mackedanz V, Stefanello FM, Scherer EB, Andreazza AC, Zanotto C, Moro AM, et al. Chronic hyperhomocysteinemia alters antioxidant defenses and increases DNA damage in brain and blood of rats: Protective effect of folic acid. *Neurochem Int* 2009; 54:7–13.

159. Selley ML, Close DR, Stern SE. The effect of increased concentrations of homocysteine on the concentration of (E)-4-hydroxy-2-nonenal in the plasma and cerebrospinal fluid of patients with Alzheimer's disease. *Neurobiol Aging* 2002; 23:383–88.

15 Folate–Vitamin B12 Interrelationships
Links to Disease Risk

Anne M. Molloy

CONTENTS

I. INTRODUCTION

The link between folate and vitamin B12 (cobalamin) metabolism has been known for decades. Early studies of the biochemistry of the sulfur-containing amino acids (cysteine, homocysteine [Hcy], and methionine) led to the discovery that transmethylation pathways exist in both rats and humans [1,2], that "biologically labile methyl groups" can be synthesized, and that the dietary requirement for methionine can be met by feeding Hcy plus folate and vitamin B12 [3,4]. The discovery, purification, and early kinetic studies of cobalamin-dependent methionine synthase (MS) were later accomplished by work from a number of laboratories, thus clarifying the metabolic connection between folate and vitamin B12 [5,6]. This chapter summarizes the research in the past decade that has led to our current understanding of the reaction synthesized by this unique enzyme.

The molecular processes leading to disruption of the uptake and flux of folate cofactors within the cell that explain why a severe vitamin B12 deficiency can be clinically manifested as a functional folate deficiency are reviewed in this chapter. There are, however, still many gaps in our understanding of the subtle influences of vitamin B12 status on the apportioning of one-carbon units across metabolic pathways within the folate metabolic axis, especially under conditions of unbalanced status. For example, the current widespread prevalence of very high blood folate concentrations, resulting from mandatory or voluntary folic acid fortification coupled with vitamin supplementation, has led to a situation in which an increased number of people have opposite extremes in terms of their folate and vitamin B12 status. Whether there are metabolic and health-related consequences of these unprecedented conditions is unknown. This chapter reviews folate and vitamin B12 interactions in the light of new evidence of associations with risk of disease.

Accumulating evidence suggests that there may be a relatively high prevalence of low vitamin B12 status among women, children, and the elderly. This chapter reviews recent literature linking folate and vitamin B12 with maternal and neonatal health as well as with the development and maintenance of bone health.

II. METABOLIC ASSOCIATIONS

A. METHIONINE SYNTHASE AND METHIONINE SYNTHASE REDUCTASE

Only two enzymes in mammalian systems are known to require vitamin B12 (cobalamin) as a cofactor: methylmalonyl CoA mutase (EC 5.4.99.2) and MS (EC 2.1.1.13). The close association of vitamin B12 with folate metabolism stems solely from its role in the function of MS because the mutase reaction has no direct links with folate pathways. Cobalamin-dependent MS uses methyl cobalamin as an intermediate methyl carrier at one active site and transfers the methyl group from cobalamin to Hcy at another active site in a mechanism that appears to be unique in biological systems [6,7]. The partial purification and early classification of the enzyme in *Escherichia coli* was carried out by Taylor and Weissbach [8–11], but in recent years extensive work from the Matthews and Ludwig laboratories on both *E. coli* and mammalian MS have identified it as a highly complex, zinc-containing enzyme, with distinct modules for binding of Hcy, 5-methyltetrahydrofolate (5-methyl-THF), cobalamin, and S-adenosylmethionine (AdoMet; also termed SAM) [12]. The enzyme undergoes dramatic conformational rearrangements during catalysis to overcome the considerable chemical and mechanistic challenges imposed by the reaction [6,13–15]. During the primary turnover of the enzyme, methylcobalamin, in the cob(III) form, is demethylated to form cob(I)alamin and then remethylated with 5-methyl-THF (Figure 15.1). Further complexity is added by the occasional oxidation of cob(I)alamin to cob(II)alamin (at an approximate rate of once in every 200–1,000 turnovers), which then requires a reductive methylation in which AdoMet rather than 5-methyl-THF supplies the methyl group, and in mammalian systems the flavoprotein MS reductase (MSR; EC 1.16.1.8; also termed MTRR) supplies the electron derived from NADP(H) [16–20] (Figure 15.1). In humans, the *MTR* gene, encoding MS, has been mapped to chromosome 1 and has been cloned by

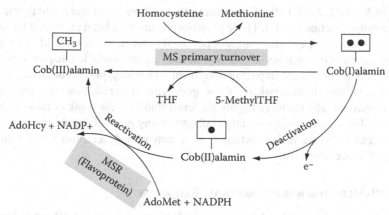

FIGURE 15.1 The cobalamin-dependent synthesis of methionine (R-S-CH₃) from homocysteine (R-S-H) and 5-methyl-THF through methionine synthase. THF (tetrahydrofolate) is the coproduct of the reaction. During the primary turnover of the enzyme, methylcobalamin (CH₃-cob(III)alamin) is demethylated to form cob(I)alamin and then remethylated with 5-methyl-THF. Oxidation of cob(I)alamin to cob(II)alamin occurs at an approximate rate of once in every 200 to 1,000 turnovers. The cofactor then requires a reductive methylation in which AdoMet (*S*-adenosylmethionine) rather than 5-methyl-THF supplies the methyl group, and the electron is supplied through the conversion of NADPH to NADP⁺ via the flavoprotein methionine synthase reductase (MSR).

several groups [21–23]. Patients with functional MS deficiency have homocystinuria and hypomethioninemia without methylmalonic aciduria. Two classes of deficiency, *CblG* and *CblE*, have been described based on complementation analysis. Defective MS protein has been identified as the underlying cobalamin-related abnormality in *CblG* patients [24–26].

The human *MTRR* gene, encoding the protein MSR, has also been cloned and has been mapped to chromosome 5 [16,27]. Recent evidence, using recombinant human MS and MSR, indicates that MSR plays an important role in stabilizing MS apoenzyme and enhancing the formation of MS holoenzyme. This seems to be achieved through MSR's additional ability to function as an aquacobalamin reductase, whereby it can convert aquacobalamin to the cob(II)alamin form, which can then be converted to enzyme-bound methylcobalamin [18]. Yamada et al. suggest that this property of the enzyme may solve an important gap in understanding the cellular formation of methylcobalamin [18]. The findings also complement earlier work identifying defective MSR protein as the underlying cause of the cobalamin disorder in *CblE* complementation patients, which causes functional MS deficiency [27,28]. Details of these properties are well described elsewhere, and the point to note for this chapter is that MSR seems to be essential for MS activity in vivo; therefore, the functions of both MS and MSR are essential to the role of vitamin B12 in folate metabolism.

Common polymorphisms have been described in the genes for both enzymes. The most widely studied of these are two nonsynonymous single nucleotide polymorphisms (SNPs), the 2756A→G (D919G) variant in *MTR* and the 66A→G (I22M) variant in *MTRR* [22,29], both of which are relatively prevalent and could potentially affect enzyme function [30,31]. These polymorphisms have been evaluated for metabolic and disease risk effects, both independently and in the context of gene–gene and gene–nutrient interactions [29,32–51]. Details are presented in Chapter 4. Briefly, there are reports of modest impacts on vitamin B12 status, plasma total Hcy (tHcy) concentration, and disease risk for these genotypes. Overall, however, the results are not consistent, and the more highly powered studies show weak or no significant effects [42,46]. Future studies on large cohorts, using more elaborate microsatellite analysis of all the genes in this metabolic axis, may provide a clearer insight into the genetic influences involved.

B.   5,10-METHYLENETETRAHYDROFOLATE REDUCTASE

The third enzyme involved in folate–vitamin B12 interactions is 5,10-methylenetetrahydrofolate reductase (MTHFR; EC 1.5.1.20), which catalyzes the reduction of 5,10-methylene-THF to 5-methyl-THF, thereby generating the methyl group substrate for MS from the folate cofactor pool (Figure 15.2). This enzyme is also a flavoprotein, containing loosely bound flavin adenine dinucleotide (FAD) that accepts reducing equivalents from NADP(H) [52]. Allosteric inhibition by AdoMet exerts an important control over activity; in mammals the enzyme exists as a homodimer of about 77 kDa, with both catalytic and AdoMet regulatory domains in each subunit

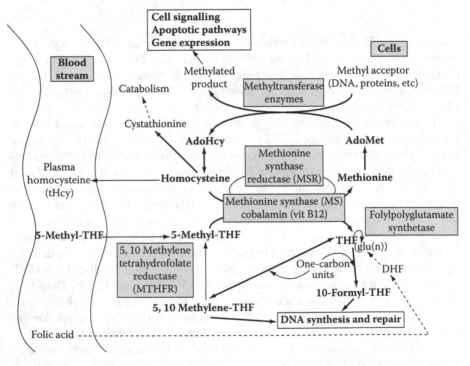

FIGURE 15.2   Folate enzymes and pathways directly influenced by vitamin B12. AdoHcy, *S*-adenosylhomocysteine; AdoMet, *S*-adenosylmethionine; DHF, dihydrofolate; Hcy, homocysteine; THF, tetrahydrofolate.

[53]. Elevated S-adenosylhomocysteine (AdoHcy; also termed SAH) can remove the inhibition by AdoMet [54], indicating that the cellular ratio of AdoMet to AdoHcy may be the most important regulatory factor and that the flux of one-carbon units through MS is controlled by the capacity to remethylate Hcy, as well as the amount of available methionine. Yamada et al. [55] showed that recombinant human MTHFR undergoes phosphorylation, resulting in a less active form that is more sensitive to inhibition by AdoMet. They proposed a dual regulation system for the mammalian enzyme, with the AdoMet/AdoHcy ratio influencing the fraction of enzyme in the active (nonphosphorylated) and inactive (phosphorylated) states. Although the implications of these new findings for MTHFR function are not understood, they give evidence of the physiological complexity of regulation over the production of 5-methyl-THF polyglutamate within the cell.

MTHFR is crucial to the balance of one-carbon units within the cell and to the efficient function of the folate–vitamin B12 metabolic axis because the formation of 5-methyl-THF from 5,10-methylene-THF is essentially irreversible under physiological conditions [56]; thus, the enzyme channels the flow of one-carbon units away from; DNA synthesis and into methionine and AdoMet synthesis (Figure 15.2). Furthermore, the reduction of 5,10-methylene-THF via MTHFR is the only biological process known to generate 5-methyl-THF [57]. The unidirectional flow and exclusive role for MTHFR in generating 5-methyl-THF, along with its potent sensitivity to AdoMet concentration, the follow-on product of methionine synthesized through MS, allows MTHFR to function as a control valve in the partitioning of folate cofactors between DNA synthesis and methylation reactions.

Genetic mutations in *MTHFR* are the most common inborn errors in folate metabolism, spanning a broad scale of disruption in enzyme activity and displaying a variety of neurological and vascular symptoms [58–60]. An important feature of mutations in *MTHFR* that give rise to less efficient function is an abnormally high tHcy level [58,59,61–63], further evidence of its role in providing methyl groups for MS. Dramatically reduced rates of methionine synthesis are also observed in tissue lines from such patients [64], and a reduced supply of methyl groups through MS for AdoMet synthesis in neurological tissue has been implicated as a mechanism for the neurological symptoms seen in these patients [65]. Kang et al. [66,67] were first to describe a "thermolabile" version of MTHFR in patients with coronary artery disease, which they predicted was caused by a genetic mutation in *MTHFR*. Goyette et al. [68] isolated the human cDNA for the enzyme, and Frosst et al. [69] reported the existence of an *MTHFR* 677C→T polymorphism that resulted in an amino acid change in the protein from alanine to valine (A222V). They also demonstrated in vitro thermolability, reduced lymphocyte enzyme activity, and elevated plasma tHcy associated with the variant, thereby making a convincing argument that it was the mutation predicted by Kang et al. Studies on the molecular effects of the mutation in *E. coli* constructs (the homologous mutant being A177V) [70] and in recombinant human enzyme [71] demonstrated that the binding affinity of the flavin cofactor for the enzyme is weakened in the presence of a valine rather than an alanine in the protein and that loss of FAD leads to structural perturbations of the enzyme, but that binding can be stabilized by the presence of a high folate concentration [70,72]. Yamada et al. [71] concluded that the variant protein is sensitive not only to low folate status but also to low riboflavin and AdoMet concentrations in vitro, and they suggested that folate, methionine, and riboflavin would all be important for maintenance of MTHFR activity in vivo. Both cell culture and human studies support these conclusions by demonstrating that riboflavin status influences plasma tHcy in subjects who are homozygous for the TT variant [73–78]. Furthermore, low vitamin B12 status may also modulate the effect of the TT genotype on plasma tHcy [78–80], suggesting that MTHFR is at the center of a "functional metabolic network" that may require correct balancing of multiple vitamins for optimal function [78]. Further characteristics of the *MTHFR* 677C→T polymorphism are discussed in Chapter 4.

C. BIOCHEMICAL UTILIZATION OF 5-METHYL-THF

As noted elsewhere, 5-methyl-THF is the predominant form of folate circulating in the blood stream and available for cellular uptake. However, the only reaction known to use 5-methyl-THF in mammalian systems is cobalamin-dependent MS. Furthermore, 5-methyl-THF is a poor substrate for folylpolyglutamate synthetase (EC 6.3.2.17), and the folate moiety must be converted to THF through the MS reaction to be incorporated into the cellular folate polyglutamate pool and participate fully in one-carbon interconversions [81,82] (Figure 15.2). The constraints imposed by 5-methyl-THF have well-described consequences for one-carbon metabolism and explain one aspect of the effect of vitamin B12 deficiency on folate metabolism (reviewed in Savage and Lindenbaum [83] and Shane and Stokstad [84]). The methyl-trap hypothesis [85,86] was put forward to describe these consequences, particularly the phenomenon of folate trapping as 5-methyl-THF. Briefly, in the absence of vitamin B12, circulating 5-methyl-THF, while available, is essentially unusable by the cell. Moreover, 5-methyl-THF polyglutamate, produced through MTHFR from THF polyglutamate cofactors already in the cell, is also blocked from further metabolism because the MTHFR reaction is irreversible (Figure 15.2). Thus, deficiency of vitamin B12 leads to an inability to incorporate new folate and a deficit of intracellular THF cofactors available for purine and pyrimidine synthesis. The metabolic and clinical consequences are similar to those seen in folate deficiency where disruption in the production of purines and pyrimidines for DNA synthesis occurs, leading in severe cases to a megaloblastic anemia (discussed in Chapter 16). The methyl-trap hypothesis has been supported in cell culture systems, animal models, and human studies [81,87–93]. Genetic disorders of enzymes involved in the folate/B12 metabolic axis also provide evidence that disruption of MS is the underlying cause of megaloblastic anemia observed in vitamin B12 deficiency [83]. The paradox of normal or high-normal serum folate in combination with deficient tissue (e.g., red blood cell) folate concentrations [83,92,94–96] may be observed in a proportion of patients with pernicious anemia and is consistent with a functional intracellular folate deficiency. Patients who have neurological manifestations of disease seem to have significantly higher serum folate compared with those who have hematological symptoms only [94,97,98], but there is no clear biological explanation for this difference.

D. REMETHYLATION OF HCY

In a vitamin B12 deficiency, disruption of Hcy remethylation results in an elevation of tissue Hcy, culminating in increased export to the plasma compartment (Figure 15.2).

Numerous studies show that an elevated plasma tHcy concentration is a highly sensitive, although nonspecific, marker of impaired vitamin B12 status [99–101]. Although intervention trials and other analyses of blood indicators show that folate status is the most powerful nutritional predictor of plasma tHcy [99,100,102–105], in situations where folate status is already optimal, such as in folic acid-fortified populations, vitamin B12 status becomes the major nutritional predictor of tHcy [106,107]. The disruption in Hcy remethylation theoretically results in reduced formation of AdoMet, thereby removing the allosteric inhibition of MTHFR activity and allowing further "trapping" of 5-methyl-THF [108]. A reduced availability of AdoMet for biological methyltransferase reactions is potentially of equal concern because methylation reactions within the cell are responsible for a variety of modifications to DNA, proteins, lipids, neurotransmitters, etc., and they function to regulate gene expression, cell signaling, and other essential cellular pathways. AdoHcy, the coproduct of these reactions, is a powerful competitive inhibitor of methyltransferase enzymes and under normal conditions is rapidly converted to adenosine and Hcy via AdoHcy hydrolase (EC 3.3.1.1) [109]. However, the AdoHcy hydrolase reaction is reversible and favors the synthesis of AdoHcy; therefore, any increase in the level of Hcy will be expected to alter the AdoHcy concentration and disturb the AdoMet/AdoHcy ratio, potentially inhibiting the activity of methyltransferase enzymes [110,111]. There is good evidence that the increase in intracellular Hcy does affect the AdoHcy concentration, and this is mirrored by strong correlations between tHcy and AdoHcy in plasma and cerebrospinal fluid (CSF) [112–114]. However, methyltransferase enzymes exhibit a range of sensitivity to AdoHcy, and theoretically a moderate increase in the level of AdoHcy might have a very variable effect on methyltransferase function, depending on the K_i for AdoHcy [113,115]. This may be an important consideration in seeking to identify changes in genomic or protein methylation status in response to mild or moderate impairment of the folate/vitamin B12 metabolic axis.

Although biologically plausible, the consequences above must be interpreted cautiously because vitamin B12 deficiency has different effects on Hcy remethylation in different tissues. In liver and kidney, for example, betaine Hcy methyltransferase (BHMT; EC 2.1.1.5) remethylates Hcy in a reaction that is folate independent and has an important sparing effect on the consequences of vitamin B12 deficiency [116–119]. Hepatic and kidney metabolic pathways are major contributors to methyl group utilization in the body, and the flux of methyl groups through AdoMet in liver is balanced by several enzymatic systems, including (1) the MAT1A form of methionine adenosyltransferase (MAT; EC 2.5.1.6), which is capable of producing very high concentrations of AdoMet with increasing concentrations of methionine [110,120]; (2) choline oxidation through betaine and BHMT, which provides an alternative source of methyl groups for Hcy remethylation [121]; and (3) glycine N-methyltransferase (EC 2.1.1.20), which may function to catabolize excess methionine and prevent wide fluctuations in AdoMet concentration [122,123]. In addition to transmethylation pathways, transsulfuration through cystathionine-β-synthase (EC 4.2.1.22) also exerts an important influence on Hcy homeostasis in these tissues [120,121] (Figure 15.2). Comprehensive reviews of these interacting systems are available elsewhere [120,121,124]. However, it must be noted that the profiles of Hcy-related metabolites in the blood circulation are largely influenced by hepatic and renal metabolism [123,125,126], and the multiplicity of pathways for maintenance of methyl group metabolism in these tissues may help to explain the inconsistent findings of studies that seek to associate disease progression or risk with plasma AdoMet and AdoHcy concentrations.

By contrast, BHMT is not expressed in neural tissue [127,128]. Therefore, the brain has an absolute requirement for cobalamin-dependent MS to remethylate Hcy [113,129,130]. Furthermore, the brain expresses the MATIIA isoform, which is inhibited by high tissue levels of AdoMet [131]. Thus, the rate of utilization of AdoMet in brain effectively controls the rate of synthesis and the level of AdoMet within brain. Animal studies indicate that the concentration of AdoMet is considerably above the K_m values of AdoMet for the vast majority of methyltransferase enzymes [132] and that the brain concentration of AdoMet is not a limiting factor for enzymatic methylation under normal conditions [115]. However, this is not necessarily the case for AdoHcy, which often has a greater affinity for methyltransferase enzymes than the substrate AdoMet, and whose level has been shown in animal studies to increase dramatically when MS activity is experimentally disrupted or in other conditions that result in elevated plasma tHcy [110,133–137]. For example, several studies have linked elevated tHcy or AdoHcy with increased concentrations of the inflammatory cytokine tumor necrosis factor α (TNFα) [138–140] and have postulated a role for AdoHcy in increasing TNFα cytotoxicity through the inhibition of specific carboxyl-O-methyltransferase enzymes [141]. Others have shown that TNFα may be a modulator of the neurological lesions seen in severe vitamin B12 deficiency both in experimental animals [142] and in human studies [143,144], but these studies did not include the measurement of AdoMet or AdoHcy.

In recent years, new methodology for the measurement of AdoMet and AdoHcy in tissues and in the blood circulation [145–149] has prompted an evaluation of these metabolites in clinical conditions, including vitamin B12 deficiency and inborn errors of the enzymes involved in the methylation of Hcy [65,97]. Elevated plasma AdoHcy was found in vitamin B12–deficient patients [150,151]. Some studies also suggested that the plasma AdoHcy level might be a more sensitive indicator of other conditions that are associated with elevated tHcy, such as cardiovascular disease [114,152–154]. Surprisingly, some studies found elevated AdoMet in serum of patients with conditions associated with elevated tHcy [97,150]. However, several workers concluded that these metabolites are strongly associated with renal function [147,150,155]; moreover, the clearance of AdoMet from plasma appears to be very different from that of AdoHcy [147]; therefore, their value in plasma as markers of hypomethylation in tissues such as the nervous system is questionable. More informative data might be obtained from measurement of AdoMet and AdoHcy in CSF [65,111,112].

E.   UTILIZATION OF FOLIC ACID

In contrast to the effect of impaired MS function on the cellular uptake and incorporation of 5-methyl-THF, folic acid is readily incorporated into the intracellular biologically active folate pool by reduction with NADPH to dihydrofolate and then THF via the enzyme dihydrofolate reductase (EC 1.5.1.3) [156,157] (Figure 15.2). As THF, it can then be used to maintain purine and pyrimidine synthesis, even in the face of impaired MS function. Thus, in theory, folic acid treatment in vitamin B12 deficiency may improve the anemia and perhaps delay the diagnosis of deficiency while allowing the neurological lesion to progress. The "masking" of the hematological disorder by treatment with folic acid while allowing the progression (and queried potential exacerbation) of the neurological signs and symptoms of vitamin B12 deficiency was originally put forward from studies between 1945 and 1950, in which large doses of folic acid (well above 1 mg/day) were used to treat pernicious anemia (reviewed in Savage and Lindenbaum [83,158] and Reynolds [98]). However, these reviewers have pointed out that the studies of that period actually showed that some neurological improvement could also occur and that both hematological and neurological relapse almost invariably ensued, but to different degrees and at different rates, which Reynolds [98] suggested might be a consequence of the specific rates of metabolism and turnover in these tissues. Savage and Lindenbaum [158] reviewed a series of patients who were treated with less than 1 mg folic acid/day, and, notwithstanding a gradual progression of disease in some of these subjects, none had the precipitous hematological or neurological responses seen after the massively large doses used in earlier studies. It is nevertheless clear that high folic acid intake is inappropriate for people with latent pernicious anemia, but the threshold of intake to cause any hazard is not known. Whether it is also hazardous for elderly people who have marginal vitamin B12 status resulting from impaired absorption of food-bound B12 to be exposed to moderately high (or even high) folic acid intake is less clear [159–161]. These issues have been hotly debated in the past decade as a potential adverse effect of high folic acid intake after the mandatory fortification of grain in the United States for the prevention of neural tube defects (NTDs) [160,162–167].

III.   POTENTIAL LINKS TO DISEASE RISK

A.   FOLATE–VITAMIN B12-RELATED METABOLITES IN SEVERE B12 DEFICIENCY

The clinical manifestations of vitamin B12 deficiency have been thoroughly reviewed elsewhere [83,98,158]. As noted above, evidence suggests that both the hematological and the neurological manifestations are largely caused by disruption of MS [98,113,158], but it is not known why the neurological and hematological consequences are so divergent from patient to patient or why metabolite changes in blood can be so varied [24,97]. In an effort to identify biochemical factors that might be selectively involved in these two processes, Carmel et al. [97] studied Hcy-related blood metabolites with regard to the presence or absence of neurological disease in 22 patients who had confirmed pernicious anemia. Plasma tHcy was similarly high in 11 patients with neurological abnormalities and 11 without neurological symptoms. No differences were observed in methionine concentrations of the two groups, but plasma AdoMet and serum folate concentrations were significantly higher and cysteine and cysteinylglycine were lower in those with neurological disease. Levels of AdoHcy were not measured. All differences were corrected with cobalamin therapy. Unfortunately, these results did not elucidate an MS-linked biochemical mechanism for the neuropathy. The authors concluded that the changes in blood may largely represent hepatic folate/B12 metabolism. Differences in renal function may also have contributed to the findings. It is not known whether measurement of such metabolites in CSF would be more informative, although this has been carried out in other neurodegenerative conditions in which the association with hyperhomocysteinemia is more tenuous [112,168–171].

B.   Folate–Vitamin B12-Related Metabolites in "Subclinical" or Moderate B12 Deficiency

It is well established that pernicious anemia is classically caused by an acquired autoimmunity to essential factors required for intestinal transport and absorption of vitamin B12. In recent years it has become clear that classical pernicious anemia, which has a low prevalence, may not be the clinical situation that is of greatest public health concern [172]. Mild or moderate B12 deficiency resulting from gastric atrophy or other conditions leading to impaired absorption of food-bound vitamin B12 is much more common, particularly among the elderly [24,159,173–176]. In this instance, a modest biochemical phenotype is usually observed, including moderate elevation of the vitamin B12 biomarkers tHcy and methylmalonic acid (MMA). An increase in plasma tHcy is often the earliest evidence of disruption in intracellular folate metabolism, even before the plasma vitamin B12 level decreases to levels that are considered to be clinically relevant [159,177]. Although researchers agree that mild or "subclinical" vitamin B12 deficiency may be widely prevalent among older persons, there is considerable debate and lack of understanding of the clinical implications of "subclinical" deficiency, which may account for up to 70% of low vitamin B12 concentrations [24,172,178]. It is also not clear to what extent these individuals might naturally progress to clinical deficiency or what type of neurological impairment might be predicted to occur, especially in older persons, in whom a number of conditions can lead to dementia and other neurological conditions. As noted below, and discussed in detail elsewhere in this book, diminished cognitive function has received particular recent attention as a potential adverse effect of low vitamin B12 status [174,179].

C.   Effects of Concomitant Low Vitamin B12 and High Folate Status

The question of the effect of high folate status on those with low vitamin B12 status is of considerable current interest. As noted above, "masking" of the anemia was rarely seen with doses of folic acid less than 1 mg/day [83], and this was considered an upper safe limit for daily consumption of free folic acid. However, the likely blood folate status that could be reached with long-term daily intake of folic acid from fortified foods and supplements was not known and is only beginning to be fully assessed. Extremely high serum folate levels (>50 nmol/L) seem to be heavily weighted toward those who take folic acid supplements [180,181], and interpretation of data on the hazards of high folic acid intake may be somewhat confounded by the lifestyle and medical reasons for why these people are taking supplements. Tucker et al. [167] assessed folate and vitamin B12 intakes and blood concentrations in 747 elderly individuals pre- and postfortification and estimated that the prevalence of combined high folate intake (>1,000 μg/day) and low plasma vitamin B12 concentration (<185 pmol/L [<250 pg/mL]) would increase from 0.1% to 0.4% after fortification. In a study of Canadian women aged 65 and older, Ray et al. [182] predicted an increase from 0.1% to 0.6% in the prevalence of people with combined blood vitamin B12 less than 150 pmol/L and serum folate greater than 45 nmol/L. Both authors raised concerns about the masking of vitamin B12 deficiency and recommended the addition of small amounts of vitamin B12 to fortified foods. Mills et al. [160] reviewed laboratory data between 1992 and 2000 from 1,573 patients with vitamin B12 levels below the normal range (<258 pmol/L) and found no evidence of an increase in the number who presented without anemia since fortification began based on hematocrit and mean cell volume (MCV) results, suggesting that masking of vitamin B12 deficiency was not a major problem. However, in a similar temporal study of 633 subjects, Wyckoff and Ganji [161] found that B12-deficient subjects postfortification were three times more likely to present with no anemia (without elevated MCV) compared with the prefortification era. These authors also found lower overall MCV values postfortification, consistent with improved folate status of the population. They, and the accompanying editorial [183], urged against the use of MCV data as a marker for vitamin B12 deficiency, but Carmel [178] defended the importance of MCV data in the clinical setting and challenged the validity of extrapolating population surveys, which may contain a high portion of individuals with "subclinical" deficiency, to form conclusions about changes in the likely manifestation of clinical vitamin B12 deficiency.

In 2005, studies on cognitive function in relation to high folate intake in the postfortification era began to emerge. Morris et al. [184] examined cognitive function in relation to folate intake in 3,718 community-dwelling older persons. Contrary to the study hypothesis, intake in the highest total folate quintile (median, 742 μg/day) was associated with faster cognitive decline over a median follow-up of approximately 6 years, but there was an interactive effect between high folate plus high vitamin B12 intake and cognition in the oldest age group, raising concern that higher folate intake might be marking poorer health. Using National Health and Nutrition Examination Survey (NHANES) data, Morris et al. [185] examined macrocytosis and impaired cognition in 1,459 elderly subjects in the context of varying extremes of folic acid intake. Significantly reduced cognitive function was observed in 45% of 42 subjects with high serum folate (>59 nmol/L) who had concomitant low vitamin B12 status (defined as either serum vitamin B12 less than 148 pmol/L or serum MMA greater than 210 nmol/L). This represented an odds ratio (OR) of 4.9 (95% confidence interval [CI], 2.6–9.2) compared with the rate of cognitive impairment (11%) in 826 subjects with normal vitamin B12 plus normal folate status. Subjects within the category of low vitamin B12 plus normal folate also had significantly increased risk of cognitive impairment (OR, 1.9; 95% CI, 1.1–3.1) but not of the same magnitude. By contrast, normal vitamin B12 plus high folate status was significantly protective (OR, 0.5; 95% CI, 0.2–0.9). The findings were exactly mirrored in relation to the presence of anemia, with the sole exception that the combination of normal vitamin B12 plus high folate was not significantly protective against anemia (OR, 0.6; 95% CI, 0.2–2.2). The article provoked considerable reaction [180,186,187]. The accompanying editorial [186] raised concerns about the current fortification policy in the United States and the implementation of similar policies in other countries, emphasizing the point that metabolic consequences of opposite extremes in the balance of folate and vitamin B12 within the cell are unknown and considering the possibility that in circumstances of very high folate status the presence of unmetabolized folic acid may be a contributing factor in determining disease risk. Berry et al. [180] provided NHANES data to point out that those in the highest folate category may be different in many ways from those in the lowest category, particularly in their use of supplements. The fact that such supplement users were also likely to be taking supplemental B12, but nevertheless had deficient B12 status, prompted Berry et al. [180] to propose that undiagnosed pernicious anemia might account for the findings. Other differences between supplement and nonsupplement users also need to be considered, such as ethnicity, education, lifestyle, and awareness of chronic disease risk—although age, race/ethnicity, and education were among adjustments in the Morris et al. [184] analysis. In response to the study, Clarke et al. [187] carried out a similar analysis on 2,559 elderly individuals with eligible data from within two population-based cohorts in the United Kingdom. In that study, low vitamin B12 status was defined as a serum holotranscobalamin less than 45 pmol/L, and high folate was categorized in two ways: as serum folate greater than 30 nmol/L and greater than 60 nmol/L. The study was limited by lower numbers in the highest at-risk category; nevertheless, the authors found that low vitamin B12 status was significantly associated with anemia and cognitive impairment, but there was no evidence that the association was negatively affected by high folate status. Selhub et al. [188] recently followed up on this topic by assessing vitamin B12 biomarkers tHcy and MMA in relation to combined vitamin B12 deficiency plus high folate status. Again using NHANES data from before (1991 to 1994) and after (1999–2002) fortification with folic acid, they categorized subjects on a serum vitamin B12 cutoff of less than 148 pmol/L for deficiency and compared trends in tHcy and MMA across folate categories, chosen to give equivalent numbers of individuals with low vitamin B12 in each category. In the 1991 to 1994 NHANES cohort, tHcy was higher in those who had low vitamin B12 status, but there was a trend toward reduction in tHcy with higher folate, both in the low and normal vitamin B12 groups. These data are consistent with the known influence of folate and vitamin B12 on tHcy status, under the relatively low blood folate conditions prevailing in the period [102]. In the postfortification cohort, the blood folate concentrations of all the subjects were much higher, such that there was little overlap between the data in the two cohorts. Plasma total Hcy was lower overall, and the effect of folate status on tHcy was greatly attenuated, also consistent with other data on postfortification determinants of tHcy [106,107]. Unexpectedly, trends toward higher tHcy and higher MMA were seen in subjects with deficient vitamin B12 status as folate levels increased, suggesting a negative interaction with both vitamin B12–dependent enzymes when the balance of folate and vitamin B12 within the cell is at opposite extremes. The metabolic mechanisms for such effects have never been previously considered. The data are intriguing, particularly with respect to MMA; however, the discrepancy in MMA values between the two cohorts makes interpretation of the trends more difficult for this metabolite. Confirmation in other studies is required, as well as further medical and lifestyle information on participants in the highest folate categories.

D. Pregnancy Complications

As discussed elsewhere in this book, folate plays a profound and wide-ranging role in maintaining healthy reproduction. By contrast, the effects of low vitamin B12 status in reproduction are not well defined, despite the close metabolic links between folate and vitamin B12. Pernicious anemia is a known cause of infertility [189–191], and severe B12 deficiency in pregnancy has also been associated with early pregnancy loss [191,192], but these conditions are extremely rare among women of reproductive age. However, it is now recognized that the global prevalence of low vitamin B12 status among women and children may be much higher than hitherto suspected [193,194], and, in parallel with effects of folate on reproduction, researchers are considering the effects of nutritional B12 deficiency on maternal and neonatal health. In one study from China, inadequate preconceptional serum vitamin B12 status (<350 pg/ml; <258 pmol/L) was associated with a 60% increased risk of preterm birth [195], and in an urban Nepalese cohort with a doubled prevalence of preeclampsia and preterm delivery, 65% of pregnant women had inadequate plasma vitamin B12, linked to elevated tHcy [196,197].

Even in well-nourished women, longitudinal studies of serum vitamin B12 concentration during normal pregnancy indicate a gradual decrease of about 30% between the first and third trimester that returns to prepregnancy levels within a few weeks postpartum [198–200]. There is little evidence of maternal tissue depletion or functional deficiency associated with these lower B12 levels in the first two trimesters [201–203], although low B12 levels in the third trimester of pregnancy seem to correlate with an increase in plasma tHcy and MMA and suggest that subclinical deficiency may start to appear at this stage, particularly in mothers on inadequate diets [199,204]. Evidence that impaired vitamin B12 status may affect MS function is also available from data showing that the plasma tHcy in neonates (measured in umbilical cords) is strongly predicted by maternal and fetal vitamin B12 rather than folate [205–208]. One possible explanation for a weaker folate relationship is the widespread folic acid supplementation to mothers in the latter part of pregnancy. However, plasma MMA, which is a marker of vitamin B12 function unrelated to folate, is also strongly associated with B12 at this time, both in mothers and infants [207,209], suggesting compromised or inefficient vitamin B12 function of neonates. Furthermore, in a randomized trial, vitamin B12 supplements corrected both the elevated MMA and tHcy in neonates [210], strengthening the argument for impaired B12 status, particularly in breast-fed infants, because infant formula is usually fortified with vitamin B12.

There is now good evidence that inadequate or deficient vitamin B12 status might be associated with NTDs. In the past decade a number of studies have shown that maternal vitamin B12 status is an independent risk factor for NTDs [211]. Two large studies, carried out during the introduction of folic acid fortification in the United States [212] and postfortification in Canada [213], found a tripling of risk between the lowest and highest quintile of serum B12 [212] or quartile of holotranscobalamin [213]. In a more recent analysis, using data from three large independent cohorts of affected mothers in a population unfortified and unsupplemented with folic acid or vitamin B12, women with early pregnancy serum vitamin B12 concentrations less than 250 ng/L (185 pmol/L) had a 2.5 to 3-fold higher risk of being the mother of an NTD-affected child, after adjusting for folate [214]. It is not known how folate and vitamin B12 might interact to affect neural tube formation, but several mechanisms are possible because B12 influences both the incorporation of folates into the cellular pool and the flux of folate-derived one-carbon units destined for DNA synthesis or for methylation reactions. Although DNA synthesis is essential for embryonic development, other factors that trigger developmental changes are likely to be influenced by methylation reactions, such as differential gene expression and activation or repression of apoptotic pathways.

E. FOLATE–VITAMIN B12 INTERACTIONS AND OSTEOPOROSIS

Osteoporotic fractures in the elderly population are a major public health problem. It is well known that classical homocystinuria is associated with skeletal deformities, and a number of researchers have hypothesized that elevated plasma tHcy might be a risk factor for osteoporotic fractures in elderly persons. In 2004, two studies concluded that increased plasma tHcy was a strong independent risk factor for osteoporotic fractures in older men and women [215,216], suggesting that nutritional and other factors influencing plasma tHcy were involved. In a number of cross-sectional and prospective studies, low serum folate concentration was associated with lower bone mineral density (BMD) [217–219] or with risk of hip fractures [220] in postmenopausal women. Low plasma vitamin B12 was also associated with lower BMD in frail elderly women [221] and with bone turnover markers in healthy elderly people [222] and in adolescents [223]. In one study involving 2,576 adults from the Framingham cohort, both men and women with plasma vitamin B12 less than 148 pmol/L had significantly lower BMD at several sites compared with those in the upper category [224]. Interestingly, there is some evidence of an association between bone mass, bone mineral density, osteoporosis, or incidence of hip fractures with the *MTHFR* 677C→T polymorphism [225–228], although not all reported studies are positive [217,220]. Associations between this variant and riboflavin, folate, and vitamin B12 status have all been cited, suggesting an important folate–vitamin B12 interaction in bone development and maintenance.

IV. SUMMARY

The interaction of folate and vitamin B12 through MS has been known for years, and the consequences of vitamin B12 deficiency on intracellular folate pathways have been studied in detail. In the past decade, considerable progress has been made in understanding the kinetic and mechanistic details of the reaction catalyzed by MS.

Information is continually expanding on genetic mutations and polymorphisms that affect the function of both MS and the enzymes MSR and MTHFR that influence, or are influenced by, MS activity. New methodologies have facilitated the analysis of downstream metabolites of MS that will hopefully elucidate the effects of impaired function of the enzyme caused by vitamin B12 deficiency. Despite this knowledge and these tools, the underlying biochemical mechanism leading to the neurological manifestation of vitamin B12 deficiency remains an enigma, and there is still little understanding of the reasons for the patient to patient differences in the clinical manifestations of deficiency, although it is believed that impairment of MS plays a dominant role. Furthermore, there is little clarity regarding the clinical consequences of "subclinical" or moderate vitamin B12 deficiencies, which are now considered to affect a substantial proportion of elderly people. The effects of mildly impaired vitamin B12 function on folate-related pathways are not known but are likely to include both molecular and epigenetic consequences. Within the past decade, the fortification of foods with folic acid has resulted in an unprecedented situation in which some elderly individuals have opposite extremes in their status of folate and vitamin B12. Further research is urgently needed to examine the impact of such extreme imbalance of nutrient status, both at a molecular level and in relation to negative health consequences.

ACKNOWLEDGMENTS

Anne Molloy is supported by the intramural research program of the Eunice Kennedy Shriver National Institute of Child Health and Human Development, National Institutes of Health (contract no. N01-HD-3-3348).

REFERENCES

1. Keller EB, Rachele JR, Du Vigneaud V. A study of transmethylation with methionine containing deuterium and C14 in the methyl group. *J Biol Chem* 1949; 177:733–38.
2. Rachele JR, Reed LJ, Kidwai AR, Ferger MF, du Vigneaud V. Conversion of cystathionine labeled with S35 to cystine in vivo. *J Biol Chem* 1950; 185:817–26.
3. du Vigneaud V, Ressler C, Rachele JR. The biological synthesis of "labile methyl group." *Science* 1950; 112:267–71.
4. Bennett MA. Utilization of homocystine for growth in presence of vitamin B12 and folic acid. *J Biol Chem* 1950; 187:751–56.
5. Weissbach H, Taylor RT. Roles of vitamin B 12 and folic acid in methionine synthesis. *Vitam Horm* 1970; 28:415–40.
6. Matthews RG. Cobalamin-dependent methionine synthase. In: Banerjee R, ed., *Chemistry and Biochemistry of B12*. New York: John Wiley and Sons, Inc, 1999:681–706.
7. Evans JC, Huddler DP, Hilgers MT, Romanchuk G, Matthews RG, Ludwig ML. Structures of the N-terminal modules imply large domain motions during catalysis by methionine synthase. *Proc Natl Acad Sci USA* 2004; 101:3729–36.
8. Taylor RT, Weissbach H. N5-Methyltetrahydrofolate-homocysteine transmethylase. Partial purification and properties. *J Biol Chem* 1967; 242:1502–08.
9. Taylor RT, Weissbach H. N5-Methyltetrahydrofolate-homocysteine transmethylase. Role of S-adenosylmethionine in vitamin B12-dependent methionine synthesis. *J Biol Chem* 1967; 242:1517–21.
10. Taylor RT, Weissbach H. N5-Methyltetrahydrofolate-homocysteine transmethylase. Propylation characteristics with the use of a chemical reducing system and purified enzyme. *J Biol Chem* 1967; 242:1509–16.
11. Taylor RT, Weissbach H. Escherichia coli B N5-methyltetrahydrofolate-homocysteine cobalamin methyltransferase: Activation with S-adenosyl-L-methionine and the mechanism for methyl group transfer. *Arch Biochem Biophys* 1969; 129:745–66.

12. Goulding CW, Postigo D, Matthews RG. Cobalamin-dependent methionine synthase is a modular protein with distinct regions for binding homocysteine, methyltetrahydrofolate, cobalamin, and adenosylmethionine. *Biochemistry* 1997; 36:8082–91.

13. Jarrett JT, Hoover DM, Ludwig ML, Matthews RG. The mechanism of adenosyl-methionine-dependent activation of methionine synthase: A rapid kinetic analysis of intermediates in reductive methylation of cob(II)alamin enzyme. *Biochemistry* 1998; 37:12649–58.

14. Bandarian V, Pattridge KA, Lennon BW, Huddler DP, Matthews RG, Ludwig ML. Domain alternation switches B(12)-dependent methionine synthase to the activation conformation. *Nat Struct Biol* 2002; 9:53–56.

15. Datta S, Koutmos M, Pattridge KA, Ludwig ML, Matthews RG. A disulfide-stabilized conformer of methionine synthase reveals an unexpected role for the histidine ligand of the cobalamin cofactor. *Proc Natl Acad Sci USA* 2008; 105: 4115–20.

16. Leclerc D, Odievre M, Wu Q,Wilson A, Huizenga JJ, Rozen R, Scherer SW, Gravel RA. Molecular cloning, expression and physical mapping of the human methionine synthase reductase gene. *Gene* 1999; 240:75–88.

17. Olteanu H, Banerjee R. Human methionine synthase reductase, a soluble P-450 reductase-like dual flavoprotein, is sufficient for NADPH-dependent methionine synthase activation. *J Biol Chem* 2001; 276:35558–63.

18. Yamada K, Gravel RA, Toraya T, Matthews RG. Human methionine synthase reductase is a molecular chaperone for human methionine synthase. *Proc Natl Acad Sci USA* 2006; 103:9476–81.

19. Leal NA, Olteanu H, Banerjee R, Bobik TA. Human ATP:Cob(I)alamin adenosyl-transferase and its interaction with methionine synthase reductase. *J Biol Chem* 2004; 279:47536–42.

20. Wolthers KR, Lou X, Toogood HS, Leys D, Scrutton NS. Mechanism of coenzyme binding to human methionine synthase reductase revealed through the crystal structure of the FNR-like module and isothermal titration calorimetry. *Biochemistry* 2007; 46:11833–44.

21. Li YN, Gulati S, Baker PJ, Brody LC, Banerjee R, Kruger WD. Cloning, mapping and RNA analysis of the human methionine synthase gene. *Hum Mol Genet* 1996; 5:1851–58.

22. Chen LH, Liu ML, Hwang HY, Chen LS, Korenberg J, Shane B. Human methionine synthase. cDNA cloning, gene localization, and expression. *J Biol Chem* 1997; 272:3628–34.

23. Leclerc D, Campeau E, Goyette P, Adjalla CE, Christensen B, Ross M, Eydoux P, Rosenblatt DS, Rozen R, Gravel RA. Human methionine synthase: cDNA cloning and identification of mutations in patients of the cblG complementation group of folate/cobalamin disorders. *Hum Mol Genet* 1996; 5:1867–74.

24. Carmel R, Green R, Rosenblatt DS, Watkins D. Update on cobalamin, folate, and homocysteine. *Hematol Am Soc Hematol Educ Prog* 2003:62–81.

25. Watkins D, Ru M, Hwang HY, Kim CD, Murray A, Philip NS, Kim W, et al. Hyperhomocysteinemia due to methionine synthase deficiency, cblG: Structure of the MTR gene, genotype diversity, and recognition of a common mutation, P1173L. *Am J Hum Genet* 2002; 71:143–53.

26. Wilson A, Leclerc D, Saberi F, Campeau E, Hwang HY, Shane B, Phillips JA 3rd, Rosenblatt DS, Gravel RA. Functionally null mutations in patients with the cblG-variant form of methionine synthase deficiency. *Am J Hum Genet* 1998; 63:409–14.

27. Leclerc D, Wilson A, Dumas R, Gafuik C, Song D, Watkins D, Heng HH, et al. Cloning and mapping of a cDNA for methionine synthase reductase, a flavoprotein defective in patients with homocystinuria. *Proc Natl Acad Sci USA* 1998; 95:3059–64.

28. Wilson A, Leclerc D, Rosenblatt DS, Gravel RA. Molecular basis for methionine synthase reductase deficiency in patients belonging to the cblE complementation group of disorders in folate/cobalamin metabolism. *Hum Mol Genet* 1999; 8:2009–16.

29. Wilson A, Platt R, Wu Q, Leclerc D, Christensen B, Yang H, Gravel RA, Rozen R. A common variant in methionine synthase reductase combined with low cobalamin (vitamin B12) increases risk for spina bifida. *Mol Genet Metab* 1999; 67:317–23.

30. Wang XL, Cai H, Cranney G, Wilcken DE. The frequency of a common mutation of the methionine synthase gene in the Australian population and its relation to smoking and coronary artery disease. *J Cardiovasc Risk* 1998; 5:289–95.

31. Morita H, Kurihara H, Sugiyama T, Hamada C, Kurihara Y, Shindo T, Oh-hashi Y, Yazaki Y. Polymorphism of the methionine synthase gene: Association with homocysteine metabolism and late-onset vascular diseases in the Japanese population. *Arterioscler Thromb Vasc Biol* 1999; 19:298–302.

32. Harmon DL, Shields DC, Woodside JV, McMaster D, Yarnell JW, Young IS, Peng K, Shane B, Evans AE, Whitehead AS. Methionine synthase D919G polymorphism is a significant but modest determinant of circulating homocysteine concentrations. *Genet Epidemiol* 1999; 17:298–309.

33. Dekou V, Gudnason V, Hawe E, Miller GJ, Stansbie D, Humphries SE. Gene-environment and gene-gene interaction in the determination of plasma homocysteine levels in healthy middle-aged men. *Thromb Haemost* 2001; 85:67–74.

34. Chen J, Stampfer MJ, Ma J, Selhub J, Malinow MR, Hennekens CH, Hunter DJ. Influence of a methionine synthase (D919G) polymorphism on plasma homocysteine and folate levels and relation to risk of myocardial infarction. *Atherosclerosis* 2001; 154:667–72.

35. Zhang Y, Zhang M, Niu T, Xu X, Zhu G, Huo Y, Chen C, et al. D919G polymorphism of methionine synthase gene is associated with blood pressure response to benazepril in Chinese hypertensive patients. *J Hum Genet* 2004; 49:296–301.

36. Ulrich CM, Curtin K, Potter JD, Bigler J, Caan B, Slattery ML. Polymorphisms in the reduced folate carrier, thymidylate synthase, or methionine synthase and risk of colon cancer. *Cancer Epidemiol Biomarkers Prev* 2005; 14:2509–16.

37. Boyles AL, Billups AV, Deak KL, Siegel DG, Mehltretter L, Slifer SH, Bassuk AG, et al. Neural tube defects and folate pathway genes: Family-based association tests of gene-gene and gene-environment interactions. *Environ Health Perspect* 2006; 114:1547–52.

38. Tsai MY, Welge BG, Hanson NQ, Bignell MK, Vessey J, Schwichtenberg K, Yang F, Bullemer FE, Rasmussen R, Graham KJ. Genetic causes of mild hyperhomocysteine-mia in patients with premature occlusive coronary artery diseases. *Atherosclerosis* 1999; 143:163–70.

39. Relton CL, Wilding CS, Pearce MS, Laffling AJ, Jonas PA, Lynch SA, Tawn EJ, Burn J. Gene-gene interaction in folate-related genes and risk of neural tube defects in a UK population. *J Med Genet* 2004; 41:256–60.

40. Doolin MT, Barbaux S, McDonnell M, Hoess K, Whitehead AS, Mitchell LE. Maternal genetic effects, exerted by genes involved in homocysteine remethylation, influence the risk of spina bifida. *Am J Hum Genet* 2002; 71:1222–26.

41. Bosco P, Gueant-Rodriguez RM, Anello G, Barone C, Namour F, Caraci F, Romano A, Romano C, Guéant JL. Methionine synthase (MTR) 2756 (A --> G) polymorphism, double heterozygosity methionine synthase 2756 AG/methionine synthase reductase (MTRR) 66 AG, and elevated homocysteinemia are three risk factors for having a child with Down syndrome. *Am J Med Genet A* 2003; 121A:219–24.

42. Jacques PF, Bostom AG, Selhub J, Rich S, Ellison RC, Eckfeldt JH, Gravel RA, Rozen R, National Heart, Lung and Blood Institute, National Institutes of Health. Effects of poly-morphisms of methionine synthase and methionine synthase reductase on total plasma homocysteine in the NHLBI Family Heart Study. *Atherosclerosis* 2003; 166:49–55.

43. Klerk M, Lievers KJ, Kluijtmans LA, LA, Blom HJ, den Heijer M, Schouten EG, Kok FJ, Verhoef P. The 2756A>G variant in the gene encoding methionine synthase: Its relation with plasma homocysteine levels and risk of coronary heart disease in a Dutch case-control study. *Thromb Res* 2003; 110:87–91.

44. De Marco P, Calevo MG, Moroni A, Arata L, Merello E, Finnell RH, Zhu H, Andreussi L, Cama A, Capra V. Study of MTHFR and MS polymorphisms as risk factors for NTD in the Italian population. *J Hum Genet* 2002; 47:319–24.

45. Yang QH, Botto LD, Gallagher M, Friedman JM, Sanders CL, Koontz D, Nikolova S, Erickson JD, Steinberg K. Prevalence and effects of gene-gene and gene-nutrient interactions on serum folate and serum total homocysteine concentrations in the United States: Findings from the third National Health and Nutrition Examination Survey DNA Bank. *Am J Clin Nutr* 2008; 88:232–46.

46. Fredriksen A, Meyer K, Ueland PM, Vollset SE, Grotmol T, Schneede J. Large-scale population-based metabolic phenotyping of thirteen genetic polymorphisms related to one-carbon metabolism. *Hum Mutat* 2007; 28:856–65.

47. Gaughan DJ, Kluijtmans LA, Barbaux S, McMaster D, Young IS, Yarnell JW, Evans A, Whitehead AS. The methionine synthase reductase (MTRR) A66G polymorphism is a novel genetic determinant of plasma homocysteine concentrations. *Atherosclerosis* 2001; 157:451–56.

48. Zhu H, Wicker NJ, Shaw GM, Lammer EJ, Hendricks K, Suarez L, Canfield M, Finnell RH. Homocysteine remethylation enzyme polymorphisms and increased risks for neural tube defects. *Mol Genet Metab* 2003; 78:216–21.

49. Vaughn JD, Bailey LB, Shelnutt KP, Dunwoody KM, Maneval DR, Davis SR, Quinlivan EP, Gregory JF 3rd, Theriaque DW, Kauwell GP. Methionine synthase reductase 66A->G polymorphism is associated with increased plasma homocysteine concentration when combined with the homozygous methylenetetrahydrofolate reductase 677C->T variant. *J Nutr* 2004; 134:2985–90.

50. O'Leary VB, Mills JL, Pangilinan F, Kirke PN, Cox C, Conley M, Weiler A, et al. Analysis of methionine synthase reductase polymorphisms for neural tube defects risk association. *Mol Genet Metab* 2005; 85:220–27.

51. O'Leary VB, Parle-McDermott A, Molloy AM, Kirke PN, Johnson Z, Conley M, Scott JM, Mills JL. MTRR and MTHFR polymorphism: Link to Down syndrome? *Am J Med Genet* 2002; 107:151–55.

52. Daubner SC, Matthews RG. Purification and properties of methylenetetrahydrofolate reductase from pig liver. *J Biol Chem* 1982; 257:140–45.

53. Matthews RG, Vanoni MA, Hainfeld JF, Wall J. Methylenetetrahydrofolate reductase. Evidence for spatially distinct subunit domains obtained by scanning transmission electron microscopy and limited proteolysis. *J Biol Chem* 1984; 259:11647–50.

54. Kutzbach C, Stokstad EL. Mammalian methylenetetrahydrofolate reductase. Partial purification, properties, and inhibition by S-adenosylmethionine. *Biochim Biophys Acta* 1971; 250:459–77.

55. Yamada K, Strahler JR, Andrews PC, Matthews RG. Regulation of human methylenetetrahydrofolate reductase by phosphorylation. *Proc Natl Acad Sci USA* 2005; 102:10454–59.

56. Green JM, Ballou DP, Matthews RG. Examination of the role of methylenetetrahydrofolate reductase in incorporation of methyltetrahydrofolate into cellular metabolism. *FASEB J* 1988; 2:42–47.

57. Rosenblatt DS, Cooper BA, Lue-Shing S, Wong PW, Berlow S, Narisawa K, Baumgartner R. Folate distribution in cultured human cells. Studies on 5,10-CH2-H4PteGlu reductase deficiency. *J Clin Invest* 1979; 63:1019–25.

58. Erbe RW. Genetic aspects of folate metabolism. *Adv Hum Genet* 1979; 9:293–354, 367–69.

59. Rosenblatt DS. Inherited disorders of folate transport and metabolism. In: Scriver CR, Beaudet AL, Sly WS, Valle D, eds., *The Metabolic and Molecular Bases of Inherited Disease*, 7th ed. New York: McGraw-Hill, 1995:3111–28.

60. Sibani S, Leclerc D, Weisberg IS, O'Ferrall E, Watkins D, Artigas C, Rosenblatt DS, Rozen R. Characterization of mutations in severe methylenetetrahydrofolate reductase deficiency reveals an FAD-responsive mutation. *Hum Mutat* 2003; 21:509–20.

61. Goyette P, Christensen B, Rosenblatt DS, Rozen R. Severe and mild mutations in cis for the methylenetetrahydrofolate reductase (MTHFR) gene, and description of five novel mutations in MTHFR. *Am J Hum Genet* 1996; 59:1268–75.

62. Goyette P, Frosst P, Rosenblatt DS, Rozen R. Seven novel mutations in the methylenetetrahydrofolate reductase gene and genotype/phenotype correlations in severe methylenetetrahydrofolate reductase deficiency. *Am J Hum Genet* 1995; 56:1052–59.

63. Chwatko G, Boers GH, Strauss KA, Shih DM, Jakubowski H. Mutations in methylenetetrahydrofolate reductase or cystathionine beta-synthase gene, or a high-methionine diet, increase homocysteine thiolactone levels in humans and mice. *FASEB J* 2007; 21:1707–13.

64. Boss GR, Erbe RW. Decreased rates of methionine synthesis by methylene tetrahydrofolate reductase-deficient fibroblasts and lymphoblasts. *J Clin Invest* 1981; 67:1659–64.

65. Surtees R, Leonard J, Austin S. Association of demyelination with deficiency of cerebrospinal-fluid S-adenosylmethionine in inborn errors of methyl-transfer pathway. *Lancet* 1991; 338:1550–54.

66. Kang SS, Wong PW, Zhou JM, Sora J, Lessick M, Ruggie N, Grcevich G. Thermolabile methylenetetrahydrofolate reductase in patients with coronary artery disease. *Metabolism* 1988; 37:611–13.

67. Kang SS, Wong PW, Susmano A, Sora J, Norusis M, Ruggie N. Thermolabile methylenetetrahydrofolate reductase: An inherited risk factor for coronary artery disease. *Am J Hum Genet* 1991;48:536–45.

68. Goyette P, Sumner JS, Milos R, Duncan AM, Rosenblatt DS, Matthews RG, Rozen R. Human methylenetetrahydrofolate reductase: Isolation of cDNA, mapping and mutation identification. *Nat Genet* 1994; 7:195–200.

69. Frosst P, Blom HJ, Milos R, et al. A candidate genetic risk factor for vascular disease: A common mutation in methylenetetrahydrofolate reductase. *Nat Genet* 1995; 10:111–13.

70. Guenther BD, Sheppard CA, Tran P, Rozen R, Matthews RG, Ludwig ML. The structure and properties of methylenetetrahydrofolate reductase from Escherichia coli suggest how folate ameliorates human hyperhomocysteinemia. *Nat Struct Biol* 1999; 6:359–65.

71. Yamada K, Chen Z, Rozen R, Matthews RG. Effects of common polymorphisms on the properties of recombinant human methylenetetrahydrofolate reductase. *Proc Natl Acad Sci USA* 2001; 98:14853–58.

72. Pejchal R, Campbell E, Guenther BD, Lennon BW, Matthews RG, Ludwig ML. Structural perturbations in the Ala --> Val polymorphism of methylenetetrahydrofolate reductase: How binding of folates may protect against inactivation. *Biochemistry* 2006; 45:4808–18.

73. Jacques PF, Kalmbach R, Bagley PJ, et al. The relationship between riboflavin and plasma total homocysteine in the Framingham Offspring cohort is influenced by folate status and the C677T transition in the methylenetetrahydrofolate reductase gene. *J Nutr* 2002; 132:283–88.

74. Hustad S, Ueland PM, Vollset SE, Zhang Y, Bjorke-Monsen AL, Schneede J. Riboflavin as a determinant of plasma total homocysteine: Effect modification by the methylenetetrahydrofolate reductase C677T polymorphism. *Clin Chem* 2000; 46:1065–71.

75. McNulty H, Dowey le RC, Strain JJ, et al. Riboflavin lowers homocysteine in individuals homozygous for the MTHFR 677C->T polymorphism. *Circulation* 2006; 113:74–80.

76. Lathrop Stern L, Shane B, Bagley PJ, Nadeau M, Shih V, Selhub J. Combined marginal folate and riboflavin status affect homocysteine methylation in cultured immortalized lymphocytes from persons homozygous for the MTHFR C677T mutation. *J Nutr* 2003; 133:2716–20.

77. McNulty H, McKinley MC, Wilson B, McPartlin J, Strain JJ, Weir DG, Scott JM. Impaired functioning of thermolabile methylenetetrahydrofolate reductase is dependent on riboflavin status: Implications for riboflavin requirements. *Am J Clin Nutr* 2002; 76:436–41.

78. Hustad S, Midttun O, Schneede J, Vollset SE, Grotmol T, Ueland PM. The methylenetetrahydrofolate reductase 677C-->T polymorphism as a modulator of a B vitamin network with major effects on homocysteine metabolism. *Am J Hum Genet* 2007; 80:846–55.

79. D'Angelo A, Coppola A, Madonna P, Fermo I, Pagano A, Mazzola G, Galli L, Cerbone AM. The role of vitamin B12 in fasting hyperhomocysteinemia and its interaction with the homozygous C677T mutation of the methylenetetrahydrofolate reductase (MTHFR) gene. A case-control study of patients with early-onset thrombotic events. *Thromb Haemost* 2000; 83:563–70.

80. Bailey LB, Duhaney RL, Maneval DR, Kauwell GP, Quinlivan EP, Davis SR, Cuadras A, Hutson AD, Gregory JF 3rd. Vitamin B-12 status is inversely associated with plasma homocysteine in young women with C677T and/or A1298C methylenetetrahydrofolate reductase polymorphisms. *J Nutr* 2002; 132:1872–78.

81. Lavoie A, Tripp E, Hoffbrand AV. The effect of vitamin B12 deficiency on methylfolate metabolism and pteroylpolyglutamate synthesis in human cells. *Clin Sci Mol Med* 1974; 47:617–30.

82. Chen L, Qi H, Korenberg J, Garrow TA, Choi YJ, Shane B. Purification and properties of human cytosolic folylpoly-gamma-glutamate synthetase and organization, localization, and differential splicing of its gene. *J Biol Chem* 1996; 271:13077–87.

83. Savage JD, Lindenbaum J. Folate-cobalamin interactions. In: Bailey LB, ed., *Folate in Health and Disease.* New York: Marcel Dekker, 1995:237–86.

84. Shane B, Stokstad EL. Vitamin B12-folate interrelationships. *Annu Rev Nutr* 1985; 5:115–41.

85. Herbert V, Zalusky R. Interrelations of vitamin B12 and folic acid metabolism: Folic acid clearance studies. *J Clin Invest* 1962; 41:1263–76.

86. Noronha JM, Silverman M. On folic acid, vitamin B12, methionine and formiminoglutamic acid metabolism. In: Heinrich HD, ed., *2nd European Symposium on Vitamin B12 and Intrinsic Factor.* Stuttgart, Germany: Enke, 1962:728–36.

87. Shane B, Watson JE, Stokstad EL. Uptake and metabolism of [3H]folate by normal and by vitamin B-12- and methionine-deficient rats. *Biochim Biophys Acta* 1977; 497:241–52.

88. Fowler B, Whitehouse C, Wenzel F, Wraith JE. Methionine and serine formation in control and mutant human cultured fibroblasts: Evidence for methyl trapping and characterization of remethylation defects. *Pediatr Res* 1997; 41:145–51.

89. Hoffbrand AV, Jackson BF. Correction of the DNA synthesis defect in vitamin B12 deficiency by tetrahydrofolate: Evidence in favour of the methyl-folate trap hypothesis as the cause of megaloblastic anaemia in vitamin B12 deficiency. *Br J Haematol* 1993; 83:643–47.

90. Gutstein S, Bernstein LH, Levy L, Wagner G. Failure of response to N5-methyltetrahydrofolate in combined folate and B 12 deficiency. Evidence in support of the "folate trap" hypothesis. *Am J Dig Dis* 1973; 18:142–46.

91. Baumgartner ER, Stokstad EL, Wick SH, Watson JE, Kusano G. Comparison of folic acid coenzyme distribution patterns in patients with methylenetetrahydrofolate reductase and methionine synthetase deficiencies. *Pediatr Res* 1985; 19:1288–92.

92. Smulders YM, Smith DE, Kok RM, Teerlink T, Swinkels DW, Stehouwer CD, Jakobs C. Cellular folate vitamer distribution during and after correction of vitamin B12 deficiency: A case for the methylfolate trap. *Br J Haematol* 2006; 132:623–29.
93. Fujii K, Nagasaki T, Huennekens FM. Accumulation of 5-methyltetrahydrofolate in cobalamin-deficient L1210 mouse leukemia cells. *J Biol Chem* 1982; 257:2144–46.
94. Waters AH, Mollin DL. Observations on the metabolism of folic acid in pernicious anaemia. *Br J Haematol* 1963; 9:319–27.
95. Cooper BA, Lowenstein L. Relative folate deficiency of erythrocytes in pernicious anemia and its correction with cyanocobalamin. *Blood* 1964; 24:502–21.
96. Chanarin I. *The Megaloblastic Anaemias,* 3rd ed. Oxford, UK: Blackwell Scientific, 1990.
97. Carmel R, Melnyk S, James SJ. Cobalamin deficiency with and without neurologic abnormalities: Differences in homocysteine and methionine metabolism. *Blood* 2003; 101:3302–08.
98. Reynolds E. Vitamin B12, folic acid, and the nervous system. *Lancet Neurol* 2006; 5:949–60.
99. Selhub J, Jacques PF, Bostom AG, Wilson PW, Rosenberg IH. Relationship between plasma homocysteine and vitamin status in the Framingham study population. Impact of folic acid fortification. *Public Health Rev* 2000; 28:117–45.
100. Selhub J, Jacques PF, Dallal G, Choumenkovitch S, Rogers G. The use of blood concentrations of vitamins and their respective functional indicators to define folate and vitamin B12 status. *Food Nutr Bull* 2008; 29:S67–73.
101. Stabler SP, Lindenbaum J, Allen RH. The use of homocysteine and other metabolites in the specific diagnosis of vitamin B-12 deficiency. *J Nutr* 1996; 126:1266S–72S.
102. Selhub J, Jacques PF, Wilson PW, Rush D, Rosenberg IH. Vitamin status and intake as primary determinants of homocysteinemia in an elderly population. *JAMA* 1993; 270:2693–98.
103. Dose-dependent effects of folic acid on blood concentrations of homocysteine: A meta-analysis of the randomized trials. *Am J Clin Nutr* 2005; 82:806–12.
104. Jacques PF, Bostom AG, Wilson PW, Rich S, Rosenberg IH, Selhub J. Determinants of plasma total homocysteine concentration in the Framingham Offspring cohort. *Am J Clin Nutr* 2001; 73:613–21.
105. Hao L, Ma J, Zhu J, Stampfer MJ, Tian Y, Willett WC, Li Z. High prevalence of hyperhomocysteinemia in Chinese adults is associated with low folate, vitamin B-12, and vitamin B-6 status. *J Nutr* 2007; 137:407–13.
106. Liaugaudas G, Jacques PF, Selhub J, Rosenberg IH, Bostom AG. Renal insufficiency, vitamin B(12) status, and population attributable risk for mild hyperhomocysteinemia among coronary artery disease patients in the era of folic acid-fortified cereal grain flour. *Arterioscler Thromb Vasc Biol* 2001; 21:849–51.
107. Quinlivan EP, McPartlin J, McNulty H, Ward M, Strain JJ, Weir DG, Scott JM. Importance of both folic acid and vitamin B12 in reduction of risk of vascular disease. *Lancet* 2002; 359:227–28.
108. Scott JM, Weir DG. The methyl folate trap. A physiological response in man to prevent methyl group deficiency in kwashiorkor (methionine deficiency) and an explanation for folic-acid induced exacerbation of subacute combined degeneration in pernicious anaemia. *Lancet* 1981; 2:337–40.
109. Clarke S, Banfield K. S-adenosylmethionine-dependent methyltransferases. In: Carmel R, Jacobsen DW, eds., *Homocysteine in Health and Disease.* Cambridge, UK: Cambridge University Press, 2001:63–78.
110. Molloy AM, Orsi B, Kennedy DG, Kennedy S, Weir DG, Scott JM. The relationship between the activity of methionine synthase and the ratio of S-adenosylmethionine to S-adenosylhomocysteine in the brain and other tissues of the pig. *Biochem Pharmacol* 1992; 44:1349–55.

111. Weir DG, Molloy AM, Keating JN, Young PB, Kennedy S, Kennedy DG, Scott JM. Correlation of the ratio of S-adenosyl-L-methionine to S-adenosyl-L-homocysteine in the brain and cerebrospinal fluid of the pig: Implications for the determination of this methylation ratio in human brain. *Clin Sci (Lond)* 1992; 82:93–97.

112. Obeid R, Kostopoulos P, Knapp JP, Kasoha M, Becker G, Fassbender K, Herrmann W. Biomarkers of folate and vitamin B12 are related in blood and cerebrospinal fluid. *Clin Chem* 2007; 53:326–33.

113. Molloy AM, Weir DG. Homocysteine and the nervous system. In: Carmel R, Jacobsen DW, eds., *Homocysteine in Health and Disease*. Cambridge, UK: Cambridge University Press, 2001:183–97.

114. Kerins DM, Koury MJ, Capdevila A, Rana S, Wagner C. Plasma S-adenosylhomocysteine is a more sensitive indicator of cardiovascular disease than plasma homocysteine. *Am J Clin Nutr* 2001; 74:723–29.

115. Paik WK, Kim S. *Protein Methylation*. New York: John Wiley & Sons, 1980.

116. Garrow TA. Purification, kinetic properties, and cDNA cloning of mammalian betaine-homocysteine methyltransferase. *J Biol Chem* 1996; 271:22831–38.

117. Chiuve SE, Giovannucci EL, Hankinson SE, Zeisel SH, Dougherty LW, Willett WC, Rimm EB. The association between betaine and choline intakes and the plasma concentrations of homocysteine in women. *Am J Clin Nutr* 2007; 86:1073–81.

118. Melse-Boonstra A, Holm PI, Ueland PM, Olthof M, Clarke R, Verhoef P. Betaine concentration as a determinant of fasting total homocysteine concentrations and the effect of folic acid supplementation on betaine concentrations. *Am J Clin Nutr* 2005; 81:1378–82.

119. Ueland PM, Holm PI, Hustad S. Betaine: A key modulator of one-carbon metabolism and homocysteine status. *Clin Chem Lab Med* 2005; 43:1069–75.

120. Finkelstein JD. Metabolic regulatory properties of S-adenosylmethionine and S-adenosylhomocysteine. *Clin Chem Lab Med* 2007; 45:1694–99.

121. Finkelstein JD. Pathways and regulation of homocysteine metabolism in mammals. *Semin Thromb Hemost* 2000; 26:219–25.

122. Mudd SH, Cerone R, Schiaffino MC, Fantasia AR, Minniti G, Caruso U, Lorini R, et al. Glycine N-methyltransferase deficiency: A novel inborn error causing persistent isolated hypermethioninaemia. *J Inherit Metab Dis* 2001; 24:448–64.

123. Mudd SH, Brosnan JT, Brosnan ME, Jacobs RL, Stabler SP, Allen RH, Vance DE, Wagner C. Methyl balance and transmethylation fluxes in humans. *Am J Clin Nutr* 2007; 85:19–25.

124. Finkelstein JD. The regulation of homocysteine metabolism. In: Graham I, Refsum H, Rosenberg IH, Ueland PM, eds., *Homocysteine Metabolism: From Basic Science to Clinical Medicine*. Boston: Kluwer Academic Publications, 1997:3–9.

125. Jacobs RL, Stead LM, Devlin C, Tabas I, Brosnan ME, Brosnan JT, Vance DE. Physiological regulation of phospholipid methylation alters plasma homocysteine in mice. *J Biol Chem* 2005; 280:28299–305.

126. Stead LM, Brosnan JT, Brosnan ME, Vance DE, Jacobs RL. Is it time to reevaluate methyl balance in humans? *Am J Clin Nutr* 2006; 83:5–10.

127. McKeever MP, Weir DG, Molloy A, Scott JM. Betaine-homocysteine methyltransferase: Organ distribution in man, pig and rat and subcellular distribution in the rat. *Clin Sci (Lond)* 1991; 81:551–56.

128. Sunden SL, Renduchintala MS, Park EI, Miklasz SD, Garrow TA. Betaine-homocysteine methyltransferase expression in porcine and human tissues and chromosomal localization of the human gene. *Arch Biochem Biophys* 1997; 345:171–74.

129. Suleiman SA, Spector R. Methionine synthetase in mammalian brain: Function, development and distribution. *Life Sci* 1980; 27:2427–32.

130. Spector R, Coakley G, Blakely R. Methionine recycling in brain: A role for folates and vitamin B-12. *J Neurochem* 1980; 34:132–37.
131. Kotb M, Kredich NM. Regulation of human lymphocyte S-adenosylmethionine synthetase by product inhibition. *Biochim Biophys Acta* 1990; 1039:253–60.
132. Gharib A, Sarda N, Chabannes B, Cronenberger L, Pacheco H. The regional concentrations of S-adenosyl-L-methionine, S-adenosyl-L-homocysteine, and adenosine in rat brain. *J Neurochem* 1982; 38:810–15.
133. Molloy AM, Weir DG, Kennedy G, Kennedy S, Scott JM. A new high performance liquid chromatographic method for the simultaneous measurement of S-adenosylmethionine and S-adenosylhomocysteine. Concentrations in pig tissues after inactivation of methionine synthase by nitrous oxide. *Biomed Chromatogr* 1990; 4:257–60.
134. Caudill MA, Wang JC, Melnyk S, Pogribny IP, Jernigan S, Collins MD, Santos-Guzman J, Swendseid ME, Cogger EA, James SJ. Intracellular S-adenosylhomocysteine concentrations predict global DNA hypomethylation in tissues of methyl-deficient cystathionine beta-synthase heterozygous mice. *J Nutr* 2001; 131:2811–18.
135. Gharib A, Chabannes B, Sarda N, Pacheco H. In vivo elevation of mouse brain S-adenosyl-L-homocysteine after treatment with L-homocysteine. *J Neurochem* 1983; 40:1110–12.
136. Selley ML. A metabolic link between S-adenosylhomocysteine and polyunsaturated fatty acid metabolism in Alzheimer's disease. *Neurobiol Aging* 2007; 28:1834–39.
137. Yi P, Melnyk S, Pogribna M, Pogribny IP, Hine RJ, James SJ. Increase in plasma homocysteine associated with parallel increases in plasma S-adenosylhomocysteine and lymphocyte DNA hypomethylation. *J Biol Chem* 2000; 275:29318–23.
138. Bogdanski P, Pupek-Musialik D, Dytfeld J, Lacinski M, Jablecka A, Jakubowski H. Plasma homocysteine is a determinant of tissue necrosis factor-alpha in hypertensive patients. *Biomed Pharmacother* 2008; 62:360–65.
139. Song Z, Zhou Z, Uriarte S, Wang L, Kang YJ, Chen T, Barve S, McClain CJ. S-adenosylhomocysteine sensitizes to TNF-alpha hepatotoxicity in mice and liver cells: A possible etiological factor in alcoholic liver disease. *Hepatology* 2004; 40:989–97.
140. Bergmann S, Shatrov V, Ratter F, Schiemann S, Schulze-Osthoff K, Lehmann V. Adenosine and homocysteine together enhance TNF-mediated cytotoxicity but do not alter activation of nuclear factor-kappa B in L929 cells. *J Immunol* 1994; 153:1736–43.
141. Ratter F, Gassner C, Shatrov V, Lehmann V. Modulation of tumor necrosis factor-alpha-mediated cytotoxicity by changes of the cellular methylation state: Mechanism and in vivo relevance. *Int Immunol* 1999; 11:519–27.
142. Buccellato FR, Miloso M, Braga M, Nicolini G, Morabito A, Pravettoni G, Tredici G, Scalabrino G. Myelinolytic lesions in spinal cord of cobalamin-deficient rats are TNF-alpha-mediated. *FASEB J* 1999; 13:297–304.
143. Peracchi M, Bamonti Catena F, Pomati M, De Franceschi M, Scalabrino G. Human cobalamin deficiency: Alterations in serum tumour necrosis factor-alpha and epidermal growth factor. *Eur J Haematol* 2001; 67:123–27.
144. Scalabrino G, Carpo M, Bamonti F, Pizzinelli S, D'Avino C, Bresolin N, Meucci G, Martinelli V, Comi GC, Peracchi M. High tumor necrosis factor-alpha [corrected] levels in cerebrospinal fluid of cobalamin-deficient patients. *Ann Neurol* 2004; 56:886–90.
145. Capdevila A, Burk RF, Freedman J, Frantzen F, Alfheim I, Wagner C. A simple rapid immunoassay for S-adenosylhomocysteine in plasma. *J Nutr Biochem* 2007; 18:827–31.
146. Melnyk S, Pogribna M, Pogribny IP, Yi P, James SJ. Measurement of plasma and intracellular S-adenosylmethionine and S-adenosylhomocysteine utilizing coulometric electrochemical detection: Alterations with plasma homocysteine and pyridoxal 5'-phosphate concentrations. *Clin Chem* 2000; 46:265–72.

147. Stabler SP, Allen RH. Quantification of serum and urinary S-adenosylmethionine and S-adenosylhomocysteine by stable-isotope-dilution liquid chromatography-mass spectrometry. *Clin Chem* 2004; 50:365–72.

148. Gellekink H, van Oppenraaij-Emmerzaal D, van Rooij A, Struys EA, den Heijer M, Blom HJ. Stable-isotope dilution liquid chromatography-electrospray injection tandem mass spectrometry method for fast, selective measurement of S-adenosylmethionine and S-adenosylhomocysteine in plasma. *Clin Chem* 2005; 51:1487–92.

149. Loehrer FM, Haefeli WE, Angst CP, Browne G, Frick G, Fowler B. Effect of methionine loading on 5-methyltetrahydrofolate, S-adenosylmethionine and S-adenosylhomocysteine in plasma of healthy humans. *Clin Sci (Lond)* 1996; 91:79–86.

150. Stabler SP, Allen RH, Dolce ET, Johnson MA. Elevated serum S-adenosylhomocysteine in cobalamin-deficient elderly and response to treatment. *Am J Clin Nutr* 2006; 84:1422–29.

151. Guerra-Shinohara EM, Morita OE, Pagliusi RA, Blaia-d'Avila VL, Allen RH, Stabler SP. Elevated serum S-adenosylhomocysteine in cobalamin-deficient megaloblastic anemia. *Metabolism* 2007; 56:339–47.

152. Wagner C, Koury MJ. Plasma S-adenosylhomocysteine versus homocysteine as a marker for vascular disease. *J Nutr* 2008; 138:980; author reply 981.

153. Wagner C, Koury MJ. S-Adenosylhomocysteine: A better indicator of vascular disease than homocysteine? *Am J Clin Nutr* 2007; 86:1581–85.

154. Loehrer FM, Tschopl M, Angst CP, et al. Disturbed ratio of erythrocyte and plasma S-adenosylmethionine/S-adenosylhomocysteine in peripheral arterial occlusive disease. *Atherosclerosis* 2001; 154:147–54.

155. Herrmann W, Schorr H, Obeid R, Makowski J, Fowler B, Kuhlmann MK. Disturbed homocysteine and methionine cycle intermediates S-adenosylhomocysteine and S-adenosylmethionine are related to degree of renal insufficiency in type 2 diabetes. *Clin Chem* 2005; 51:891–97.

156. Wright AJ, Finglas PM, Dainty JR, Wolfe CA, Hart DJ, Wright DM, Gregory JF. Differential kinetic behavior and distribution for pteroylglutamic acid and reduced folates: A revised hypothesis of the primary site of PteGlu metabolism in humans. *J Nutr* 2005; 135:619–23.

157. Wright AJ, Dainty JR, Finglas PM. Folic acid metabolism in human subjects revisited: Potential implications for proposed mandatory folic acid fortification in the UK. *Br J Nutr* 2007; 98:667–75.

158. Savage DG, Lindenbaum J. Neurological complications of acquired cobalamin deficiency: Clinical aspects. *Baillieres Clin Haematol* 1995; 8:657–78.

159. Stabler SP, Lindenbaum J, Allen RH. Vitamin B-12 deficiency in the elderly: Current dilemmas. *Am J Clin Nutr* 1997; 66:741–49.

160. Mills JL, Von Kohorn I, Conley MR, Zeller JA, Cox C, Williamson RE, Dufour DR. Low vitamin B-12 concentrations in patients without anemia: The effect of folic acid fortification of grain. *Am J Clin Nutr* 2003; 77:1474–77.

161. Wyckoff KF, Ganji V. Proportion of individuals with low serum vitamin B-12 concentrations without macrocytosis is higher in the post folic acid fortification period than in the pre folic acid fortification period. *Am J Clin Nutr* 2007; 86:1187–92.

162. Herbert V, Bigaouette J. Call for endorsement of a petition to the Food and Drug Administration to always add vitamin B-12 to any folate fortification or supplement. *Am J Clin Nutr* 1997; 65:572–73.

163. Mills JL. Fortification of foods with folic acid—How much is enough? *N Engl J Med* 2000; 342:1442–45.

164. Reynolds E. Folic acid fortification: Clarify the neurological risks. *BMJ* 2007; 335:171.

165. Oakley GP Jr. Let's increase folic acid fortification and include vitamin B-12. *Am J Clin Nutr* 1997; 65:1889–90.

166. Dickinson CJ. Does folic acid harm people with vitamin B12 deficiency? *QJM* 1995; 88:357–64.

167. Tucker KL, Mahnken B, Wilson PW, Jacques P, Selhub J. Folic acid fortification of the food supply. Potential benefits and risks for the elderly population. *JAMA* 1996; 276:1879–85.

168. Di Rocco A, Bottiglieri T, Werner P, Geraci A, Simpson D, Godbold J, Morgello S. Abnormal cobalamin-dependent transmethylation in AIDS-associated myelopathy. *Neurology* 2002; 58:730–35.

169. Obeid R, Kasoha M, Knapp JP, Kostopoulos P, Becker G, Fassbender K, Herrmann W. Folate and methylation status in relation to phosphorylated tau protein(181P) and beta-amyloid(1–42) in cerebrospinal fluid. *Clin Chem* 2007; 53:1129–36.

170. Bottiglieri T, Laundy M, Crellin R, Toone BK, Carney MW, Reynolds EH. Homocysteine, folate, methylation, and monoamine metabolism in depression. *J Neurol Neurosurg Psychiatry* 2000; 69:228–32.

171. Serot JM, Barbe F, Arning E, Bottiglieri T, Franck P, Montagne P, Nicolas JP. Homocysteine and methylmalonic acid concentrations in cerebrospinal fluid: Relation with age and Alzheimer's disease. *J Neurol Neurosurg Psychiatry* 2005; 76:1585–87.

172. Carmel R. Efficacy and safety of fortification and supplementation with vitamin B12: Biochemical and physiological effects. *Food Nutr Bull* 2008; 29:S177–87.

173. Clarke R, Grimley Evans J, Schneede J, Nexo E, Bates C, Fletcher A, Prentice A, et al. Vitamin B12 and folate deficiency in later life. *Age Ageing* 2004; 33:34–41.

174. Hin H, Clarke R, Sherliker P, Atoyebi W, Emmens K, Birks J, Schneede J, et al. Clinical relevance of low serum vitamin B12 concentrations in older people: The Banbury B12 study. *Age Ageing* 2006; 35:416–22.

175. Dharmarajan TS, Kanagala MR, Murakonda P, Lebelt AS, Norkus EP. Do acid-lowering agents affect vitamin B12 status in older adults? *J Am Med Dir Assoc* 2008; 9:162–67.

176. Dharmarajan TS, Adiga GU, Norkus EP. Vitamin B12 deficiency. Recognizing subtle symptoms in older adults. *Geriatrics* 2003; 58:30–34, 37–38.

177. Green R. Indicators for assessing folate and vitamin B12 status and for monitoring the efficacy of intervention strategies. *Food Nutr Bull* 2008; 29:S52–63; discussion S64–66.

178. Carmel R. Mean corpuscular volume and other concerns in the study of vitamin B-12 deficiency: Epidemiology with pathophysiology. *Am J Clin Nutr* 2008; 87:1962–63; author reply 1963–64.

179. Clarke R, Birks J, Nexo E, Ueland PM, Schneede J, Scott J, Molloy A, Evans JG. Low vitamin B-12 status and risk of cognitive decline in older adults. *Am J Clin Nutr* 2007; 86:1384–91.

180. Berry RJ, Carter HK, Yang Q. Cognitive impairment in older Americans in the age of folic acid fortification. *Am J Clin Nutr* 2007; 86:265–67; author reply 267–69.

181. Yeung L, Yang Q, Berry RJ. Contributions of total daily intake of folic acid to serum folate concentrations. *JAMA* 2008; 300:2486–87.

182. Ray JG, Vermeulen MJ, Langman LJ, Boss SC, Cole DE. Persistence of vitamin B12 insufficiency among elderly women after folic acid food fortification. *Clin Biochem* 2003; 36:387–91.

183. Brouwer I, Verhoef P. Folic acid fortification: Is masking of vitamin B-12 deficiency what we should really worry about? *Am J Clin Nutr* 2007; 86:897–98.

184. Morris MC, Evans DA, Bienias JL, Tangney CC, Hebert LE, Scherr PA, Schneider JA. Dietary folate and vitamin B12 intake and cognitive decline among community-dwelling older persons. *Arch Neurol* 2005; 62:641–45.

185. Morris MS, Jacques PF, Rosenberg IH, Selhub J. Folate and vitamin B-12 status in relation to anemia, macrocytosis, and cognitive impairment in older Americans in the age of folic acid fortification. *Am J Clin Nutr* 2007; 85:193–200.

186. Smith AD. Folic acid fortification: The good, the bad, and the puzzle of vitamin B-12. *Am J Clin Nutr* 2007; 85:3–5.

187. Clarke R, Sherliker P, Hin H, Molloy AM, Nexo E, Ueland PM, Emmens K, Scott JM, Evans JG. Folate and vitamin B12 status in relation to cognitive impairment and anaemia in the setting of voluntary fortification in the UK. *Br J Nutr* 2008; 100:1054–59.

188. Selhub J, Morris MS, Jacques PF. In vitamin B12 deficiency, higher serum folate is associated with increased total homocysteine and methylmalonic acid concentrations. *Proc Natl Acad Sci USA* 2007; 104:19995–20000.

189. Jackson IM, Doig WB, McDonald G. Pernicious anaemia as a cause of infertility. *Lancet* 1967; 2:1159–60.

190. Hall M, Davidson RJ. Prophylactic folic acid in women with pernicious anaemia pregnant after periods of infertility. *J Clin Pathol* 1968; 21:599–602.

191. Bennett M. Vitamin B12 deficiency, infertility and recurrent fetal loss. *J Reprod Med* 2001; 46:209–12.

192. Reznikoff-Etievant MF, Zittoun J, Vaylet C, Pernet P, Milliez J. Low vitamin B(12) level as a risk factor for very early recurrent abortion. *Eur J Obstet Gynecol Reprod Biol* 2002; 104:156–59.

193. McLean E, de Benoist B, Allen LH. Review of the magnitude of folate and vitamin B12 deficiencies worldwide. *Food Nutr Bull* 2008; 29:S38–51.

194. Ray JG, Goodman J, O'Mahoney PR, Mamdani MM, Jiang D. High rate of maternal vitamin B12 deficiency nearly a decade after Canadian folic acid flour fortification. *QJM* 2008; 101:475–77.

195. Ronnenberg AG, Goldman MB, Chen D, Aitken IW, Willett WC, Selhub J, Xu X. Preconception homocysteine and B vitamin status and birth outcomes in Chinese women. *Am J Clin Nutr* 2002; 76:1385–91.

196. Bondevik GT, Lie RT, Ulstein M, Kvale G. Maternal hematological status and risk of low birth weight and preterm delivery in Nepal. *Acta Obstet Gynecol Scand* 2001; 80:402–08.

197. Bondevik GT, Schneede J, Refsum H, Lie RT, Ulstein M, Kvale G. Homocysteine and methylmalonic acid levels in pregnant Nepali women. Should cobalamin supplementation be considered? *Eur J Clin Nutr* 2001; 55:856–64.

198. Bruinse HW, van den Berg H. Changes of some vitamin levels during and after normal pregnancy. *Eur J Obstet Gynecol Reprod Biol* 1995; 61:31–37.

199. Murphy MM, Molloy AM, Ueland PM, Fernandez-Ballart JD, Schneede J, Arija V, Scott JM. Longitudinal study of the effect of pregnancy on maternal and fetal cobalamin status in healthy women and their offspring. *J Nutr* 2007; 137:1863–67.

200. Koebnick C, Heins UA, Dagnelie PC, Wickramasinghe SN, Ratnayaka ID, Hothorn T, Pfahlberg AB, Hoffmann I, Lindemans J, Leitzmann C. Longitudinal concentrations of vitamin B(12) and vitamin B(12)-binding proteins during uncomplicated pregnancy. *Clin Chem* 2002; 48:928–33.

201. Hibbard ED, Spencer WJ. Low serum B12 levels and latent Addisonian anaemia in pregnancy. *J Obstet Gynaecol Br Commonw* 1970; 77:52–57.

202. Metz J, McGrath K, Bennett M, Hyland K, Bottiglieri T. Biochemical indices of vitamin B12 nutrition in pregnant patients with subnormal serum vitamin B12 levels. *Am J Hematol* 1995; 48:251–55.

203. Pardo J, Peled Y, Bar J, Hod M, Sela BA, Rafael ZB, Orvieto R. Evaluation of low serum vitamin B(12) in the non-anaemic pregnant patient. *Hum Reprod* 2000; 15:224–26.

204. Chery C, Barbe F, Lequere C, Abdelmouttaleb I, Gérard P, Barbarino P, Boutroy JL, Guéant JL. Hyperhomocysteinemia is related to a decreased blood level of vitamin B12 in the second and third trimester of normal pregnancy. *Clin Chem Lab Med* 2002; 40:1105–08.

205. Minet JC, Bisse E, Aebischer CP, Beil A, Wieland H, Lutschg J. Assessment of vitamin B-12, folate, and vitamin B-6 status and relation to sulfur amino acid metabolism in neonates. *Am J Clin Nutr* 2000; 72:751–57.

206. Molloy AM, Mills JL, McPartlin J, Kirke PN, Scott JM, Daly S. Maternal and fetal plasma homocysteine concentrations at birth: The influence of folate, vitamin B12, and the 5,10-methylenetetrahydrofolate reductase 677C-->T variant. *Am J Obstet Gynecol* 2002; 186:499–503.

207. Bjorke Monsen AL, Ueland PM, Vollset SE, Guttormsen AB, Markestad T, Solheim E, Refsum H. Determinants of cobalamin status in newborns. *Pediatrics* 2001; 108:624–30.

208. Obeid R, Morkbak AL, Munz W, Nexo E, Herrmann W. The cobalamin-binding proteins transcobalamin and haptocorrin in maternal and cord blood sera at birth. *Clin Chem* 2006; 52:263–69.

209. Bjorke Monsen AL, Ueland PM. Homocysteine and methylmalonic acid in diagnosis and risk assessment from infancy to adolescence. *Am J Clin Nutr* 2003; 78:7–21.

210. Bjorke-Monsen AL, Torsvik I, Saetran H, Markestad T, Ueland PM. Common metabolic profile in infants indicating impaired cobalamin status responds to cobalamin supplementation. *Pediatrics* 2008; 122:83–91.

211. Ray JG, Blom HJ. Vitamin B12 insufficiency and the risk of fetal neural tube defects. *QJM* 2003; 96:289–95.

212. Suarez L, Hendricks K, Felkner M, Gunter E. Maternal serum B12 levels and risk for neural tube defects in a Texas-Mexico border population. *Ann Epidemiol* 2003; 13:81–88.

213. Ray JG, Wyatt PR, Thompson MD, Vermeulen MJ, Meier C, Wong PY, Farrell SA, Cole DE. Vitamin B12 and the risk of neural tube defects in a folic-acid-fortified population. *Epidemiology* 2007; 18:362–66.

214. Molloy AM, Kirke PN, Troendle JF, Burke H, Sutton M, Brody LC, Scott JM, Mills JL. Maternal vitamin B12 status and risk of neural tube defects in a population with high neural tube defect prevalence and no folic acid fortification. *Pediatrics* 2009; 123:917–23..

215. McLean RR, Jacques PF, Selhub J, Tucker KL, Samelson EJ, Broe KE, Hannan MT, Cupples LA, Kiel DP. Homocysteine as a predictive factor for hip fracture in older persons. *N Engl J Med* 2004; 350:2042–49.

216. van Meurs JB, Dhonukshe-Rutten RA, Pluijm SM, van der Klift M, de Jonge R, Lindemans J, de Groot LC. Homocysteine levels and the risk of osteoporotic fracture. *N Engl J Med* 2004; 350:2033–41.

217. Baines M, Kredan MB, Usher J, Davison A, Higgins G, Taylor W, West C, Fraser WD, Ranganath LR. The association of homocysteine and its determinants MTHFR genotype, folate, vitamin B12 and vitamin B6 with bone mineral density in postmenopausal British women. *Bone* 2007; 40:730–36.

218. Cagnacci A, Bagni B, Zini A, Cannoletta M, Generali M, Volpe A. Relation of folates, vitamin B12 and homocysteine to vertebral bone mineral density change in postmenopausal women. A five-year longitudinal evaluation. *Bone* 2008; 42:314–20.

219. Gjesdal CG, Vollset SE, Ueland PM, Refsum H, Meyer HE, Tell GS. Plasma total homocysteine level and bone mineral density: The Hordaland Homocysteine Study. *Arch Intern Med* 2006; 166:88–94.

220. Gjesdal CG, Vollset SE, Ueland PM, Refsum H, Meyer HE, Tell GS. Plasma homocysteine, folate, and vitamin B 12 and the risk of hip fracture: The Hordaland Homocysteine Study. *J Bone Miner Res* 2007; 22:747–56.

221. Dhonukshe-Rutten RA, Lips M, de Jong N, Chin A Paw MJ, Hiddink GJ, van Dusseldorp M, De Groot LC, van Staveren WA. Vitamin B-12 status is associated with bone mineral content and bone mineral density in frail elderly women but not in men. *J Nutr* 2003; 133:801–07.

222. Dhonukshe-Rutten RA, Pluijm SM, de Groot LC, Lips P, Smit JH, van Staveren WA. Homocysteine and vitamin B12 status relate to bone turnover markers, broadband ultrasound attenuation, and fractures in healthy elderly people. *J Bone Miner Res* 2005; 20:921–29.

223. Dhonukshe-Rutten RA, van Dusseldorp M, Schneede J, de Groot LC, van Staveren WA. Low bone mineral density and bone mineral content are associated with low cobalamin status in adolescents. *Eur J Nutr* 2005; 44:341–47.

224. Tucker KL, Hannan MT, Qiao N, Jacques PF, Selhub J, Cupples LA, Kiel DP. Low plasma vitamin B12 is associated with lower BMD: The Framingham Osteoporosis Study. *J Bone Miner Res* 2005; 20:152–58.

225. Abrahamsen B, Jorgensen HL, Nielsen TL, Andersen M, Haug E, Schwarz P, Hagen C, Brixen K. MTHFR c.677C>T polymorphism as an independent predictor of peak bone mass in Danish men—Results from the Odense Androgen Study. *Bone* 2006; 38:215–19.

226. Abrahamsen B, Madsen JS, Tofteng CL, Stilgren L, Bladbjerg EM, Kristensen SR, Brixen K, Mosekilde L. Are effects of MTHFR (C677T) genotype on BMD confined to women with low folate and riboflavin intake? Analysis of food records from the Danish osteoporosis prevention study. *Bone* 2005; 36:577–83.

227. Macdonald HM, McGuigan FE, Fraser WD, New SA, Ralston SH, Reid DM. Methylenetetrahydrofolate reductase polymorphism interacts with riboflavin intake to influence bone mineral density. *Bone* 2004; 35:957–64.

228. Steer C, Emmett P, Lewis S, Smith GD, Tobias J. The methylenetetrahydrofolate reductase (MTHFR) C677T polymorphism is associated with spinal BMD in nine-year-old children. *J Bone Miner Res* 2009; 24:117–24.

16 Clinical Folate Deficiency

Sally P. Stabler

CONTENTS

I. INTRODUCTION

Because folates are required for the synthesis of RNA and DNA precursors, provide methyl groups and other one-carbon units, and are important in the metabolism of amino acids, it is not surprising that folate deficiency impacts the rapidly proliferating tissues such as bone marrow and mucous membranes, the gastrointestinal tract, and the reproductive system [1–3]. The focus of this chapter is clinical folate deficiency, including its role in the etiology of megaloblastic anemia, the conditions in which it occurs, diagnosis, and treatment.

II. CLINICAL FOLATE DEFICIENCY

A. MEGALOBLASTIC ANEMIA

1. Hematological Changes Associated with Megaloblastic Anemia Resulting from Folate Deficiency

Severe folate deficiency causes pancytopenia or anemia described as megaloblastic because of characteristic pathological features of the hematopoietic cell nuclei with classical abnormalities described in Table 16.1 [1,2,4,5]. Decreased DNA synthesis leads to impaired maturation of the nuclei of erythropoietic precursors, resulting in larger than normal red blood cells (RBCs), i.e., macrocytes or macroovalocytes, and therefore a gradual increase in the mean cell volume (MCV). The hypercellular bone marrow with large erythroblasts with abnormally open, uncondensed chromatin can suggest a misdiagnosis of acute leukemia in severe megaloblastic anemia. Many of these megaloblasts die before maturation and release from the bone marrow. This condition of ineffective erythropoiesis or intramedullary hemolysis can be confused with hemolytic anemia because of clinical chemistry findings of increased indirect bilirubin, lactate dehydrogenase, and decreased serum haptoglobin [5,6]. Occasionally, the reticulocyte count is even mildly increased. There are often fragmented and malformed cells observed in the peripheral blood smear as well as large variation in size and shape, anisocytosis, and poikilocytosis. The MCV may not be increased to more than 100 fL if fragmentation is severe, but the red cell distribution width (RDW) will often be very high [6]. The white blood cell and platelet count may also be decreased in severe cases. Larger than normal white blood cell precursors are present in the marrow (especially giant bands and metamyelocytes). The hypersegmented neutrophil has been used as a characteristic marker for megaloblastic hematopoiesis [2]. Hypersegmentation, however, is subject to interpretation by different observers with different definitions of the separations between lobes ranging from less than one-third the size of the lobe to only the size of a thread. A widely used definition requires one 6-lobed or five 5-lobed neutrophils per 100 cells [1,2,5]. The bone marrow often shows dysplastic hematopoiesis with abnormal erythroid

TABLE 16.1

Hematological Abnormalities in Megaloblastic Anemia[a]

Megaloblastic Morphology

Peripheral Blood

Macrocytosis[b]
Hypersegmentation
Anemia
Leukopenia
Thrombocytopenia

Bone Marrow

Hypercellular
Nuclear-cytoplasmic dysynchrony
Immature nuclear chromatin pattern
Giant bands and metamyelocytes

Ineffective Erythropoiesis

Increased iron turnover
Dysplasia
Nuclear karyorrhexis
Leukoerythroblastic peripheral blood
Increased indirect bilirubin
Increased lactate dehydrogenase
Decreased haptoglobin

[a] Observed in either folate or cobalamin deficiency.
[b] Macrocytosis affected by iron deficiency, thalassemia, and anemia of chronic disease.

nuclei undergoing karyorrhexis and those with nuclear remnants. As the anemia worsens, there may be a release of immature white blood cells such as metamyelocytes, as well as myelocytes and nucleated RBCs with megaloblastic morphology, known as leukoerythroblastic changes, in the peripheral blood smear. Cytogenetic studies can reveal fragmented chromosomes, fragile site breaks, and even clonal disorders [7].

2. Other Nutrient Deficiencies That May Affect Diagnosis Based on Hematological Indices

The megaloblastic anemia of either folate or vitamin B12 deficiencies is indistinguishable with identical abnormalities, which can only be distinguished by comparing vitamin or vitamin-dependent metabolite concentrations or the clinical response to small amounts of individual vitamins. The metabolic interrelationship between folate and vitamin B12 that provides an explanation for the shared hematological abnormalities associated with a deficiency of either nutrient is the topic of Chapter 15. A common clinical practice is to treat megaloblastic anemia with both vitamins, further confusing the interpretation of clinical response. Folic acid can improve megaloblastic anemia resulting from vitamin B12 deficiency, although eventually the patients relapse (see the extensive discussion in the previous edition of this book by Savage and Lindenbaum [3]). Treatment of the vitamin B12–deficient patient with folic acid does not cure or prevent central nervous system disease; thus, it is important to either make a specific diagnosis or provide long-term therapy with both vitamins. Vitamin B12 deficiency anemia may occur in persons of normal health on a B12-sufficient diet as a result of the autoimmune lack of intrinsic factor, thus providing a specific model for isolated vitamin B12 deficiency. In contrast, a common cause of folate deficiency is alcohol abuse with its attendant toxicities and multiple nutrient deficiencies, as described in Chapter 17. Other major causes such as malabsorption and food deprivation also lead to multiple nutrient deficiencies; thus, it has been difficult to study "pure" cases of folate deficiency [1,2,4].

Sideroblastic anemia (reduced incorporation of iron into heme), possibly associated with a deficiency of pyridoxine (required for heme synthesis), or toxicity resulting from alcohol itself, may coexist in about 50% of the patients [8]. Iron deficiency, characterized by a reduction in MCV, caused by bleeding or consumption of an iron-deficient diet that is common in those with alcoholism, will mask the macrocytosis of folate deficiency. Likewise, iron deficiency usually coexists with folate deficiency associated with chronic inflammatory bowel diseases.

The low MCV in thalassemia will increase with megaloblastic anemia but rarely exceeds 100 fL [9]. Protein-calorie malnutrition may cause serous fat atrophy of the bone marrow and hypoplasia, which could mask megaloblastic changes observed in folate deficiency. Acute bacterial infections (which bring patients to medical care) will cause the release of hyposegmented band forms of neutrophils and can mask hypersegmentation in a folate deficiency. All the examples above illustrate the difficulties in determining from the pathological and clinical features whether the anemia in an individual patient is exclusively caused by folate deficiency. Even lack of response to folic acid cannot be used to rule out folate deficiency if iron or erythropoietin deficiencies coexist.

B. MEGALOBLASTIC CHANGES IN OTHER TISSUES

Megaloblastic changes can occur in other tissues with high cellular turnover such as the mucous membranes of the mouth, leading to glossitis of the tongue, and of the intestinal tract, resulting in malabsorbtion, discussed later in this chapter. The reproductive system may also be negatively impacted by megaloblastic abnormalities resulting from a folate deficiency, which have been linked to infertility [1,2].

C. PATHOPHYSIOLOGY OF MEGALOBLASTIC ANEMIA

1. Use of Animal Models to Study Pathophysiology

It has been difficult to study the pathophysiology of megaloblastic anemia in folate-deficient animals because of the lack of bone marrow or peripheral blood abnormalities similar to those observed in folate-deficient humans [10]. Because animal RBCs are much smaller than human RBCs—30 to 50 fL versus 90 to 100 fL— the parameters used by clinical pathologists are not practical for diagnostic purposes in other mammals. Likewise, the neutrophil nuclei are often morphologically different between species. For example, rodents have a ribbon-shaped nucleus, which does not lend itself well to interpretation of hypersegmentation. An amino acid–based folate-deficient rodent diet has been used to cause folate-deficient anemia and leukopenia in rats, although the MCV does not increase [11,12]. A useful mouse model of folate deficiency (in which the animals are infected with the Friend virus) has been developed that causes an acute erythroblastosis phase accentuating megaloblastic erythropoiesis [10].

2. Impaired DNA Synthesis

Laser-scanning cytometry was recently used to show that hypersegmented neutrophils in peripheral blood had a normal average value of DNA ploidy of 2.0 but that the giant metamyelocytes and neutrophils from bone marrow of patients with megaloblastic anemia had increased ploidy, with mean values of 3 to 3.5 N [13]. The megaloblasts had an increased proportion of cells in the S phase; however, their DNA content was not increased over normal cells [13]. Other investigations have provided evidence that megaloblastic cells also have impaired incorporation of tritiated thymidine into DNA [10,14]. The presumed decrease in DNA synthesis and repair may cause DNA damage, which could lead to apoptosis of the hematopoietic precursors, which is clinically documented by ineffective erythropoiesis [10,14]. Some [14–16], but not all [17], studies show increased incorporation of uracil into DNA. A wide variety of cells have been evaluated in different studies, including those from human bone marrow, peripheral blood white blood cells, cells in culture, or isolated erythroblasts from folate-deficient rats, which could explain reported differences.

The trigger for apoptosis of bone marrow precursors is not understood, although DNA damage caused by double strand breaks from uracil misincorporation may play a role [10]. An in vitro model of folate-deficient erythropoiesis provided evidence that the erythroblasts underwent apoptosis in S phase and required purines and thymidine [18]. Apparently both purine and thymidine synthesis are important in preventing megaloblastic cell death [18].

3. Impaired Methylation

Because of the block in methionine synthase, decreased S-adenosylmethionine (SAM)–dependent methylation of DNA or other molecules may occur as a result of a folate deficiency. However, methionine is not deficient in patients with folate-deficient megaloblastic anemia [19]. S-Adenosylhomocysteine (SAH) was elevated twofold in the serum of severely vitamin B12–deficient megaloblastic anemia patients, but SAM was not low [20]. Also, SAH hydrolase deficiency, with severe impairment of methylation of choline and creatine, has not been associated with megaloblastic or other types of anemia [21]. In addition, it seems unlikely that direct toxicity of homocysteine (Hcy) could be the culprit because cystathionine-β-synthase (CBS) deficiency and severe methylene tetrahydrofolate (THF) deficiency do not cause anemia. There is evidence that inflammatory cytokine cascades may be important in vitamin B12–deficient megaloblastic anemia because elevated serum tumor necrosis factor α and epidermal growth factor concentrations were found in humans and corrected after treatment [22].

III. METABOLITE ABNORMALITIES IN FOLATE AND COBALAMIN DEFICIENCY

A. Hcy and Methylmalonic Acid

The pattern of folate-dependent metabolites has been studied in a cohort of well-documented patients with folate-deficient megaloblastic anemia collected by Lindenbaum and Savage from two hospitals in New York before food folic acid fortification in the United States [23]. The cohort included all cases of vitamin B12 and folate deficiency between July 1968 and June 1989. The serum folate concentration was measured either by milk binder radioassays or by microbiological assay with *Lactobacillus casei*. The cases were defined by a diagnostic megaloblastic bone marrow or changes on peripheral blood smear, serum folate less than 4 ng/mL, serum vitamin B12 greater than 300 pg/mL, underlying consistent disorder, and in 76%, a documented response to folic acid treatment. The underlying causes were alcoholism in 86%, malnutrition in 9%, and single cases of tropical sprue, sickle cell anemia, pregnancy, malabsorption, and oral contraceptive use. By definition, all the folate-deficient patients were anemic, and 75% had an MCV greater than 100 and 55% greater than 110 fL. Leukopenia was present in 18%, thrombocytopenia in 66% and pancytopenia in 18%; and lactate dehydrogenase was greater than 1,000 U/L in 29%. Atrophic glossitis was present in 22%, and 29% had peripheral neuropathy, ataxia, and/or cerebral dysfunction. The serum total Hcy (tHcy) concentration is shown plotted against the serum methylmalonic acid (MMA) in Figure 16.1 for the folate-deficient subjects and in Figure 16.2 for a concurrent series of vitamin B12–deficient subjects with megaloblastic anemia [23]. The tHcy ranged from approximately 15 μmol/L to more than 250 μmol/L in the folate-deficient subjects with 91% over a 3-SD cut-off point of 21.3 μmol/L. The tHcy concentration was also elevated in the vast majority of vitamin B12–deficient subjects. However, the vitamin B12–deficient subjects had elevated MMA, usually over 500 nmol/L, consistent with impairment of the vitamin B12–dependent enzyme L-methylmalonyl CoA mutase. In contrast, the serum MMA was elevated in 12% of the folate-deficient subjects, of whom 14 of 15 had renal dysfunction. Thus, it is readily apparent that elevated Hcy cannot be used to differentiate between a folate and vitamin B12 deficiency. In contrast, when MMA is elevated (especially when elevated over 1,000 nmol/L and any elevated level in the absence of renal impairment), vitamin B12 deficiency is likely present. If MMA is not elevated, it is extremely unlikely that a significant vitamin B12 deficiency is present. These metabolites are useful diagnostically because of the problem of lack of sensitivity and specificity of serum vitamin B12 and serum folate concentrations. For example, serum folate concentration was between 2.1 and 3.9 ng/mL in 24 of the folate-deficient subjects depicted in Figure 16.1 despite clear evidence for hyperhomocysteinemia and megaloblastic anemia. Serum tHcy concentration decreases promptly on replacement with folic acid [19] and thus must be measured before treatment with vitamins or a nutritionally adequate diet. In subjects with misdiagnosed vitamin B12 deficiency who are treated with folic acid, serum tHcy concentration does not fall into the normal range [24]. This unfortunate situation can also be avoided by measuring serum MMA to rule out vitamin B12–deficiency before

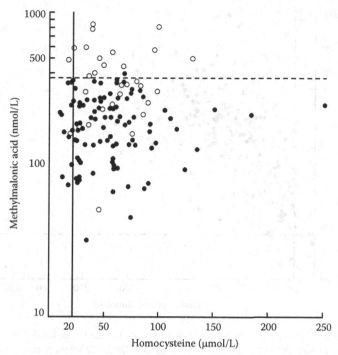

FIGURE 16.1 Serum concentrations of total homocysteine and methylmalonic acid in 123 episodes of megaloblastic anemia resulting from folate deficiency. Open circles indicate patients with elevated serum creatinine. Reference lines indicate methylmalonic acid (376 nmol/L) and total homocysteine (21.3 μmol/L), both 3 SD above the mean in controls. (Adapted from Savage DG, Lindenbaum J, Stabler SP, Allen RH, *Am J Med* 1994; 96:239–46. With permission.)

starting folic acid therapy. Two vitamin B12–deficient patients have been described who had hematological responses after folic acid treatment despite no correction of elevated Hcy concentration [24].

B.   OTHER FOLATE AND COBALAMIN-DEPENDENT METABOLITES

The other serum metabolites that have been found to be abnormal in folate and vitamin B12 deficiency are included in Table 16.2. The subjects studied were subgroups of the large cohorts of Lindenbaum and Savage described above [23]. Data for both folate- and vitamin B12–deficiency are shown because there are some interesting differences. Both folate- and vitamin B12–deficient subjects frequently have elevated cystathionine [25] despite the expectation that transsulfuration would be decreased if there were impaired remethylation. The elevated cystathionine in combination with high tHcy virtually rules out CBS-deficient homocystinuria and is diagnostically useful [26].

Hcy can be methylated by betaine Hcy methyltransferase in hepatic and renal tissues in a reaction that does not require folate. The demethylated product of this reaction, *N,N*-dimethylglycine, requires THF to be demethylated to

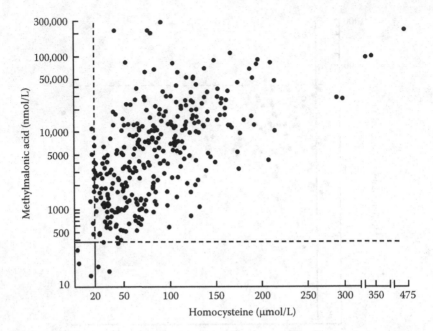

FIGURE 16.2 Serum concentrations of methylmalonic acid and total homocysteine in 313 episodes of megaloblastic anemia caused by cobalamin deficiency. Reference lines are described in the Figure 16.1 legend. (Adapted from Savage DG, Lindenbaum J, Stabler SP, Allen RH, *Am J Med* 1994; 96:239–46. With permission.)

TABLE 16.2
Metabolic Abnormalities in Megaloblastic Anemia[a,b]

Serum Metabolite	Folate Deficiency	Cobalamin Deficiency
Homocysteine [19]	↑↑↑	↑↑↑
Methylmalonic acid [23]	N	↑↑↑
Cystathionine [25]	↑↑	↑↑
N,N-Dimethylglycine [27]	↑↑	↑
N-Methylglycine [27]	↑↑	N
Betaine [27]	N	N
S-Adenosylhomocysteine [20]	↑[c]	↑↑
S-Adenosylmethionine [20]	N	N, ↑
Methionine [19]	N	N
Cysteine [19]	N	N

[a] ↑ indicates increase in serum metabolite concentration, the number of arrows indicates the magnitude of the increase relative to other metabolites.

[b] N indicates no change in metabolite concentration.

[c] Only one subject.

N-methylglycine (sarcosine). N-methylglycine also requires THF to be demethylated to glycine [26]. Some of the folate-deficient patients were found to have elevated N,N-dimethylglycine and N-methylglycine. A few vitamin B12–deficient subjects had elevated N, N-dimethylglycine but not elevated N-methylglycine [27]. N-Methylglycine is not only formed from the demethylation of N,N-dimethylglycine but also by the SAM-dependent methylation of glycine by glycine N-methyltransferase. This protein is highly abundant in liver and is thought to regulate the SAM/SAH ratio by removing excess SAM [28]. The enzyme is inhibited by methyl-THF, which could explain why N-methylglycine is not increased in a vitamin B12 deficiency. Perhaps lack of inhibition of glycine N-methyltransferase in folate deficiency may cause "wasting" of SAM in a folate deficiency.

The excretion of 5-formiminoglutamic acid (FIGLU) after a histidine load was widely evaluated in the 1960s and appears to be increased in patients with folate deficiency. However, there were problems with its specificity because it was elevated in vitamin B12 deficiency and in hospitalized patients [1,2].

IV. EXPERIMENTAL FOLATE DEFICIENCY

A. SEVERE DIETARY FOLATE DEFICIENCY

Herbert self-induced folate deficiency by consuming a triple-boiled diet over 20 weeks [29]. Unexpected problems with study design such as the development of hypokalemia and iron deficiency resulting from extensive phlebotomy makes interpretation of the timeline for the development of the folate deficiency difficult to delineate. Although it has been quoted that the neutrophil lobe average increased by 7 weeks, inspection of the reported data suggests that there were wide fluctuations until a sustained increase at about 18 weeks of deficiency. Likewise, the red blood cell MCV fell with iron deficiency and responded to iron therapy and also correlated with increases in the reticulocyte count, but definitely increased by 18 to 20 weeks. The bone marrow was considered clearly megaloblastic after 19 weeks. Serum folate (*L. casei*) fell within 2 weeks and reached the lower limit of the assay by 6 weeks. The initial RBC folate value was 150 ng/mL and decreased to less than 20 ng/mL by 18 weeks. The urinary FIGLU response to histidine loading became abnormal at 13 to 16 weeks. Anemia took approximately 18 weeks to develop, although interpretation is confusing because of phlebotomy and iron therapy. There were no megaloblastic changes noted in either the stomach or small intestine. Irritability was also reported by Herbert, in addition to forgetfulness late in the course of deficiency. The bone marrow was normoblastic 48 hours after treatment with 250 µg of folic acid. The reticulocyte count increased at 24 hours, and the serum iron concentration decreased [29].

Three healthy, young females were treated with the same folate-deficient diet as that consumed by Herbert and repleted with 25, 50, or 100 µg folic acid/day for 6 weeks [30]. Serum folate concentration decreased to about 50% of the starting value of 9 ng/mL with no hematological abnormalities in the subjects taking 25 and 50 µg/day. The subject taking 100 µg had a higher starting serum folate concentration and a subsequent reduction of only 2 ng/mL, suggesting a minimum requirement between 50 and 100 µg/day. When the same diet was fed to two folate-repleted alcoholic subjects, one developed bone marrow megaloblastic changes in 5 to 6 weeks, but the other subject required 9 weeks for the same changes to occur. Serum folate concentration decreased to less than 2 ng/mL at 3 weeks in one subject and 4 weeks in the other, and RBC folate values decreased after 7 weeks to less than 100 ng/mL [31]. The effects of consumption of a controlled low-folate diet coupled with large doses of alcohol have also been evaluated [32]. Concurrent consumption of alcohol and a folate-deficient diet produced a more severe folate deficiency than diet alone, as evidenced by the observation that serum folate concentrations fell within 3 days, and megaloblastic erythropoiesis was observed as early as 7 days [32].

B. CONTROLLED FOLATE FEEDING STUDIES

A series of controlled feeding studies during the past 20 years has also shown that serum or plasma folate concentration decreases within 3 weeks of the initiation of folate-deficient diets [33–36]. The period of severe deficiency must be continued for more than approximately 7 weeks to observe subtle increases in hypersegmentation of neutrophils, and there are usually no changes in MCV or hemoglobin [33]. Interestingly, the DU suppression test became abnormal at about 5 to 7 weeks in one study, with an increased ratio of deoxyuridine 5'-triphosphate/thymidine 5'-triphosphate in mitogen-stimulated lymphocyte DNA after 10 weeks of severe to moderate depletion [35]. After tHcy was recognized as a sensitive marker of folate status [37], it was used to monitor depletion and repletion [34–36,38]. At the same time, the methodology for determining folate content of food changed, resulting in an approximate threefold increase in the estimated quantity of natural food folate (e.g., 50 µg/day dietary folate was estimated to be ~150 µg with new methodology [39]).

It is also recognized that the bioavailability of folic acid is much higher than that of natural food folates [40–42]. A definition of dietary folate equivalents is used in the most recent literature to describe intake [40]. Needless to say, this makes interpreting the older studies of severe depletion for prolonged periods difficult to interpret in light of newer investigations of shorter intervals using improved analytical methodology with higher estimates of intake. It is clear, however, that a prolonged period of severe depletion is needed to cause megaloblastic anemia, with hypersegmentation and macrocytosis appearing only after 15 to 20 weeks. It is also recognized that serum tHcy is extremely sensitive to the quantity of absorbed folate and will increase and decrease as folate intake is manipulated.

V. ALCOHOL AND FOLATE DEFICIENCY

A. ALCOHOL-RELATED SYNDROMES

Alcohol abuse is likely the most common cause of folate deficiency anemia and has been investigated intensively for more than 50 years. The myriad ways in which alcohol affects folate metabolism and depletes the body of folate are described in Chapter 17. Megaloblastic changes occur much faster with folate depletion when there is concurrent high alcohol intake [32]. Because the majority of patients with severe folate-deficient megaloblastic anemia are alcohol abusers [23], it can be difficult to attribute aspects of the clinical syndrome to folate deficiency versus alcohol toxicity or coexisting nutrient deficiencies (i.e., thiamine or pyridoxine). The fact that the majority of patients with severe folate deficiency are also high alcohol consumers who may be deficient in multiple nutrients is particularly pertinent to the debate about whether folate deficiency causes neurological disease. Most series of studies of alcoholic subjects describe one-third or more of patients with a largely axonal peripheral neuropathy [23]. Other reported neurological lesions include cortical and subcortical brain atrophy, especially atrophic changes in the cerebellum [43]. Of note is the fact that the syndrome of subacute combined degeneration of the spinal cord does not appear to occur in folate deficiency, with rare exceptions (congenital folate malabsorption).

B. ALCOHOL AND MEGALOBLASTIC ANEMIA

One of the anticipated benefits of food folic acid fortification in the United States was the elimination of severe "alcoholic" megaloblastic anemia, but there are insufficient data currently to evaluate the postfortification effects on this condition. Anecdotally, this author is still consulting on folate-deficient anemic alcoholic patients in a university hospital. Either the increased folate intake from fortification is not enough to counteract alcohol-induced depletion/destruction of folate or, even more likely, alcoholic subjects do not consume an adequate diet. Macrocytosis has long been used as a marker of high alcohol intake in populations. In a study conducted in Finland, 40% of patients who were referred for a bone marrow biopsy because of abnormal peripheral blood counts were found to be alcoholics [44]. The MCV was higher in these patients; however, the RBC folate concentration did not differ between the alcoholic and nonalcoholic groups [44]. Liver disease without folate deficiency or megaloblastic bone marrow can also cause macrocytosis in alcoholic subjects [45]. Both nonalcoholic and alcoholic cirrhotic patients from Japan had elevated MCV [46]. Macrocytosis was marginally significantly related to alcohol intake ($P = .06$) in elderly persons even after folic acid fortification in the United States [47]. Chronic hyperhomocysteinemia has been associated with a series of abnormalities in alcoholism. There was a strong correlation between the blood alcohol concentration and the plasma tHcy value on admission to a German hospital even though the mean serum folate concentration was normal [48]. Elevated tHcy predicted a decrease in hippocampal brain volume in a group of subjects with chronic alcoholism as compared with normal control subjects [49] and was a risk factor for cognitive impairment in those with chronic alcoholism admitted for withdrawal [50]. The median tHcy concentration was 15.4 μmol/L (some >40 μmol/L) with a mean RBC folate concentration of 262 ng/mL (593 nmol/L) in 51 subjects admitted to the hospital for alcohol detoxification in New Zealand [51].

C. ALCOHOL AND HYPERHOMOCYSTEINEMIA

The fact that tHcy is more likely to be abnormal than serum folate in alcoholism complicates the interpretation of folate status and attribution of anemia to folate deficiency. There will be many more patients with alcoholism with elevated tHcy than have megaloblastic bone marrow [2]. Anemia will not respond to folate replacement solely, unless iron deficiency, sideroblastic anemia, or other pathology is treated. Conversely, the presence of unexpected hyperhomocysteinemia in someone on a normal diet, once vitamin B12 deficiency is eliminated, is highly suggestive of high chronic alcohol intake. More research is clearly needed regarding the amount of folate intake that would prevent hyperhomocysteinemia and alcohol-related complications.

VI. MALABSORPTION OF FOLATES AND OTHER CAUSES OF DEFICIENCY

A. POSTGASTRECTOMY

In patients who have undergone total or subtotal gastrectomy, folate deficiency rarely occurs, in contrast to the iron and vitamin B12 deficiencies that are common [52,53]. Laparoscopic Roux-en-Y gastric bypass was not associated with a folate deficiency in any of 30 vitamin-supplemented patients at 3 years postsurgery [54]. There have been no reports of the effects of gastric bypass surgery on patients not receiving supplemental vitamins.

B. TROPICAL SPRUE AND GLUTEN ENTEROPATHY

Tropical sprue is a chronic diarrheal disease of unknown etiology that causes progressive small intestinal villus atrophy and megaloblastic anemia [55]. Patients respond to folic acid (often high oral doses) with or without vitamin B12 supplementation and broad-spectrum antibiotics [55].

Gluten enteropathy (celiac disease) causes villous atrophy of the upper small intestine and has long been known to cause folate deficiency. In a study from Italy [56], the median serum folate concentration was 3.4 versus 6.0 ng/mL (patients vs. controls), and 42.5% of the patients had folate deficiency. The median plasma Hcy concentration was also higher, 11.1 versus 8.9 µmol/L and elevated (>13.9, 18.7 µmol/L for females and males, respectively) in 20% of the patients. Folate deficiency is common in gluten enteropathy both at diagnosis and in patients not taking supplemental vitamins on a gluten-free diet [57]. Anemias are common, but the widespread prevalence of iron deficiency in these patients often masks the macrocytic features associated with folate deficiency [57]. Macrocytic anemia with folate deficiency was less common in a group of patients diagnosed in New York, which could possibly be the result of fortification, because folic acid has also been added to nonwheat flour products [58]. It should also be remembered that there is a substantial lifetime risk of pernicious anemia in patients with gluten enteropathy; thus, screening for vitamin B12 deficiency should be done [59].

C. INFLAMMATORY BOWEL DISEASE

Impaired nutrition is very common in inflammatory bowel disease (both Crohn's disease and ulcerative colitis). The restrictive diet in addition to involvement of the upper small bowel, affecting iron and folate absorption, or terminal ileum, affecting vitamin B12 absorption, and surgical resections all contribute. Steger et al. [60]

found that a folate absorption test was abnormal in patients with Crohn's disease. Numerous investigators have reported elevated tHcy with lower serum folate and/or vitamin B12 levels in patients with inflammatory bowel disease and short bowel syndrome [61,62]. Food folic acid fortification may have had a positive impact in patients with inflammatory bowel disease, as evidenced by findings from a US clinical study in which the median folate value was twice that reported in European studies and hyperhomocysteinemia was attributed to vitamin B12 deficiency [63].

D. CLINICAL CONDITIONS THAT MAY INCREASE CELLULAR FOLATE REQUIREMENTS

1. Hemolytic Anemia and Psoriasis

Hemolytic anemia may cause increased folate utilization [1]. In addition, it appears that subjects with proliferative skin diseases such as psoriasis may have hyperhomocysteinemia and impaired folate status [64].

2. Sickle Cell Disease

Supplementation with folic acid in sickle cell disease is unpredictable [65]. Evaluation of hyperhomocysteinemia shows complex relationships between age (children vs. adults) and presence of chronic kidney disease, which develops in many older patients with sickle cell disease [66]. A combination of folic acid (700 μg) with vitamin B12 (600 μg) and vitamin B6 (6 mg) was shown to give a maximum decrease of tHcy in patients with sickle cell disease [67].

3. Renal Dialysis

The tHcy concentration is elevated in those with chronic kidney disease and even higher in dialysis patients. This hyperhomocysteinemia is partially responsive to high-dose folic acid; however, very few subjects achieve normal tHcy values even with massive quantities of vitamins [68]. During dialysis, folate and vitamin B6, as well as other water-soluble vitamins, are lost; thus, it has been common practice to use a replacement multivitamin, which has been shown to lower tHcy [69]. High-dose oral folic acid, vitamin B6, and vitamin B12 were used in a recent trial of Hcy lowering in a large cohort of dialysis patients in the United States, which lowered Hcy 25% but did not have an effect on mortality [70].

4. Drugs Inducing Folate Deficiency

Drugs that have been found to cause folate deficiency and/or hyperhomocysteinemia are listed in Table 16.3. Numerous studies have evaluated the influence of these drugs (e.g., [71–75]). A key point is that the prevalence of hyperhomocysteinemia or even megaloblastic anemia will be dependent on the folate intake of the individual. It is common practice in the United States to give folic acid supplementation to patients on anticonvulsants and those being treated with methotrexate for rheumatological diseases [76]. The multitargeted antifols used in cancer chemotherapy, such as pemetrexed, were associated with severe toxicity until it was demonstrated that the patients with underlying folate and/or vitamin B12 deficiency, demonstrated by hyperhomocysteinemia and/or elevated MMA, were at greatest risk for neutropenia and mucositis. The drugs are now given with folic acid and vitamin B12 supplementation, with reduced toxicity [77].

TABLE 16.3
Drugs Interfering with Folate Metabolism

Anticonvulsants
Carbamazepine
Phenytoin
Valproic acid
Lamotrigine
Primidone
Phenobarbital

Antifolates
Methotrexate
Pemetrexed
Trimethoprim
Pyrimethamine
Proguanil
Triamterene
Sulfasalazine

Disturbance of Methyl Balance
Levodopa
Niacin

VII. DIAGNOSIS AND TREATMENT OF FOLATE DEFICIENCY

A. BLOOD FOLATE CONCENTRATION

The time-honored starting point for the diagnosis of folate deficiency has been vitamin concentrations in plasma, serum, or RBCs. Assays have evolved from microbiological to radiodilution to newer methodologies, which are addressed in detail in Chapter 21 of this book. Suffice to say, different assays in different laboratories will have varying normal ranges. In addition, the RBC folate assays in many clinical labs have technical problems. RBC folate is frequently low in severe vitamin B12–deficient megaloblastic anemia [1]; thus, it is not a good discriminant between the two major causes. Serum folate concentration can be low in subjects with vitamin B12 deficiency and lead to the incorrect vitamin diagnosis [1–3]. Further complicating the assessment of serum folate levels is that there is an inverse relationship between serum folate and tHcy concentrations that encompasses ranges of what is considered low to normal to high folate status. This makes arbitrary cut points for "normal" concentrations somewhat meaningless, and the concept of folate "deficiency" is in many ways a relative term. All the reasons cited above make it difficult to recommend a lower "cutoff" or normal level for serum folate. In a study from New York, many folate-deficient megaloblastic anemic patients with hyperhomocysteinemia who responded to folic acid had serum folate between 2 and 4 ng/mL [23]. However, increasing the lower limit of normal serum folate to 4 or 6 ng/mL will only decrease the predictive value for anemia. A low serum folate concentration is rarely encountered in populations with food folic acid fortification, and concentrations of less than 3 ng/mL is usually associated with alcoholism, disease of the gastrointestinal tract, eating disorders, medications, or hemolytic anemias.

B. Hcy Measurements for Diagnosis of Folate Status

The tHcy concentration is such a sensitive indicator of folate status that one can almost predict the mean folate intake of a population based on the mean tHcy value. However, Hcy is also affected by age, with small children in a fortified population having very low values. It is sensitive to the creatinine clearance; thus, minor decrements in kidney function will increase the serum tHcy concentration [78]. Low tHcy (<10 µmol/L) would rarely be associated with megaloblastic anemia, but the clinical situation must be considered. The most serious error is to diagnose folate deficiency based on an elevated serum tHcy when it is caused by vitamin B12 deficiency. A serum vitamin B12 concentration in the range of 100 to 300 pg/mL has such poor sensitivity and specificity that attribution of hyperhomocysteinemia to folate or vitamin B12 or both deficiencies is hazardous without either measurement of MMA or treating with either vitamin to test response [24].

C. Attributing Anemia to Folate Deficiency

All the above comments about Hcy are appropriate when attributing anemia or pancytopenia (reduction in number of red and white blood cells and platelets) to a folate deficiency. In addition to folate depletion, other etiologies that may affect hematopoietic processes should be considered, including alcohol consumption, which can cause toxicity to hematopoietic precursors, iron deficiency, sideroblastosis (may result from a vitamin B6 deficiency), and pernicious anemia resulting from vitamin B12 malabsorption [1,8]. The anemias associated with gastrointestinal diseases are almost always multifactorial with iron deficiency complicating most folate-deficient gluten enteropathy or inflammatory bowel diseases. Chronic inflammatory diseases and chronic kidney disease cause erythropoietin deficiency, which frequently coexists with aging, drug-induced, and vitamin deficiency–induced anemia. Even a "pure" megaloblastic anemia caused by folate or vitamin B12 deficiency can be difficult to recognize if the hematological picture is dominated by intramedullary hemolysis, rather than easily recognized macrocytosis [5,6].

D. Folic Acid Therapy

Folic acid given orally is the most common and least expensive way to correct a folate deficiency [1,2,4]. Other forms of oral folate such as leucovorin (folinic acid) and methyl-THF are available and also have Hcy-lowering effects. Folic acid in doses of 1 mg/day has been widely used to treat and prophylax against folate deficiency in alcoholism, gut disease, and in patients treated with drugs such as methotrexate and anticonvulsants. Intravenous folic acid, often combined with intravenous multivitamins, is commonly used in emergency rooms for treatment of patients who appear to be alcohol abusers; this can affect later assessment of folate status. Intramuscular folic acid was used in large doses in the past but is rarely used now except perhaps for congenital folate malabsorption.

The type and dose of vitamins needed for Hcy lowering have been extensively investigated [79]. It appears that 800 µg of folic acid orally will give the maximum Hcy lowering that can be achieved with folate alone [79]. If elevated Hcy is caused by vitamin B12 deficiency, folic acid alone will not correct the condition [24]. However, high-dose oral vitamin B12 (2.5 mg) combined with 400 µg of folic acid and vitamin B6 (2 mg) achieved remarkable tHcy lowering in elderly subjects, including those with mild renal impairment [80]. The response of megaloblastic anemia caused by "pure" folate deficiency is fairly rapid with folate replacement. If iron, erythropoietin, vitamin B12, and vitamin B6 status are all satisfactory, then the serum iron will decrease promptly, the reticulocyte count will increase within days, and hemoglobin concentration will correct over 1 to 4 weeks with a decrease in MCV. The hypersegmentation will disappear in approximately 1 to 2 weeks.

VIII. SUMMARY

Severe deficiency of folate causes harm to rapidly proliferative tissues such as the bone marrow, the gastrointestinal tract, and the reproductive system. Severe deficiency (usually induced by alcoholism) causes megaloblastic anemia, with the first signs occurring within 4 months. Megaloblastic anemia caused by folate deficiency is rare in the absence of alcohol, drugs, or malabsorption. Total Hcy measurements appear to be the most sensitive indicator of folate status; however, folate deficiency is often accompanied by drug and alcohol toxicities or other micronutrient deficiencies; therefore, its specific predictive value for anemia is probably limited.

REFERENCES

1. Antony AC. Megaloblastic anemias. In: Hoffman R, Benz EJ Jr, Shattil SJ, Furie B, Cohen HJ, eds., *Hematology, Basic Principles and Practice*. New York: Churchill Livingston, 1990:392–421.
2. Lindenbaum J, Allen RHA. Clinical spectrum and diagnosis of folate deficiency. In: Bailey LB, ed., *Folate in Health and Disease*. New York: Marcel Dekker, 1995:43–73.
3. Savage DG, Lindenbaum J. Folate-cobalamin interactions. In: Bailey LB, ed., *Folate in Health and Disease*. New York: Marcel Dekker, 1995:237–85.
4. Stabler SP. Megaloblastic anemias: Pernicious anemia and folate deficiency. In: Young NS, Green SL, High KA, eds., *Clinical Hematology*. Philadelphia: Mosby Elsevier, 2006:242–51.
5. Wickramasinghe SN. Diagnosis of megaloblastic anaemias. *Blood Rev* 2006; 20:299–318.
6. Sekhar J, Stabler SP. Life-threatening megaloblastic pancytopenia with normal mean cell volume: Case series. *Eur J Intern Med* 2007; 18:548–50.
7. Heath CW Jr. Cytogenetic observations in vitamin B12 and folate deficiency. *Blood* 1966; 27:800–15.
8. Savage D, Lindenbaum J. Anemia in alcoholics. *Medicine (Baltimore)* 1986; 65:322–38.
9. Green R, Kuhl W, Jacobson R, Johnson C, Carmel R, Beutler E. Masking of macrocytosis by alpha-thalassemia in blacks with pernicious anemia. *N Engl J Med* 1982; 307:1322–25.

10. Koury MJ, Ponka P. New insights into erythropoiesis: The roles of folate, vitamin B12, and iron. *Annu Rev Nutr* 2004; 24:105–31.
11. Bills ND, Koury MJ, Clifford AJ, Dessypris EN. Ineffective hematopoiesis in folate-deficient mice. *Blood* 1992; 79:2273–80.
12. Stabler SP, Sampson DA, Wang, L, Allen RH. Elevations of serum cystathionine and total homocysteine in pyridoxine, folate and cobalamin deficient rats. *Nutr Biochem* 1997; 8:279–89.
13. Tsujioka T, Tochigi A, Kishimoto M, Kondo T, Tasaka T, Wada H, Sugihara T, Yoshida Y, Tohyama K. DNA ploidy and cell cycle analyses in the bone marrow cells of patients with megaloblastic anemia using laser scanning cytometry. *Cytometry B Clin Cytom* 2008; 74:104–09.
14. Wickramasinghe SN. The wide spectrum and unresolved issues of megaloblastic anemia. *Semin Hematol* 1999; 36:3–18.
15. Wickramasinghe SN, Fida S. Bone marrow cells from vitamin B12- and folate-deficient patients misincorporate uracil into DNA. *Blood* 1994; 83:1656–61.
16. Mashiyama ST, Courtemanche C, Elson-Schwab I, Crott J, Lee BL, Ong CN, Fenech M, Ames BN. Uracil in DNA, determined by an improved assay, is increased when deoxynucleosides are added to folate-deficient cultured human lymphocytes. *Anal Biochem* 2004; 330:58–69.
17. Ren J, Ulvik A, Refsum H, Ueland PM. Uracil in human DNA from subjects with normal and impaired folate status as determined by high-performance liquid chromatography-tandem mass spectrometry. *Anal Chem* 2002; 74:295–99.
18. Koury MJ, Price JO, Hicks GG. Apoptosis in megaloblastic anemia occurs during DNA synthesis by a p53-independent, nucleoside-reversible mechanism. *Blood* 2000; 96:3249–55.
19. Stabler SP, Marcell PD, Podell ER, Allen RH, Savage DG, Lindenbaum J. Elevation of total homocysteine in the serum of patients with cobalamin or folate deficiency detected by capillary gas chromatography-mass spectrometry. *J Clin Invest* 1988; 81:466–74.
20. Guerra-Shinohara EM, Morita OE, Pagliusi RA, Blaia-d'Avila VL, Allen RH, Stabler SP. Elevated serum S-adenosylhomocysteine in cobalamin-deficient megaloblastic anemia. *Metabolism* 2007; 56:339–47.
21. Baric I, Fumic K, Glenn B, Cuk M, Schulze A, Finkelstein JD, James SJ, et al. S-adenosylhomocysteine hydrolase deficiency in a human: A genetic disorder of methionine metabolism. *Proc Natl Acad Sci USA* 2004; 101:4234–39.
22. Peracchi M, Bamonti Catena F, Pomati M, De Franceschi M, Scalabrino G. Human cobalamin deficiency: Alterations in serum tumour necrosis factor-alpha and epidermal growth factor. *Eur J Haematol* 2001; 67:123–27.
23. Savage DG, Lindenbaum J, Stabler SP, Allen RH. Sensitivity of serum methylmalonic acid and total homocysteine determinations for diagnosing cobalamin and folate deficiencies. *Am J Med* 1994; 96:239–46.
24. Allen RH, Stabler SP, Savage DG, Lindenbaum J. Diagnosis of cobalamin deficiency I: Usefulness of serum methylmalonic acid and total homocysteine concentrations. *Am J Hematol* 1990; 34:90–98.
25. Stabler SP, Lindenbaum J, Savage DG, Allen RH. Elevation of serum cystathionine levels in patients with cobalamin and folate deficiency. *Blood* 1993; 81:3404–13.
26. Mudd SH, Levy HL, Svoby F. Disorders of transsulfuration. In: Scriver CR, Beaudet AL, Sly WS, Valle D, eds., *The Metabolic and Molecular Bases of Inherited Disease,* 8th ed. New York: McGraw-Hill, 2001:2007–56.
27. Allen RH, Stabler SP, Lindenbaum J. Serum betaine, N,N-dimethylglycine and N-methylglycine levels in patients with cobalamin and folate deficiency and related inborn errors of metabolism. *Metabolism* 1993; 42:1448–60.
28. Cook RJ, Wagner C. Glycine N-methyltransferase is a folate binding protein of rat liver cytosol. *Proc Natl Acad Sci USA* 1984; 81:3631–34.

29. Herbert V. Experimental nutritional folate deficiency in man. *Trans Assoc Am Physicians* 1962; 75:307–20.
30. Herbert V. Minimal daily adult folate requirement. *Arch Intern Med* 1962; 110:649–52.
31. Eichner ER, Pierce HI, Hillman RS. Folate balance in dietary-induced megaloblastic anemia. *N Engl J Med* 1971; 284:933–38.
32. Eichner ER, Hillman RS. The evolution of anemia in alcoholic patients. *Am J Med* 1971; 50:218–32.
33. Sauberlich HE, Kretsch MJ, Skala JH, Johnson HL, Taylor PC. Folate requirement and metabolism in nonpregnant women. *Am J Clin Nutr* 1987; 46:1016–28.
34. O'Keefe CA, Bailey LB, Thomas EA, Hofler SA, Davis BA, Cerda JJ, Gregory JF 3rd. Controlled dietary folate affects folate status in nonpregnant women. *J Nutr* 1995; 125:2717–25.
35. Jacob RA, Gretz DM, Taylor PC, James SJ, Pogribny IP, Miller BJ, Henning SM, Swendseid ME. Moderate folate depletion increases plasma homocysteine and decreases lymphocyte DNA methylation in postmenopausal women. *J Nutr* 1998; 128:1204–12.
36. Jacob RA, Wu MM, Henning SM, Swendseid ME. Homocysteine increases as folate decreases in plasma of healthy men during short-term dietary folate and methyl group restriction. *J Nutr* 1994; 124:1072–80.
37. Stabler SP, Marcell PD, Podell ER, Allen RH. Quantitation of total homocysteine, total cysteine, and methionine in normal serum and urine using capillary gas chromatography-mass spectrometry. *Anal Biochem* 1987; 162:185–96.
38. Yang TL, Hung J, Caudill MA, Urrutia TF, Alamilla A, Perry CA, Li R, Hata H, Cogger EA. A long-term controlled folate feeding study in young women supports the validity of the 1.7 multiplier in the dietary folate equivalency equation. *J Nutr* 2005; 135:1139–45.
39. Tamura T, Mizuno Y, Johnston KE, Jacob RA. Food folate assay with protease, beta-amylase, and folate conjugase treatments. *J Agric Food Chem* 1997; 45:135–39.
40. Sanderson P, McNulty H, Mastroiacovo P, McDowell IF, Melse-Boonstra A, Finglas PM, Gregory JF 3rd, UK Food Standards Agency. Folate bioavailability: UK Food Standards Agency workshop report. *Br J Nutr* 2003; 90:473–79.
41. Cuskelly GJ, McNulty H, Scott JM. Effect of increasing dietary folate on red-cell folate: Implications for prevention of neural tube defects. *Lancet* 1996; 347:657–59.
42. Hung J, Yang TL, Urrutia TF, Li R, Perry CA, Hata H, Cogger EA, Moriarty DJ, Caudill MA. Additional food folate derived exclusively from natural sources improves folate status in young women with the MTHFR 677 CC or TT genotype. *J Nutr Biochem* 2006; 17:728–34.
43. Bönsch D, Lenz B, Reulbach U, Kornhuber J, Bleich S. Homocysteine associated genomic DNA hypermethylation in patients with chronic alcoholism. *J Neural Transm* 2004; 111:1611–16.
44. Latvala J, Parkkila S, Niemelä O. Excess alcohol consumption is common in patients with cytopenia: Studies in blood and bone marrow cells. *Alcohol Clin Exp Res* 2004; 28:619–24.
45. Savage DG, Ogundipe A, Allen RH, Stabler SP, Lindenbaum J. Etiology and diagnostic evaluation of macrocytosis. *Am J Med Sci* 2000; 319:343–52.
46. Maruyama S, Hirayama C, Yamamoto S, Koda M, Udagawa A, Kadowaki Y, Inoue M, Sagayama A, Umeki K. Red blood cell status in alcoholic and non-alcoholic liver disease. *J Lab Clin Med* 2001; 138:332–37.
47. Morris MS, Jacques PF, Rosenberg IH, Selhub J. Folate and vitamin B-12 status in relation to anemia, macrocytosis, and cognitive impairment in older Americans in the age of folic acid fortification. *Am J Clin Nutr* 2007; 85:193–200.
48. Bleich S, Carl M, Bayerlein K, Reulbach U, Biermann T, Hillemacher T, Bönsch D, Kornhuber J. Evidence of increased homocysteine levels in alcoholism: The Franconian alcoholism research studies (FARS). *Alcohol Clin Exp Res* 2005; 29:334–36.

49. Bleich S, Bandelow B, Javaheripour K, Müller A, Degner D, Wilhelm J, Havemann-Reinecke U, Sperling W, Rüther E, Kornhuber J. Hyperhomocysteinemia as a new risk factor for brain shrinkage in patients with alcoholism. *Neurosci Lett* 2003; 335:179–82.

50. Wilhelm J, Bayerlein K, Hillemacher T, Reulbach U, Frieling H, Kromolan B, Degner D, Kornhuber J, Bleich S. Short-term cognition deficits during early alcohol withdrawal are associated with elevated plasma homocysteine levels in patients with alcoholism. *J Neural Transm* 2006; 113:357–63.

51. Robinson G, Narasimhan S, Weatherall M, Beasley R. Raised plasma homocysteine levels in alcoholism: Increasing the risk of heart disease and dementia? *N Z Med J* 2005; 118:U1490.

52. Sumner AE, Chin MM, Abrahm JL, Berry GT, Gracely EJ, Allen RH, Stabler SP. Elevated methylmalonic acid and total homocysteine levels show high prevalence of vitamin B12 deficiency after gastric surgery. *Ann Intern Med* 1996; 124:469–76.

53. Beyan C, Beyan E, Kaptan K, Ifran A, Uzar AI. Post-gastrectomy anemia: Evaluation of 72 cases with post-gastrectomy anemia. *Hematology* 2007; 12:81–84.

54. Vargas-Ruiz AG, Hernández-Rivera G, Herrera MF. Prevalence of iron, folate, and vitamin B12 deficiency anemia after laparoscopic Roux-en-Y gastric bypass. *Obes Surg* 2008; 18:288–93.

55. Westergaard H. Tropical sprue. *Curr Treat Options Gastroenterol* 2004; 7:7–11.

56. Saibeni S, Lecchi A, Meucci G, Cattaneo M, Tagliabue L, Rondonotti E, Formenti S, De Franchis R, Vecchi M. Prevalence of hyperhomocysteinemia in adult gluten-sensitive enteropathy at diagnosis: Role of B12, folate, and genetics. *Clin Gastroenterol Hepatol* 2005; 3:574–80.

57. Tikkakoski S, Savilahti E, Kolho KL. Undiagnosed coeliac disease and nutritional deficiencies in adults screened in primary health care. *Scand J Gastroenterol* 2007; 42:60–65.

58. Harper JW, Holleran SF, Ramakrishnan R, Bhagat G, Green PH. Anemia in celiac disease is multifactorial in etiology. *Am J Hematol* 2007; 82:996–1000.

59. Dahele A, Ghosh S. Vitamin B12 deficiency in untreated celiac disease. *Am J Gastroenterol* 2001; 96:745–50.

60. Steger GG, Mader RM, Vogelsang H, Schöfl R, Lochs H, Ferenci P. Folate absorption in Crohn's disease. *Digestion* 1994; 55:234–38.

61. Oldenburg B, Fijnheer R, van der Griend R, vanBerge-Henegouwen GP, Koningsberger JC. Homocysteine in inflammatory bowel disease: A risk factor for thromboembolic complications? *Am J Gastroenterol* 2000; 95:2825–30.

62. Chowers Y, Sela BA, Holland R, Fidder H, Simoni FB, Bar-Meir S. Increased levels of homocysteine in patients with Crohn's disease are related to folate levels. *Am J Gastroenterol* 2000; 95:3498–502.

63. Vasilopoulos S, Saiean K, Emmons J, Berger WL, Abu-Hajir M, Seetharam B, Binion DG. Terminal ileum resection is associated with higher plasma homocysteine levels in Crohn's disease. *J Clin Gastroenterol* 2001; 33:132–36.

64. Gisondi P, Fantuzzi F, Malerba M, Girolomoni G. Folic acid in general medicine and dermatology. *J Dermatol Treat* 2007; 18:138–46.

65. Wang WC. Role of nutritional supplement in sickle cell disease. *J Pediatr Hematol Oncol* 1999; 21:176–78.

66. Dhar M, Bellevue R, Brar S, Carmel R. Mild hyperhomocysteinemia in adult patients with sickle cell disease: A common finding unrelated to folate and cobalamin status. *Am J Hematol* 2004; 76:114–20.

67. van der Dijs FP, Fokkema MR, Dijck-Brouwer DA, Niessink B, van der Wal TI, Schnog JJ, Duits AJ, Muskiet FD, Muskiet FA. Optimization of folic acid, vitamin B(12), and vitamin B(6) supplements in pediatric patients with sickle cell disease. *Am J Hematol* 2002; 69:239–46.

68. Cianciolo G, La Manna G, Colì L, Donati G, D'Addio F, Persici E, Comai G, et al. 5-Methyltetrahydrofolate administration is associated with prolonged survival and reduced inflammation in ESRD patients. *Am J Nephrol* 2008; 28:941–48.

69. House AA, Donnelly JG. Effect of multivitamins on plasma homocysteine and folate levels in patients on hemodialysis. *ASAIO J* 1999; 45:94–97.

70. Jamison RL, Hartigan P, Kaufman JS, Goldfarb DS, Warren SR, Guarino PD, Gaziano JM, Veterans Affairs Site Investigators. Effect of homocysteine lowering on mortality and vascular disease in advanced chronic kidney disease and end-stage renal disease: A randomized controlled trial. *JAMA* 2007; 298:1163–70.

71. Dierkes J, Westphal S. Effect of drugs on homocysteine concentrations. *Semin Vasc Med* 2005; 5:124–39.

72. Stebbins R, Scott J, Herbert V. Drug-induced megaloblastic anemias. *Semin Hematol* 1973; 10:235–51.

73. Elliott JO, Jacobson MP, Haneef Z. Cardiovascular risk factors and homocysteine in epilepsy. *Epilepsy Res* 2007; 76:113–23.

74. Huemer M, Ausserer B, Graninger G, Hubmann M, Huemer C, Schlachter K, Tscharre A, Ulmer H, Simma B. Hyperhomocysteinemia in children treated with antiepileptic drugs is normalized by folic acid supplementation. *Epilepsia* 2005; 46:1677–83.

75. Haagsma CJ, Blom HJ, van Riel PL, van't Hof MA, Giesendorf BA, van Oppenraaij-Emmerzaal D, van de Putte LB. Influence of sulphasalazine, methotrexate, and the combination of both on plasma homocysteine concentrations in patients with rheumatoid arthritis. *Ann Rheum Dis* 1999; 58:79–84.

76. Visser K, Katchamart W, Loza E, Martinez-Lopez JA, Salliot C, Trudeau J, Bombardier C, et al. Multinational evidence-based recommendations for the use of methotrexate in rheumatic disorders with a focus on rheumatoid arthritis: Integrating systematic literature research and expert opinion of a broad international panel of rheumatologists in the 3E Initiative. *Ann Rheum Dis* 2009; 68:1086–93.

77. Niyikiza C, Baker SD, Seitz DE, Walling JM, Nelson K, Rusthoven JJ, Stabler SP, Paoletti P, Calvert AH, Allen RH. Homocysteine and methylmalonic acid: Markers to predict and avoid toxicity from pemetrexed therapy. *Mol Cancer Ther* 2002; 1:545–52.

78. Stabler SP, Allen RH, Fried LP, Pahor M, Kittner SJ, Penninx BW, Guralnik JM. Racial differences in prevalence of cobalamin and folate deficiencies in disabled elderly women. *Am J Clin Nutr* 1999; 70:911–19.

79. Homocysteine Lowering Trialists' Collaboration. Dose-dependent effects of folic acid on blood concentrations of homocysteine: A meta-analysis of the randomized trials. *Am J Clin Nutr* 2005; 82:806–12.

80. Johnson MA, Hawthorne NA, Brackett WR, Fischer JG, Gunter EW, Allen RH, Stabler SP. Hyperhomocysteinemia and vitamin B-12 deficiency in elderly using Title IIIc nutrition services. *Am J Clin Nutr* 2003; 77:211–20.

17 Influence of Alcohol on Folate Status and Methionine Metabolism in Relation to Alcoholic Liver Disease

Charles H. Halsted, Valentina Medici, and Farah Esfandiari

CONTENTS

I. INTRODUCTION

Alcoholic beverages are consumed to some extent by about two-thirds of the US population over age 14. Alcohol abuse, defined roughly as chronic usage affecting patterns of daily living including health, legal, or societal problems, is found in about 5% of the US population, with greater prevalence in men (7%) than in women (2.5%) and in those aged 18 to 44 years [1]. Alcoholic liver disease (ALD), the principal medical complication of chronic alcoholism, occurs in about 20% of persons with chronic alcoholism, has an overall mortality of 9.6 in 100,000, and is the 12th leading cause of death in the United States [2]. The risk of ALD is dependent on a daily intake of more than 30 g of alcohol, as found in two shots of 80-proof liquor, two glasses of wine, or two cans of beer, for at least 10 years [2]. In addition, ALD patients typically exhibit multiple vitamin deficiencies, most commonly those of folate, thiamin, and vitamin B6 [3]. As discussed in this chapter, folate deficiency is prevalent among persons with chronic alcoholism and, through its effects on aberrant methionine metabolism in the liver, may play a central role in the pathogenesis of ALD.

II. FOLATE DEFICIENCY IN CHRONIC ALCOHOLISM

A. INCIDENCE

Before the mandatory US governmental institution of folic acid fortification of grains at a level of 140 µg/100 g in 1998, the incidence of low serum folate concentration in chronic derelict alcoholic patients was as high as 80% [4], and a similar percentage of low serum folate concentrations was found in sequential ALD patients with cirrhosis admitted to large US municipal hospitals [5]. Low red blood cell (RBC) folate concentrations with megaloblastic anemia, a sign of tissue folate deficiency, were found in approximately 40% of patients with chronic alcoholism with low hemoglobin concentrations who were admitted to a large municipal hospital in New York City [6]. Among the entire US population, the policy of folic acid fortification reduced the prevalence of folate deficiency over a 5-year period to less than 5% [7]. In contrast, the incidence of folate deficiency was 11.1% among 36 patients admitted to a US hospital with an alcohol-related illness after the initiation of folic acid fortification [8].

B. CLINICAL MANIFESTATIONS OF FOLATE DEFICIENCY IN PATIENTS
WITH CHRONIC ALCOHOLISM

1. Anemia

Anemia is common in persons with chronic alcoholism, and its etiologies are multifactorial. Among 121 consecutive patients with anemia and alcoholism admitted to a large US municipal hospital before folic acid fortification of the US diet, 34% had megaloblastic bone marrow consistent with folate deficiency, 23% had sidero-blastosis of bone marrow consistent with vitamin B6 deficiency, and iron stores were absent from the bone marrow in 13% [6].

2. Hyperhomocysteinemia

The association of hyperhomocysteinemia with alcoholism was first reported from an alcohol detoxification center in Sweden in 1993, where mean homocysteine (Hcy) concentrations were increased twofold in a group of 42 patients admitted for alcohol detoxification compared with concentrations in a group of control subjects and a group of abstinent persons with alcoholism [9]. A comprehensive Portuguese study of 32 people with chronic alcoholism and matching control subjects confirmed the significant effects of alcohol use on the risk of hyperhomocysteinemia. Whereas 65% of the people with chronic alcoholism had low RBC folate concentrations, there was no correlation of folate and Hcy concentrations, thus ruling out low folate status as a principal cause of hyperhomocysteinemia [10]. In a more recent German study, elevated Hcy concentrations were found in more than 100 actively drinking people with alcoholism, which correlated with blood alcohol concentrations and which normalized with 10 days of abstinence [11]. Evaluating potential effects of ALD, a Spanish study of more than 200 people with chronic alcoholism found that Hcy concentrations were higher in 111 patients with laboratory evidence of ALD than in 117 patients without liver disease. In this study, the incidence of folate deficiency was greater in those with ALD (62.3%) than in the people with chronic alcoholism without liver disease (33.3%), whereas plasma Hcy concentrations were closely correlated with serum folic acid concentrations [12]. According to results from a study of ethanol-fed rats, the mechanism for hyperhomocysteinemia in actively drinking subjects with alcoholism is the inhibitory effect of acetaldehyde, the initial metabolite of ethanol, on the activity of hepatic methionine synthase (MS), which transmethylates Hcy in the synthesis of endogenous methionine [13]. Summarizing the data from these European studies, it appears that plasma Hcy is commonly elevated in actively drinking people with alcoholism in relation to blood ethanol concentrations, whereas the presence of liver dysfunction is an additional contributing factor, in part through its effects on lowering folate concentrations in the liver. Because these studies were all reported from countries without dietary folic acid fortification, the data on hyperhomocysteinemia in relation to folate deficiency cannot be applied predictably to people with alcoholism in the United States.

3. Colorectal Cancer and Folate Deficiency in PATIENTS with Chronic Alcoholism

Chronic alcoholism is associated with increased incidences of several cancers, including oropharyngeal, esophageal, liver, breast, and colorectal. The acetaldehyde product of alcohol metabolism is a likely etiological factor for cancers of the oropharynx, esophagus, and colorectum in people with alcoholism and has been found in increased concentrations at these sites, possibly because of bacterial metabolism of alcohol in saliva and in the lumen of the colon [14]. Other evidence identifies folate deficiency as important in the etiology of colorectal cancer.

One large study of more than 25,000 men and women undergoing colonoscopy screening found an increased incidence of adenomatous precancerous colonic polyps in those consuming more than moderate amounts of alcohol daily, which was three times greater in drinkers with low folate intake than in nondrinkers with normal to high folate intake [15]. A case-control study of more than 800 subjects associated low folate intake with increased risk of rectal but not colon cancer [16]. The propensity for dietary folate deficiency to induce colon cancer was demonstrated in a rat model treated with the carcinogen dimethylhydrazine [17]. In patients undergoing sigmoidoscopic evaluations, lower rectal mucosal folate concentrations were found in patients with adenomatous polyps with correlations observed between colonic mucosal folate and blood folate and Hcy concentrations [18]. A recent study linked dietary folate intake to levels of DNA methylation of a tumor suppressor gene in the colonic mucosa of aging rats [19]. A clinical study with more than 100 patients with sporadic colorectal cancer found that promoter regions in DNA of genes relevant to carcinogenesis were hypermethylated in patients consuming low folate diets with high alcohol intakes compared with patients consuming high folate diets with low ethanol intakes [20]. Together, these studies suggest links between acetaldehyde, a product of ethanol metabolism and inhibitor of MS [13], and folate deficiency, with altered methionine metabolism resulting in changes in gene methylation relevant to increased cancer risk.

III. ETIOLOGIES OF FOLATE DEFICIENCY IN PEOPLE WITH CHRONIC ALCOHOLISM

The etiology of folate deficiency in chronic alcoholism with or without ALD is multifactorial, in part because of dietary inadequacy but also based on the potential effects of short- and/or long-term use of ethanol on mechanisms of folate homeostasis that include intestinal absorption of dietary pteroylpolyglutamyl and pteroyl-monoglutamyl folate, altered uptake and metabolism of 5-methyltetrahydrofolate (5-methyl-THF) in the liver and biliary circulation, and effects on the renal excretion of 5-methyl-THF. In addition, ethanol or its metabolite acetaldehyde may have direct destructive oxidative effects on the folate molecule. Figure 17.1 depicts pathways for normal folate homeostasis and can be used as a reference for following the potential effects of chronic ethanol exposure.

A. DIETARY INSUFFICIENCY

There is little or no folate in alcoholic beverages with the exception of beer, in which concentrations vary according to brand [21]. Because alcoholics who are binge drinkers generally restrict their usual dietary intake, they are less likely to consume adequate amounts of folate-containing foods. In addition, decreased folate stores place patients with ALD at increased risk of developing dietary folate deficiency [22]. Early reports ascribed folate deficiency among derelict people with chronic alcoholism to dietary inadequacy [3,4], whereas others found little evidence for folate deficiency in well-nourished patients with alcoholism [23]. As indicated, there

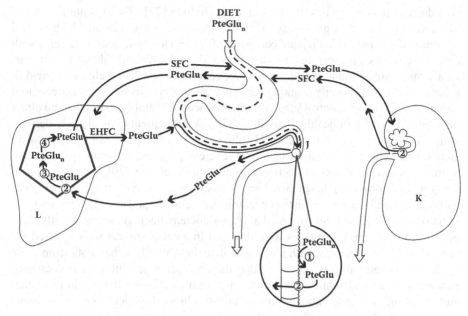

FIGURE 17.1   Folate homeostasis. See Section III, Etiologies of Folate Deficiency in People with Chronic Alcoholism, for details. PteGlu$_n$, pteroylpolyglutamates as found in diet and liver folate storage; PteGlu, pteroylglutamate, found as folic acid in diet and supplements and as 5-methyltetrahydrofolate in diet, liver, bile, and portal and systemic circulation; J, jejunum, L, liver; K, kidney; SFC, systemic folate circulation; EHFC, enterohepatic folate circulation. 1, glutamate carboxypeptidase II, required for hydrolysis of dietary PteGlu$_n$; 2, PteGlu transporter, candidates including folate-binding protein (FBP), reduced folate carrier (RFC1), or proton coupled folate transporter (PCFT); 3, pteroylpolyglutamate synthetase; 4, intracellular folate hydrolase.

are no current data on the potential for folic acid fortification of the US grain supply to improve folate status among people with chronic alcoholism.

B.   INTESTINAL MALABSORPTION

The potential for direct effects of ethanol on folate absorption can be placed in context of the known concentration of ethanol at 2 g/100 mL in the proximal jejunum after the rapid ingestion of an ethanol solution equivalent to three drinks [24], whereas megaloblastic changes can be found in the absorbing intestinal cells, or enterocytes, of folate-deficient people with alcoholism [25]. The intestinal absorption of dietary folate requires the initial stage of hydrolysis of dietary pteroylpolyglutamyl folates (PteGlu$_n$) to their pteroylmonoglutamyl (PteGlu) derivatives, which are subsequently transported across the brush-border and basolateral membranes of the enterocytes to the portal vein (Figure 17.1). Jejunal perfusion studies in normal human subjects provided evidence that the absorption of labeled PteGlu$_n$ is limited by the requirement for initial hydrolysis [26], whereas the extent of hydrolysis of perfused PteGlu$_n$

was decreased in a pig model of chronic alcoholism [27]. The potential effect of alcoholism on the intestinal uptake of the PteGlu derivative was studied by both oral tolerance and triple-lumen jejunal perfusion of ^{3}H-labeled folic acid in patients with chronic alcoholism presenting with alcohol withdrawal after binge drinking. The earliest clinical study found that the timed appearance of the ^{3}H-labeled folic acid in serum and urine of recently drinking persons with chronic alcoholism was decreased compared with that in control subjects, whereas acute alcohol ingestion had no effect on folate absorption in healthy individuals [28]. A subsequent clinical study demonstrated decreased jejunal uptake of ^{3}H-folic acid of recently drinking patients with alcoholism, with lowest values in folate-deficient patients, whereas uptakes were normalized after 2 weeks of abstinence and a hospital diet [29]. Another clinical study was performed on hospitalized and 2-week-abstinent volunteers with alcoholism with normalized serum folate concentrations; jejunal uptake of ^{3}H-folic acid was reduced in two subjects who ingested a folate-deficient diet together, with daily alcohol for 6 weeks, but no changes were detected in another subject who ingested the same daily dose of alcohol with a normal folate diet [30]. Together, data from these studies in human subjects suggested that the absorption of folic acid is decreased in malnourished and folate-deficient patients with alcoholism but not in recovered and nutritionally replete patients with alcoholism. In a subsequent study of macaque monkeys fed ethanol with adequate dietary folate for 2 years, folate malabsorption was demonstrated by greater fecal excretion and reduced urine excretion of the tritium label after gastric gavage administration of ^{3}H-folic acid [31].

Potential mechanisms for the effect of long-term alcohol exposure on reducing folate absorption may relate to its effects on regulatory enzymes and transporters in the intestinal mucosa. Glutamate carboxypeptidase (GCPII), the enzyme that hydrolyzes dietary PteGlu$_n$, is predominantly present in the brush-border membrane of duodenum and jejunum of humans and pigs with a pH optimum of 5.5 and K_m of 0.6 μM [32,33], and its activity was reduced in jejunal brush-border vesicles by long-term ethanol feeding of micropigs [34]. At least three candidate genes regulate the transport of PteGlu across the brush-border and basolateral membranes of the absorbing enterocytes of the jejunum: the folate receptor or folate-binding protein (FBP), the reduced folate carrier (RFC1), and the recently discovered proton-coupled folate transporter (PCFT). A study that used immunohistochemical techniques demonstrated the absence of FBP from micropig intestine [35], confirming previous findings in other species [36]. On the other hand, transcripts of RFC1 are present on the pig jejunal brush border, but at lower levels than in liver and kidney, and kinetic studies showed that RFC1 V_{max} was twofold lower in jejunum from ethanol-fed micropigs than for controls [37]. More recently, PCFT was identified as the more likely physiological transporter of PteGlu in the intestine because, in contrast to the neutral pH optimum of RFC1, the optimal pH for PCFT is 5.5, consistent with the known acid microclimate that exists at the jejunal brush border [38]. The specificity of PCFT for PteGlu transport was shown by finding that a loss of function mutation of this gene is the cause of human hereditary folate malabsorption [39]. Further, PCFT protein is highly expressed in duodenal and jejunal brush-border membranes, and its mRNA expression in these tissues was increased more than 10-fold in response to a folate-deficient diet [38]. The finding of similar distributions of RFC1 and PCFT in mouse duodenum and jejunum suggests a cooperative function of both proteins, where PCFT transports PteGlu at the normal acid microclimate, and RFC1 activity is optimal at neutral pH [38]. Whereas hereditary folate malabsorption was ascribed to a loss of function mutation of PCFT [39], there are no studies to date on the potential effect of long-term ethanol exposure on the expression or kinetics of PCFT in the mammalian intestine.

C.   HEPATIC UPTAKE AND METABOLISM OF FOLATE

Following transport across membranes of the absorbing enterocytes, PteGlu in the 5-methyl-THF form circulates to the liver in the portal vein and is transported across basolateral cell membranes into metabolically active hepatocytes, where it is stored and metabolized in the $PteGlu_n$ form. Subsequent release of endogenous folate to the circulation involves intracellular hydrolysis to the 5-methyl-THF form. In addition, a significant fraction of the total body folate pool is excreted as 5-methyl-THF into bile, then reabsorbed in an enterohepatic folate cycle [40]. Hepatic folate storage is decreased in patients with ALD, as shown by a twofold accelerated development of folate deficiency when these patients were placed on low folate diets [22], as compared with an observed 22-week time to folate deficiency in a healthy subject [41]. In a primate model following exposure to 2 years of ethanol, liver folate concentrations were lower, together with an about one-third decrease in hepatic uptake of parenterally administered folic acid. However, hepatic folate metabolism was unchanged according to chromatographic patterns of labeled $PteGlu_n$ and PteGlu folate metabolites [42]. Causes of the observed decreased retention of labeled folate could include decrease in cell uptake or increased biliary excretion. In contrast, lower biliary excretion, i.e., greater hepatic retention, of labeled folate in ethanol-fed rodents was observed in another study [43]. Together these observations suggest that decreased transport of folates across the basolateral hepatocyte membranes is the main regulatory process for decreased hepatic folate stores in the monkey model of ALD.

Studies in micropigs demonstrated the immunological presence of FBP in the basolateral membrane of pig hepatocytes [35], as well as hepatic transcripts and basolateral membrane activity of RFC1 [37], whereas others demonstrated PCFT transcripts in mouse liver [38]. Although previous primate studies by our research group suggested that long-term ethanol feeding impairs hepatocyte uptake of PteGlu [42], liver RFC1 transcripts and basolateral membrane transport were not affected by ethanol feeding in the micropig [37]. A previous study demonstrated that transport of 5-methyl-THF into isolated rat hepatocytes is optimal at acid pH [44], now known to be consistent with PCFT activity, and a more recent study using cultured human hepatoma cells found a similar acid pH optimum for folic acid transport that was unaffected by knockdown of RFC1 [45]. Thus, similar to transport of monoglutamyl folate across the intestinal brush-border membrane, it is possible that both RFC1 and PCFT interact at neutral and acid pH optima for folate transport across the hepatocyte basolateral membrane. Whether FPB also plays an interactive role in basolateral membrane transport is not clear, but transcripts of this protein were found to be absent from human liver [35]. There are no available data on the potential effect of ethanol exposure on the hepatic expression of PCFT or the kinetics of its activity in hepatocyte basolateral membranes.

D. Increased Renal Excretion of Folate

The kidney is the principal route of folate elimination from the body by a mechanism that includes initial glomerular filtration and then regulated proximal renal tubular cell reabsorption. In clinical studies, the excretion of labeled folate was increased by up to 40% in persons with chronic alcoholism after 2 weeks of controlled consumption of alcohol [46]. This observation has been confirmed in ethanol-fed rat models [47], whereas a study of ethanol-fed monkeys demonstrated increased urinary excretion of labeled folic acid as a significant mechanism for the decrease in the body folate pool [48]. Both FBP and RFC1 are present in proximal renal tubular cells [35,37], but long-term ethanol feeding of micropigs had no effect on the transcript expression of RFC1 [37]. However, short-term ethanol exposure in a rat model reduced proximal tubular membrane transport of folic acid, although longer exposure up-regulated the protein expressions of both RFC1 and FBP with lesser effects on transport, suggestive of an overall adaptive response [49]. Others found no effect of long-term ethanol exposure in rats on binding of 5-methyl-THF to isolated renal brush-border vesicles [50]. PCFT transcript expression has also been identified in kidneys, although its relative role compared with the other transport proteins and potential regulation by ethanol exposure have not been clarified [38].

E. Oxidative Destruction of Folate

Two clinical observations suggest that ethanol and/or its metabolite acetaldehyde may have a direct destructive effect on folate. Four decades ago, a classical clinical investigation by Sullivan and Herbert [51] demonstrated in two folate-deficient persons with alcoholism and megaloblastic anemia that the repeated oral administration of ethanol rapidly inhibited the erythropoietic response of the bone marrow to small doses of oral or parenteral folic acid. A study in volunteers with alcoholism demonstrated that the serum folate concentration decreases precipitously in response to the acute ingestion of ethanol [52]. Although these observations could reflect an inhibitory effect of ethanol on release of endogenous folate from its hepatic stores, others found that folate catabolites could be produced by the in vitro incubation of 5-methyl-THF with the ethanol metabolite acetaldehyde, iron, and xanthine oxidase in a reaction that was inhibited by the addition of superoxide dismutase [53]. In contrast, the urinary excretion of folate catabolites was unchanged in long-term ethanol-fed mice [54].

IV. HEPATIC FOLATE-DEPENDENT METHIONINE METABOLISM AND INTERACTIONS WITH ETHANOL EXPOSURE

As depicted in Figure 17.2, both dietary and endogenous folate play significant roles in hepatic methionine metabolism, which in turn regulates Hcy turnover, antioxidant defenses, DNA assembly, lipid export, and all epigenetic methylation reactions that regulate selected gene expressions. The principal methionine metabolite S-adenosylmethionine (SAM), which is synthesized at a rate of 6 to 8 g/day in the human liver, is integral to antioxidant defense and substrate for all methylation reactions, is dependent on folate supply, and is reduced by long-term ethanol exposure [55].

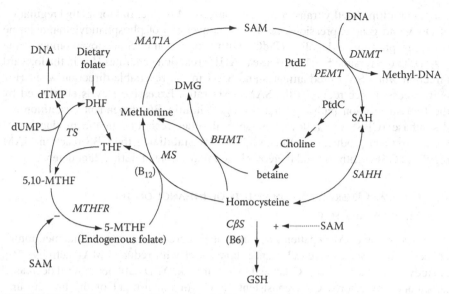

FIGURE 17.2 Folate and methionine metabolism. See Section IV, Hepatic Folate-Dependent Methionine Metabolism and Interactions with Ethanol Exposure, for details. 5-MTHF, methyltetrahydrofolate; 5,10-MTHF, 5,10 methylenetetrahydrofolate; BHMT, betaine homocysteine methyltransferase; CBS, cystathionine-β-synthase; DHF, dihydrofolate; DMG, dimethyl glycine; DNMT, DNA methyltransferase(s); dTMP, deoxythymidine monophosphate; dUMP, deoxyuridine monophosphate; GSH, glutathione; MAT1A, methionine adenosyltransferase 1A; MS, methionine synthase; MTHFR, methylene tetrahydrofolate reductase; PEMT, phosphatidylethanolamine methyltransferase; PtdC, phosphatidylcholine, PtdE, phosphatidylethanolamine, SAH, S-adenosylhomocysteine; SAHH, S-adenosylhomocysteine hydrolase; SAM, S-adenosylmethionine; THF, tetrahydrofolate, TS, thymidine synthase.

A. NORMAL INTERACTIONS OF FOLATE AND METHIONINE METABOLISM

Briefly, dietary folates are absorbed or undergo metabolism in the liver and other tissues to 5-methyl-THF, which is a substrate for MS in conversion of Hcy to methionine, with the additional production of THF and 5,10-methylene-THF (Figure 17.2). In the presence of an adequate SAM concentration, 5,10-methylene-THF reacts with thymidine synthase (TS) for regulation of uridine to thymidine conversion and ultimately DNA nucleotide balance. However, reduced SAM promotes the methyltetrahydrofolate reductase (MTHFR) reaction that uses 5,10-methylene-THF substrate to increase endogenous 5-methyl-THF. At the same time, this pathway reduces the availability of 5,10-methylene-THF for the TS reaction, thereby enhancing DNA nucleotide imbalance. In transmethylation reactions, methionine, the product of MS, is the substrate for endogenous SAM production through methionine adenosyl transferase (MAT), which is encoded in the liver by the gene *MAT1A*. In the liver and kidney, methionine and SAM are also generated from Hcy by betaine Hcy methyltransferase (BHMT), which uses betaine that is available sparingly in the diet and endogenously from its substrate choline. As the methyl donor in multiple methyltransferase reactions, SAM is essential for methyl regulation of DNA and gene expressions, as well as conversion of phosphatidylethanolamine (PtdE) to phosphatidylcholine (PtdC), with production of S-adenosylhomocysteine (SAH). The reversible SAH hydrolase (SAHH) reaction generates Hcy in the forward direction when SAH predominates and SAH in the reversible direction when Hcy is in excess, hence reducing the SAM/SAH ratio. Excessive Hcy is eliminated by the transsulfuration pathway, first through vitamin B6–dependent cystathionine-β-synthase (CBS) and followed by several other reactions in the production of the antioxidant product glutathione (GSH). By stabilizing the CBS reaction, SAM regulates GSH synthesis and thereby plays a major role in antioxidant defense.

B. CLINICAL OBSERVATIONS ON EFFECTS OF ETHANOL ON THE METHIONINE CYCLE

A clinical study of ALD patients demonstrated increased fasting plasma methionine concentrations and delayed clearance, consistent with reduced MAT activity [56]. A study of the turnover of ^{13}C-labeled methionine in ALD patients showed decreased appearance of labeled CO_2, consistent also with impairment of the transsulfuration excretion pathway [57]. Other studies showed reduced SAM and transcript levels of MAT1A, MS, BHMT, and CBS in liver biopsies from patients with ALD [58–61], complemented by studies in the ethanol-fed micropig model documenting decreased transcripts of MTHFR, MS, MAT1A, and SAHH [62]. A comprehensive study established a link between abnormal methionine metabolism and the clinical severity of ALD, finding increased plasma concentrations of methionine, Hcy, and cystathionine in 81 patients with moderate to severe cirrhosis compared with 55 healthy control subjects, consistent with impaired SAM production and a block in the transsulfuration pathway at a level downstream of the CBS enzyme. Of significance, plasma concentrations of these metabolites were correlated with concentrations of liver disease serum markers albumin, bilirubin, and prothrombin time [63]. Two European studies demonstrated a positive effect of SAM supplementation in treatment of moderately severe ALD, with an increase in liver GSH in one study [64], and in the other, a reduction in mortality or liver transplant requirement from 30% in the placebo group to 16% in the SAM group [65].

C. EFFECTS OF ETHANOL EXPOSURE ON METHIONINE METABOLISM AND INTERACTIONS WITH ALCOHOLIC LIVER DISEASE

Multiple interacting pathways contribute to the pathogenesis of ALD [66]. The recognized mechanisms of oxidative liver injury with steatosis in ALD include increased intestinal permeation of luminal lipopolysaccharide, which in turn stimulates hepatic Kupffer cells to release proinflammatory cytokines, such as tumor necrosis factor α (TNFα), and to promote the induction of oxidant free radicals through nicotinamide-adenine dinucleotide phosphate, reduced form (NADPH) oxidase [67]. At the same time, ethanol up-regulation of hepatocyte cytochrome P450 2E1 (CYP2E1) produces hydroxyethanol radicals, which induce oxidative stress [68]. Apoptotic hepatocyte death is initiated though ethanol and related effects on caspases, including those generated through the endoplasmic reticulum (ER) stress pathway [69]. Steatosis, or increased hepatocellular triglyceride, provides a platform for the generation of lipid oxidant products and represents the net effects of de novo lipogenesis, reduced fatty acid oxidation, and reduced transport of triglyceride from the liver [70]. Hepatic lipid metabolism is regulated through both the adiponectin and ER stress pathways [70,71]. Studies in animal models have shown that long-term ethanol exposure has significant influences on several regulatory pathways and mediators of hepatic methionine metabolism. Two independent groups demonstrated that long-term ethanol-fed rats develop reduced hepatic SAM concentrations with reduced MS activity and increased compensatory activity of BHMT [72,73]. Ethanol-fed baboons demonstrated reduced hepatic levels of GSH, which were corrected by SAM supplementation together with improved microscopic changes of ALD [74]. Intragastric ethanol-fed mice demonstrated decreased SAM and SAM/SAH ratio, together with decreased MAT activity and increased DNA strand breaks [75]. Changes in methionine metabolism may also predispose to malignant degeneration in the liver. After intragastric ethanol feeding for 9 weeks, a switch in MAT expression and synthesis was observed, with rapid hepatic growth, global DNA hypomethylation, increased c-myc expression, and genome-wide DNA strand breaks consistent with increased propensity for the development of hepatocellular carcinoma [75]. Reduced synthesis of MAT that regulates SAM production may be a result of post-transcriptional oxidant modification of a cysteine 121 amino acid residue [76]. Ethanol consumption also results in increased hepatocellular levels of SAH, which results from Hcy accumulation with consequent increased reverse activity of SAH hydrolase in the SAH synthesis direction. In a study of hepatocytes isolated from ethanol-fed rats, SAH concentrations were elevated together with increased hepatocyte apoptosis, which is typically associated with alcohol toxicity, as well as increased caspase-3 activity and DNA fragmentation. Coincubation with betaine led to a significant decrease in DNA fragmentation to almost control levels [77]. In another study from the same group, betaine supplementation in ethanol-fed rats maintained the SAM/SAH ratio and normalized the activity of phosphatidylethanolamine methyltransferase, significantly preventing fatty infiltration associated with ethanol feeding [78]. Others found that an increase in SAH concentration was associated with an increase in hepatic TNFα concentrations, caspase-8 activity, and cell death in ethanol-fed mice, whereas hepatocytes, when exposed to SAH-enhancing agents, were sensitized to TNFα killing. These results demonstrate that elevated SAH potentiates TNFα toxicity in ALD [79] by a mechanism that may involve blockage by SAH of the mitochondrial transport of SAM [80]. A mouse *MAT1A* knockout model developed features of ALD together with reduced SAM and GSH concentrations [81]. Other studies in the intragastric ethanol-fed mouse model found that significant perturbations of the ER stress pathways of hepatocyte apoptosis and steatosis were associated with aberrant methionine metabolism. In these experiments, ethanol feeding resulted in elevated Hcy in association with increased hepatocellular apoptosis and steatosis, with enhanced expressions of relevant regulatory ER proteins, all prevented by the addition of betaine to the feeding regimen [82,83]. Summarizing, SAM deficiency and Hcy elevation are promoted by ethanol through acetaldehyde inhibition of MS activity, reduction of MAT1A expression, and hepatocyte accumulation of SAH.

SAM deficiency contributes to depletion of the mitochondrial antioxidant GSH, whereas elevated SAH may prevent transport of SAM into mitochondria.

V. ETHANOL-INDUCED ABERRANT METHIONINE METABOLISM IN THE PATHOGENESIS OF ALCOHOLIC LIVER DISEASE

Because chronic alcoholism perturbs hepatic methionine metabolism by increasing Hcy concentrations and decreasing the SAM/SAH ratio together with reduced antioxidant defense and altered gene expression, we postulated that ethanol-induced aberrant methionine metabolism could play a central role in the pathogenesis of ALD. Initial studies established the model of ALD and the effects of ethanol feeding on aberrant methionine metabolism in the micropig, a species that ingests ethanol voluntarily and completely in the diet. All histopathological features of ALD, including fat accumulation (steatosis), inflammation, hepatocyte necrosis, and fibrosis, could be induced by feeding ethanol at 40% of kilocalorie in a pro-oxidant diet high in polyunsaturated corn oil for 12 months [84]. Additional findings in a subsequent study included increased hepatocellular apoptosis with progressive increase in serum Hcy and reduction of methionine concentrations, reduced hepatic SAM/SAH ratio, and DNA instability as shown by an increased ratio of nucleotides uridine to thymidine [85]. We then tested the premise that aberrant methionine metabolism contributed to the development of ALD by evaluating potential interactive or additional effects of folate deficiency, which is known to perturb methionine metabolism and is common in persons with chronic alcoholism as described above. After just 14 weeks of feeding, micropigs fed combined ethanol and folate-deficient diets had maximal serum Hcy concentrations and demonstrated the lowest hepatic SAM/SAH ratio and lowest GSH concentrations, together with histopathology of ALD, which was absent in controls fed normal or folate-deficient diets or ethanol with normal folate diets [86]. The hepatic concentrations of SAM were highly correlated with those of GSH, underscoring the regulatory role of SAM in the transsulfuration pathway for reduction in Hcy and production of GSH (Figure 17.2). Consistent with previous observations on DNA instability, micropigs fed combined folate-deficient and ethanol diets also showed increased DNA oxidation and strand breaks [86] that were associated with increased hepatocellular apoptosis [87]. To study mechanistic interactions, liver specimens from this study were used for measurements of signals and gene expressions of liver injury that were then correlated with liver SAM and SAH. Each metabolite and their ratio were correlated with hepatic transcript and protein levels of CYP2E1, which metabolizes ethanol while promoting the production of reactive oxygen species. This study also correlated SAM, SAH, and their ratios with ER stress signals, including glucose-related protein 78 and sterol regulatory element binding protein (SREBP) 1-c, and with transcript levels of lipid-synthesizing enzymes fatty acid synthase (FAS), acetyl-CoA carboxylase (ACC), and stearoyl-CoA desaturase [87].

The potential effect of SAM supplementation in the prevention of ALD in the micropig model was then investigated, as a further test of the hypothesis that the pathogenesis of ALD is mediated through the effects of ethanol on methionine metabolism. In these experiments micropigs were fed one of three diets: folate-deficient diets as control, folate deficient diets with ethanol, and folate deficient diets with ethanol and SAM supplementation for 14 weeks. Whereas ethanol feeding resulted in significant steatosis and oxidative damage, SAM supplementation maintained liver histopathology at control levels while normalizing liver Hcy, SAM/SAH ratio, and antioxidant GSH levels [88,89]. Similarly, SAM supplementation prevented ethanol-induced pathways of steatosis, including serum adiponectin, liver adenosine monophosphate kinase, SREBP 1-c, ACC, FAS, and glycerol-3-phosphate acyltransferase [88]. Evaluating effects on oxidative liver injury, SAM supplementation prevented ethanol-induced elevations in CYP2E1, NADPH oxidase, and inducible nitric oxide synthase activities [89].

VI. POTENTIAL EPIGENETIC EFFECTS OF ETHANOL AND FOLATE DEFICIENCY ON DEVELOPMENT OF ALCOHOLIC LIVER DISEASE

Epigenetic research is the study of postsynthetic modification of either DNA or proteins that associate with DNA as the key mediators of downstream biological effects. Gene expression is regulated at different levels, one of which is the methylation of DNA, and the other is the remodeling of chromatin, which is the complex of DNA, histone, and nonhistone proteins. Research during the past few years has shown the effects of external factors such as diet and toxins on epigenetic processes that may regulate the development of chronic diseases, potentially including ethanol-induced hepatic injury. The methylation of transcriptional control regions in the specific CpG-rich regions of DNA, called CpG islands, plays a fundamental role in the regulation of gene expression. Methylation of gene promoter-related CpG islands is an epigenetic modification of DNA that can inappropriately suppress gene expression and could have deleterious effects if the targeted genes function in a regulatory capacity. Conversely, hypomethylation could lead to accentuated expression of selected genes, which, for example in ALD, could promote pathways of steatosis and other aspects of liver injury. In the context of hepatic methionine metabolism, the level of substrate SAM is critical for the function of DNA methyltransferases (DNMTs), which transfer a methyl group from SAM to cytosine in CpG dinucleotides while generating its product SAH. At the same time, SAH is a potent inhibitor of DNMT reactions [90], with K_i 1.4 μM that is similar to the K_m for SAM [91]. Therefore, the SAM/SAH ratio is a practical index of methylation capacity [55]. In recent studies in the micropig model, the relationships of decreased SAM/SAH ratio to increased expressions of genes associated with liver injury and steatosis, such as *CYP2E1*, *SREBP 1-c*, and *FAS* [87], and their corrections by SAM supplementation [88,89] suggest a mechanism of specific gene regulation by hypomethylation that is induced by combinations of ethanol feeding and folate deficiency. Previous studies in a rat model of hepatocarcinogenesis provided evidence that a folate-, choline-, and methionine-deficient diet induced significant reductions in the hepatic SAM/SAH ratio together with genome-wide DNA hypomethylation and differential expressions of DNMTs and methylated DNA binding proteins [92,93]. Chromatin remodeling can be initiated by the addition of methyl groups to DNA or by post-translational modifications of the amino acids that make up histones. The fundamental unit of chromatin is the polymer nucleosome, which is composed of 147 base pairs of DNA wrapped around an octamer of histone core proteins [94]. There are several types of post-translational modifications of histones, including acetylation and methylation of position-specific lysine residues of histones H3 and H4, which serve as markers of either transcriptional-competent euchromatin or silent heterochromatin [95–97]. Histone H3 and H4 hyperacetylation in promoter regions is closely associated with gene activation or transcriptionally active euchromatin. Furthermore, lysine residues can be mono-, di-, or trimethylated with subsequent functional responses, thus providing another layer of complexity in gene regulation. H3K9 trimethylation is one of the most important repressive markers for the maintenance of inactive heterochromatin [96,98,99].

Several studies have demonstrated ethanol modification of histones, although potential histone modification by the combination of folate deficiency and ethanol exposure has not been evaluated. Feeding rats ethanol orally caused chromatin condensation in the liver, followed by specific changes in the nonhistone nuclear pool [100]. Exposure of primary rat hepatocytes to ethanol caused opposing changes in methylation of histone H3, including reduced H3K9 methylation with a subsequent increase of H3K4 methylation in the regulatory region of the up-regulated genes [101]. Intragastric administration of ethanol increased acetylation of H3K9 in rat liver but had no effect on other lysine residues [102]. In another study, feeding ethanol to rats by intragastric infusion at a constant rate for 1 month increased histone acetyltransferase and acetylated H3K9 levels [103]. The significance of these modifications to expressions of genes relevant to liver injury is unknown.

VII. SUMMARY AND FUTURE RESEARCH NEEDS

Chronic alcoholism both increases risks for folate deficiency and impairs folate and methionine metabolism. The multiple causes of folate deficiency in chronic alcoholism include poor diet, intestinal malabsorption, impaired hepatic uptake with reduced storage of endogenous folates, and enhanced renal excretion. Chronic alcoholism is a cause of hyperhomocysteinemia owing to both effects of deficiency of folate substrate and effects of ethanol on MS. Folate deficiency is a leading cause of anemia in chronic alcoholism, and folate deficiency and chronic alcoholism together also increase the risk of colorectal cancer. Ethanol exposure reduces the expressions and activities of many regulatory enzymes in the methionine cycle, and folate deficiency has an additive effect in disruption of methionine metabolism with resultant low SAM, elevated SAH and Hcy, and reduced SAM/SAH ratio. Reduced SAM increases the risk of ALD by decreasing antioxidative defenses, and increased SAH and Hcy are associated with increased signals of ER stress that enhance lipogenesis and apoptosis.

Compelling evidence suggests that aberrant methionine metabolism that results from the combination of long-term ethanol exposure and folate deficiency plays a central role in the pathogenesis of ALD. Future research needs to be directed at defining mechanisms for this hypothesis. The profound effects of experimental ethanol exposure and chronic alcoholism on hepatic methionine metabolism suggest a mechanism of altered epigenetic control of the expressions of genes relevant to the development of ALD.

REFERENCES

1. Grant BF DD, Stinson FS, Chou P, Dufour MC, Pickering MS. The 12-month prevalence and trends in DSM-IV Alcohol Abuse and Dependence: United States, 1991–1992 and 2001–2002. *Alcohol Res Health* 2006; 29:79–93.
2. Mann R, Smart RG, Govoni R. The epidemiology of alcoholic liver disease. *Alcohol Res Health* 2003; 27:209–19.
3. Leevy CM, Baker H, Tenhove W, Frank O, Cherrick GR. B-complex vitamins in liver disease of the alcoholic. *Am J Clin Nutr* 1965; 16:339–46.
4. Herbert V, Zalusky R, Davidson CS. Correlation of folate deficiency with alcoholism and associated macrocytosis, anemia, and liver disease. *Ann Intern Med* 1963; 58:977–88.
5. Baker H, Frank O, Ziffer H, Goldfarb S, Leevy CM, Sobotka H. Effect of hepatic disease on liver B-complex vitamin titers. *Am J Clin Nutr* 1964; 14:1–6.
6. Savage D, Lindenbaum J. Anemia in alcoholics. *Medicine (Baltimore)* 1986; 65:322–38.
7. Pfeiffer CM, Johnson CL, Jain RB, Yetley EA, Picciano MF, Rader JI, Fisher KD, Mulinare J, Osterloh JD. Trends in blood folate and vitamin B-12 concentrations in the United States, 1988 2004. *Am J Clin Nutr* 2007; 86:718–27.
8. Fernando OV, Grimsley EW. Prevalence of folate deficiency and macrocytosis in patients with and without alcohol-related illness. *South Med J* 1998; 91:721–25.
9. Hultberg B, Berglund M, Andersson A, Frank A. Elevated plasma homocysteine in alcoholics. *Alcohol Clin Exp Res* 1993; 17:687–89.
10. Cravo ML, Gloria LM, Selhub J, Nadeau MR, Camilo ME, Resende MP, Cardoso JN, Leitao CN, Mira FC. Hyperhomocysteinemia in chronic alcoholism: Correlation with folate, vitamin B-12, and vitamin B-6 status. *Am J Clin Nutr* 1996; 63:220–24.
11. Bleich S, Carl M, Bayerlein K, Reulbach U, Biermann T, Hillemacher T, Bonsch D, Kornhuber J. Evidence of increased homocysteine levels in alcoholism: The Franconian alcoholism research studies (FARS). *Alcohol Clin Exp Res* 2005; 29:334–36.
12. Blasco C, Caballeria J, Deulofeu R, Lligona A, Pares A, Lluis JM, Gual A, Rodes J. Prevalence and mechanisms of hyperhomocysteinemia in chronic alcoholics. *Alcohol Clin Exp Res* 2005; 29:1044–48.
13. Kenyon SH, Nicolaou A, Gibbons WA. The effect of ethanol and its metabolites upon methionine synthase activity in vitro. *Alcohol* 1998; 15:305–09.
14. Seitz HK BP. Alcohol metabolism and cancer risk. *Alcohol Res Health* 2007; 30:38–47.
15. Giovannucci E, Stampfer MJ, Colditz GA, Rimm EB, Trichopoulos D, Rosner BA, Speizer FE, Willett WC. Folate, methionine, and alcohol intake and risk of colorectal adenoma. *J Natl Cancer Inst* 1993; 85:875–84.
16. Freudenheim JL, Graham S, Marshall JR, Haughey BP, Cholewinski S, Wilkinson G. Folate intake and carcinogenesis of the colon and rectum. *Int J Epidemiol* 1991; 20:368–74.
17. Cravo ML, Mason JB, Dayal Y, Hutchinson M, Smith D, Selhub J, Rosenberg IH. Folate deficiency enhances the development of colonic neoplasia in dimethylhydrazine-treated rats. *Cancer Res* 1992; 52:5002–06.
18. Kim YI, Fawaz K, Knox T, Lee YM, Norton R, Arora S, Paiva L, Mason JB. Colonic mucosal concentrations of folate correlate well with blood measurements of folate status in persons with colorectal polyps. *Am J Clin Nutr* 1998; 68:866–72.
19. Keyes MK, Jang H, Mason JB, Liu Z, Crott JW, Smith DE, Friso S, Choi SW. Older age and dietary folate are determinants of genomic and p16-specific DNA methylation in mouse colon. *J Nutr* 2007; 137:1713–17.
20. van Engeland M, Weijenberg MP, Roemen GM, Brink M, de Bruine AP, Goldbohm RA, van den Brandt PA, Baylin SB, de Goeij AF, Herman JG. Effects of dietary folate and alcohol intake on promoter methylation in sporadic colorectal cancer: The Netherlands cohort study on diet and cancer. *Cancer Res* 2003; 63:3133–37.

21. Darby W. The nutrient contributions of fermented beverages. In: Gastineau CH, Darby W, Turner TB, eds., *Fermented Food Beverages in Nutrition*. New York: Academic Press, 1979:61–79.

22. Eichner ER, Hillman RS. The evolution of anemia in alcoholic patients. *Am J Med* 1971; 50:218–32.

23. Neville JN, Eagles JA, Samson G, Olson RE. Nutritional status of alcoholics. *Am J Clin Nutr* 1968; 21:1329–40.

24. Halsted CH, Robles EA, Mezey E. Distribution of ethanol in the human gastrointestinal tract. *Am J Clin Nutr* 1973; 26:831–34.

25. Hermos JA, Adams WH, Liu YK, Sullivan LW, Trier JS. Mucosa of the small intestine in folate-deficient alcoholics. *Ann Intern Med* 1972; 76:957–65.

26. Halsted CH, Baugh CM, Butterworth CE Jr. Jejunal perfusion of simple and conjugated folates in man. *Gastroenterology* 1975; 68:261–69.

27. Reisenauer AM, Buffington CA, Villanueva JA, Halsted CH. Folate absorption in alcoholic pigs: In vivo intestinal perfusion studies. *Am J Clin Nutr* 1989; 50:1429–35.

28. Halsted CH, Griggs RC, Harris JW. The effect of alcoholism on the absorption of folic acid (H3-PGA) evaluated by plasma levels and urine excretion. *J Lab Clin Med* 1967; 69:116–31.

29. Halsted CH, Robles EA, Mezey E. Decreased jejunal uptake of labeled folic acid (3 H-PGA) in alcoholic patients: Roles of alcohol and nutrition. *N Engl J Med* 1971; 285:701–06.

30. Halsted CH, Robles EA, Mezey E. Intestinal malabsorption in folate-deficient alcoholics. *Gastroenterology* 1973; 64:526–32.

31. Romero JJ, Tamura T, Halsted CH. Intestinal absorption of [3H]folic acid in the chronic alcoholic monkey. *Gastroenterology* 1981; 80:99–102.

32. Chandler CJ, Wang TT, Halsted CH. Pteroylpolyglutamate hydrolase from human jejunal brush borders. Purification and characterization. *J Biol Chem* 1986; 261:928–33.

33. Chandler CJ, Harrison DA, Buffington CA, Santiago NA, Halsted CH. Functional specificity of jejunal brush-border pteroylpolyglutamate hydrolase in pig. *Am J Physiol* 1991; 260:G865–72.

34. Naughton CA, Chandler CJ, Duplantier RB, Halsted CH. Folate absorption in alcoholic pigs: In vitro hydrolysis and transport at the intestinal brush border membrane. *Am J Clin Nutr* 1989; 50:1436–41.

35. Villanueva J, Ling EH, Chandler CJ, Halsted CH. Membrane and tissue distribution of folate binding protein in pig. *Am J Physiol* 1998; 275:R1503–10.

36. Weitman SD, Lark RH, Coney LR, Fort DW, Frasca V, Zurawski VR Jr, Kamen BA. Distribution of the folate receptor GP38 in normal and malignant cell lines and tissues. *Cancer Res* 1992; 52:3396–401.

37. Villanueva JA, Devlin AM, Halsted CH. Reduced folate carrier: Tissue distribution and effects of chronic ethanol intake in the micropig. *Alcohol Clin Exp Res* 2001; 25:415–20.

38. Qiu A, Min SH, Jansen M, Malhotra U, Tsai E, Cabelof DC, Matherly LH, Zhao R, Akabas MH, Goldman ID. Rodent intestinal folate transporters (SLC46A1): Secondary structure, functional properties, and response to dietary folate restriction. *Am J Physiol Cell Physiol* 2007; 293:C1669–78.

39. Qiu A, Jansen M, Sakaris A, Min SH, Chattopadhyay S, Tsai E, Sandoval C, Zhao R, Akabas MH, Goldman ID. Identification of an intestinal folate transporter and the molecular basis for hereditary folate malabsorption. *Cell* 2006; 127:917–28.

40. Steinberg SE, Campbell CL, Hillman RS. Kinetics of the normal folate enterohepatic cycle. *J Clin Invest* 1979; 64:83–88.

41. Herbert V. Experimental nutritional folate deficiency in man. *Trans Assoc Am Physicians* 1962; 75:307–20.

42. Tamura T, Romero JJ, Watson JE, Gong EJ, Halsted CH. Hepatic folate metabolism in the chronic alcoholic monkey. *J Lab Clin Med* 1981; 97:654–61.
43. Hillman RS, McGuffin R, Campbell C. Alcohol interference with the folate enterohepatic cycle. *Trans Assoc Am Physicians* 1977; 90:145–56.
44. Horne DW. Na+ and pH dependence of 5-methyltetrahydrofolic acid and methotrexate transport in freshly isolated hepatocytes. *Biochim Biophys Acta* 1990; 1023:47–55.
45. Zhao R, Hanscom M, Goldman ID. The relationship between folate transport activity at low pH and reduced folate carrier function in human Huh7 hepatoma cells. *Biochim Biophys Acta* 2005; 1715:57–64.
46. Russell RM, Rosenberg IH, Wilson PD, Iber FL, Oaks EB, Giovetti AC, Otradovec CL, Karwoski PA, Press AW. Increased urinary excretion and prolonged turnover time of folic acid during ethanol ingestion. *Am J Clin Nutr* 1983; 38:64–70.
47. McMartin KE, Collins TD, Eisenga BH, Fortney T, Bates WR, Bairnsfather L. Effects of chronic ethanol and diet treatment on urinary folate excretion and development of folate deficiency in the rat. *J Nutr* 1989; 119:1490–97.
48. Tamura T, Halsted CH. Folate turnover in chronically alcoholic monkeys. *J Lab Clin Med* 1983; 101:623–28.
49. Romanoff RL, Ross DM, McMartin KE. Acute ethanol exposure inhibits renal folate transport, but repeated exposure upregulates folate transport proteins in rats and human cells. *J Nutr* 2007; 137:1260–65.
50. Ross DM, McMartin KE. Effect of ethanol on folate binding by isolated rat renal brush border membranes. *Alcohol* 1996; 13:449–54.
51. Sullivan LW, Herbert V. Suppression of hematopoiesis by ethanol. *J Clin Invest* 1964; 43:2048–62.
52. Eichner ER, Hillman RS. Effect of alcohol on serum folate level. *J Clin Invest* 1973; 52:584–91.
53. Shaw S, Jayatilleke E, Herbert V, Colman N. Cleavage of folates during ethanol metabolism. Role of acetaldehyde/xanthine oxidase-generated superoxide. *Biochem J* 1989; 257:277–80.
54. Kelly D, Reed B, Weir D, Scott J. Effect of acute and chronic alcohol ingestion on the rate of folate catabolism and hepatic enzyme induction in mice. *Clin Sci (Lond)* 1981; 60:221–24.
55. Mato JM CF, Pajares MA. S-adenosylmethionine and the liver. In: Arias IM, Fausto N, Jacoby WB, Schachter DA, Shafritz DA, eds., *The Liver: Biology and Pathobiology*, 3rd ed. New York: Raven Press, 1994:461–70.
56. Marchesini G, Bugianesi E, Bianchi G, Fabbri A, Marchi E, Zoli M, Pisi E. Defective methionine metabolism in cirrhosis: Relation to severity of liver disease. *Hepatology* 1992; 16:149–55.
57. Russmann S, Junker E, Lauterburg BH. Remethylation and transsulfuration of methionine in cirrhosis: Studies with L-[H3-methyl-1-C]methionine. *Hepatology* 2002; 36:1190–96.
58. Avila MA, Berasain C, Torres L, Martin-Duce A, Corrales FJ, Yang H, Prieto J, et al. Reduced mRNA abundance of the main enzymes involved in methionine metabolism in human liver cirrhosis and hepatocellular carcinoma. *J Hepatol* 2000; 33:907–14.
59. Cabrero C, Duce AM, Ortiz P, Alemany S, Mato JM. Specific loss of the high-molecular-weight form of S-adenosyl-L- methionine synthetase in human liver cirrhosis. *Hepatology* 1988; 8:1530–34.
60. Duce AM, Ortíz P, Cabrero C, Mato JM. S-Adenosyl-L-methionine synthetase and phospholipid methyltransferase are inhibited in human cirrhosis. *Hepatology* 1988; 8:65–68.
61. Lee TD, Sadda MR, Mendler MH, Bottiglieri T, Kanel G, Mato JM, Lu SC. Abnormal hepatic methionine and glutathione metabolism in patients with alcoholic hepatitis. *Alcohol Clin Exp Res* 2004; 28:173–81.

62. Villanueva JA, Halsted CH. Hepatic transmethylation reactions in micropigs with alcoholic liver disease. *Hepatology* 2004; 39:1303–10.

63. Look MP, Riezler R, Reichel C, Brensing KA, Rockstroh JK, Stabler SP, Spengler U, Berthold HK, Sauerbruch T. Is the increase in serum cystathionine levels in patients with liver cirrhosis a consequence of impaired homocysteine transsulfuration at the level of gamma-cystathionase? *Scand J Gastroenterol* 2000; 35:866–72.

64. Vendemiale G, Altomare E, Trizio T, Le Grazie C, Di Padova C, Salerno MT, Carrieri V, Albano O. Effects of oral S-adenosyl-L-methionine on hepatic glutathione in patients with liver disease. *Scand J Gastroenterol* 1989; 24:407–15.

65. Mato JM, Camara J, Fernandez de Paz J, Caballeria L, Coll S, Caballero A, Garcia-Buey L, et al. S-Adenosylmethionine in alcoholic liver cirrhosis: A randomized, placebo-controlled, double-blind, multicenter clinical trial. *J Hepatol* 1999; 30:1081–89.

66. Day CP. Pathogenesis of steatohepatitis. *Best Pract Res Clin Gastroenterol* 2002; 16:663–78.

67. Tilg H, Diehl AM. Mechanisms of disease: Cytokines in alcoholic and nonalcoholic steatohepatitis. *N Engl J Med* 2000; 343:1467–76.

68. Arteel GE. Oxidants and antioxidants in alcohol-induced liver disease. *Gastroenterology* 2003; 124:778–90.

69. Ji C, Kaplowitz N. Hyperhomocysteins, ER stress and alcoholic liver injury. *World J Gastroenterol* 2004; 10:1699–708.

70. You M, Crabb DW. Recent advances in alcoholic liver disease. II. Minireview: Molecular mechanisms of alcoholic fatty liver. *Am J Physiol Gastrointest Liver Physiol* 2004; 287:G1–6.

71. Kaplowitz N, Ji C. Unfolding new mechanisms of alcoholic liver disease in the endoplasmic reticulum. *J Gastroenterol Hepatol* 2006; 21(Suppl 3):S7–9.

72. Barak AJ, Beckenhauer HC, Tuma DJ, Badakhsh S. Effects of prolonged ethanol feeding on methionine metabolism in rat liver. *Biochem Cell Biol* 1987; 65:230–33.

73. Trimble KC, Molloy AM, Scott JM, Weir DG. The effect of ethanol on one-carbon metabolism: Increased methionine catabolism and lipotrope methyl-group wastage. *Hepatology* 1993; 18:984–89.

74. Lieber CS, Casini A, DeCarli LM, Kim CI, Lowe N, Sasaki R, Leo MA. S-Adenosyl-L-methionine attenuates alcohol-induced liver injury in the baboon. *Hepatology* 1990; 11:165–72.

75. Lu SC, Huang ZZ, Yang H, Mato JM, Avila MA, Tsukamoto H. Changes in methionine adenosyltransferase and S-adenosylmethionine homeostasis in alcoholic rat liver. *Am J Physiol Gastrointest Liver Physiol* 2000; 279:G178–85.

76. Avila MA, Mingorance J, Martinez-Chantar ML, Casado M, Martin-Sanz P, Bosca L, Mato JM. Regulation of rat liver S-adenosylmethionine synthetase during septic shock: Role of nitric oxide. *Hepatology* 1997; 25:391–96.

77. Kharbanda KK, Rogers DD 2nd, Mailliard ME, Siford GL, Barak AJ, Beckenhauer IIC, Sorrell MF, Tuma DJ. Role of elevated S-adenosylhomocysteine in rat hepatocyte apoptosis: Protection by betaine. *Biochem Pharmacol* 2005; 70:1883–90.

78. Kharbanda KK, Mailliard ME, Baldwin CR, Beckenhauer HC, Sorrell MF, Tuma DJ. Betaine attenuates alcoholic steatosis by restoring phosphatidylcholine generation via the phosphatidylethanolamine methyltransferase pathway. *J Hepatol* 2007; 46:314–21.

79. Song Z, Zhou Z, Uriarte S, Wang L, Kang YJ, Chen T, Barve S, McClain CJ. S-Adenosylhomocysteine sensitizes to TNF-alpha hepatotoxicity in mice and liver cells: A possible etiological factor in alcoholic liver disease. *Hepatology* 2004; 40:989–97.

80. Song Z, Zhou Z, Song M, Uriarte S, Chen T, Deaciuc I, McClain CJ. Alcohol-induced S-adenosylhomocysteine accumulation in the liver sensitizes to TNF hepatotoxicity: Possible involvement of mitochondrial S-adenosylmethionine transport. *Biochem Pharmacol* 2007; 74:521–31.

81. Lu SC, Alvarez L, Huang ZZ, Chen L, An W, Corrales FJ, Avila MA, Kanel G, Mato JM. Methionine adenosyltransferase 1A knockout mice are predisposed to liver injury and exhibit increased expression of genes involved in proliferation. *Proc Natl Acad Sci USA* 2001; 98:5560–65.

82. Ji C, Chan C, Kaplowitz N. Predominant role of SREBP lipogenic pathways in hepatic steatosis in the murine intragastric ethanol feeding model. *J Hepatol* 2006; 45: 717–24.

83. Ji C, Kaplowitz N. Betaine decreases hyperhomocysteinemia, endoplasmic reticulum stress, and liver injury in alcohol-fed mice. *Gastroenterology* 2003; 124:1488–99.

84. Halsted CH, Villanueva J, Chandler CJ, Ruebner B, Munn RJ, Parkkila S, Niemela O. Centrilobular distribution of acetaldehyde and collagen in the ethanol-fed micropig. *Hepatology* 1993; 18:954–60.

85. Halsted CH, Villanueva J, Chandler CJ, Stabler SP, Allen RH, Muskhelishvili L, James SJ, Poirier L. Ethanol feeding of micropigs alters methionine metabolism and increases hepatocellular apoptosis and proliferation. *Hepatology* 1996; 23:497–505.

86. Halsted CH, Villanueva JA, Devlin AM, Niemela O, Parkkila S, Garrow TA, Wallock LM, Shigenaga MK, Melnyk S, James SJ. Folate deficiency disturbs hepatic methionine metabolism and promotes liver injury in the ethanol-fed micropig. *Proc Natl Acad Sci USA* 2002; 99:10072–77.

87. Esfandiari F, Villanueva JA, Wong DH, French SW, Halsted CH. Chronic ethanol feeding and folate deficiency activate hepatic endoplasmic reticulum stress pathway in micropigs. *Am J Physiol Gastrointest Liver Physiol* 2005; 289:G54–63.

88. Esfandiari F, You M, Villanueva JA, Wong DH, French SW, Halsted CH. S-Adenosylmethionine attenuates hepatic lipid synthesis in micropigs fed ethanol with a folate-deficient diet. *Alcohol Clin Exp Res* 2007; 31:1231–39.

89. Villanueva JA, Esfandiari F, White ME, Devaraj S, French SW, Halsted CH. S-Adenosylmethionine attenuates oxidative liver injury in micropigs fed ethanol with a folate-deficient diet. *Alcohol Clin Exp Res* 2007; 31:1934–43.

90. Yi P, Melnyk S, Pogribna M, Pogribny IP, Hine RJ, James SJ. Increase in plasma homocysteine associated with parallel increases in plasma S-adenosylhomocysteine and lymphocyte DNA hypomethylation. *J Biol Chem* 2000; 275:29318–23.

91. Clarke S, Banfield, K. S-Adenosylmethionine-dependent methyltransferases. In: Carmel R, Jacobsen D, eds., *Homocysteine in Health and Disease.* Cambridge, UK: Cambridge University Press, 2001:63–68.

92. Ghoshal K, Li X, Datta J, Bai S, Pogribny I, Pogribny M, Huang Y, Young D, Jacob ST. A folate- and methyl-deficient diet alters the expression of DNA methyltransferases and methyl CpG binding proteins involved in epigenetic gene silencing in livers of F344 rats. *J Nutr* 2006; 136:1522–27.

93. Esfandiari F, Green R, Cotterman RF, Pogribny IP, James SJ, Miller JW. Methyl deficiency causes reduction of the methyl-CpG-binding protein, MeCP2, in rat liver. *Carcinogenesis* 2003; 24:1935–40.

94. Kouzarides T. Chromatin modifications and their function. *Cell* 2007; 128:693–705.

95. Bernstein BE, Meissner A, Lander ES. The mammalian epigenome. *Cell* 2007; 128:669–81.

96. Vakoc CR, Sachdeva MM, Wang H, Blobel GA. Profile of histone lysine methylation across transcribed mammalian chromatin. *Mol Cell Biol* 2006; 26:9185–95.

97. Wu J, Wang SH, Potter D, Liu JC, Smith LT, Wu YZ, Huang TH, Plass C. Diverse histone modifications on histone 3 lysine 9 and their relation to DNA methylation in specifying gene silencing. *BMC Genomics* 2007; 8:131.

98. Barski A, Cuddapah S, Cui K, Roh TY, Schones DE, Wang Z, Wei G, Chepelev I, Zhao K. High-resolution profiling of histone methylations in the human genome. *Cell* 2007; 129:823–37.

99. Hake SB, Xiao A, Allis CD. Linking the epigenetic "language" of covalent histone modifications to cancer. *Br J Cancer* 2004; 90:761–69.
100. Mahadev K, Vemuri MC. Ethanol-induced changes in hepatic chromatin and nonhistone nuclear protein composition in the rat. *Alcohol* 1998; 15:207–11.
101. Pal-Bhadra M, Bhadra U, Jackson DE, Mamatha L, Park PH, Shukla SD. Distinct methylation patterns in histone H3 at Lys-4 and Lys-9 correlate with up- & down-regulation of genes by ethanol in hepatocytes. *Life Sci* 2007; 81:979–87.
102. Kim JS, Shukla SD. Acute in vivo effect of ethanol (binge drinking) on histone H3 modifications in rat tissues. *Alcohol Alcohol* 2006; 41:126–32.
103. Bardag-Gorce F, French BA, Joyce M, Baires M, Montgomery RO, Li J, French S. Histone acetyltransferase p300 modulates gene expression in an epigenetic manner at high blood alcohol levels. *Exp Mol Pathol* 2007; 82:197–202.

18 Folate and Choline Interrelationships

Metabolic and Potential Health Implications

Marie A. Caudill

CONTENTS

I. INTRODUCTION

The nutritional importance of choline was recognized in 1932 by Charles Best, codiscoverer of the hormone insulin. In a series of elegant experiments, Best et al. [1–3] demonstrated the essential role of choline in the prevention of fatty liver in rodents and depancreatized dogs. A decade later, Schaefer et al. [4] provided evidence of the metabolic intermingling of choline and folate by demonstrating that folate had a choline-sparing effect in rats and chicks. The term *lipotropic* was subsequently coined to describe dietary agents such as choline and folate that prevented or reduced accumulation of fat in liver [5,6]. More recently, the possible use of choline as a homocysteine (Hcy)-lowering agent [7,8] and the establishment of a dietary recommendation [9] have stimulated immense interest in choline, its interplay with folate, and its role in disease prevention. The objectives of this chapter are to provide an overview of the metabolism, function, and essentiality of choline; describe the interrelationship between folate and choline; and consider the potential health implications of this reciprocal relationship.

II. CHOLINE CHEMISTRY, METABOLISM, AND FUNCTION

Choline, a methyl-rich quaternary amine with the chemical formula $(CH_3)_3N^+CH_2CH_2OH$, functions as a precursor for several important compounds: the phospholipids phosphatidylcholine (the primary phospholipid of all classes of lipoproteins in mammals) and sphingomyelin; the cholinergic neurotransmitter acetylcholine; and the methyl group donor and osmolyte betaine (Figure 18.1). In addition, critical cellular signaling molecules (i.e., platelet-activating factor, diacylglycerol, ceramide, and sphingosine) are derived from the catabolism of choline phospholipids. As such, choline and its metabolites are important for the structural integrity and signaling functions of cells, the transport and metabolism of lipids, the transmission of nerve impulses, and the remethylation of Hcy to methionine [10].

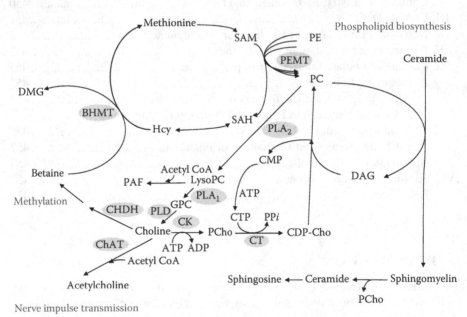

FIGURE 18.1 Choline metabolism. Relevant enzymes are highlighted in gray. ADP, adenine diphosphate; ATP, adenine triphosphate; BHMT, betaine homocysteine methyltransferase; CDP-Cho, cytidine diphosphate – choline; ChAT, choline acetyltransferase; CHDH, choline dehydrogenase; CK, choline kinase; CMP, cytidine monophosphate; CT, cytidylyl transferase; CTP, cytidine triphosphate; DAG, diacylglycerol; DMG, dimethylglycine; GPC, glycerophosphocholine; Hcy, homocysteine; PAF, platelet-activating factor; PC, phosphatidylcholine; PCho, phosphocholine; PE, phosphatidylethanolamine; PEMT, phosphatidylethanolamine methyltransferase; PL, phospholipase; PPi, inorganic pyrophosphate; SAM, *S*-adenosylmethionine; SAH, *S*-adenosylhomocysteine.

In mammalian cells, choline metabolism to phosphatidylcholine occurs in the cytidine diphosphate (CDP)-choline pathway in which cytidylyl transferase serves as the rate-limiting and regulating enzyme [11]. In a subsequent reaction, phosphatidylcholine may be used for the biosynthesis of sphingomyelin. Otherwise, choline may be converted to acetylcholine by choline acetyltransferase or oxidized to betaine in a two-step reaction catalyzed by choline dehydrogenase, the rate-limiting enzyme, and betaine aldehyde dehydrogenase. The biologically labile methyl groups of betaine may be used for the remethylation of Hcy to methionine in a reaction catalyzed by betaine Hcy N-methyltransferase, an enzyme found primarily in liver and kidney [12]. Alternatively, this reaction may be carried out by methionine synthase (MS), a ubiquitously expressed enzyme that requires cobalamin (i.e., methylcobalamin) as the coenzyme and 5-methyltetrahydrofolate (5-methyl-THF) as the source of labile methyl groups. Methionine may then be activated to S-adenosylmethionine (SAM), and the folate (or betaine)-derived methyl group may be used for the provision of carbons for more than 50 additional transmethylation reactions.

An auxiliary pathway enabling de novo biosynthesis of phosphatidylcholine exists in liver and a few other tissues [13]. Phosphatidylethanolamine N-methyltransferase (PEMT) catalyzes the sequential transfer of three methyl groups from SAM to phosphatidylethanolamine to generate phosphatidylcholine and S-adenosylhomocysteine (SAH). It is estimated that about 30% of phosphatidylcholine is synthesized via the PEMT pathway, with the remaining 70% coming from the CDP-choline pathway [14]. These pathways are exquisitely regulated to ensure that phosphatidylcholine homeostasis is maintained [15]. As a major consumer of methyl groups, PEMT is also a major producer of Hcy [16–18]. In this regard, PEMT deficiency is associated with a 50% reduction in plasma Hcy concentrations in mice [16].

Although the PEMT pathway has traditionally been viewed as a back-up pathway for the CDP-choline pathway and is most active when dietary choline intake is low [19], heterogeneity in the fatty acid profiles of the phosphatidylcholine molecule derived from the PEMT versus the CDP-choline pathway suggests that the two pathways have distinct physiological roles. Phosphatidylcholine molecules produced from the PEMT pathway are composed of long-chain polyunsaturated fatty acids (PUFA), whereas phosphatidylcholine derived from the CDP-choline pathway is composed mainly of medium-chain, saturated fatty acids [20]. Studies performed in *pemt*-deficient mice suggest that the PEMT pathway is critical for the mobilization of docosahexaenoic acid (DHA; 22:6(n-3)) and arachidonic acid (20:4(n-6)) into plasma with subsequent usage by peripheral tissues [21].

III. CHOLINE DEFICIENCY

In addition to humans, several different mammals require an exogenous source of choline, including the guinea pig, rat, hamster, swine, chicken, dog, and rhesus monkey. The major phenotype of choline deficiency is the accumulation of lipid in the liver and hepatic steatosis. In healthy male volunteers consuming a semisynthetic diet devoid of choline for 3 weeks, plasma choline and phosphatidylcholine concentrations decreased by about 30%, serum cholesterol decreased by 15%, and serum alanine aminotransferase increased; no such changes occurred in the control group [22]. These findings were corroborated in a subsequent study involving patients receiving parenteral nutrition. In this regard, hepatic steatosis resolved completely in all patients who received choline and in none of the patients who did not receive choline [23].

The fatty liver and hepatic steatosis are likely caused by inadequate phosphatidylcholine synthesis required for the secretion of very-low-density lipoproteins (VLDLs) from liver and the subsequent export of triglycerides [24]. However, gender differences have been described. Specifically, in *Pemt*-deficient mice, VLDL secretion was inhibited in male but not female mice [25]. In addition, female mice showed a marked 40% decrease in plasma phosphatidylcholine and cholesterol in high-density lipoproteins; reductions of 19% to 25% were observed in the males [25]. Choline insufficiency also results in a decreased phosphatidylcholine/phosphatidylethanolamine ratio in hepatic plasma lipid bilayers, a change that adversely affects membrane integrity and results in liver damage [26].

IV. NUTRITIONAL IMPORTANCE OF CHOLINE DURING PREGNANCY

The importance of choline in fetal development is suggested by the observations that the fetus receives a large supply of choline during gestation [27]; maternal plasma choline concentrations are elevated throughout the later portion of pregnancy [28,29]; pregnancy causes depletion of hepatic choline pools in rats consuming a normal diet [30,31]; and the human neonate is born with blood levels that are at least three times higher than maternal blood concentrations [29]. During pregnancy, choline is actively taken up by placental tissue against a concentration gradient [32], with the majority of placental choline transfer to the developing fetus occurring throughout the third trimester. The heavy reliance on maternal stores of choline for fetal development is supported by the apparent absence/insignificant quantities of PEMT activity in placental tissue and fetal liver [32–34]. Hence the observed increase in serum choline concentrations in pregnant women may reflect a mechanism for ensuring an adequate supply of choline to the fetus. Importantly, giving supplemental choline to pregnant rats protects them from depleting their choline reserves, increases phosphocholine concentrations in the fetus, and decreases apoptotic cell death in fetal brain [35,36].

The developing brain, particularly basal forebrain cholinergic neurons and their projection systems, the hippocampus and the frontal cortex, appears to be especially sensitive to choline availability based on the results of rodent studies [37]. Variation in maternal choline intake produces life-long effects on memory and attentional function of the offspring, functions that are subserved by the hippocampus and frontal cortex, respectively. Notably, supplementing the maternal diet with excess choline (approximately three times higher than normal dietary intake) produces lasting improvements in these cognitive functions in young animals and reduces cognitive decline during aging [38–43]. Although the mechanisms underlying these effects are poorly understood, choline availability appears to be required for the structural development of the hippocampus and may modulate the activities of enzymes involved in acetylcholine metabolism in offspring [37,44–46]. Taken together, these studies suggest that choline plays a critical role in fetal development and that pregnancy represents a time of markedly increased maternal choline requirements.

V. DIETARY RECOMMENDATIONS FOR CHOLINE

In 1998, the Institute of Medicine established the first choline dietary intake recommendations, 425 and 550 mg/day for women and men, respectively, based on the estimated level of choline intake required to prevent liver damage [9]. For pregnant women, the adequate intake was increased to 450 mg/day; the 25-mg/day increase during pregnancy was based on fetal and placental accumulation of choline derived primarily from studies conducted in animal models. The highest level of daily choline intake that was estimated to pose no adverse health effects (i.e., hypotension, fishy body odor), referred to as the Tolerable Upper Intake Level, is 3,500 mg/day.

In food (both plant and animal products), choline exists as free choline (small amounts) or as derivatives of choline, including phosphatidylcholine (most abundant), phosphocholine, sphingomyelin, and glycerophosphocholine [47]. Eggs, liver, organ/muscle meats, wheat germ, legumes, and cauliflower are good sources of food choline [48]. Betaine is also found in food, but in contrast to the compounds mentioned above, it cannot be converted back to choline and thus is not included in the "total" choline content estimate of one's diet. Nevertheless, existing data suggest that although betaine cannot serve as a substitute for choline, it may spare choline for phospholipid synthesis, thereby decreasing choline requirements as was recently shown in an animal model [49]. Wheat bran, shrimp, spinach, wheat bread, and pretzels are good sources of betaine [48]. Habitual choline intake ranges from about 100 to 850 mg/day [50] with an estimated mean intake of about 300 mg/day [8,50–55].

VI. CHOLINE AND FOLATE INTERRELATIONSHIP

A. METABOLIC IMPLICATIONS

It is likely that the dietary requirement for choline is affected by folate and possibly the intake of other methyl donors. The interrelationship between choline and folate arises from the participation of these nutrients in one-carbon metabolism (Figure 18.2). In liver and kidney tissue, either folate or betaine may serve as methyl donors for the conversion of Hcy to methionine. Thus, deficiency of one nutrient may increase the demand for the other. Further, hepatic biosynthesis of phosphatidylcholine through the PEMT pathway is a major consumer of one-carbon units [18,56]. Thus, 5-methyl-THF, as a primary source of methyl groups for PEMT, is integral to de novo biosynthesis of choline. Finally, the catabolism of choline provides one-carbon units that ultimately feed into folate-mediated one-carbon metabolism as formate [57,58]. However, the quantitative significance of the choline oxidation pathway to one-carbon metabolism is uncertain.

1. Folate Intake and Biomarkers of Choline Status

The choline-sparing effect and the lipotropic properties of folate depend on its possession of biologically labile methyl groups that may be used for the biosynthesis

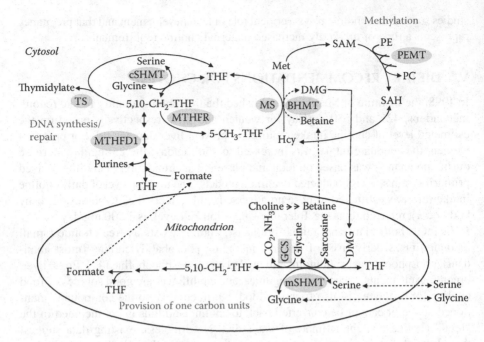

FIGURE 18.2 The interrelationship of choline and folate arises from the participation of both nutrients in one-carbon metabolism. In this regard, (1) betaine is an alternative source of methyl groups for the remethylation of homocysteine to methionine; (2) the labile methyl groups of dimethylglycine (DMG) enter cytosolic folate-mediated one-carbon metabolism as formate; and (3) the hepatic biosynthesis of phosphatidylcholine from phosphatidyleth-anolamine is a major consumer of folate derived one-carbon moieties. Relevant enzymes are highlighted in gray. BHMT, betaine homocysteine methyltransferase; cSHMT, cystolic serine hydroxyl methyltransferase; DMG, dimethylglycine; GCS, glycine cleavage system, Hcy, homocysteine; MTHFD1, 5,10-methylenetetrahydrofolate dehydrogenase, mSHMT, mitochondrial serine hydroxyl methyltransferase; MTHFR, 5,10-methylenetetrahydrofolate reductase; MS, methionine synthetase; PC, phosphatidylcholine; PE, phosphatidyletha-nolamine; PEMT, phosphatidylethanolamine methyltransferase; SAM, S-adenosylmethionine; SAH, S-adenosylhomocysteine THF, tetrahydrofolate; TS, thymidylate synthetase.

of choline (i.e., phosphatidylcholine) through the PEMT pathway. Evidence of interplay between folate and choline was demonstrated by showing perturbed choline metabolism, as assessed by abnormalities in hepatic betaine concentrations, in rats following the administration of the folate antagonist methotrexate [59]. Subsequent work showed that rats made severely folate deficient had 65% to 80% lower hepatic choline and phosphocholine concentrations than did folate-adequate controls; moderately folate-deficient rats had a 36% ($P < .09$) reduction in hepatic choline [60]. Investigations with healthy male [61] and female [62–64] study participants have also demonstrated an effect of folate intake on biomarkers of choline status. In premenopausal Mexican American (MA) women consuming a constant intake of choline (i.e., 349 mg/day), plasma phosphatidylcholine decreased in response to folate restriction (i.e., 135 μg of dietary folate equivalents [DFE]/day) and increased

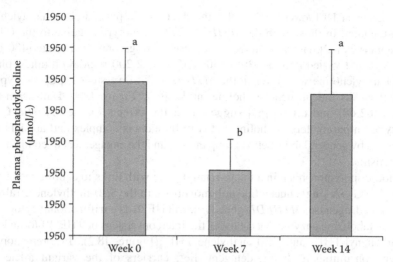

FIGURE 18.3 Plasma phosphatidylcholine (mean ± SEM) at baseline (week 0), after 7 weeks of folate restriction with 135 μg/day as dietary folate equivalents (DFE; week 7), and after 7 weeks of folate treatment with 800 μg of DFE/day (week 14). Throughout the 14-week study, choline intake remained constant at 349 mg/day. Identical letters indicate no significant difference ($P > .05$). (Adapted from Abratte CM, Wang W, Li R, Moriarty DJ, Caudill MA, *J Nutr Biochem* 2008; 19:158–65.)

in response to folate treatment with 800 μg of DFE/day [62] (Figure 18.3). These findings are consistent with the important role of folate in providing labile methyl groups required for de novo biosynthesis of phosphatidylcholine through the PEMT pathway.

2. Genetic Variation in Folate-Metabolizing Enzymes and Biomarkers of Choline Status

Effects of genetic variation in folate-metabolizing enzymes on biomarkers of choline status have also been demonstrated. In liver tissue from methylenetetrahydrofolate reductase (*MTHFR*) knockout mice, betaine, phosphocholine, and glycerophosphocholine were lowest in the nullizygotes, intermediate in heterozygotes, and highest in wild-type mice; no significant effects of genotype were detected on choline or phosphatidylcholine [65]. Like folate deficiency, impaired MTHFR activity may disturb de novo choline synthesis by decreasing the availability of methyl groups and/ or by increasing the demand for betaine as a methyl donor. In humans, the *MTHFR* 677C→T genetic variant is associated with reduced enzyme activity [66], decreased serum folate (i.e., 5-methyl-THF) and increased plasma total Hcy concentrations, particularly under conditions of suboptimal folate intake [67]. To date, several controlled feeding studies [62,63,68] and one large epidemiological study [69] have assessed the relationship between the *MTHFR* C677T genotype and biomarkers of choline status. The controlled feeding studies demonstrated an effect of the *MTHFR* C677T genotype on plasma concentrations of phosphatidylcholine with evidence for gender differences. In premenopausal MA women consuming a folate-restricted diet (135 μg of DFE/day) for 7 weeks, the decrease in plasma phosphatidylcholine was attenuated in those with the *MTHFR* 677TT genotype relative to the CT and CC genotypes [62]. However, in MA men consuming controlled folate (400 μg of DFE/day) and varied choline (300, 550, 1,100, or 2,200 mg/day) intakes, plasma phosphatidylcholine was lower in the *MTHFR* 677TT versus 677CC genotype, an effect that was independent of choline intake [68] (Figure 18.4). Data from these studies [62,68] and others [63] suggest that the effects of the *MTHFR* C677T genotype on parameters of choline status in humans is complex and appears to be influenced by gender, labile methyl group intake, and the engagement of compensatory mechanisms.

Another polymorphism in a folate-related gene with links to choline metabolism is the 1958G→A single nucleotide polymorphism in the 5,10-methylenetetrahydrofolate dehydrogenase (*MTHFD1*) gene [70]. MTHFD1 is a trifunctional cytoplasmic folate-metabolizing enzyme that catalyzes the interconversions of THF, 10-formyl-THF, 5,10-methenyl-THF, and 5,10-methylene-THF (Figure 18.2). In premenopausal women consuming a choline-deficient diet, carriers of the variant allele were 15 times more likely than noncarriers to develop choline deficiency [70]. MTHFD1 deficiency may reduce the pool of 5,10-methylene-THF and 5-methyl-THF, which in turn may lead to decreased availability of methyl groups for phosphatidylcholine biosynthesis through PEMT and to increased choline demand for Hcy remethylation. The biological feasibility of this hypothesis is supported by recent findings in MA women showing a greater increase ($P = .086$) in plasma total Hcy after a 7-week period of folate restriction in the *MTHFD1* 1958AA genotype relative to the 1958GA and 1958GG genotypes [71].

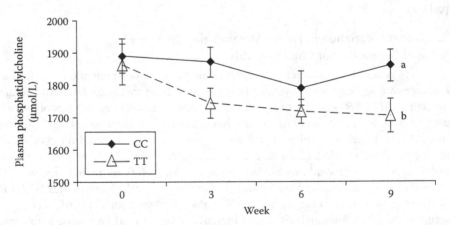

FIGURE 18.4 Plasma phosphatidylcholine (mean ± SEM) in Mexican American men differing in methylenetetrahydrofolate reductase (*MTHFR*) C677T genotype in response to controlled choline and folate intakes. Throughout the study, men with the *MTHFR* 677TT genotype had lower concentrations ($P < .05$) relative to those with the 677CC genotype regardless of choline intake as indicated by the different letters. (Adapted from Veenema K, Solis C, Li R, Wang W, Maletz CV, Abratte CF, Caudill MA, *Am J Clin Nutr* 2008; 88:685–92.)

3. Choline Intake and Biomarkers of Folate Status

Effects of choline intake on biomarkers of folate status (and one-carbon metabolism) have also been demonstrated. In rodents, short-term (≤ 3 weeks) choline deficiency resulted in decreased hepatic folate content, decreased tissue concentrations of SAM, decreased global DNA methylation, and/or increased Hcy concentrations [72–76]. These alterations may arise from increased utilization of folate as a methyl donor, reduced hepatic betaine and impaired betaine-dependent methionine synthesis, and/ or increased endogenous production of phosphatidylcholine through the PEMT pathway. In chronically (12 months) choline-deficient rats, hepatic total folate concentration was not altered; however, polyglutamation was elevated possibly because of increased conservation of the folate coenzymes [77].

In humans with severe metabolic disturbances in cystathionine-β-synthase or remethylation defects resulting from MS or MTHFR deficiencies, pharmacological doses of betaine lowered plasma total Hcy by varying degrees [78–82]. In healthy human volunteers with mildly elevated plasma Hcy concentrations, daily supplementation with betaine (1.5, 3, and 6 g) for 6 weeks resulted in fasting plasma total Hcy concentrations that were 12%, 15%, and 20% less ($P < .01$) than in the placebo group, respectively [83]. Further, supplementation with phosphatidylcholine (34 g containing 2.6 g of choline) for 2 weeks reduced fasting plasma Hcy concentrations by 18% [7]. However, in a 12-week controlled feeding study involving healthy MA men with decreased folate stores, choline intakes ranging from 300 to 2,200 mg/day were ineffective in attenuating the increase in fasting plasma total Hcy, particularly in those with the *MTHFR* 677TT genotype [84].

Data derived from tracer studies using [U-^{13}C$_5$]methionine and [3-^{13}C$_5$]serine suggest that serine (rather than betaine) is the major source of methyl groups for total body Hcy remethylation in a nonsupplemented, unchallenged state [85]. In this regard, serine was calculated to contribute about 100% of the methyl groups used for total-body Hcy remethylation [85]. However, the importance of betaine/choline as a source of one-carbon moieties appears to increase under conditions of enhanced Hcy production. Specifically, supplementation with choline-related supplements (i.e., betaine, phosphatidylcholine, or choline) for at least 2 weeks suppressed the increase in plasma total Hcy following the administration of a methionine load by 23% to 40% [7,68,83]. Further, clinically choline-depleted men had post–methionine load plasma Hcy concentrations that were 35% greater than those in men not choline depleted [74].

Additional conditions in which methyl groups derived from choline may be particularly important for one-carbon metabolism include cystic fibrosis [86–88] and pregnancy [29,30,89]. In children with cystic fibrosis, supplementation with betaine, choline, or phosphatidylcholine improved abnormal concentrations of plasma methionine, SAM, SAH, and the SAM/SAH ratio [87]. In pregnancy, betaine (rather than folate) was the strongest predictor of plasma Hcy throughout the second half of gestation, suggesting that conserving methionine via a folate-independent route may be beneficial [89].

Only a few studies have examined the effect of supplemental choline on blood folate concentrations in humans. Steenge et al. [90] administered betaine (6 g/day) for 6 weeks to 36 men and women and reported no effect on serum folate comprised primarily of

5-methyl-THF. Similarly, administration of choline at intake levels ranging from 300 to 2,200 mg/day for 12 weeks had no main effect on serum folate or RBC folate [68], although 2,200 mg/day appeared to mitigate the decrease in serum folate.

B. POTENTIAL HEALTH IMPLICATIONS

Suboptimal folate status is linked to a number of developmental and chronic diseases, including cardiovascular disease, certain cancers, cognitive impairment, pregnancy complications, and birth anomalies, including neural tube defects (NTDs) [91–94]. The mechanism by which folate modulates disease risk is not clearly defined but likely involves aberrations in methylation reactions, both globally and locally, with ramifications on gene expression, and/or impairments in nucleotide synthesis with effects on DNA repair and integrity [92,94]. Like folate, these events may also be modified by choline. For example, in cultured human neuroblastoma cells and in rodent models, choline deficiency altered both global and gene-specific DNA methylation and the expression of these genes [95,96]. In human lymphocytes, choline deficiency increased DNA damage [97] and influenced lymphocyte gene expression [98].

Not surprisingly, overlaps between choline and certain folate-related diseases/conditions and vice versa have been identified. Recent work suggests that suboptimal maternal choline intake may have adverse effects on fetal development. Shaw et al. [99] reported an increased risk of NTDs in infants of mothers who had lower intakes of dietary choline relative to those with higher intakes. Data from animal models support this relationship: Inhibition of choline uptake and metabolism during murine neurulation resulted in growth retardation and developmental defects, including an increase in the prevalence of NTDs in mouse embryos [100]. Further, genetic polymorphisms in choline-metabolizing genes are associated with altered risk of spina bifida in human newborns [101]. However, there are examples of an apparent divergence between choline and folate-related diseases. In US women enrolled in the Nurses' Health Study, higher choline intake was associated with an increased risk of colorectal adenoma [55]. A potential explanation for this unexpected finding may reside in the critical role of choline in carcinogenesis. Specifically, once a tumor is initiated, growth into a detectable tumor depends in part on choline availability because choline is required for membrane biosynthesis [55]. Similar analogies have been raised regarding the possible tumor-promoting role of folic acid [102,103].

An interesting metabolic link between choline, folate, and DHA has also emerged. In liver, the conversion of phosphatidylethanolamine to phosphatidylcholine via the PEMT pathway is critical for DHA mobilization from the liver into plasma. When this reaction does not occur normally, as seen in *pemt* knockout mice, plasma concentrations of DHA are decreased [21]. Folate intake also appears to modulate PEMT activity and thus may affect DHA mobilization from liver to plasma. In this regard, Durand et al. [104] reported that folate deficiency in rats resulted in a marked decrease in long chain (n-3) fatty acids; Umhau et al. [105] reported a significant positive relationship between RBC folate and plasma DHA ($r = 0.57$; $P = .005$) in men with aggressive and hostile traits, and Krauss-Etschmann et al. [106] reported that folic acid supplementation from gestation week 22 until delivery improves fetal n-3 long-chain PUFA status and attenuates depletion of maternal stores. Finally, Selley et al. [107] reported an inverse relationship between plasma Hcy and DHA composition of erythrocyte phosphatidylcholine concentrations in 26 patients with Alzheimer's disease. However, in a randomized clinical trial involving 253 healthy men aged 65 years, daily supplementation with 1,000 μg of folic acid, 500 μg of vitamin B12, and 10 mg of vitamin B6 had no effect on the proportion of n-3 long-chain PUFA (including DHA) in plasma phosphatidylcholine [108]. A possible explanation for the seemingly discrepant findings may lie in the folate status of the subjects. That is, supplementation with folic acid may only benefit individuals whose PEMT activity is compromised as a result of folate insufficiency. In this regard, pregnancy and alcoholism (as observed in the hostile men study) are associated with increased requirements of folate and are populations that are more likely to have an inadequate folate intake/status.

VII. SUMMARY AND CONCLUSIONS

The interplay between folate and choline was recognized more than 50 years ago when the choline-sparing effect of folate was noted in animal models of fatty liver. The metabolic intermingling of choline and folate arises from their participation in one-carbon metabolism. Suboptimal folate intake/status results in aberrations in choline metabolism likely caused by decreased phosphatidylcholine biosynthesis through the PEMT pathway. Similarly, choline deficiency adversely influences biomarkers of one-carbon metabolism, particularly after a methionine load and in certain physiological states. Because of the interrelationship between folate and choline, it may be prudent to consider both nutrients in studies aimed at elucidating their roles in human health.

REFERENCES

1. Best CH, Hershey JM. Further observations on the effects of some component of crude lecithine on depancreatized animals. *J Physiol* 1932; 75:49–55.
2. Best CH, Hershey JM, Huntsman ME. The effect of lecithine on fat deposition in the liver of the normal rat. *J Physiol* 1932; 75:56–66.
3. Best CH, Huntsman ME. The effects of the components of lecithine upon deposition of fat in the liver. *J Physiol* 1932; 75:405–12.
4. Schaefer AE, Salmon WD, Strength DR, Copeland DH. Interrelationship of folacin, vitamin B12 and choline; Effect on hemorrhagic kidney syndrome in the rat and on growth of the chick. *J Nutr* 1950; 40:95–111.
5. Best CH, Lucas CC, Ridout JH. The lipotropic factors. *Ann N Y Acad Sci* 1954; 57:646–53.
6. Kelley B, Totter JR, Day PL. The lipotropic effect of folic acid on rats receiving various purified diets. *J Biol Chem* 1950; 187:529–35.
7. Olthof MR, Brink EJ, Katan MB, Verhoef P. Choline supplemented as phosphatidylcholine decreases fasting and postmethionine-loading plasma homocysteine concentrations in healthy men. *Am J Clin Nutr* 2005; 82:111–17.
8. Chiuve SE, Giovannucci EL, Hankinson SE, Zeisel SH, Dougherty LW, Willett WC, Rimm EB. The association between betaine and choline intakes and the plasma concentrations of homocysteine in women. *Am J Clin Nutr* 2007; 86:1073–81.

9. Institute of Medicine. National Academy of Sciences USA. *Dietary Reference Intakes for Thiamin, Riboflavin, Niacin, Vitamin B6, Folate, Vitamin B12, Pantothenic Acid, Biotin, and Choline.* Washington, DC: National Academy Press, 1998.

10. Zeisel SH. Dietary choline: Biochemistry, physiology, and pharmacology. *Annu Rev Nutr* 1981; 1:95–121.

11. Kent C. Regulatory enzymes of phosphatidylcholine biosynthesis: A personal perspective. *Biochim Biophys Acta* 2005; 1733:53–66.

12. Sunden SLF, Renduchintala MS, Park EI, Miklasz SD, Garrow TA. Betaine-homocysteine methyltransferase expression in porcine and human tissues and chromosomal localization of the human gene. *Arch Biochem Biophys* 1997; 345:171–74.

13. Vance DE, Ridgway ND. The methylation of phosphatidylethanolamine. *Prog Lipid Res* 1988; 27:61–79.

14. Reo NV, Adinehzadeh M, Foy BD. Kinetic analyses of liver phosphatidylcholine and phosphatidylethanolamine biosynthesis using (13)C NMR spectroscopy. *Biochim Biophys Acta* 2002; 1580:171–88.

15. Kulinski A, Vance DE, Vance JE. A choline-deficient diet in mice inhibits neither the CDP-choline pathway for phosphatidylcholine synthesis in hepatocytes nor apolipoprotein B secretion. *J Biol Chem* 2004; 279:23916–24.

16. Noga AA, Stead LM, Zhao Y, Brosnan ME, Brosnan JT, Vance DE. Plasma homocysteine is regulated by phospholipid methylation. *J Biol Chem* 2003; 278:5952–55.

17. Jacobs RL, Stead LM, Devlin C, Tabas I, Brosnan ME, Brosnan JT, Vance DE. Physiological regulation of phospholipid methylation alters plasma homocysteine in mice. *J Biol Chem* 2005; 280:28299–305.

18. Stead LM, Brosnan JT, Brosnan ME, Vance DE, Jacobs RL. Is it time to reevaluate methyl balance in humans? *Am J Clin Nutr* 2006; 83:5–10.

19. Walkey CJ, Yu L, Agellon LB, Vance DE. Biochemical and evolutionary significance of phospholipid methylation. *J Biol Chem* 1998; 273:27043–46.

20. DeLong CJ, Shen YJ, Thomas MJ, Cui Z. Molecular distinction of phosphatidylcholine synthesis between the CDP-choline pathway and phosphatidylethanolamine methylation pathway. *J Biol Chem* 1999; 274:29683–88.

21. Watkins SM, Zhu X, Zeisel SH. Phosphatidylethanolamine-N-methyltransferase activity and dietary choline regulate liver-plasma lipid flux and essential fatty acid metabolism in mice. *J Nutr* 2003; 133:3386–91.

22. Zeisel SH, Da Costa KA, Franklin PD, Alexander EA, Lamont JT, Sheard NF, Beiser A. Choline, an essential nutrient for humans. *FASEB J* 1991; 5:2093–98.

23. Buchman AL, Ament ME, Sohel M, Dubin M, Jenden DJ, Roch M, Pownall H, Farley W, Awal M, Ahn C. Choline deficiency causes reversible hepatic abnormalities in patients receiving parenteral nutrition: Proof of a human choline requirement: A placebo-controlled trial. *J Parenter Enteral Nutr* 2001; 25:260–68.

24. Yao ZM, Vance DE. The active synthesis of phosphatidylcholine is required for very low density lipoprotein secretion from rat hepatocytes. *J Biol Chem* 1988; 263:2998–3004.

25. Noga AA, Vance DE. A gender-specific role for phosphatidylethanolamine N-methyltransferase-derived phosphatidylcholine in the regulation of plasma high density and very low density lipoproteins in mice. *J Biol Chem* 2003; 278:21851–59.

26. Li Z, Agellon LB, Allen TM, Umeda M, Jewell L, Mason A, Vance DE. The ratio of phosphatidylcholine to phosphatidylethanolamine influences membrane integrity and steatohepatitis. *Cell Metab* 2006; 3:321–31.

27. Zeisel SH. Choline: Critical role during fetal development and dietary requirements in adults. *Annu Rev Nutr* 2006; 26:229–50.

28. Ilcol YO, Uncu G, Ulus IH. Free and phospholipid-bound choline concentrations in serum during pregnancy, after delivery and in newborns. *Arch Physiol Biochem* 2002; 110:393–400.

29. Molloy AM, Mills JL, Cox C, Daly SF, Conley M, Brody LC, Kirke PN, Scott JM, Ueland PM. Choline and homocysteine interrelations in umbilical cord and maternal plasma at delivery. *Am J Clin Nutr* 2005; 82:836–42.
30. Zeisel SH, Mar MH, Zhou Z, da Costa KA. Pregnancy and lactation are associated with diminished concentrations of choline and its metabolites in rat liver. *J Nutr* 1995; 125:3049–54.
31. Gwee MC, Sim MK. Free choline concentration and cephalin-N-methyltransferase activity in the maternal and foetal liver and placenta of pregnant rats. *Clin Exp Pharmacol Physiol* 1978; 5:649–53.
32. Gwee MC, Sim MK. Changes in the concentration of free choline and cephalin-N-methyltransferase activity of the rat material and foetal liver and placenta during gestation and of the maternal and neonatal liver in the early postpartum period. *Clin Exp Pharmacol Physiol* 1979; 6:259–65.
33. Welsch F, Wenger WC, Stedman DB. Choline metabolism in placenta: Evidence for the biosynthesis of phosphatidylcholine in microsomes via the methylation pathway. *Placenta* 1981; 2:211–21.
34. Sweiry JH, Yudilevich DL. Characterization of choline transport at maternal and fetal interfaces of the perfused guinea-pig placenta. *J Physiol* 1985; 366:251–66.
35. Garner SC, Mar MH, Zeisel SH. Choline distribution and metabolism in pregnant rats and fetuses are influenced by the choline content of the maternal diet. *J Nutr* 1995; 125:2851–58.
36. Albright CD, Tsai AY, Friedrich CB, Mar MH, Zeisel SH. Choline availability alters embryonic development of the hippocampus and septum in the rat. *Brain Res Dev Brain Res* 1999; 113:13–20.
37. Meck WH, Williams CL. Metabolic imprinting of choline by its availability during gestation: Implications for memory and attentional processing across the lifespan. *Neurosci Biobehav Rev* 2003; 27:385–99.
38. McCann JC, Hudes M, Ames BN. An overview of evidence for a causal relationship between dietary availability of choline during development and cognitive function in offspring. *Neurosci Biobehav Rev* 2006; 30:696–712.
39. Meck WH, Smith RA, Williams CL. Pre- and postnatal choline supplementation produces long-term facilitation of spatial memory. *Dev Psychobiol* 1988; 21:339–53.
40. Meck WH, Williams CL. Characterization of the facilitative effects of perinatal choline supplementation on timing and temporal memory. *Neuroreport* 1997; 8:2831–35.
41. Meck WH, Williams CL. Perinatal choline supplementation increases the threshold for chunking in spatial memory. *Neuroreport* 1997; 8:3053–59.
42. Meck WH, Williams CL. Simultaneous temporal processing is sensitive to prenatal choline availability in mature and aged rats. *Neuroreport* 1997; 8:3045–51.
43. Tees RC, Mohammadi E. The effects of neonatal choline dietary supplementation on adult spatial and configural learning and memory in rats. *Dev Psychobiol* 1999; 35:226–40.
44. Cermak JM, Holler T, Jackson DA, Blusztajn JK. Prenatal availability of choline modifies development of the hippocampal cholinergic system. *FASEB J* 1998; 12:349–57.
45. Mellott TJ, Follettie MT, Diesl V, Hill AA, Lopez-Coviella I, Blusztajn JK. Prenatal choline availability modulates hippocampal and cerebral cortical gene expression. *FASEB J* 2007; 21:1311–23.
46. Sanders LM, Zeisel SH. Choline: Dietary requirements and role in brain development. *Nutr Today* 2007; 42:181–86.
47. Koc H, Mar MH, Ranasinghe A, Swenberg JA, Zeisel SH. Quantitation of choline and its metabolites in tissues and foods by liquid chromatography/electrospray ionization-isotope dilution mass spectrometry. *Anal Chem* 2002; 74:4734–40.
48. Zeisel SH, Mar MH, Howe JC, Holden JM. Concentrations of choline-containing compounds and betaine in common foods. *J Nutr* 2003; 133:1302–07.

49. Dilger RN, Garrow TA, Baker DH. Betaine can partially spare choline in chicks but only when added to diets containing a minimal level of choline. *J Nutr* 2007; 137:2224–28.

50. Detopoulou P, Panagiotakos DB, Antonopoulou S, Pitsavos C, Stefanadis C. Dietary choline and betaine intakes in relation to concentrations of inflammatory markers in healthy adults: The ATTICA study. *Am J Clin Nutr* 2008; 87:424–30.

51. Cho E, Zeisel SH, Jacques P, Selhub J, Dougherty L, Colditz GA, Willett WC. Dietary choline and betaine assessed by food-frequency questionnaire in relation to plasma total homocysteine concentration in the Framingham Offspring Study. *Am J Clin Nutr* 2006; 83:905–11.

52. Dalmeijer GW, Olthof MR, Verhoef P, Bots ML, van der Schouw YT. Prospective study on dietary intakes of folate, betaine, and choline and cardiovascular disease risk in women. *Eur J Clin Nutr* 2008; 62:386–94.

53. Bidulescu A, Chambless LE, Siega-Riz AM, Zeisel SH, Heiss G. Usual choline and betaine dietary intake and incident coronary heart disease: The Atherosclerosis Risk in Communities (ARIC) study. *BMC Cardiovasc Disord* 2007; 7:20.

54. Cho E, Holmes M, Hankinson SE, Willett WC. Nutrients involved in one-carbon metabolism and risk of breast cancer among premenopausal women. *Cancer Epidemiol Biomarkers Prev* 2007; 16:2787–90.

55. Cho E, Willett WC, Colditz GA, Fuchs CS, Wu K, Chan AT, Zeisel SH, Giovannucci EL. Dietary choline and betaine and the risk of distal colorectal adenoma in women. *J Natl Cancer Inst* 2007; 99:1224–31.

56. Mudd SH, Brosnan JT, Brosnan ME, Jacobs RL, Stabler SP, Allen RH, Vance DE, Wagner C. Methyl balance and transmethylation fluxes in humans. *Am J Clin Nutr* 2007; 85:19–25.

57. Cook R. Folate metabolism. In: Carmel R, Jacobsen DW, eds., *Homocysteine in Health and Disease.* New York: Cambridge University Press, 2001:113–34.

58. Gregory JF 3rd, Cuskelly GJ, Shane B, Toth JP, Baumgartner TG, Stacpoole PW. Primed, constant infusion with [2H3]serine allows in vivo kinetic measurement of serine turnover, homocysteine remethylation, and transsulfuration processes in human one-carbon metabolism. *Am J Clin Nutr* 2000; 72:1535–41.

59. Barak AJ, Kemmy RJ. Methotrexate effects on hepatic betaine levels in choline-supplemented and choline-deficient rats. *Drug Nutr Interact* 1982; 1:275–78.

60. Kim YI, Miller JW, da Costa KA, Nadeau M, Smith D, Selhub J, Zeisel SH, Mason JB. Severe folate deficiency causes secondary depletion of choline and phosphocholine in rat liver. *J Nutr* 1994; 124:2197–203.

61. Jacob RA, Jenden DJ, Allman-Farinelli MA, Swendseid ME. Folate nutriture alters choline status of women and men fed low choline diets. *J Nutr* 1999; 129:712–17.

62. Abratte CM, Wang W, Li R, Moriarty DJ, Caudill MA. Folate intake and the MTHFR C677T genotype influence choline status in young Mexican American women. *J Nutr Biochem* 2008; 19:158–65.

63. Abratte CM, Wang W, Li R, Axume J, Moriarty DJ, Caudill MA. Choline status is not a reliable indicator of moderate changes in dietary choline consumption in premenopausal women. *J Nutr Biochem* 2009; 20:62–69.

64. Hung J, Abratte CM, Wang W, Li R, Moriarty DJ, Caudill MA. Ethnicity and folate intake influence choline status in young women consuming controlled nutrient intakes. *J Am Coll Nutr* 2008; 27:253–59.

65. Schwahn BC, Chen Z, Laryea MD, Wendel U, Lussier-Cacan S, Genest J Jr, Mar MH, et al. Homocysteine-betaine interactions in a murine model of 5,10-methylenetetrahydrofolate reductase deficiency. *FASEB J* 2003; 17:512–14.

66. Frosst P, Blom HJ, Milos R, Goyette P, Sheppard CA, Matthews RG, Boers GJ, den Heijer M, Kluijtmans LA, Rozen R. A candidate genetic risk factor for vascular disease: A common mutation in methylenetetrahydrofolate reductase. *Nat Genet* 1995; 10:111–13.

67. Guinotte CL, Burns MG, Axume JA, Hata H, Urrutia TF, Alamilla A, McCabe D, Singgih A, Cogger EA, Caudill MA. Methylenetetrahydrofolate reductase 677C→T variant modulates folate status response to controlled folate intakes in young women. *J Nutr* 2003; 133:1272–80.
68. Veenema K, Solis C, Li R, Wang W, Maletz CV, Abratte CF, Caudill MA. Choline intakes at AI levels are sufficient in preventing elevations in serum markers of liver dysfunction but are not optimal in minimizing plasma total homocysteine increases after a methionine load. *Am J Clin Nutr* 2008; 88:685–92.
69. Holm PI, Hustad S, Ueland PM, Vollset SE, Grotmol T, Schneede J. Modulation of the homocysteine-betaine relationship by methylenetetrahydrofolate reductase 677 C→T genotypes and B-vitamin status in a large-scale epidemiological study. *J Clin Endocrinol Metab* 2007; 92:1535–41.
70. Kohlmeier M, da Costa KA, Fischer LM, Zeisel SH. Genetic variation of folate-mediated one-carbon transfer pathway predicts susceptibility to choline deficiency in humans. *Proc Natl Acad Sci USA* 2005; 102:16025–30.
71. Ivanov AA, Nash-Barboza S, Hinkis S, Caudill MA. Genetic variants in phosphatidyle-thanolamine N-methyltransferase (PEMT) and methylenetetrahydrofolate dehydrogenase (MTHFD1) influence biomarkers of choline metabolism when folate intake is restricted. *J Am Diet Assoc* 2009; 139:727–33.
72. Selhub J, Seyoum E, Pomfret EA, Zeisel SH. Effects of choline deficiency and methotrex-ate treatment upon liver folate content and distribution. *Cancer Res* 1991; 51:16–21.
73. Varela-Moreiras G, Ragel C, Perez de Miguelsanz J. Choline deficiency and methotrexate treatment induces marked but reversible changes in hepatic folate concentrations, serum homocysteine and DNA methylation rates in rats. *J Am Coll Nutr* 1995; 14:480–85.
74. da Costa KA, Gaffney CE, Fischer LM, Zeisel SH. Choline deficiency in mice and humans is associated with increased plasma homocysteine concentration after a methionine load. *Am J Clin Nutr* 2005; 81:440–44.
75. Svardal AM, Ueland PM, Berge RK, Aarsland A, Aarsaether N, Lonning PE, Refsum H. Effect of methotrexate on homocysteine and other sulfur compounds in tissues of rats fed a normal or a defined, choline-deficient diet. *Cancer Chemother Pharmacol* 1988; 21:313–18.
76. Pomfret EA, daCosta KA, Zeisel SH. Effects of choline deficiency and methotrexate treatment upon rat liver. *J Nutr Biochem* 1990; 1:533–41.
77. Varela-Moreiras G, Selhub J, daCosta K-A, Zeisel SH. Effect of chronic choline defi-ciency in rats on liver folate content and distribution. *J Nutr Biochem* 1992; 3:519–22.
78. Wilcken DE, Wilcken B, Dudman NP, Tyrrell PA. Homocystinuria—The effects of betaine in the treatment of patients not responsive to pyridoxine. *N Engl J Med* 1983; 309:448–53.
79. Wendel U, Bremer HJ. Betaine in the treatment of homocystinuria due to 5,10-methyl-enetetrahydrofolate reductase deficiency. *Eur J Pediatr* 1984; 142:147–50.
80. Holme E, Kjellman B, Ronge E. Betaine for treatment of homocystinuria caused by methylenetetrahydrofolate reductase deficiency. *Arch Dis Child* 1989; 64:1061–64.
81. Kishi T, Kawamura I, Harada Y, Eguchi T, Sakura N, Ueda K, Narisawa K, Rosenblatt DS. Effect of betaine on S-adenosylmethionine levels in the cerebrospinal fluid in a patient with methylenetetrahydrofolate reductase deficiency and peripheral neuropathy. *J Inherit Metab Dis* 1994; 17:560–65.
82. Singh RH, Kruger WD, Wang L, Pasquali M, Elsas LJ 2nd. Cystathionine beta-synthase deficiency: Effects of betaine supplementation after methionine restriction in B6-nonresponsive homocystinuria. *Genet Med* 2004; 6:90–95.
83. Olthof MR, van Vliet T, Boelsma E, Verhoef P. Low dose betaine supplementation leads to immediate and long term lowering of plasma homocysteine in healthy men and women. *J Nutr* 2003; 133:4135–38.

84. Solis C, Veenema K, Ivanov AA, Tran S, Li R, Wang W, Moriarty DJ, Maletz CV, Caudill MA. Folate intake at RDA levels is inadequate for Mexican American men with the methylenetetrahydrofolate reductase 677TT genotype. *J Nutr* 2008; 138:67–72.

85. Davis SR, Stacpoole PW, Williamson J, Kick LS, Quinlivan EP, Coats BS, Shane B, Bailey LB, Gregory JF 3rd. Tracer-derived total and folate-dependent homocysteine remethylation and synthesis rates in humans indicate that serine is the main one-carbon donor. *Am J Physiol Endocrinol Metab* 2004; 286:E272–79.

86. Innis SM, Davidson AG, Chen A, Dyer R, Melnyk S, James SJ. Increased plasma homocysteine and S-adenosylhomocysteine and decreased methionine is associated with altered phosphatidylcholine and phosphatidylethanolamine in cystic fibrosis. *J Pediatr* 2003; 143:351–56.

87. Innis SM, Davidson AG, Melynk S, James SJ. Choline-related supplements improve abnormal plasma methionine-homocysteine metabolites and glutathione status in children with cystic fibrosis. *Am J Clin Nutr* 2007; 85:702–08.

88. Innis SM, Hasman D. Evidence of choline depletion and reduced betaine and dimethylglycine with increased homocysteine in plasma of children with cystic fibrosis. *J Nutr* 2006; 136:2226–31.

89. Velzing-Aarts FV, Holm PI, Fokkema MR, van der Dijs FP, Ueland PM, Muskiet FA. Plasma choline and betaine and their relation to plasma homocysteine in normal pregnancy. *Am J Clin Nutr* 2005; 81:1383–89.

90. Steenge GR, Verhoef P, Katan MB. Betaine supplementation lowers plasma homocysteine in healthy men and women. *J Nutr* 2003; 133:1291–95.

91. Vollset SE, Refsum H, Irgens LM, Emblem BM, Tverdal A, Gjessing HK, Monsen AL, Ueland PM. Plasma total homocysteine, pregnancy complications, and adverse pregnancy outcomes: The Hordaland Homocysteine study. *Am J Clin Nutr* 2000; 71:962–68.

92. Caudill M. The role of folate in reducing chronic and developmental disease risk: An overview. *J Food Sci* 2004; 69:SNQ55–60.

93. Miller JW. Folate, cognition, and depression in the era of folic acid fortification. *J Food Sci* 2004; 69:SNQ61–67.

94. McCabe DC, Caudill MA. DNA methylation, genomic silencing, and links to nutrition and cancer. *Nutr Rev* 2005; 63:183–95.

95. Niculescu MD, Yamamuro Y, Zeisel SH. Choline availability modulates human neuroblastoma cell proliferation and alters the methylation of the promoter region of the cyclin-dependent kinase inhibitor 3 gene. *J Neurochem* 2004; 89:1252–59.

96. Niculescu MD, Craciunescu CN, Zeisel SH. Dietary choline deficiency alters global and gene-specific DNA methylation in the developing hippocampus of mouse fetal brains. *FASEB J* 2006; 20:43–49.

97. da Costa KA, Niculescu MD, Craciunescu CN, Fischer LM, Zeisel SH. Choline deficiency increases lymphocyte apoptosis and DNA damage in humans. *Am J Clin Nutr* 2006; 84:88–94.

98. Niculescu MD, da Costa KA, Fischer LM, Zeisel SH. Lymphocyte gene expression in subjects fed a low-choline diet differs between those who develop organ dysfunction and those who do not. *Am J Clin Nutr* 2007; 86:230–39.

99. Shaw GM, Carmichael SL, Yang W, Selvin S, Schaffer DM. Periconceptional dietary intake of choline and betaine and neural tube defects in offspring. *Am J Epidemiol* 2004; 160:102–09.

100. Fisher MC, Zeisel SH, Mar MH, Sadler TW. Inhibitors of choline uptake and metabolism cause developmental abnormalities in neurulating mouse embryos. *Teratology* 2001; 64:114–22.

101. Enaw JO, Zhu H, Yang W, Lu W, Shaw GM, Lammer EJ, Finnell RH. CHKA and PCYT1A gene polymorphisms, choline intake and spina bifida risk in a California population. *BMC Med* 2006; 4:36.

102. Ulrich CM, Potter JD. Folate supplementation: Too much of a good thing? *Cancer Epidemiol Biomarkers Prev* 2006; 15:189–93.
103. Kim YI. Folate: A magic bullet or a double edged sword for colorectal cancer prevention? *Gut* 2006; 55:1387–89.
104. Durand P, Prost M, Blache D. Pro-thrombotic effects of a folic acid deficient diet in rat platelets and macrophages related to elevated homocysteine and decreased n-3 polyunsaturated fatty acids. *Atherosclerosis* 1996; 121:231–43.
105. Umhau JC, Dauphinais KM, Patel SH, Nahrwold DA, Hibbeln JR, Rawlings RR, George DT. The relationship between folate and docosahexaenoic acid in men. *Eur J Clin Nutr* 2006; 60:352–57.
106. Krauss-Etschmann S, Shadid R, Campoy C, Hoster E, Demmelmair H, Jimenez M, Gil A, et al. Effects of fish-oil and folate supplementation of pregnant women on maternal and fetal plasma concentrations of docosahexaenoic acid and eicosapentaenoic acid: A European randomized multicenter trial. *Am J Clin Nutr* 2007; 85:1392–400.
107. Selley ML. A metabolic link between S-adenosylhomocysteine and polyunsaturated fatty acid metabolism in Alzheimer's disease. *Neurobiol Aging* 2007; 28:1834–39.
108. Crowe FL, Skeaff CM, McMahon JA, Williams SM, Green TJ. Lowering plasma homocysteine concentrations of older men and women with folate, vitamin B-12, and vitamin B-6 does not affect the proportion of (n-3) long chain polyunsaturated fatty acids in plasma phosphatidylcholine. *J Nutr* 2008; 138:551–55.

19 Folate

Recommended Intakes, Consumption, and Status

Gail P. A. Kauwell, Megan L. Diaz,
Quanhe Yang, and Lynn B. Bailey

CONTENTS

I. INTRODUCTION

Intake recommendations are targeted to provide adequate folate to support critical metabolic functions. A brief overview of the approaches used to establish the Dietary Reference Intakes (DRIs) for folate for different life-stage groups in the United States and Canada is presented in this chapter, along with specific intake recommendations established by the Institute of Medicine (IOM), Food and Agriculture Organization (FAO)/World Health Organization (WHO), and countries in various parts of the world. Although there is considerable overlap in the DRI standards worldwide, there are distinct differences, including the fact that not all countries express folate intake recommendations as dietary folate equivalents (DFEs).

Suboptimal folate status was identified as a public health concern as a result of reports generated from the 1976 through 1980 and 1988 through 1994 National Health and Nutrition Examination Surveys (NHANES) [1]. It was, however, the findings of randomized controlled trials showing that periconceptional intake of folic acid reduced neural tube defect (NTD) risk [2,3] that provided the impetus for mandating folic acid fortification of enriched cereal grain products in the United States [4] and issuing the recommendation that all women of child-bearing age consume 400 μg of folic acid every day [5,6]. The effectiveness of folic acid fortification in improving the folate status of all life-stage groups in the United States and reducing the prevalence of low blood folate concentrations is evident from comparisons of NHANES data collected before and after folic acid fortification [1,7]. This chapter summarizes these findings, along with the impact on folate status of exposure to an increasing number of sources of folic acid.

Estimation of the worldwide prevalence of folate deficiency is a research challenge with major public health implications. Although the evidence available suggests that folate deficiency is prevalent worldwide, the extent of the problem is yet to be determined because of limitations of existing data as highlighted in this chapter.

II. DIETARY FOLATE SOURCES

A. NATURALLY OCCURRING FOOD FOLATE

A relatively small number of foods are concentrated sources of naturally occurring folate (i.e., food folate), including dark green vegetables, orange juice, legumes, nuts, and seeds (Table 19.1). Meat is not a nutrient-dense source of folate, except for liver. Substantial losses of this vitamin can occur during the cooking process as a result of the combination of thermal degradation and leaching into the cooking water [8,9].

B. FOLIC ACID IN FORTIFIED FOODS

Folic acid is added to food in the United States as a result of two Food and Drug Administration (FDA) regulations: (1) mandatory fortification of enriched cereal grain products through a standards of identity regulation at 1.4 mg/kg flour or cereal grain product [4], and (2) optional fortification of ready-to-eat (RTE) products such as breakfast cereals with up to 400 μg of folic acid/serving through a food additive regulation [10].

The mandatory folic acid fortification of enriched cereal grain products beginning in the late 1990s in the United States and Canada has increased the folate content of staple foods such as bread, rice, and pasta, as well as thousands of mixed food items (Table 19.1) [4,11]. In addition to enriched cereal grain products, fortified RTE cereals are another important dietary source of folic acid with the majority of products providing 100 μg/serving and many contributing an amount comparable to the dosage found in supplements (i.e., 400 μg/serving) (Table 19.1). Folic acid is also

TABLE 19.1
Folate/Folic Acid Content of Selected Foods[a,b,c,d,e]

Foods (weight; average serving size)	Folic Acid	Food Folate	DFE
	μg/average serving		
I. Excellent Folate Sources (≥ 80 μg DFE/average serving)			
A. Meat			
Beef, liver, braised (85 g; 3 oz)	0	215	215
B. Legumes			
Pinto beans, cooked, boiled (86 g; 1/2 cup)	0	147	147
Black beans, cooked, boiled (86 g; 1/2 cup)	0	128	128
C. Vegetables			
Asparagus, cooked, boiled (90 g; 1/2 cup)	0	134	134
Spinach, cooked, boiled (90 g; 1/2 cup)	0	131	131
D. Fruit			
Orange juice, frozen concentrated diluted w/3 volumes of water (249 g; 1 cup)	0	110	110
E. Ready-To-Eat Cereals (RTE)			
Selected RTE Cereals Fortified with 100% of Daily Value Folic Acid (400 μg)			
Cap'N Crunch, Quaker (27 g; 3/4 cup)	415	4	710
Whole Grain TOTAL, General Mills (30 g; 3/4 cup)	394	6	676
Special K, Kellogg (31 g; 1 cup)	394	6	676
Selected RTE Cereals Fortified with ≥ 25% of Daily Value Folic Acid (100 μg)			
Cheerios, General Mills (30 g; 1 cup)	287	6	493
Post Raisin Bran, Kraft (56 g; 1 cup)	180	11	317
Rice Krispies, Kellogg (28 g; 1 cup)	150	1	256
F. Enriched Cereal Grain Products and Bakery and Snack Products Made with Enriched Flour			
Egg noodles, cooked, enriched (160 g; 1 cup)	123	11	221
Macaroni, cooked, enriched (140 g; 1 cup)	92	10	167
Rice, white, long-grain, regular, cooked, enriched (158 g;1 cup)	87	5	153
Bagel, plain, enriched (57 g; 3" diameter)	66	17	129
White bread, commercial prep (60 g; 2 slices)	52	15	103
Pretzels, hard, enriched (28 g; 1 oz)	40	12	81

continued

TABLE 19.1 (continued)
Folate/Folic Acid Content of Selected Foods[a,b,c,d,e]

Foods (weight; average serving size)	Folic Acid	Food Folate	DFE
	μg/average serving		
II. Good Folate Sources (40–79 μg DFE/average serving)			
A. Fruit			
Oranges, raw, navels (140 g; 2-7/8" diameter)	0	48	48
B. Vegetables			
Lettuce, romaine (47 g; 1 cup shredded)	0	64	64
Spinach, raw (30 g; 1 cup)	0	58	58
Broccoli, flowerets, raw (71 g; 1 cup)	0	50	50
Peas, green, frozen, cooked, boiled (80 g; 1 cup)	0	47	47
C. Nuts and Seeds			
Sunflower seed kernels, dry roasted (28 g; 1 oz)	0	67	67
Peanuts, dry roasted (28 g; 1 oz)	0	41	41
D. Bakery and Snack Products Made with Enriched Flour			
Flour tortilla (46 g; 1 tortilla-7–8")	42	6	77
Rolls, hamburger or hotdog, plain (43 g; 1 whole roll)	36	12	73
Pancake, buttermilk (114 g; 3 pancakes, 4" diameter)	28	15	64
Saltine crackers (30 g; 10 crackers)	32	9	64
Biscuit, plain or buttermilk (51 g; 1 medium)	32	4	58
III. Moderate Folate Sources (20–39 μg DFE/average serving)			
A. Vegetables			
Potato, baked, flesh and skin (138 g; 1 small)	0	39	39
Corn, yellow, sweet, canned (82 g; 1/2 cup)	0	35	35
Broccoli, frozen, spears, cooked, boiled (92 g; 1/2 cup)	0	28	28
Beans, snap, green, canned (78 g; 1/2 cup)	0	25	25
French fries, frozen, oven heated (67 g; 5 steak fries)	0	21	21
Lettuce, iceberg (72 g; 1 cup shredded)	0	21	21
B. Fruit			
Strawberries, raw (144 g; 1 cup whole)	0	35	35
Cantaloupe, raw (160 g; 1 cup of cubes)	0	34	34
Bananas, raw (136 g; 1 large-8–8-7/8" long)	0	27	27
C. Nuts and Seeds			
Walnuts, English (28 g; 1 oz)	0	28	28
Peanut butter (32 g; 2 tbsp)	0	24	24
D. Seafood			
Salmon, Atlantic, cooked (85 g; 3 oz)	0	25	25
E. Eggs and Dairy			
Egg, whole, fried (46 g; 1 large)	0	23	23
Yogurt, nonfat, fruit variety (245 g; 1 cup)	0	22	22
F. Bakery Products Made with Enriched Flour			
Whole-wheat bread, commercial prep (56 g; 2 slices)	0	28	28

TABLE 19.1 (continued)
Folate/Folic Acid Content of Selected Foods[a,b,c,d,e]

Foods (weight; average serving size)	Folic Acid	Food Folate	DFE
	μg/average serving		
G. Snacks			
Potato chips (28 g; 1 oz)	0	21	21
IV. Fair–Poor Folate Sources (<20 μg DFE/average serving)			
A. Fruit			
Apples, raw, with skin (149 g; 1 small, 2-3/4" diameter)	0	4	4
Grapes, European type, red or green (151 g; 1 cup)	0	3	3
B. Vegetables			
Carrots, raw (91.5 g; 1/2 cup strips or slices)	0	17	17
Tomatoes, red, raw (91 g; 1 small whole, 2–2/5" diameter)	0	14	14
C. Dairy			
Milk, low-fat 1%, fluid (244 g; 1 cup)	0	12	12
Cheddar cheese (28 g; 1 oz)	0	5	5
Ice cream, vanilla (66 g; 1/2 cup)	0	3	3
D. Meat and Seafood			
Beef, ground, 85% lean, cooked (85 g; 3 oz)	0	8	8
Chicken, dark meat only, roasted (85 g; 3 oz)	0	7	7
Beef, porterhouse steak, cooked (85 g; 3 oz)	0	6	6
Pork, loin, chop, cooked (85 g; 3 oz)	0	3	3
Tuna, light, canned (58 g; 2 oz)	0	2	2

[a] Foods sorted within each category from highest to lowest folate/folic acid content.

[b] Daily Values (DVs) are a set of reference values, including the reference daily intake (RDI), on food labels used to compare the amount of a nutrient in a serving of food with the amount recommended for daily consumption. The RDI for folate is 400 μg.

[c] Foods listed in this table are classified as excellent or good sources of folate using the definitions established by the FDA for nutrient content claims on food labels. Foods classified as an "excellent source of folate" must contain 20% or more of the folate DV (≥80 μg DFE/serving); foods classified as "good source of folate" must contain 10% to 19% of the DV for folate (40–79 μg DFE/serving). The FDA nutrient content claims do not include specific definitions for foods that do not qualify as excellent or good sources. To assist in classifying key foods based on folate content, "moderate" and "fair-poor" folate sources have been defined in this table as 5% to 9% of the folate DV (20–39 μg DFE/serving) and less than 5% of DV for folate (<20 μg DFE/serving), respectively. Source: Center for Food Safety and Applied Nutrition Food and Drug Administration—Office of Nutritional Products Labeling and Dietary Supplements [homepage on the Internet]. *A Food Labeling Guide.* Available at http://www.cfsan.fda. gov/~dms/2lg-toc.html; accessed June 16, 2008.

[d] Government Printing Office [homepage on the Internet]. *Electronic Code of Federal Regulations— Reference Amounts Customarily Consumed per Eating Occasion: General Food Supply. Title 21-Food and Drugs Part 101-Food Labeling Subpart A-General Provisions Section 101-12,* Available at http:// ecfr.gpoaccess.gov/cgi/t/text/text- idx?c=ecfr;sid=1e06c5b0786822ff75468318ccdd506b;rgn=div8;vie w=text;node=21%3A2.0.1.1.2.1.1.8;idno=21;cc=ecfr; accessed July 1, 2008.

[e] *USDA National Nutrient Database for Standard Reference, Release 21, 2008* [online database]. US Department of Agriculture and Agricultural Research Service. Beltsville, MD, Available at Nutrient Data Laboratory Home Page, http://www.ars.usda.gov/ba/bhnrc/ndl; accessed September 29, 2008.

an ingredient in meal replacement foods, infant formulas, and an ever-increasing number of snack food items such as "nutrient bars."

Folic acid was selected as the form of the vitamin used for food fortification because of its excellent stability characteristics [12,13]. The retention of folic acid in vitamin-mineral premixes used for food fortification and in RTE cereals has been examined with evidence of little or no loss during storage for up to 6 months [14,15], and folic acid stability during baking of bread products has been reported to be high [14–16].

III. DIETARY REFERENCE INTAKE STANDARDS

A. INSTITUTE OF MEDICINE: NATIONAL ACADEMY OF SCIENCES

The IOM established the DRIs, which include a series of reference values for folate intake, including the Estimated Average Requirement (EAR), Recommended Dietary Allowance (RDA), Adequate Intake (AI), and the Tolerable Upper Intake Level (UL) [6]. The EAR is defined as the median usual intake of folate needed to meet the requirements of 50% of the population. The RDA is estimated from the EAR by correcting for population variance and represents the average daily dietary intake level sufficient to meet the nutrient requirement of approximately 98% of the population (Table 19.2). The AI, defined as the quantity of folate consumed by a group with no evidence of folate inadequacy, was estimated when there were insufficient data on which to derive an EAR (Table 19.2). The UL pertains specifically to folic acid (rather than food folate) and is characterized as the maximum daily *usual* intake at which no risk of adverse health effects would be expected when consumed over long periods (Table 19.2) [6]. The appropriate application of these values in dietary assessment was the focus of a subsequent IOM report [17].

1. Dietary Folate Equivalents

To account for the higher bioavailability of folic acid compared with naturally occurring food folate, the folic acid content of fortified foods is converted to an equivalent amount of food folate using the following equation: (1.7 × μg folic acid in the fortified food) + μg naturally occurring food folate. The resulting value is referred to as micrograms DFE. The DRIs for folate, except for the UL, are expressed as micrograms per day DFE [6].

2. Dietary Reference Intakes for Different Life-Stage Groups

a. Infancy

An AI for folate was set for infants because there were insufficient data on which to base an EAR. The AI was estimated from the mean folate intake of infants principally fed human milk (i.e., volume of milk consumed × folate concentration). No UL was set for infants [6].

TABLE 19.2
Selected Examples of Folate Intake Recommendations Worldwide[a]

Age/Gender/Life-Stage Category	Dietary Reference Intakes, US and Canada, Institute of Medicine[b] RDA/AI[c] µg/d DFE	Recommended Nutrient Intake FAO/WHO[d] RNI µg/d DFE	Nutrient Reference Values, Australia/New Zealand[e] RDI/AI[c] µg/d DFE	Dietary Reference Value, United Kingdom[f] RNI µg/d folate	Recommended Dietary Allowances, Ireland[g] RDA µg/d folate	Reference Values for Nutrient Intake, Germany, Switzerland, Austria[h] RI µg/d DFE	Dietary Reference Values, the Netherlands[i] RDA/AI[c] µg/d DFE	Recommended Intake, Nordic Countries[j] RI µg/d folate	Recommended Dietary Allowances, Southeast Asia[k] RDA µg/d folate
Infants (mo)									
0–6	65[c]	80	65[c]	50	50	(<4 mo) 60	(0–5 mo) 50[c]	None set	(0–5 mo) 80
7–12	80[c]	80	80[c]	50	50	(4–11 mo) 80	(6–11 mo) 60[c]	50	(6–11 mo) 80
Children (y)									
1–3	150	160	150	70	100	(1–4 y) 200	85[c]	(12–23 mo) 60 (2–5 y) 80	160
4–8	200	(4–6 y) 200 (7–9 y) 300	200	(4–6 y) 100 (7–10 y) 150	(4–10 y) 200	(4–9 y) 300	150[c]	(6–9 y) 130	(4–6 y) 200 (7–9 y) 300
Males (y)									
9–13	300	(≥10 y) 400	300	(≥11 y) 200	(≥11 y) 300	(≥10 y) 400	225[c]	(10–13 y) 200	(≥10 y) 400
≥14	400		400				(14–18 y) 300[c] (≥19 y) 300[c]	(≥14 y) 300	
Females (y)									
9–13	300	(≥10 y) 400	300	(≥11 y) 200	(≥11 y) 300	(≥10 y) 400	225[c]	(10–13 y) 200	(≥10 y) 400
≥14	400		400				(14–18 y) 300[c] (≥19 y) 300[c]	(14–17 y) 300 (18–30 y) 400 (≥30 y) 300	

continued

TABLE 19.2 (continued)
Selected Examples of Folate Intake Recommendations Worldwide[a]

Age/Gender/Life-Stage Category	Dietary Reference Intakes, US and Canada Institute of Medicine[b] RDA/AI[c] µg/d DFE	Recommended Nutrient Intake FAO/WHO[d] RNI µg/d DFE	Nutrient Reference Values, Australia/New Zealand[e] RDI/AI[c] µg/d DFE	Dietary Reference Value, United Kingdom[f] RNI µg/d folate	Recommended Dietary Allowances, Ireland[g] RDA µg/d folate	Reference Values for Nutrient Intake, Germany, Switzerland, Austria[h] RI µg/d DFE	Dietary Reference Values, the Netherlands[i] RDA/AI[c] µg/d DFE	Recommended Intake, Nordic Countries[j] RI µg/d folate	Recommended Dietary Allowances, Southeast Asia[k] RDA µg/d folate
Pregnancy (all ages)	600	600	600	300	(2nd half) 500	600	400[c]	500	600
Lactation (all ages)	500	500	500	260	(1st 6 mo) 400	600	400[c]	500	500

Note: RDA, RNI, RDI, and RI are defined as the average daily dietary intake level that is sufficient to meet the nutrient requirements of nearly all (97%–98%) healthy individuals in a particular life stage and gender group. RDA, recommended dietary allowance; AI, adequate intake; RNI, recommended dietary intake; RDI, recommended nutrient intake; RI, recommended intake.

[a] Note that units used to express recommended intake levels differ among countries.

[b] Institute of Medicine, *Dietary Reference Intakes for Thiamin, Riboflavin, Niacin, Vitamin B6, Folate, Vitamin B12, Pantothenic Acid, Biotin, and Choline,* National Academy Press, Washington, DC, 1998.

[c] Indicates value is an Adequate Intake (AI). The AI is believed to cover needs of all individuals in the group, but lack of data or uncertainty in the data prevents being able to specify with confidence the percentage of individuals covered by this intake.

d Food and Agriculture Organization: World Health Organization: United Nations. *Report of a Joint FAO/WHO Expert Consultation. Folate and Folic Acid. Human Vitamin and Mineral Requirements.* FAO/WHO, Rome, Italy, 2004.

e Australian National Health and Medical Research Council, New Zealand Ministry of Health. *Nutrient Reference Values for Australia and New Zealand Including Recommended Dietary Intakes*, National Health and Medical Research Council, Canberra, Australia, 2006.

f Department of Health, *Dietary Reference Values for Food Energy and Nutrients for the United Kingdom. Report of the Panel on Dietary Reference Values of the Committee on Medical Aspects of Food Policy. Report on Health and Social Subjects, No. 41*, HMSO, London, UK, 1991; Scientific Advisory Committee on Nutrition 2006. *Folate and Disease Prevention.* The Stationery Office, Norwich, UK, 2006.

g Food Safety Authority of Ireland RDA Working Group, *Recommended Dietary Allowances for Ireland*, Food Safety Authority of Ireland, Dublin, Ireland: 1999.

h German Nutrition Society, Austrian Nutrition Society, Swiss Society for Nutrition Research, Swiss Nutrition Association, *Reference Values for Nutrient Intake* (1st English ed.), Umschau Braus GmbH/German Nutrition Society, Frankfurt/Main, Germany, 2002.

i Health Council of the Netherlands, *Towards an Optimal Use of Folic Acid*, Health Council of the Netherlands, The Hague, Netherlands, 2008: publication no. 2008/02E.

j Nordic Council of Ministers, *Nordic Nutrition Recommendations 2004: Integrating Nutrition and Physical Activity*, 4th ed., Nordic Council of Ministers, Copenhagen, Denmark, 2005.

k Barba CV, Cabrera MI, *Asia Pac J Clin Nutr* 2008; 17(Suppl 2): 405–08

b. Children and Adolescents

The EAR for children was extrapolated from adult values for each of the following age categories: 1 to 3, 4 to 8, 9 to 13, and 14 to 18 years. The RDA, which is the same for both genders, was set using the respective EAR for each age category plus twice the coefficient of variation (CV). Although there were no reports of adverse effects from high levels of intake in these age groups, the ULs for folic acid for children and adolescents were derived from the adult value by adjusting for differences in body weight [6].

c. Adult Males and Nonpregnant Females ≥19 Years

The primary indicator used to evaluate adequacy of folate intake to maintain status, and on which the EAR and RDA were based, was red blood cell (RBC) folate concentration, an index of tissue stores, and long-term status [6]. Ancillary biomarkers included serum folate and homocysteine concentrations. The EAR for adults was based primarily on data from controlled metabolic studies in which folate response to defined diets was determined [18–22]. Additional supporting evidence included data from epidemiological studies in which folate intake was estimated in conjunction with status indicators [23–29]. Similar to the approach used for children and adolescents, a 10% CV was assumed, and the RDA (400 µg/day DFE) was set using the EAR plus twice the 10% CV.

The UL (1,000 µg/day) for folic acid was based primarily on case reports of individuals with known pernicious anemia who experienced neurological complications while taking oral folic acid supplements. Treatment of these patients with high doses of folic acid (≥5 mg/day in most cases) reversed the anemia (when present) in the majority of patients, but not the neurological symptoms, thus delaying the diagnosis of vitamin B12 deficiency. In an excellent review, Savage and Lindenbaum [30] summarized and critiqued all the reported studies on which the UL was based. There were no reported adverse effects of consumption of food folate at any level of intake; thus, the UL applies exclusively to folic acid [6].

d. Pregnancy

Folate requirements are greater during pregnancy to meet the needs for increased cell division and metabolism associated with placental and fetal development, uterine enlargement, and maternal blood volume expansion. The primary indicator used to assess adequacy of folate intake during pregnancy is RBC folate concentration [6]. The RDA for pregnant women (600 µg/day DFE) is based on data from a controlled metabolic study [31] and a series of population-based studies in which dietary folate intake was reported [32–37]. NTD risk reduction was not considered as a basis for estimating adequacy of folate intake for pregnant women. Women carrying more than one fetus may require intakes higher than the RDA [6]. Approaches to meet the intake recommendation for pregnant women through dietary and supplemental means have been addressed [38]. The UL for folic acid is the same (1,000 µg/day) for pregnant and lactating women 19 years of age and older as it is for nonpregnant women.

e. Lactation

The EAR for lactating women is based on the amount of folate necessary to replace the folate secreted daily in human milk plus the amount required to maintain maternal folate status [6]. To determine the additional quantity of folate needed during lactation, the average volume of milk produced (0.78 L) was multiplied by the folate concentration of breast milk (85 μg/L), and this quantity was multiplied by a bioavailability correction factor of 2. This amount (133 μg) was added to the EAR for nonpregnant, nonlactating women to derive the RDA (500 μg/day DFE). Women nursing more than one infant may require intakes higher than the RDA [6].

B. Food and Agriculture Organization/World Health Organization

The FAO/WHO Expert Consultation agreed that the 1998 IOM DRIs were the best available estimates of folate intake recommendations based on current published studies, and therefore adopted those RDAs as the basis for the Recommended Nutrient Intakes (RNIs) (Table 19.2) [39]. In reference to ULs, the FAO/WHO report supports the conclusions regarding the IOM's UL of 1,000 μg/day for folic acid for adults [6,39].

C. Australia and New Zealand

The Australian and New Zealand governments have worked collaboratively over the years to develop nutrition recommendations for their countries (Table 19.2) [40]. The 2006 recommendations issued by these countries were developed using the approach taken by the IOM. The terminology differs as follows: (1) their set of reference values is referred to as Nutrient Reference Values (NRV) instead of DRIs; and (2) although defined the same, the term Recommended Dietary Intake (RDI) is used in place of RDA. With the exception of the UL, which is expressed in micrograms per day folic acid, the NRVs are expressed as micrograms per day DFEs.

D. European Countries and Regions

1. United Kingdom

Similar to the United States, the United Kingdom (UK) has developed a series of recommendations for the amount of nutrients needed by different groups of healthy people. These estimates, collectively referred to as the Dietary Reference Values, include three types of values: Reference Nutrient Intakes (RNIs), EARs, and Lower Reference Nutrient Intakes. The RNIs are estimates of the amount of nutrient intakes that should meet the needs of most healthy people in a particular group. The RNIs for folate, which are considerably below those of a number of other countries, were agreed on by the Committee on Medical Aspects of Food and Nutrition Policy in 1991 (Table 19.2) [41]. The basis of the UK RNI was the amount of dietary folate intake associated with normal RBC folate concentration (>150 ng/mL; >340 nmol/L) or autopsied liver folate concentrations (>3 μg/g) [41]. The UK Expert Group on Vitamins and Minerals estimated a guidance level (1,000 μg/day folic acid) for adults in 2003 that represents an approximate indication of an intake that would not be expected to cause adverse effects [42]. The basis for the guidance level was the same as that used by the IOM [6]. Because there were no data providing evidence for an adverse effect in children and adolescents, guidance levels were not set for these age groups.

2. Ireland

Using the same definition as the IOM, the folate RDA for Ireland was updated in 1999 by a working group appointed by the Nutrition Sub-committee of the Food Safety Authority of Ireland (Table 19.2) [43]. The revisions were based on reviews of reports compiled by the United States [6], the UK [41], and the European Union [44], in combination with newer research findings and the prevailing Irish conditions [43]. The recommendations are expressed in micrograms per day folate instead of DFEs.

3. The Netherlands

The Health Council of the Netherlands' definitions of the terms AI and RDA agree with those used by the IOM, and these recommendations are expressed as DFEs (Table 19.2) [45]. Adults are the only group for whom an RDA was established. AIs were set for the remaining life-stage groups [45]. The recommended intake levels set by the Netherlands are lower than other countries' values with the exception of the UK. The UL for folic acid for adults (1,000 µg/day) is in agreement with that of the IOM [6,45].

4. Germany, Austria, and Switzerland

The Reference Values for Nutrient Intakes for Germany, Austria, and Switzerland represent a combined effort of the nutrition societies from these countries [46]. The recommended intake level is equivalent, by definition, to the IOM's RDA and is expressed in micrograms per day DFEs (Table 19.2).

5. Nordic Countries

A collaborative committee of scientists from Denmark, Sweden, Norway, Iceland, and Finland reviewed data from intervention and observational studies to establish the folate intake recommendations for those countries (Table 19.2) [47]. With the exception of women 18 to 30 years of age, nonpregnant women of reproductive age, and pregnant and lactating women, the Recommended Intake for adult males and females is 300 µg/day folate. UL values are similar to the IOM, with values extrapolated for children based on body weight [6,47].

E. SOUTHEAST ASIA

The Southeast Asia RDAs (Table 19.2) were derived through a collaborative endeavor by a committee with representatives from Indonesia, Malaysia, Philippines, Singapore, Thailand, and Vietnam [48]. The committee based its report primarily on external data sources and reports, including the IOM report [6] and the Report of the Joint FAO/WHO Expert Consultation on Human Vitamin and Mineral Requirements [39]. The Southeast Asia RDAs are expressed as micrograms per day instead of micrograms per day DFE.

IV. FOLIC ACID INTAKE NEURAL TUBE DEFECT RECOMMENDATIONS

Clinical trials demonstrating the effectiveness of folic acid supplementation in reducing the number of NTDs [2,3] prompted the US Public Health Service

(USPHS) in 1992 [5] to issue a recommendation that all women of child-bearing age consume 400 µg of folic acid daily to reduce their chance of having an NTD-affected pregnancy. Although not an RDA, the IOM issued a similar recommendation in 1998 advising that all women capable of becoming pregnant consume 400 µg/day folic acid from supplements, fortified foods, or both *in addition to* a varied diet [6]. The evidence on which the USPHS and IOM recommendations are based supports the conclusion that supplemental folic acid (400 µg/day) consumed in addition to naturally occurring food folate is associated with NTD risk reduction [6]. Other countries (e.g., Australia/New Zealand, UK, Ireland, the Netherlands, and Germany/Austria/Switzerland) have similar recommendations for periconceptional folic acid supplemental intake [40,43,45,46,49], with some specifying specific time intervals before and after conception [40,45,49]. It has been shown in a number of investigations that the establishment of policies recommending supplemental folic acid to women of child-bearing age has not generally been associated with a reduction in NTD prevalence, providing a rationale for folic acid fortification programs [50,51].

V. FOLATE/FOLIC ACID USUAL INTAKE ESTIMATES IN THE UNITED STATES

In the United States, total dietary folate intake includes food folate plus folic acid from enriched cereal grain products (140 µg/100 g flour) and fortified RTE cereals, including those with up to 400 µg/serving [4]. Estimates of dietary folate intake (µg/day) can be determined and categorized as (1) food folate, (2) folic acid, (3) total folate, (4) and total folate as DFEs using the US Department of Agriculture Food and Nutrient Database for Dietary Studies (version 1), which has been used to estimate intake in the US starting with NHANES 2001–2002 [52]. Table 19.3 summarizes the median usual folate/folic acid intake estimates for children, adolescents, and adults (nonsupplement and supplement users) who participated in the 2003–2004 and 2005–2006 NHANES with reliable 2-day dietary recall data. In addition to the contribution of folic acid from enriched cereal grain products and RTE cereals, it is very important to consider the contribution of supplements to total folate/folic acid intake. In NHANES, an estimated 38% of adults 19 years of age and older reported regular use of a folic acid–containing supplement, with other surveys suggesting a similar prevalence rate for children [53]. Although the data presented for supplement users (Table 19.3) do not distinguish between folic acid derived from dietary (fortified) sources of folic acid versus supplements, the median folic acid intake of supplement users was at least 2.5-fold higher than nonsupplement users. The median total folate and DFE intake for children (1–8 years) was approximately twofold higher for supplement users compared with nonsupplement users. These data indicate that folic acid–containing supplements contribute a substantial proportion to total folate intake in the United States.

Median folic acid intake for nonsupplement-using adolescent and adult women of reproductive potential (excluding lactating women) was less than half the amount recommended (i.e., 400 µg/day) by the USPHS [5] and the IOM [6] for NTD risk reduction. In contrast, use of folic acid–containing supplements by women of reproductive

TABLE 19.3

Usual Folate Intake (Median [25th, 75th Percentiles]) for Nonsupplement and Supplement Users in the United States[a,b,c,d,e]

Life-Stage Group	Folic Acid µg/day	Food Folate µg/day	Total Folate µg/day	Dietary Folate Equivalents µg/day DFE
Nonsupplement users				
Children (males and females)				
1–3 y ($n = 1,119$)	190 (150, 249)	176 (148, 208)	384 (321, 456)	519 (432, 625)
4–6 y ($n = 664$)	189 (151, 244)	178 (146, 213)	387 (317, 453)	517 (425, 629)
7–8 y ($n = 447$)	186 (150, 239)	168 (144, 211)	377 (314, 453)	505 (429, 627)
Adolescents (males)				
9–13 y ($n = 788$)	183 (142, 230)	167 (134, 205)	365 (308, 442)	492 (408, 598)
14–18 y ($n = 1,101$)	192 (144, 244)	174 (138, 222)	390 (304, 467)	527 (409, 631)
Adolescents (females)				
9–13 y ($n = 813$)	195 (149, 241)	183 (153, 229)	394 (322, 456)	531 (433, 627)
14–18 y ($n = 1,037$)	181 (141, 254)	171 (141, 217)	374 (307, 460)	503 (409, 637)
Adults (males)				
19–30 y ($n = 761$)	195 (153, 254)	179 (141, 224)	387 (318, 469)	525 (427, 648)
31–50 y ($n = 924$)	194 (149, 246)	181 (148, 223)	388 (325, 456)	527 (434, 628)
51–70 y ($n = 681$)	192 (143, 251)	176 (141, 216)	384 (315, 450)	517 (424, 623)
>70 y ($n = 417$)	196 (139, 250)	175 (143, 212)	383 (329, 446)	516 (441, 620)
Adults (females)				
19–30 y ($n = 636$)	180 (139, 232)	165 (139, 207)	355 (311, 427)	481 (411, 586)
31–50 y ($n = 853$)	184 (143, 243)	170 (137, 215)	372 (311, 437)	498 (415, 608)
51–70 y ($n = 632$)	180 (143, 247)	179 (142, 221)	378 (315, 458)	508 (420, 629)
>70 y ($n = 373$)	186 (145, 245)	177 (138, 225)	378 (313, 444)	504 (420, 608)
Pregnant women				
All ages ($n = 143$)	216 (157, 282)	196 (156, 252)	438 (344, 531)	595 (440, 725)
Lactating women				
All ages ($n = 42$)	261 (207, 294)	188 (139, 240)	434 (398, 517)	610 (553, 707)
Supplement users				
Children (males and females)				
1–3 y ($n = 284$)	541 (387, 675)	198 (160, 228)	753 (593, 876)	1,137 (869, 1,343)
4–6 y ($n = 349$)	505 (378, 632)	195 (157, 227)	712 (587, 870)	1,070 (850, 1,320)
7–8 y ($n = 137$)	528 (398, 622)	187 (167, 229)	727 (598, 840)	1,097 (881, 1,292)
Adolescents (males)				
9–13 y ($n = 173$)	521 (401, 693)	178 (147, 204)	738 (587, 906)	1,097 (831, 1,384)
14–18 y ($n = 145$)	541 (423, 739)	204 (158, 251)	725 (646, 982)	1,104 (927, 1,518)
Adolescents (females)				
9–13 y ($n = 177$)	474 (351, 652)	209 (172, 276)	716 (561, 911)	1,056 (821, 1,388)
14–18 y ($n = 164$)	481 (283, 578)	196 (150, 239)	667 (530, 769)	1,016 (721, 1,180)

TABLE 19.3 (continued)
Usual Folate Intake (Median [25th, 75th Percentiles]) for Nonsupplement and Supplement Users in the United States[a,b,c,d,e]

	Folic Acid µg/day	Food Folate µg/day	Total Folate µg/day	Dietary Folate Equivalents µg/day DFE
		Supplement users		
Adults (males)				
19–30 y (n = 193)	479 (304, 642)	207 (161, 252)	680 (552, 868)	1,001 (796, 1,328)
31–50 y (n = 396)	510 (424, 629)	198 (165, 240)	716 (601, 860)	1,077 (912, 1,282)
51–70 y (n = 439)	521 (410, 625)	194 (160, 230)	729 (603, 890)	1,095 (906, 1,298)
>70 y (n = 332)	511 (415, 646)	184 (153, 230)	711 (610, 860)	1,069 (919, 1,322)
Adults (females)				
19–30 y (n = 245)	484 (371, 669)	178 (141, 236)	679 (531, 864)	1,024 (789, 1,357)
31–50 y (n = 445)	505 (382, 625)	196 (153, 239)	701 (585, 855)	1,055 (863, 1,303)
51–70 y (n = 570)	502 (391, 626)	198 (156, 242)	705 (600, 833)	1,062 (872, 1,260)
>70 y (n = 361)	504 (428, 607)	202 (168, 246)	723 (604, 872)	1,091 (915, 1,316)
Pregnant women				
All ages (n = 446)	846 (543, 1,184)	203 (169, 250)	1,076 (764, 1,362)	1,675 (1,123, 2,184)
Lactating women				
All ages (n = 55)	812 (646, 891)	170 (129, 230)	974 (873, 1,106)	1,550 (1,301, 1,747)

[a] Intake data collected by the National Center for Health Statistics, Centers for Disease Control and Prevention (CDC) for NHANES 2003–2004 and 2005–2006. Refer to http://www.cdc.gov/nchs/nhanes. htm for detailed information on NHANES surveys and data collection procedures. Data analysis by coauthor Q. Yang (unpublished).

[b] Supplement use defined as consumption of a folic acid–containing supplement at least one time in the past month.

[c] *Usual* folate and folic acid intakes were estimated using the Software for Intake Distribution Estimation (PC-SIDE version 1.0, 2003) developed by the Department of Statistics, Iowa State University, which requires that some of the respondents have multiple days of nutrient values to provide a within-person estimate of variation (Dodd KW, *A User's Guide to C-SIDE: Software for Intake Distribution Estimation Version 1.0. CARD Technical Report 96-TR31.* Ames, IA: Center for Agriculture and Rural Development, Iowa State University, 1996; Carriquiry AL. *J Nutr* 2003; 133:601S–08S.) We selected all participants in NHANES 2003–2006 who had reliable 2-day dietary recall data and used PC-SIDE with Jackknife replication weights to estimate the usual folate and folic acid intakes for each individual. The estimates of usual intakes were conducted for folic acid–containing supplement users and nonusers separately. The outputs of usual folate and folic acid intakes for each individual from PC-SIDE were then analyzed using SUDAAN 10.0 (RTI, Research Triangle Park, NC) that takes into account the complex sampling design of NHANES to obtain the median and 25th and 75th percentile distribution of usual intakes by different age groups for nonsupplement and supplement users.

[d] Government Printing Office [homepage on the Internet]. *Electronic Code of Federal Regulations— Reference Amounts Customarily Consumed per Eating Occasion: General Food Supply. Title 21-Food and Drugs Part 101-Food Labeling Subpart A-General Provisions Section 101-12.* Available at http:// ecfr.gpoaccess.gov/cgi/t/text/text-idx?c=ecfr;sid=1e06c5b0786822ff75468318ccdd506b;rgn=div8; view=text;node=21%3A2.0.1.1.2.1.1.8;idno=21;cc=ecfr; accessed July 1, 2008.

[e] *USDA National Nutrient Database for Standard Reference, Release 21, 2008* [database on the Internet]. Beltsville, MD: US Department of Agriculture and Agricultural Research Service. Available at Nutrient Data Laboratory Home Page, http://www.ars.usda.gov/ba/bhnrc/ndl; accessed September 29, 2008.

potential was associated with median folic acid intakes that meet the USPHS and IOM recommendation for NTD risk reduction (Table 19.3).

VI. FOLATE STATUS IN THE UNITED STATES

A. INFLUENCE OF FORTIFICATION ON BLOOD FOLATE CONCENTRATIONS

Folate status is continually monitored in the United States by the National Center for Health Statistics at the Centers for Disease Control and Prevention (CDC). Low folate status was noted as a public health concern in early NHANES reports (i.e., NHANES II 1976–1980 and NHANES III 1988–1994), which made monitoring this nutrient a priority [1]. The addition of folic acid to the food supply, which was fully implemented in 1998 [4], and the ongoing NHANES monitoring system provide the opportunity to assess the impact of the folic acid fortification program by comparing folate status of the population pre- and postfortification (i.e., NHANES III 1988–1994 vs. NHANES 1999–2000 and beyond).

Serum and RBC folate data categorized by race/ethnicity, age, and gender for 1999–2002 NHANES participants (≥3 years) were released in a report issued by the CDC in 2008 [54]. Figure 19.1 shows the geometric mean serum folate concentrations in the United States for the total population (≥3 years) and population subgroups [54]. Although serum folate concentrations increased in all categories postfortification, they were highest in children (3–11 years) and older adults (≥60 years). The higher blood folate concentrations of children and older adults may be associated with the more frequent use of multivitamins in these age groups [53]. For example, Yu et al. [55] reported that 46.5% of 8,285 3-year-old children in the United States were given a multivitamin/mineral supplement based on data collected for the 1991

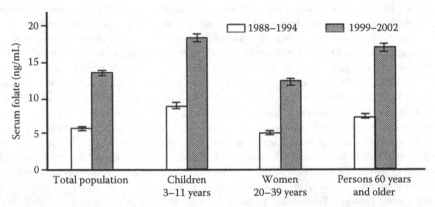

FIGURE 19.1 Geometric mean concentrations (95% CI) for serum folate in the total US population (≥3 years) and in population subgroups. To convert to SI units (nmol/L), multiply folate values by 2.266. (From McDowell MA, et al., *Blood Folate Levels: The latest NHANES Results. NCHS Data Briefs, No. 6*, National Center for Health Statistics, Hyattsville, MD: 2008. Available at http://www.cdc.gov/nchs/data/databriefs/db06.pdf; accessed September 14, 2008.)

Longitudinal Follow-up to the 1988 National Maternal and Infant Health Survey, a nationally representative sample. Among adults, multivitamin/mineral supplement use in the NHANES 1999–2000 was positively associated with age [56].

Blood folate concentrations, postfortification (NHANES 1999–2002), for US females by age group are illustrated in Figure 19.2. Folate status was adequate for the majority (>95%) of females; however, adolescent girls (12–19 years) and adult women (20–59 years), age groups for which optimal folate status is most critical, had lower geometric mean serum folate concentrations than females in other age categories. Adolescent females also had the lowest RBC folate concentrations [54].

The impact of folic acid fortification on blood folate concentrations is further illustrated by frequency distributions for serum and RBC folate for the total 1998–2004 NHANES population (≥4 years) (Figure 19.3). Pfeiffer et al. [1] determined time trends for serum and RBC folate by comparing values from about 23,000 participants obtained during the prefortification NHANES III (1988–1994) periods with those of about 8,000 participants from three postfortification NHANES periods (together covering 1999–2004) [1]. Median serum folate concentrations increased approximately threefold for the population from 5.5 ng/mL (12.5 nmol/L) in 1988–1994 (prefortification) to 14.1 ng/mL (32 nmol/L) during the first postfortification survey period (1999–2000) (Figure 19.3, top) [1,7]. Following this, modest decreases occurred during the next two postfortification survey periods (2001–2002 and 2003–2004). The 2005–2006 NHANES median serum folate estimate (12.2 ng/mL; 27.6 nmol/L; not included in figure) indicates no change from the 2003–2004 estimate [7]. Similar trends were observed for RBC folate concentrations (Figure 19.3, bottom), where the median value increased about 60%, from 174 ng/mL (394 nmol/L) to 276 ng/mL (625 nmol/L) between 1988–1994 (prefortification) and 1999–2000 (postfortification), decreased slightly from 2001–2002 to 2003–2004 [1], and has remained constant through 2005–2006 [7].

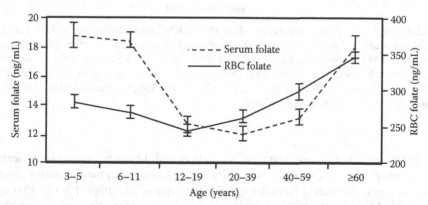

FIGURE 19.2 Cross-sectional age pattern showing geometric mean concentrations (95% CI) for serum and RBC folate in females. To convert to SI units (nmol/L), multiply folate values by 2.266. (From McDowell MA, et al., *Blood Folate Levels: The latest NHANES Results. NCHS Data Briefs, No. 6,* National Center for Health Statistics, Hyattsville, MD: 2008. Available at http://www.cdc.gov/nchs/data/databriefs/db06.pdf; accessed September 14, 2008.)

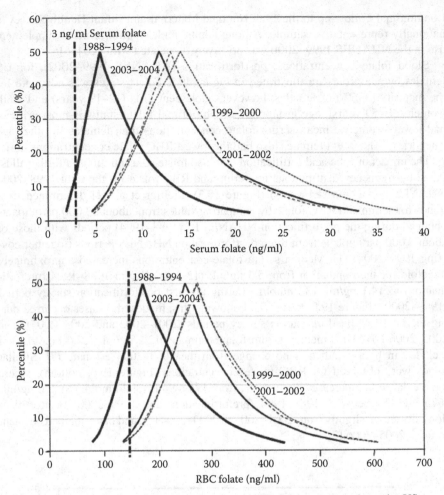

FIGURE 19.3 Frequency distribution of serum and RBC folate among the entire US population (≥4 years) according to the National Health and Nutrition Examination Surveys spanning 1988–1994, 1999–2000, 2001–2002, and 2003–2004. The vertical dotted lines indicate the cutoff for low serum folate and RBC folate concentrations, respectively. To convert to SI units (nmol/L), multiply folate values by 2.266. (Reprinted from Pfeiffer CM, et al., *Am J Clin Nutr* 2007; 86:718–27. With permission.)

Improvements in folate status of women of child-bearing age (15–45 years) mimic the pattern observed for the total US population, with median serum folate concentrations increasing from 4.8 ng/mL (10.9 nmol/L) in 1988–1994 to 13.0 ng/mL (29.5 nM) in 1999–2000 and median RBC folate concentrations increasing 65% from 160 ng/mL (363 nmol/L) to 264 ng/mL (599 nmol/L) during the same time frame. The NHANES 2005–2006 median serum and RBC folate concentrations were 11.4 ng/mL (25.8 nmol/L) and 257 ng/mL (582 nmol/L), respectively [7]. Folate status of women of child-bearing age also has improved in Canada, where folic acid fortification of enriched cereal grain products was implemented concurrent with implementation in the United States [57].

The observed increase in blood folate concentration postfortification was greater than expected, and based on the analysis of a large number of enriched foods, it has been attributed to overages by the food industry [58]. Two research groups using different approaches [59,60] estimated the increase in folic acid intake during the early postfortification period to be approximately 200 μg/day, higher than originally predicted by the FDA [4]. Although there has been no systematic evaluation of enriched foods in the marketplace, recent analysis of select foods suggests that the amount currently added to these foods does not exceed federal guidelines [61,62]. Thus, it is possible that the observed decrease in blood folate concentration following the initial postfortification increase was caused by a subsequent reduction by manufacturers in the amount of folic acid added to enriched cereal grain products. A second possibility is that consumers reduced their intake of enriched cereal grain products with the advent of the low carbohydrate diet trend that became popular sometime after the first postfortification period (1999–2000) [1,63].

Trends in the prevalence of low blood folate concentrations in the US population 4 years of age and older and in special populations, such as women of reproductive potential, have also been monitored using the NHANES data. The prevalence of low serum folate (<3 ng/mL; 6.8 nmol/L) in the US population 4 years of age and older decreased from 15.5% in 1988–1994 to 0.5% in 1999–2000, and rates have remained less than 1% up through and including the NHANES 2005–2006, the most recent data available [7]. A decrease in the prevalence of low RBC folate concentrations (<140 ng/ml; 317 nmol/L) (30.4% in 1988–1994 to 2.8% in 1999–2000) was observed for the US population, with the rates remaining low through 2005–2006 [7]. The prevalence of low blood folate concentrations in women of child-bearing age (15–45 years) also has decreased since the initiation of fortification, from 20.6% in 1988–1994 to 0.8% in 1999–2000 for serum folate and from 37.6% to 5.1% for RBC folate during the same periods.

B. INFLUENCE OF SPECIFIC FOLIC ACID SOURCES ON BLOOD FOLATE CONCENTRATIONS

Yeung et al. [64] estimated the contribution of specific folic acid sources to serum folate concentrations using NHANES 2001–2004 data (n = 8,655, nonpregnant participants ≥19 years who had both intake and blood values) [64]. Participants were categorized by serum folate quintile, and differences across quintiles for each folic acid source were determined. When the intake of folic acid from enriched cereal grain products was compared across the quintiles, consumption was relatively constant (~140 μg/day) (Figure 19.4). In contrast, folic acid intake ranged from 14 to 107 μg/day from the first to the fifth quintile for RTE cereals and from 42 to 392 μg/day from supplements (Figure 19.4). The mean total folic acid intake in the highest serum folate quintile was 643 μg/day. In this quintile, 75% of the subjects took folic acid–containing supplements contributing 61% of the total folic acid intake, and enriched cereal grain products contributed 32%. These data illustrate that higher blood folate

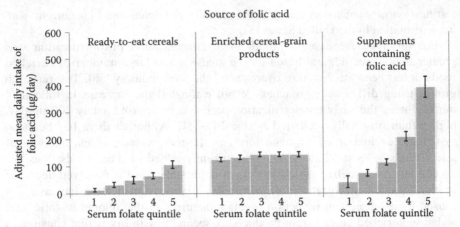

FIGURE 19.4 Estimated daily intake of folic acid by serum folate quintile data were obtained from the National Health and Nutrition Examination Survey (NHANES) 2001–2004 for 8,655 nonpregnant adults aged 19 years and older. For ready-to-eat cereals, $P < 0.001$; for enriched cereal grain products, $P = 0.01$; and for supplements, $P < 0.001$ (Satterthwaite adjusted F statistic). All the analyses were adjusted for age, sex, and race/ethnicity. Error bars indicate 95% CI. (Reprinted from Yeung L, Yang Q, Berry RJ, *JAMA* 2008; 300:2486–87. With permission.)

concentrations in the US can be attributed primarily to the use of supplements containing folic acid [64].

VII. FOLATE STATUS OF POPULATIONS IN OTHER COUNTRIES

In an attempt to characterize the magnitude of folate deficiencies worldwide, McLean et al. [65] reviewed all accessible reports of status assessment studies conducted during the past decade (1995–2005). Definitive conclusions regarding the extent of folate deficiencies globally could not be drawn because of limitations of the data, including (1) the paucity of population-based studies designed to assess folate status at the national or regional level; (2) variation in the life-stage groups (e.g., children, pregnant women) evaluated in different countries, with very few surveys designed to assess the folate status in the general population; (3) use of different analytical methods to measure serum and RBC folate, which raises concern regarding assay variability and validity, an issue discussed in Chapter 21 by Pfeiffer and coauthors; and (4) use of poorly defined and inconsistent cutoff values to define folate deficiency based on serum and/or RBC folate concentrations [65]. It was possible, however, to provide some indication based on this extensive evaluation of available data that in the majority of countries for which there are national survey data, folate deficiency appears to be a public health problem [65]. There is a pressing need for further studies to address the limitations of the folate assessment data, which will facilitate planning for appropriate public health intervention strategies in specific countries around the world [65].

VIII. SUMMARY

DRI standards have been developed by countries in many regions of the world. Among the countries whose dietary intake recommendations are included in this chapter, there is variability with regard to the nomenclature used to define recommendations, the units used to express intake recommendations (i.e., µg/day folate, µg/day DFE), and the level of recommended intake, although with regard to the latter, there is considerable overlap with regard to recommended intake levels. Most countries included in this chapter have a separate recommendation for women of reproductive potential to consume periconceptional folic acid to reduce the risk of an NTD-affected pregnancy.

The impact of folic acid fortification in the US is evident from comparisons of intake and status data collected pre- and postfortification. Enriched cereal grain products and foods made with these, which formerly provided only a very small amount of naturally occurring food folate, now make an important contribution to total folate intake. Other sources of folic acid, such as folic acid–fortified RTE cereals and supplements, also make important contributions to total folic acid intake in consumers who use these products. In fact, intake data comparing supplement users to nonusers suggest that folic acid–containing supplements contribute a substantial proportion to total folate intake in children, adolescents, and adults.

Consistent with increases in folate intake among population subgroups, folate status in the US has improved more than expected postfortification. Furthermore, prevalence estimates of low serum and RBC folate concentrations for the US population 4 years of age and older decreased to extremely low levels immediately following the initiation of folic acid fortification and did not change in subsequent surveys. In examining the relationship between folate status and intake, the data reviewed in this chapter illustrate that the highest blood folate concentrations in the US can be attributed primarily to the use of folic acid–containing supplements.

Research studies need to be designed to provide more definitive data on which to base conclusions regarding the magnitude of folate deficiencies worldwide. Once folate status has been characterized in specific countries, appropriate intervention strategies can be designed and implemented in an effort to prevent the well-known health-related consequences of insufficient folate intake.

REFERENCES

1. Pfeiffer CM, Johnson CL, Jain RB, Yetley EA, Picciano MF, Rader JI, Fisher KD, Mulinare J, Osterloh J. Trends in blood folate and vitamin B-12 concentrations in the United States, 1988 2004. *Am J Clin Nutr* 2007; 86:718–27.
2. MRC Vitamin Study Research Group. Prevention of neural tube defects: Results of the Medical Research Council Vitamin Study. *Lancet* 1991; 338:131–37.
3. Czeizel AE, Dudas I. Prevention of the first occurrence of neural-tube defects by periconceptional vitamin supplementation. *N Engl J Med* 1992; 327:1832–35.
4. Food and Drug Administration. Food standards: Amendment of standards of identity for enriched grain products to require addition of folic acid, Final Rule. 21 CFR Parts 136, 137, and 139. *Fed Reg* 1996; 64:8781–97.

5. US Centers for Disease Control and Prevention. Recommendations for the use of folic acid to reduce the number of cases of spina bifida and other neural tube defects. *Morbid Mortal Wkly Rep* 1992; 41:001.
6. Institute of Medicine. *Dietary Reference Intakes for Thiamin, Riboflavin, Niacin, Vitamin B6, Folate, Vitamin B12, Pantothenic Acid, Biotin, and Choline.* Washington, DC: National Academy Press, 1998.
7. McDowell MA, Lacher DA, Pfeiffer CM, Mulinare J, Picciano MF, Rader JI, Yetley EA, Kennedy-Stephenson J, Johnson CL. *Blood Folate Levels: The latest NHANES Results. NCHS Data Briefs, No. 6.* Hyattsville, MD: National Center for Health Statistics, 2008. Available at http://www.cdc.gov/nchs/data/databriefs/db06.pdf; accessed September 14, 2008.
8. Eitenmiller RR, Landen Jr WO. Folate. In Eitenmiller RR, Landen WO Jr, eds., *Vitamin Analysis for the Health and Food Sciences.* Boca Raton, FL: CRC Press, 1999:411–65.
9. Gregory JF 3rd. Chemical and nutritional aspects of folate research: Analytical procedures, methods of folate synthesis, stability, and bioavailability of dietary folates. *Adv Food Nutr Res* 1989; 33:1–101.
10. Food and Drug Administration. Food additives permitted for direct addition to food for human consumption; Folic acid (folacin), final rule. *Fed Reg* 1996; 64:8797–807.
11. Lewis CJ, Crane NT, Wilson DB, Yetley EA. Estimated folate intakes: Data updated to reflect food fortification, increased bioavailability, and dietary supplement use. *Am J Clin Nutr* 1999; 70:198–207.
12. O'Broin JD, Temperley IJ, Brown JP, Scott JM. Nutritional stability of various naturally occurring monoglutamate derivatives of folic acid. *Am J Clin Nutr* 1975; 28:438–44.
13. Temple CT, Montgomery JA. Chemical and physical properties of folic acid and reduced derivatives. In: Blakley RL, Benkovic SJ, eds., *Folates and Pterins, vol. I, Chemistry and Biochemistry of Folates*, 2nd ed. New York: John Wiley and Sons, 1984:61–120.
14. Anderson R, Maxwell D, Mulley A, Fritsch C. Effects of processing and storage on micronutrients in breakfast cereals. *Food Technol* 1976; 30:110–14.
15. Cort WM, Borenstein B, Harley JH, Oscadca M, Scheiner M. Nutrient stability of fortified cereal products. *Food Technol* 1976; 30: 52–62.
16. Rubin SH, Emodi A, Scialpi L. Micronutrient additions to cereal grain products. *Cereal Chemistry* 1977; 54:895–904.
17. Institute of Medicine. *Dietary Reference Intakes: Applications in Dietary Assessment.* Washington, DC: National Academy Press, 2000.
18. Milne DB, Johnson LK, Mahalko JR, Sandstead HH. Folate status of adult males living in a metabolic unit: Possible relationships with iron nutriture. *Am J Clin Nutr* 1983; 37:768–73.
19. Sauberlich HE, Kretsch MJ, Skala JH, Johnson HL, Taylor PC. Folate requirement and metabolism in nonpregnant women. *Am J Clin Nutr* 1987; 46:1016–28.
20. Jacob RA, Wu MM, Henning SM, Swendseid ME. Homocysteine increases as folate decreases in plasma of healthy men during short-term dietary folate and methyl group restriction. *J Nutr* 1994; 124:1072–80.
21. O'Keefe CA, Bailey LB, Thomas EA, Hofler SA, Davis BA, Cerda JJ, Gregory JF 3rd. Controlled dietary folate affects folate status in nonpregnant women. *J Nutr* 1995; 125:2717–25.
22. Jacob RA, Gretz DM, Taylor PC, James SJ, Pogribny IP, Miller BJ, Henning SM, Swendseid ME. Moderate folate depletion increases plasma homocysteine and decreases lymphocyte DNA methylation in postmenopausal women. *J Nutr* 1998; 128:1204–12.
23. Jagerstad M. Folate intake and blood folate in elderly subjects, a study using the double sampling portion technique. *Nutr Metab* 1977; 21(Suppl 1):29–31.
24. Bates CJ, Fleming M, Paul AA, Black AE, Mandal AR. Folate status and its relation to vitamin C in healthy elderly men and women. *Age Ageing* 1980; 9:241–48.

25. Garry PJ, Goodwin JS, Hunt WC, Hooper EM, Leonard AG. Nutritional status in a healthy elderly population: Dietary and supplemental intakes. *Am J Clin Nutr* 1982; 36:319–31.
26. Garry PJ, Goodwin JS, Hunt WC. Folate and vitamin B12 status in a healthy elderly population. *J Am Geriatr Soc* 1984; 32:719–26.
27. Sahyoun NR, Otradovec CL, Hartz SC, Jacob RA, Peters H, Russell RM, McGandy RB. Dietary intakes and biochemical indicators of nutritional status in an elderly, institutionalized population. *Am J Clin Nutr* 1988; 47:524–33.
28. Selhub J, Jacques PF, Wilson PW, Rush D, Rosenberg IH. Vitamin status and intake as primary determinants of homocysteinemia in an elderly population. *JAMA* 1993; 270:2693–98.
29. Koehler KM, Romero LJ, Stauber PM, Pareo-Tubbeh SL, Liang HC, Baumgartner RN, Garry PJ, Allen RH, Stabler SP. Vitamin supplementation and other variables affecting serum homocysteine and methylmalonic acid concentrations in elderly men and women. *J Am Coll Nutr* 1996; 15:364–76.
30. Savage DG, Lindenbaum J. Folate-cobalamin interactions. In: Bailey LB, ed., *Folate in Health and Disease*. New York: Marcel Dekker, 1995:237–85.
31. Caudill MA, Cruz AC, Gregory JF 3rd, Hutson AD, Bailey LB. Folate status response to controlled folate intake in pregnant women. *J Nutr* 1997; 127:2363–70.
32. Dawson DW. Microdoses of folic acid in pregnancy. *J Obstet Gynaecol Br Commonw* 1966; 73:44–48.
33. Lowenstein L, Cantlie G, Ramos O, Brunton L. The incidence and prevention of folate deficiency in a pregnant clinic population. *Can Med Assoc J* 1966; 95:797–806.
34. Willoughby ML, Jewell FJ. Investigation of folic acid requirements in pregnancy. *BMJ* 1966; 2:1568–71.
35. Chanarin I, Rothman D, Ward A, Perry J. Folate status and requirement in pregnancy. *BMJ* 1968; 2:390–94.
36. Willoughby ML, Jewell FG. Folate status throughout pregnancy and in postpartum period. *BMJ* 1968; 4:356–60.
37. Colman N, Larsen JV, Barker M, Barker EA, Green R, Metz J. Prevention of folate deficiency by food fortification. III. Effect in pregnant subjects of varying amounts of added folic acid. *Am J Clin Nutr* 1975; 28:465–70.
38. Bailey LB. New dietary folate intake standard for pregnant women. *Am J Clin Nutr* 2000; 71:1304S–07S.
39. Food and Agriculture Organization: World Health Organization: United Nations. *Report of a Joint FAO/WHO Expert Consultation. Folate and Folic Acid. Human Vitamin and Mineral Requirements*. Rome, Italy: FAO/WHO, 2004.
40. Australian National Health and Medical Research Council, New Zealand Ministry of Health. *Nutrient Reference Values for Australia and New Zealand Including Recommended Dietary Intakes*. Canberra, Australia: National Health and Medical Research Council, 2006.
41. Department of Health. *Dietary Reference Values for Food Energy and Nutrients for the United Kingdom. Report of the Panel on Dietary Reference Values of the Committee on Medical Aspects of Food Policy. Report on Health and Social Subjects, No. 41*. London: HMSO, 1991.
42. Expert Group on Vitamins and Minerals. *Safe Upper Levels of Vitamins and Minerals*. London: Food Standards Agency, 2003.
43. Food Safety Authority of Ireland RDA Working Group. *Recommended Dietary Allowances for Ireland*. Dublin, Ireland: Food Safety Authority of Ireland, 1999.
44. Scientific Committee for Food and Commission of the European Communities. *Nutrient and Energy Intakes for the European Community. Reports of the Scientific Committee for Food, 31st Series*. Luxembourg: Office for Official Publications of the European Communities, 1993.

45. Health Council of the Netherlands. *Towards an Optimal Use of Folic Acid*. The Hague, the Netherlands: Health Council of the Netherlands, 2008: publication no. 2008/02E.

46. German Nutrition Society, Austrian Nutrition Society, Swiss Society for Nutrition Research, Swiss Nutrition Association. *Reference Values for Nutrient Intake*, 1st English ed. Frankfort/Main, Germany: Umschau Braus GmbH/German Nutrition Society, 2002.

47. Nordic Council of Ministers. *Nordic Nutrition Recommendations 2004: Integrating Nutrition and Physical Activity*, 4th ed. Copenhagen, Denmark: Nordic Council of Ministers, 2004.

48. Barba CV, Cabrera MI. Recommended dietary allowances harmonization in Southeast Asia. Asia Pac *J Clin Nutr* 2008; 17(Suppl 2):405–08.

49. Scientific Advisory Committee on Nutrition 2006. Folate and Disease Prevention. Norwich, UK: The Stationery Office, 2006.

50. Busby A, Abramsky L, Dolk H, Armstrong B. Preventing neural tube defects in Europe: Population based study. *BMJ* 2005; 330:574–75.

51. Botto LD, Lisi A, Robert-Gnansia E, Erickson JD, Vollset SE, Mastroiacovo P, Botting B, et al. International retrospective cohort study of neural tube defects in relation to folic acid recommendations: Are the recommendations working? *BMJ* 2005; 330:571–73.

52. *USDA Food and Nutrient Database for Dietary Studies, version 1.0.* [database on the Internet]. Beltsville, MD: US Department of Agriculture and Agricultural Research Service, Food Surveys Research Group, 2004. Available at http://www.ars.usda.gov/services/docs.htm?docid=7673; accessed August 5, 2008.

53. Rock CL. Multivitamin-multimineral supplements: Who uses them? *Am J Clin Nutr* 2007; 85:277S–79S.

54. US Centers for Disease Control and Prevention. *National Report on Biochemical Indicators of Diet and Nutrition in the US Population 1999–2002*. Atlanta, GA: National Center for Environmental Health, 2008.

55. Yu SM, Kogan MD, Gergen P. Vitamin-mineral supplement use among preschool children in the United States. *Pediatrics* [serial online] 1997; 100:e4. Available at http://pediatrics.aappublications.org/content/vol100/issue5/index.shtml; accessed October 20, 2008.

56. Radimer K, Bindewald B, Hughes J, Ervin B, Swanson C, Picciano MF. Dietary supplement use by US adults: Data from the National Health and Nutrition Examination Survey, 1999–2000. *Am J Epidemiol* 2004; 160:339–49.

57. Ray JG, Vermeulen MJ, Boss SC, Cole DE. Increased red cell folate concentrations in women of reproductive age after Canadian folic acid food fortification. *Epidemiology* 2002; 13:238–40.

58. Rader JI, Weaver CM, Angyal G. Total folate in enriched cereal-grain products in the United States following fortification. *Food Chem* 2000; 70:275–89.

59. Quinlivan EP, Gregory JF 3rd. Reassessing folic acid consumption patterns in the United States (1999 2004): Potential effect on neural tube defects and overexposure to folate. *Am J Clin Nutr* 2007; 86:1773–79.

60. Choumenkovitch SF, Selhub J, Wilson PW, Rader JI, Rosenberg IH, Jacques PF. Folic acid intake from fortification in United States exceeds predictions. *J Nutr* 2002; 132:2792–98.

61. Johnston KE, Tamura T. Folate content in commercial white and whole wheat sandwich breads. *J Agric Food Chem* 2004; 52:6338–40.

62. Poo-Prieto R, Haytowitz DB, Holden JM, Rogers G, Choumenkovitch SF, Jacques PF, Selhub J. Use of the affinity/HPLC method for quantitative estimation of folic acid in enriched cereal-grain products. *J Nutr* 2006; 136:3079–83.

63. Bailey LB. The rise and fall of blood folate in the United States emphasizes the need to identify all sources of folic acid. *Am J Clin Nutr* 2007; 86:528–30.

64. Yeung L, Yang Q, Berry RJ. Contributions of total daily intake of folic acid to serum folate concentrations. *JAMA* 2008; 300:2486–87.

65. McLean E, de Benoist B, Allen LH. Review of the magnitude of folate and vitamin B12 deficiencies worldwide. *Food Nutr Bull* 2008; 29:S38–51.

20 Kinetics of Folate and One-Carbon Metabolism

*Jesse F. Gregory III, Vanessa R. da Silva,
and Yvonne Lamers*

CONTENTS

I. INTRODUCTION

Kinetics is the study of rates. In the context of this chapter, we focus on the rates of processes by which folate undergoes absorption, distribution, and metabolism and through which it functions in one-carbon metabolism. Most research studies and clinical assessments in nutrition involve the use of biomarkers on which to draw inferences about nutritional status. Biomarkers are constituents of accessible body fluids, cells, or tissues that respond in a manner that reflects a metabolic or physiological response and thus can be used as quantitative or diagnostic tools.

These also yield information about the metabolic consequences of dietary interventions, nutritional supplements, physiological changes, genetics, and a wide range of genetic variables. Even the simultaneous analysis of many biomarkers (as in modern metabolomics) may provide little information about the mechanisms involved. Well-designed kinetic studies often can provide more mechanistic insight.

The objective of this chapter is to review several aspects of folate kinetics. These include (1) kinetic aspects of changes in folate nutritional status in response to changes in the intake of unlabeled folate from supplemental or dietary sources; (2) experimental approaches and results from isotopic studies of folate metabolism and inferences from these studies; (3) approaches to and inferences from the mathematical modeling of folate metabolism and folate-dependent one-carbon metabolism; and (4) approaches and results of isotopic studies of one-carbon metabolism.

II. KINETIC ASPECTS OF INTERVENTION STUDIES WITH CONTROLLED DIETS OR FOLATE SUPPLEMENTS

Human intervention trials using unlabeled sources of folates provide information about the dose-response relationships between level of folate intake and steady-state concentrations of indicators such as serum or plasma folate and red blood cell (RBC) folate and plasma total homocysteine (Hcy) concentrations. In addition, such studies yield important information regarding the rate of attainment of the new steady state following initiation or termination of a dietary treatment or supplement. Such studies also provide information about the linearity of dose dependence. This kind of information is directly applicable in predicting and interpreting the impact of dietary interventions and supplementation regimens.

A. CONTROLLED DIETS

O'Keefe et al. [1] reported a study in which three groups of healthy women were fed a controlled diet providing total folate intakes of either 319, 489, or 659 μg/day dietary folate equivalent (DFE; 30 μg of dietary folate plus [170, 270, and 370 μg of folic acid × 1.7]) for 8 weeks. This was the first controlled dietary intervention trial providing evidence that a folate intake (319 μg/day DFE) above the former recommended daily allowance (RDA) of 180 μg/day was not sufficient to maintain an adequate folate status in the majority of a group [1]. Caudill et al. [2] reported that a total folate intake of 681 μg/day DFE (120 μg of dietary folate plus [330 μg of folic acid × 1.7]) in pregnant women was sufficient to maintain an adequate folate status reflected by serum and RBC folate concentrations (>13.6 nmol/L and >363 nmol/L, respectively) after 12 weeks of controlled dietary intake. This confirms the adequacy of the current RDA for pregnant women of 600 μg/day DFE. Kauwell et al. [3] determined that about 500 μg/day DFE total folate was more adequate in restoring normal folate status postdepletion in older adults than about 200 μg/day DFE. Further studies investigating the adequacy of the RDA provided evidence that 400 μg/day DFE was adequate to maintain normal folate status independent of genotype for the methylenetetrahydrofolate reductase (MTHFR) 677C→T polymorphism [4] and race and ethnicity [5]. Data at intermediate time points were also generated in most of these studies, which would allow analysis of the rates of change of the various biomarkers evaluated.

Changes in serum or plasma folate and RBC folate concentrations reflect adjustment to altered folate intake. In response to dietary folate depletion (135 µg/day), serum folate concentrations decreased continuously over 7 weeks of intervention without reaching a plateau [5]. In view of the very long mean residence time of whole-body folate at low intakes (e.g., approaching 200 days at 200 µg/day intake [6]), this observation is not unexpected. Reduction in serum folate concentration caused by low folate intake and increased serum folate concentration in response to a high-folate diet stabilized after 8 and 9 weeks, respectively, in a 12-week intervention [2]. In contrast, RBC folate concentration did not reach steady state during 12 weeks of increased dietary folate intake [2]. RBC folate turnover is much slower than that of serum folate as only 1% of erythrocytes is replaced per day and folate is only incorporated during erythropoiesis. Shelnutt et al. [4] found that RBC folate concentration decreased after 7 weeks of folate depletion (115 µg/day) and continued to decrease even during an ensuing 7-week repletion period with 400 µg/day DFE intake. This illustrates the fact that RBC folate concentration is a good indicator of long-term folate nutriture but a poor indicator of recent changes in folate intake.

B.   UNLABELED SUPPLEMENTS

1.   Short-Term Kinetics

As previously reviewed [7], short-term folate kinetics often have been examined using a single folate dose administered orally or intravenously followed by serial measurements of either total folate or individual folate forms in serum or plasma [8–11]. One notable and currently relevant aspect of short-term kinetic studies involved the measurement of plasma folate clearance rate following an intravenous injection of folic acid. Chanarin et al. [12] observed that the clearance rate of serum folate following folic acid injection was greater in vitamin B12–deficient megaloblastic anemia patients than in normal control subjects. Metz et al. [13] reported that elevated plasma folate clearance rate after folic acid injection is an indicator both of vitamin B12 deficiency and of folate deficiency in megaloblastic anemia. Although this phenomenon is undoubtedly attributable to accelerated folate turnover resulting from the methyl trap in vitamin B12 deficiency, the mechanism responsible in folate deficiency is unclear. Contrasting observations were reported by Gregory et al. [14], who showed that urinary excretion of labeled folate from a single oral dose of deuterium-labeled folic acid increases in proportion to folate intake over the range of 200 to 400 µg/day.

It is important to recognize the strengths and limitations of high-dose clinical studies in terms of their limited relevance to metabolic patterns under more typical nutritional situations. Examples of such studies are the examinations of plasma area-under-the curve (AUC) response of 5-formyltetrahydrofolate (5-formyl-THF) and other plasma folates in response to oral high-dose leucovorin (125–500 mg/m^2) as used in certain cancer chemotherapy regimens [11,15]. Nonlinear dose-response for the AUC values of plasma 5-formyl-THF suggested a saturable absorptive process irrespective of the fact that these doses were well above the range of saturation of more physiological absorption processes. In addition, the patterns of conversion from 5-formyl-THF to 5-methyltetrahydrofolate (5-methyl-THF) and other metabolically active folates demonstrate that high leucovorin doses provide gradual conversion to metabolically active folate species. This observation also raises the question of whether the transiently high concentration of cellular 5-formyl-THF, an inhibitory folate species, may perturb one-carbon metabolism in addition to its role as a precursor to other folates. Whereas the AUC values and rate constants for folate absorption, interconversion, and elimination processes from such studies are fully relevant to applications of high-dose leucovorin, these results almost assuredly do not reflect more typical in vivo kinetics of folate metabolism.

2. Long-Term Kinetics

The relation between the change in steady-state serum or plasma folate concentration to change in folate intake was described by Quinlivan and Gregory [16], who summarized data from 11 intervention studies. This regression model showed a linear relation between serum folate concentration and folate intake and predicts an incremental response of serum or plasma folate concentration by 2.7 ng/mL (or 6.1 nmol/L) for each increase in folate intake of 100 µg/day DFE [16,17]. Thus, the daily folate intake or change induced by supplementation or food fortification can be estimated on a population basis by monitoring serum folate concentrations if the comparison is based on values that have reached a plateau concentration [16]. Wald et al. [18] determined dose dependence between oral folic acid administration in dosages of 200, 400, 600, 800, and 1,000 µg of folic acid/day for 3 months and serum folate concentration in patients with ischemic heart disease. In a dose-response trial by van Oort et al. [19], serum and RBC folate concentrations increased linearly with increasing doses of folic acid provided as daily doses containing 50, 100, 200, 400, 600, or 800 µg of folic acid over 12 weeks. Also Daly et al. [20] reported that changes in RBC folate concentration are proportional to folate intake after a 6-month consumption of folic acid–fortified foods providing 100, 200, or 400 µg of folic acid/day.

Several studies revealed that a plateau in serum or plasma folate concentration is achieved after 12 to 14 weeks of folate supplementation independent of folate form or dosage [21–24]. This length of time required to reach the full effect of supplementation must be recognized in designing and interpreting supplementation trials and other nutritional interventions. In addition, this moderately slow response of plasma folate illustrates that plasma folate concentration not only reflects recent intake (as is conventional dogma) but also is in equilibrium with and governed by cellular folate concentration [7]. Plasma folate concentration also was shown to decrease after cessation of folic acid supplementation but did not reach baseline conditions at 3 months (~12 weeks) after the dosage was terminated [18,24]. As described above, RBC folate has a slower turnover and response to altered folate intake than serum or plasma folate as a result of the approximately 120-day lifespan of RBCs and because folate is mostly incorporated during erythropoiesis [25]. In supplementation studies with various folate dosages ranging from 100 to 4,000 µg/day, RBC folate concentrations did not plateau within the duration of the 12- to 24-week observation periods

[22–24,26] regardless of folate form or dosage. At 3 months after cessation of intervention with 400 µg/day and 4,000 µg/day folic acid, RBC folate concentrations remained higher than at baseline [24], whereas, in contrast, RBC folate concentration returned to baseline 3 months after dosage termination in subjects receiving 100 µg of folic acid/day or 4,000 µg of folic acid once weekly [24]. These data indicate that a 400-µg/day supplementation regimen provides at least some lingering benefit for 3 months, assuming that RBC folate concentration provides some indication of prolonged elevation of retained tissue folate. Pietrzik et al. [26] developed a working kinetic model based on the simplified assumption that RBC folate kinetics could be approximated as behaving in first-order kinetic fashion despite the finite life of the cells. Based on this assumption and half-lives derived from long-term folate supplementation studies, these investigators estimated that RBC folate appearance and elimination would reach steady state about 40 weeks after the start or following cessation of supplement usage [26].

Plasma total Hcy concentration can serve as a functional indicator of folate metabolism, but the nonlinear relation between folate intake and plasma total Hcy must be recognized [18,19,27–29]. In a meta-analysis of supplementation trials using daily 100- to 10,000-µg folic acid doses, the greatest Hcy-lowering effect was suggested to occur from daily supplementation of 800 µg or more of folic acid [29]. The Hcy-lowering effect of dietary folate or folic acid not only depends on the dosage but also on factors such as baseline plasma total Hcy concentration [29,30], plasma or serum folate concentration [29], and duration of supplementation [27]. Further determinants of Hcy concentration are age, gender, smoking status, serum creatinine levels, renal function, and caffeine consumption [31,32]. In their dose-response trial, van Oort et al. [19] observed that daily supplements providing 400 µg of folic acid over 12 weeks provided more than 90% of the maximal reduction of plasma Hcy in healthy adults aged 50 to 75 years with baseline plasma total Hcy concentrations of 11.5 µmol/L. In healthy women with a mean age of 23 years and mean baseline total Hcy concentration of 8.5 µmol/L, 4 weeks of supplementation with either 400 µg/day folic acid or equimolar amount of 5-methyl-THF yielded steady-state conditions with no further change over an additional intervention period of 4 weeks [33] and 20 weeks [34], respectively. The impact of the duration of supplementation was shown in a study by Ward et al. [27]. After 12 weeks of folic acid supplementation with 100 and 200 µg/day folic acid (each 6 weeks), no further Hcy-lowering effect was observed with a 14-week additional supplementation of 400 µg/day folic acid in healthy men (34–65 years and 9 µmol/L baseline plasma total Hcy concentration) [27].

With respect to periodicity of supplementation, weekly high-dose folic acid regimens were shown to be less effective in increasing folate status and decreasing plasma total Hcy than daily supplements of one-seventh of this dosage. For example, daily supplementation of 400 µg of folic acid led to higher plasma and RBC folate concentrations than a 2,800-µg folic acid supplement given once weekly over 12 weeks [35]. A weekly supplement of 4,000 µg of folic acid was less effective in increasing blood folate and decreasing plasma total Hcy than 400 µg of folic acid/day [24]. These effects presumably occurred as a result of a saturation of metabolic capacity and renal reabsorption shortly after the very high dose. Although weekly supplementation may have practical advantages in aspects of international nutrition programs, its efficacy does not equate to that of more conventional administration of daily doses for these kinetic and metabolic reasons. However, there is no advantage to administration of moderate doses of supplemental folic acid more often than once per day. Hao et al. [24] showed that blood folate and plasma total Hcy responses were similar for the same daily amount of folic acid (25 μg of folic acid four times daily versus 100 μg/day folic acid and 100 μg of folic acid four times daily versus 400 μg/day folic acid).

The conversion of folic acid to 5-methyl-THF occurs by saturable metabolic processes. When administered as a single 500- to 1,000-μg oral dose, folic acid is absorbed largely through the intestine and converted to 5-methyl-THF primarily in the liver [36,37]. This observation was confirmed in a short-term study using oral doses of stable-isotopically labeled folates [38]. Unmetabolized folic acid has been detected in plasma at folic acid consumption greater than 200 μg/day [33,39,40], and the proportion of folic acid increases with increasing total plasma folate concentration [41,42]. Kalmbach et al. [42] determined a positive linear association between folic acid intake and circulating folic acid concentrations in a cohort of healthy men and women who were exposed to folic acid–fortified food and self-selected supplements for more than a year. The proportion of folic acid from total folate would undoubtedly vary as a function of time after dose, but these relationships have not been thoroughly examined. The impact of unmetabolized folic acid on human health and disease is not fully elucidated. Besides the beneficial role of folic acid in the prevention of neural tube defects (NTDs) and maintaining overall nutritional adequacy, the specific benefits and risks of folic acid versus high folate intake remain controversial [43].

Short-term AUC studies have shown that oral 5-methyl-THF exhibits approximately equivalent bioavailability as folic acid in healthy men and women [44,45]. Long-term supplementation studies showed similar effects of 5-methyl-THF and folic acid on the increase in RBC and plasma folate concentrations in young women [22,23,46]. In a report by Venn et al. [23], daily supplementation with 100 μg of folic acid and the equimolar amount of 5-methyl-THF increased blood folate concentrations equally. In a study by Lamers et al. [22], RBC folate concentration increased more after 416 μg/day 5-methyl-THF supplementation than after supplementation with equimolar amounts of folic acid (400 μg/day); however, the increase in plasma folate concentration was equivalent. Houghton et al. [46] observed a greater effect of 5-methyl-THF supplements than folic acid supplements for maintaining RBC folate concentration in lactating women. In similar studies, 5-methyl-THF supplements were slightly more effective than [47] or equally effective as [34] equimolar amounts of folic acid in lowering plasma total Hcy in healthy individuals. Both folate forms were equally effective in Hcy reduction after a 12-week supplementation with 17 mg/day 5-methyl-THF and equimolar folic acid in long-term hemodialysis patients [48].

The racemic form of 5-methyl-THF is predictably half as effective as the equivalent amount of folic acid to lower plasma total Hcy concentrations in young women [33]. Mader et al. [49] evaluated plasma and renal clearance of single intravenous infusions of different dosages of racemic [6R,S]-5-methyl-THF (100,

200, 300, 400, 500, 600 mg/m²) in patients with advanced colorectal cancer. The nonphysiological, metabolically inactive [6R]-5-methyl-THF component of racemic supplements exhibited greater protein binding in plasma and led to a higher renal clearance of [6S]-5-methyl-THF [49]. The maximal plasma concentration of [6R]-5-methyl-THF was twice that of [6S]-5-methyl-THF, and the AUC was threefold greater for plasma [6R]-5-methyl-THF than for plasma [6S]-5-methyl-THF. One week after administration of a single oral dose of 5 mg of [6R,S]-5-methyl-THF, residual [6R]-5-methyl-THF form was observed in plasma [50]. The metabolic significance of [6R]-5-methyl-THF in racemic preparations is unclear, but such observations raise concern.

III. KINETIC ANALYSIS WITH ISOTOPIC TRACERS

A. EXPERIMENTAL APPROACHES AND RATIONALE

The use of radioactive and stable isotopes facilitates the evaluation of nutrient absorption, distribution, metabolism, and disappearance in cells, tissues, organs, and/or the whole body. Investigations using isotopic tracers provide assurance that any labeled compound in blood, tissues, or excreta is derived from the administered dose. This specificity constitutes an important attribute in metabolic protocols. In addition, the use of isotopic tracers facilitates the calculation of rates of metabolic and physiological processes and often contributes to mechanistic interpretations that may not otherwise be feasible from the results of nonisotopic protocols. Finally, the results of isotopic studies often allow the development of mathematical models of the metabolic and physiological processes involved. These models not only give basic quantitative information but also provide important tools for use in simulations of the effects of nutritional, physiological, and genetic variables not readily tested experimentally.

Two approaches are available for isotopic studies relevant to folate metabolism and folate-dependent one-carbon metabolism. The first of these involves the administration of a folate dose (folic acid or other folate species) labeled with radioisotope such as tritium (^{3}H) or ^{14}C or with nonradioactive stable isotopes such as deuterium (^{2}H) or ^{13}C. Protocols using radioisotopically labeled folates led to the initial understanding of whole-body folate turnover in animals and, to a lesser extent, in humans. Such protocols often involved administration of a single bolus oral or injected tracer dose, followed by analysis of total radioactivity or, following chromatographic separation, the profile of folates and folate metabolites in tissues, blood, and excreta. Collection of samples over a sufficient range of sampling times allows kinetic analysis of tracer distribution, metabolism, and turnover. Because of the high specific radioactivity of ^{3}H-labeled folates and the resulting ability to detect labeled products in tissue and excreta by liquid scintillation counting, studies with [^{3}H]folates were feasible following just a single tracer dose (e.g., Russell et al. [51]). The use of folates labeled with ^{14}C was less frequent in metabolic protocols because of the lower specific radioactivity of that radionuclide. Thus, multiple doses of the tracer were necessary in some protocols to achieve sufficient initial labeling of body folate to allow appropriate kinetic analysis of its elimination [52]. An alternative technique allows radiologically insignificant doses of ^{14}C-folate (~35 µg, 100 nCi) that are enabled through the high sensitivity of accelerator mass spectrometry (MS) for the measurement of changes over time in ^{14}C content of tracer-derived folates and catabolites in serum, erythrocytes, and excreta [53,54]. Unless coupled with appropriate chromatography to aid in the identification of the various folate species and catabolic products, all techniques for the measurement of ^{3}H or ^{14}C are ambiguous because the identity of the labeled compound(s) is unknown.

The experimental use of folates labeled with the stable isotopes, primarily ^{2}H and ^{13}C, provides a valuable alternative to radiolabeled folate tracers for kinetic studies (for reviews, see Gregory and Quinlivan [7], Pfeiffer and Gregory [55], and Gregory [56]). Essentially all forms of folate can be prepared in [2]H- or [13]C- labeled form (see review, Gregory [56]), and ^{13}C-labeled folic acid and various reduced folates now are available commercially. Aside from obviating concerns about radiochemical use in human subjects, disposal costs and the regulatory issues of radiochemical use also are minimized or eliminated. Quantification in the use of stable isotopically labeled folates relies almost exclusively on mass spectrometric determination of isotopic enrichment of the folates and catabolic products in blood and excreta. Initial investigations with stable isotopically labeled folates were limited by analytical sensitivity and the laborious multistep procedure to prepare samples for gas chromatography/mass spectrometry (GC/ MS) analysis [57], but this method provided a viable approach for many studies of folate bioavailability, metabolism, requirements, and in vivo kinetics largely involving analysis of urinary folates and catabolites [6,58–62]. Modern liquid chromatography/mass spectrometry and tandem mass spectrometry instruments (LC/MS/MS) exhibit lower detection limits and thus extend the range of protocols (e.g., Wright et al. [38,63]).

An analytical principle that must be considered in planning metabolic studies with stable-isotopically labeled folates is that the limit of detection above background enrichment from natural abundance of stable isotopes with typical quadrupole-based mass spectrometric techniques (GC/MS, LC/MS, or LC/MS/MS) is generally no lower than 0.1 to 0.2 mol% excess (i.e., 1–2 labeled molecules/1,000). Considering the fact that kinetic investigations involve the analysis of change of enrichment with time, doses must be used of sufficient quantity or with repeated dosage schedules needed to achieve labeling of folate pools into the reliably measurable range of isotopic enrichment. For this reason, long-term protocols with chronic repeated doses of labeled folate are often advantageous (e.g., Gregory et al. [14], Stites et al. [61], and Caudill et al. [64]). Furthermore, such long-term dosage protocols also can be conducted under steady-state conditions to view the decrease in labeling of folate pools simply by terminating the administration of the labeled folate dose and replacing it with an equivalent unlabeled folate.

Recent data regarding the short-term kinetics of folate absorption and metabolism suggest that much of oral folic acid doses (in the range of several hundred micrograms) enters the portal blood in unreduced form, with metabolic processing in the liver or other tissues [38,63]. The analysis of urinary folates in protocols involving the administration of similar quantities of labeled folic acid has shown no unreduced folic acid [14,64], which indicates that postabsorptive metabolism is rapid and complete in this range. Depending on the objectives of the study, the selection of reduced folates (e.g., 5-methyl-THF or 5-formyl-THF) should be considered for kinetic studies.

B. KNOWLEDGE OF FOLATE METABOLISM DERIVED FROM STUDIES USING FOLATE TRACERS

1. Physiological Aspects

Many studies with radiolabeled folates in animals (e.g., Bhandari and Gregory [65], Lakshmaiah and Bamji [66], Murphy and Scott [67], and Pheasant et al. [68]) and humans (e.g., Russell et al. [51], Krumdieck et al. [52], and Butterworth et al. [69]) have provided evidence for whole-body kinetics that could be described readily by a two-pool kinetic model characterized by fast- and slow-turnover processes (Figure 20.1A). In such a two-pool analysis [65], whole-body retention of the tracer (R_t) could be described by the following equation with two exponential terms: $R_t = A \cdot e^{-\alpha t} + B \cdot e^{-\beta t}$, where t = time after administration of labeled folate, α = first-order rate constant for rapid-turnover phase, β = first-order rate constant for slow-turnover phase, A = content at $t = 0$ of the rapid-turnover pool, and B = content at $t = 0$ of the slow-turnover component.

Although such an analysis has provided a simple working model and initial framework for investigation of in vivo folate processing, this approach is clearly an oversimplification. For example, a protocol that involved long-term administration of ^{2}H-labeled folate along with analysis of folates and folate catabolic products in urine provided unambiguous evidence for the existence of at least three identifiable pools: one rapid turnover and two slow turnover [6]. The existence of more than two pools was shown in this study by differences in profiles of labeling in urinary folates and folate catabolites [6]. A simplified version of this compartmental model is presented in Figure 20.1B. Others have reported a more extensive compartmental model [54] based on data generated using analysis of labeled folate-derived constituents in blood and excreta.

For greatest physiological relevance to whole-body in vivo folate metabolism, a mathematical model should have the following characteristics. First, the mass of folate pools should increase as a nonlinear function of folate intake [70] and not simply expand linearly as a function of intake. The rate of turnover of the various folate pools and whole-body folate also should increase as a function of intake, as seen in human folate kinetics studies [6]. In addition, a realistic model should have provisions for urinary, catabolic, and fecal losses as routes of folate turnover. Finally, the kinetic properties of the various pools of a model should reflect the large disparity in turnover rate and mass between the smaller, kinetically fast pools and the much larger, slower-turnover tissue folate pools. The models developed by Gregory et al. [6] and Lin et al. [54] meet most of these criteria and provide similar overall estimates of systemic folate kinetics despite very different compartmental structures.

The folate pools that exhibit fastest turnover in whole-body kinetic studies typically have half-lives of a few hours or less. Although predicting the anatomical locus of kinetically identifiable pools can be tenuous, it appears likely that the fast-turnover folates are composed mostly of monoglutamyl species primarily in plasma,

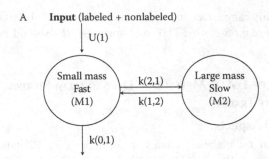

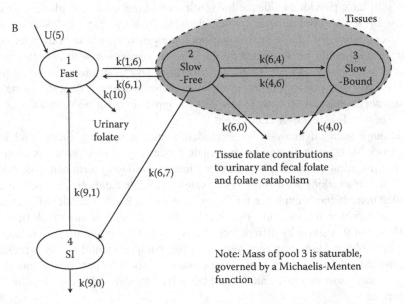

FIGURE 20.1 Compartmental models used in analysis of folate kinetics data. A, two-pool model: first-order outputs nonsaturable. Typical two-pool model composed of a small, fast-turnover compartment and a larger, slow-turnover compartment (e.g., Bhandari and Gregory [65]). B, multicompartmental model of in vivo folate metabolism. Expanded, more physiologically accurate compartmental model consisting of a small, fast-turnover pool, a small, fast-turnover nonsaturable tissue folate pool, and a large, saturable tissue folate pool. The recirculation from tissue pool 6 to pool 1 represents the folate enterohepatic cycle. (B redrawn in simplified form from Gregory JF, Williamson J, Liao JF, Bailey LB, Toth JP, *J Nutr* 1998; 128:1896–906.)

including newly absorbed folate and 5-methyl-THF transported among tissues and perhaps folates involved in enterohepatic circulation. The far slower-turnover folate pools often exhibit half-lives on the order of months and are composed of mostly polyglutamyl folates in tissues. Some of these polyglutamyl folates serve as regulatory molecules tightly bound to enzymes of one-carbon metabolism (e.g., serine hydroxymethyltransferases and glycine *N*-methyltransferase), such that their turnover would be expected to be slow. However, such results also imply that the polyglutamyl folates dynamically involved in one-carbon metabolism also exhibit slow turnover of the folate moieties even though the various one-carbon units undergo biochemical processing and interchange at a much higher rate. Extended in vivo retention undoubtedly is attributable to cellular trapping by polyglutamylation and protein binding. In addition, surprisingly high stability of folates in tissues also may be attributable to effective oxidant defense and protection contributed by protein binding. Tracer studies in rats [65–68] show substantially faster turnover of whole-body folate pools than observed in comparable human studies [6,52,54]; however, the reasons for this discrepancy are unclear.

Tracer studies have identified the urine as the primary excretory route for folate and its catabolic products after administration of the radiolabeled folate dose in rats and humans [52,54,65]. Typically 20% to 30% of the tracer from an administered oral dose of labeled folate appears in the feces, although the chemical identity of the excreted label is unknown. Balance calculations from a metabolic study in young women suggested that fecal excretion approaches 50% of the labeled dose [6]. This hypothesis was based on the observation that the urinary excretion of labeled intact folate plus labeled folate catabolites only accounted for approximately half of the ingested folate. These contradictory findings have not been resolved. Urinary excretion of tracer-derived folates and catabolic products includes intact folate molecules that escape the renal reabsorption mechanism and facile, more extensive urinary excretion of folate catabolites. Quantification of fecal excretion of tissue-derived folates is complicated by the contribution of folate produced by colonic bacteria; thus, balance studies involving the measurement of unlabeled folate and catabolites are not informative. The urinary folate catabolites are formed by cleavage of the C9-N10 bond by nonspecific oxidative cleavage and possibly specific enzymatically mediated processes [71–73] to yield one or more pterins and para-aminobenzoylglutamate (pABG). The latter undergoes extensive acetylation to para-acetamidobenzolyglutamate (ApABG) and is excreted in the urine. The excretion of total pABG (free and acetylated) has been shown to exceed urinary folate and respond weakly to increased folate intake [60,74,75]. However, urinary folate excretion has been shown to be more intake dependent than urinary ApABG [6,60].

The expanded kinetic models described require an estimation of the rate of enterohepatic circulation of folates. Most absorbed folate is extensively recycled by the bile and eventually eliminated in the urine or feces. Bile folate concentration was determined to be 2 to 10 times that of plasma folate after ingestion of 1 mg of ^{3}H-labeled folic acid [76]. The flux of visceral pteroylmonoglutamate to the gastrointestinal tract via bile was estimated to be 5,351 nmol/day in modeling by Lin et al. [54], which was 24 times higher than the 227 nmol/day determined by Herbert [77]. This value was almost 90 times higher than the assumed 60 nmol/day used in modeling by Gregory [6], which was derived from published analyses of bile folate and bile flow rates. In light of the importance of enterohepatic circulation in folate metabolism, these discrepancies should be resolved.

2. Clinical Applications of Folate Kinetics in Human Nutrition

The classic study by Krumdieck et al. [52] was conducted in a human subject who was a Hodgkin's disease patient in remission, with a total of 320 μg (40 μCi) of

[14]C-labeled folic acid administered as four doses in succession. As described earlier in this chapter, the pattern of urinary radioactivity elimination suggested the existence of a short-lived pool ($t_{1/2}$, 31.5 hours) and a long-lived pool ($t_{1/2}$, 100 days). In view of the similarity of these results with those based on other isotopic protocols in humans [6,54,58], it appears that the Hodgkin's disease status had little impact on the results.

A qualitatively similar pattern of urinary excretion was observed by Russell et al. [51], who studied the effects of ethanol on folate kinetics in five patients with chronic alcoholism. Their results differed quantitatively because the subjects were given 5 mg of folic acid daily to increase their folate status before a single dose of ^{3}H-labeled folic acid was administered. Ethanol intake did not affect the half-life of the short-lived pool ($t_{1/2}$, ~9 hours). However, ethanol consumption significantly altered the half-life of the long-lived pool in these subjects with alcoholism, with a half-life of 63.7 days when subjects were consuming ethanol and 9.6 days when subjects abstained from drinking. The mechanism responsible for this unexpected effect is unclear, with interpretation probably complicated by the use of the 5-mg/day flushing dose and effects of alcoholism on its processing.

3. Stable Isotopic Investigations of Folate Kinetics

Although the use of stable isotopes in metabolic studies was pioneered in the early 20th century, their extensive use in folate research did not begin until the advances in MS occurred in the late 1980s. Initial kinetic evaluation of folate metabolism using stable isotope labeling of a folic acid tracer was conducted in normal humans under conditions of long-term folic acid supplementation [62]. In this study, six men were supplemented with 1.6 mg/day [2]H-labeled folic acid for 4 weeks, followed by 3.5 months without supplementation. Urine was collected weekly during supplementation and bimonthly postsupplementation. Using a two-pool model for overall metabolism and distribution of folate, the half-life of the slow-turnover pool was calculated to be 18.7 days. The systemic fractional turnover rate (also termed fractional catabolic rate, which refers to the fraction of the whole-body folate pool that is excreted or catabolized per day) was 0.045 day[-1]; thus, 4.5% of total-body folate was excreted daily in intact or catabolized form. The applicability of these results in predicting folate turnover in nonsupplemented individuals is limited because of the high intake and non–steady-state design.

A much lower folate turnover rate was found when using a more physiological folate intake. Gregory et al. [78] maintained a single female on a controlled diet that consisted of a 2-week equilibration period taking 190 µg/day folic acid, followed by an 8-week administration of 190 µg/day deuterium-labeled folic acid. In this study, the systemic fractional catabolic rate was 0.55% of whole-body folate per day (0.0055 day[-1]). The slow-turnover pool exhibited a half-life of 95 days, in close agreement with the 100 days reported by Krumdieck et al. [52]. This protocol was repeated with four male subjects and extended to 10 weeks. The extended two-pool model includes provisions for folate turnover by urinary intact folate excretion and by fecal excretion and catabolic processes [61]. Two weeks of daily administration of 200 µg of unlabeled folic acid were followed by 8 weeks of 100 µg of unlabeled plus 100 µg/day deuterium-labeled folic acid, then 8 more weeks of 200 µg/day unlabeled folic acid. Based on analysis of urinary folate enrichment alone, this model yielded predictions of total-body folate mass of 59 mg with a systemic fractional catabolic rate of 0.008 day^{-1} (i.e., 0.8%/day).

In an expanded study [14], nonpregnant women ($n = 17$) were maintained on controlled regimens of 200, 300, or 400 µg/day total folate (not converted to DFEs) consumed for 10 weeks. This controlled dietary protocol involved a low-folate basal diet (~30 µg/day from food) plus intake twice daily of supplemental folic acid to achieve the desired total intake, with a portion of the folic acid dose in deuterium-labeled form from weeks 3 to 10 to achieve constant intake of the tracer. Kinetic modeling was based on analysis of isotopic enrichment of urinary folate and the primary folate catabolite ApABG, which led to the development of the compartmental model described earlier (Figure 20.1B). Data from this study were the first to suggest that a 200-µg/day folate intake did not maintain adequate folate status [1]. Systemic fractional catabolic rates were 0.0047 day^{-1}, 0.006 day^{-1}, and 0.008 day^{-1}, and mean residence times for whole-body folate were 212 ± 8, 169 ± 12, and 124 ± 7 days for the intakes of 200, 300, or 400 µg/day folate, respectively. These findings indicated clearly that the rates of folate turnover change markedly with increasing folate intake even within the range of typical dietary intake. It also should be noted that plasma Hcy concentration was increased in subjects consuming the 200-µg/day intake level, which was indicative of suboptimal folate status. However, there was no obvious breakpoint at which folate kinetics changed over the range of adequate to insufficient intakes. This illustrates a limitation of such kinetic analysis; that is, modeling can provide a wealth of quantitative information, but these analyses lack functional evidence regarding nutritional adequacy.

To assess whether folate catabolism and body pools are affected by pregnancy, Caudill et al. [64] conducted a 12-week study of controlled folate intake in second-trimester pregnant women and nonpregnant control subjects. From days 1 to 41 of the study, subjects were given 120 µg/day folate from food plus supplemental folic acid that was 15% labeled, providing a total intake of 450 or 850 µg/day (not converted to DFEs). From days 42 to 84, the folic acid supplements continued but in a totally unlabeled form. The kinetic analysis was based on data obtained following withdrawal of the tracer when conditions approximated a steady state of folate status [58]. Pregnant women exhibited slightly greater whole-body folate pool mass than nonpregnant control subjects when expressed on a total body weight basis or per kilogram of body weight, although the differences did not reach significance (Table 20.1). Also, most aspects of excretion of labeled urinary folate and catabolites did not differ among pregnant women and nonpregnant control subjects [58]. Enrichment data for urinary folate catabolites indicate that pABG is derived from intracellular catabolism rather than being derived from oxidative degradation of urinary folate and that pABG appears to arise from different tissue pools than ApABG and at a different turnover rate [58]. The excretion of intact urinary folate appears to be affected to a greater extent than folate catabolites by folate intake [2,6,58–60,64]. For reasons that remain unclear, these results contrast from those of McPartlin et al. [79,80], who reported greater folate catabolism during pregnancy. Although it was suggested that the difference was the result of analytical issues, this was ruled out in a direct comparative study of blinded urine samples from the study of Caudill

TABLE 20.1

Estimated Body Folate Pool Size in Second-Trimester Pregnant Women and Nonpregnant Controls[a]

Folate Pool Size	Nonpregnant, 450 µg/day Intake	Pregnant, 450 µg/day Intake	Nonpregnant, 850 µg/day Intake	Pregnant, 850 µg/day Intake	Standard Error of Least Square Mean
Total µmol folate	49.5	58.5	69.0	94.0	21.4
µmol folate/kg body weight	0.835	0.955	1.09	1.41	0.344

Source: Adapted from Gregory JF, Caudill MA, Opalko FJ, Bailey LB. *J Nutr* 2001; 131:1928–37. With permission.

[a] Effects of pregnancy status and folate intake were not significant with the limited sample size of this study (*n* = 3 per treatment group). Controlled folate intakes were either 450 or 850 µg/day. Pool sizes are expressed both as total micromole and micromole per kilogram body weight.

et al. [58,81]. A possible explanation was that these studies examined different stages because of differences in defining trimesters of pregnancy [81].

Whole-body folate mass in humans has not been accurately determined, and differences in reported values are caused by differences in estimation methods used, as well as variations in study protocols, assumptions, and kinetic models developed from them. Estimates for the total in vivo folate mass range from about 7.5 to 100 mg (17–225 µmol) [6,54,58,61,82]. In addition, the in vivo pool size associated with adequate nutritional status has not been determined.

All the kinetic data for human folate metabolism reported thus far have been derived using labeled folic acid as the tracer. Although the focus of the preceding discussion has been on long-term folate kinetics relevant to whole-body folate turnover and metabolism, it is important to make a side note regarding short-term folate kinetics. Wright et al. [63] evaluated short-term kinetics of changes in labeled and unlabeled forms of plasma 5-methyl-THF following single $^{13}C_6$-labeled doses of folic acid (*n* = 12) or 5-formyl-THF (*n* = 10) given to fasted subjects. The dose of 5-formyl-THF induced a faster increase in plasma 5-methyl-THF than did folic acid, with strong evidence that most of the metabolic processing of folic acid occurred after intestinal absorption [38,63]. No tracer studies have compared long-term kinetics of different folate forms in humans. However, short-term studies in folate-pretreated humans compared various deuterium-labeled folate forms at doses similar to those used by Wright et al. [63]. The studies by Wright et al. [38,63] confirmed the previously reported evidence of different in vivo processing of folic acid compared with reduced folates in response to doses of several hundred micrograms [83]. In contrast, the rat study by Bhandari and Gregory [65] compared very small tracer doses of ^3H-labeled folic acid, [6S]-5-methyl-THF, and [6S]-5-formyl-THF and showed identical intestinal absorption, in vivo distribution, and whole-body kinetics.

IV. MATHEMATICAL MODELS OF ONE-CARBON METABOLISM

A major current research focus concerning folate nutrition and metabolism is the application of modeling and related tracer kinetics to clarify and extend our knowledge of the functional aspects of folate-dependent one-carbon metabolism and to clarify the influence of genetic and nutritional variables. Mathematical models provide a description that allows simulation of the dynamic biological systems, which permits investigators to modify variables and predict the effects on the system. Mathematical models of complex systems such as folate-dependent one-carbon metabolism are especially useful in identifying specific interactions that are worth investigating in vivo, generating hypotheses for experimental testing, and conducting "in silico" experiments that cannot otherwise be performed.

Folate is vital to one-carbon metabolism by facilitating the delivery of one-carbon units into biochemical reactions related to methylation, amino acid metabolism, and nucleotide synthesis. Folate-mediated one-carbon metabolism is characterized by several interconnected cycles and is involved in the etiology of several diseases, such as NTDs, several forms of cancer, and cardiovascular disease [84]. The modeling of this complex system can help elucidate how dietary and genetic factors can influence health and the risk of disease. Such modeling also is an important tool in evaluating nutritional interrelationships affecting folate-dependent one-carbon metabolism, including effects of methionine intake, and nutritional status with respect to other vitamins, such as B6, B12, and riboflavin.

An early attempt to use a mathematical model to better understand cellular folate metabolism was made by Jackson and Harrap in 1973 [85]. This model was based on data derived from studies with L1210 mouse leukemia cells and included enzyme kinetic parameters and cellular substrate and cofactor concentrations. One outcome predicted by the model was a lack of changes in flux through rate-limiting reactions after partial inhibition of dihydrofolate reductase (DHFR).

Several other mathematical models were subsequently developed that focused mostly on the effects and interactions of antifolate drugs [86–90]. Additional modeling permitted investigation of regulatory events in methionine metabolism [91,92]. Another model of the cytosolic folate cycle [93], based on biochemical properties of the various enzymes, led to predictions that closely corresponded to properties of folate metabolism derived experimentally. For example, the predicted half-life of 89 days of the slow-turnover folate pool agrees with the approximately 100 days calculated after tracer studies [52,78]. The cytosolic folate cycle model also determined that variation in enzyme parameters mainly affected only local velocities and pool sizes. For example, the model showed that very extensive variation of the activities of thymidylate synthase and DHFR had little effect on the rest of folate metabolism [93].

The model for the folate cycle was expanded and combined with one developed for the methionine cycle [94]. This approach resulted in a mathematical model of the complete cytosolic folate-mediated one-carbon metabolism, which included expanded examination of both the roles of folate substrate concentration and that of allosteric regulation [95]. The predictions made with the expanded model agreed with experimental data. For example, the inverse association between folate and

Hcy was greatest at very low folate levels, whereas at high folate concentration no association was seen. Changes in folate pool size did not affect DNA methylation reaction rates to a great extent; however, at very high folate concentrations, enzyme velocities were shown to decrease as a result of the regulatory role of folate binding to enzymes such as serine hydroxymethyltransferase, glycine N-methyltransferase, and MTHFR [95].

The combined mathematical model described above was further extended to account for mitochondrial in addition to cytosolic one-carbon metabolism [96]. Changes include the addition of mitochondrial folate substrates and enzymes, as well as sarcosine and dimethylglycine. The addition of the folate mitochondrial cycle allowed investigators to examine the contribution of mitochondrial reactions to overall one-carbon metabolism. When all mitochondrial reactions were eliminated (by setting their velocities to zero), the levels of S-adenosylmethionine and methionine showed no great change; in fact, most of the methionine cycle was unaffected. However, eliminating mitochondrial reactions did have a major effect on the rates of thymidylate and purine synthesis, both of which decreased. This model also yielded the unexpected prediction that the mitochondrial glycine cleavage system is a major source of one-carbon units entering folate-dependent one-carbon metabolism as 5,10-methylene-THF.

Another aspect of one-carbon metabolism research in which mathematical models can be particularly useful is in providing preliminary predictions of the effects of genetic polymorphisms on disease risk biomarkers. Polymorphisms that have not been well defined can be examined under simulated effects of normal and low folate status. To that end, Ulrich et al. [97] used the model developed by Reed et al. [95] to investigate the predicted effect of known and potential polymorphisms in folate-mediated one-carbon metabolism. The functional effect of hypothetical polymorphisms on genes of other one-carbon metabolism enzymes was predicted by increasing activity by 50% or decreasing by 40% or 70% compared with wild type (100%). All predictions were modeled both at normal/high and low folate status. Modeled predictions of polymorphisms in MTHFR and thymidylate synthase were consistent with published data. Overall the model reflected the robustness of one-carbon metabolism toward variation in single-enzyme function. It did, nonetheless, predict sites where polymorphisms might have a stronger effect, such as 10-formyltetrahydrofolate dehydrogenase, 10-formyltetrahydrofolate synthase, 5,10-methenyltetrahydrofolate cyclohydrolase, and methionine synthase (MS) reductase, whose changed activity, especially at low folate status, affected nucleotide synthesis [97].

In conclusion, mathematical models of folate-mediated one-carbon metabolism are powerful tools in predicting effects of variations in nutritional and genetic factors on mechanisms relevant to disease risk. They allow investigators to pinpoint areas of relevance and facilitate the development of hypotheses in the design of in vivo studies.

V. STABLE ISOTOPE TRACER STUDIES FOR QUANTIFICATION OF THE FOLATE-DEPENDENT ONE-CARBON METABOLISM

The pioneering isotope studies of Vernon Young's laboratory provided the conceptual framework for the quantification of the folate-dependent methionine cycle in humans

[98,99]. Vernon Young was a leading scientist in the research and assessment of protein and amino acid requirements using stable isotope tracer techniques [100]. The tracer model his group designed for quantification of multiple aspects of methionine metabolism uses differently labeled methionine isotopomers, either as individual tracers [methyl-$^2H_3$]methionine and [1-^{13}C]methionine [98] or as dual tracer [1-^{13}C; methyl-$^2H_3$]methionine [98,99]. The loss of enrichment of the methyl label relative to the carboxyl label is an index for the recycling of the methionine molecule in the reaction of Hcy remethylation. The dual tracer protocol allows quantification of whole-body methyl-labeled methionine flux (Q_m) and whole-body carboxyl-labeled methionine flux (Q_c). The difference between the fluxes provides direct measurement of the remethylation flux (RM = $Q_m - Q_c$) [98]. The only outflow of the carboxyl label is via transsulfuration, the irreversible breakdown of Hcy to cysteine, the oxidation of which can be quantified by measuring breath $^{13}CO_2$ enrichment. This process has been loosely termed as methionine oxidation. The transmethylation rate, i.e., the rate of transfer of the methionine methyl group (as S-adenosylmethionine) to a one-carbon acceptor, is the sum of the remethylation and the transsulfuration rates accounting for both possible fates of Hcy after transmethylation [98]. Further, this protocol allows quantification of the disappearance of methionine into protein synthesis and its appearance from protein breakdown [98]. In this tracer model, the remethylation flux is an aggregate of reactions catalyzed by MS (i.e., folate- and vitamin B12–dependent remethylation) and that catalyzed by betaine-Hcy methyltransferase (i.e., independent of both folate and vitamin B12).

With the use of this novel tracer model, Hcy remethylation was three times greater at fed state (5.7 μmol·kg^{-1}·h^{-1}) compared with postabsorptive state (1.8 μmol·kg^{-1}·h^{-1}) in healthy young men [98]. As shown later by others, remethylation in healthy humans under normal nutritional conditions primarily occurs by the vitamin-dependent MS process [101,102]. The transsulfuration rate was 8.3 μmol·kg^{-1}·h^{-1} at fed state and half that at fasting state [98]. The transmethylation rate was 14 μmol·kg^{-1}·h^{-1} in the fed state and accounted for 35% of whole-body methionine flux [98].

Further studies of Young's laboratory used this dual methionine tracer approach for assessment of the methionine-sparing effect by cysteine [99,103], methionine requirement [104,105], and the usage of cysteine as a marker of sulfur amino acid loss [106]. Van Guldener et al. [107] performed the dual tracer protocol in patients with end-stage renal disease of which most develop hyperhomocysteinemia. Although the transsulfuration rate was unaffected, patients with end-stage renal disease showed a 30% lower Hcy remethylation and 24% lower transmethylation rate than healthy control subjects [107].

Most tracer protocols provide the tracer(s) intravenously, with relatively few using oral administration. Storch et al. [108] investigated the effect of supplementation of betaine, a one-carbon donor, on dynamics of methionine metabolism with the use of the dual tracer method. For example, Storch et al. [108] found that 3 g/day of betaine supplementation had no effect on the methionine cycle as assessed with intravenous methionine tracers; however, the betaine supplement yielded significantly higher trans-sulfuration and transmethylation rate as determined using oral methionine tracers in healthy young men. This observation can be explained by the organ-specific distribution of betaine Hcy methyltransferase, which has its main activity in the liver.

The dual tracer protocol for quantification of the methionine cycle was improved by MacCoss et al. [109]. Storch et al. [98] measured plasma methionine enrichment for estimation of whole-body methionine flux and corrected it for an assumed intracellular dilution by 20%. Alternatively, MacCoss et al. [109] used plasma Hcy enrichment as a more direct surrogate marker of intracellular methionine enrichment.

To date, no direct application of the dual methionine tracer model has been reported for determination of the folate dependence of the methionine cycle, but variations have been used. The impact of folate deficiency on methionine kinetics was investigated by Cuskelly et al. [110]. Instead of the dual methionine tracer, [1-^{13}C] methionine and [2,3,3-^{2}H$_3$]serine were used for quantification of the remethylation rate in vivo [110,111]. Subjects were in adequate nutritional status or were deficient in folate or vitamin B6. Hcy remethylation from serine-derived one-carbon units was 39% lower in folate deficiency compared with adequate status under the conditions of this study. Davis et al. [101,102,112] used a fully labeled methionine tracer, [U-^{13}C]methionine, in conjunction with [3-^{13}C]serine for quantification of the folate-dependent remethylation and the Hcy synthesis rate in vivo. This approach showed that serine is the main one-carbon donor for folate-dependent Hcy remethylation [102]. Most one-carbon units for serine synthesis recently were shown to derive from glycine cleavage [113], confirming a prediction from mathematical modeling mentioned previously. The impact of folate on remethylation and Hcy synthesis rates was determined before and after subjects underwent a dietary folate restriction [112]. In the absence of dietary methionine intake, total remethylation flux was unaffected by dietary folate restriction or *MTHFR* 677C→T polymorphism [112]. This indicates that, even in folate deficiency, there is enough folate for the metabolic processes of the folate-dependent enzymes serine hydroxymethyltransferase, MTHFR, and MS. This study also showed that the mild homocysteinemia from folate deficiency is attributable to greater production of Hcy, rather than the previously hypothesized impairment in remethylation [112]. This appears to be because folate depletion relieves the inhibition of glycine *N*-methyltransferase by 5-methyl-THF that leads to greater utilization of *S*-adenosylmethionine, ultimately yielding more Hcy.

Besides Hcy remethylation, folate serves as a one-carbon carrier for the synthesis of nucleotides and for cellular methylation reactions. Another aspect of the Davis et al. study [112] was the examination of nucleotide metabolism [114]. Based on analysis of labeling of monocyte DNA, the results suggested that moderate folate deficiency did not significantly affect purine or thymidylate synthesis but that the *MTHFR* 677TT genotype favored greater synthesis of thymidylate [114].

The interactive effects of vitamin B6 status on folate-dependent one-carbon metabolism have also been investigated because of the role of pyridoxal 5′-phosphate as coenzyme in cystathionine-β-synthase (CBS), cystathionine-γ-lyase, serine hydroxymethyltransferase, and glycine decarboxylase in the mitochondrial glycine cleavage system. Stable isotope tracer studies revealed that Hcy remethylation rate was only slightly and nonsignificantly depressed by vitamin B6 deficiency [101,110]. Vitamin B6 deficiency tended to increase the cytosolic synthesis of methionine (i.e., by Hcy remethylation) from serine [110], which may be caused by the increased serine synthesis from glycine in marginal vitamin B6 deficiency [115]. Glycine concentrations increase during vitamin B6 deficiency [101,115,116] possibly because of reduced activity of the glycine cleavage system. Despite the reduced maximum velocity of serine hydroxymethyltransferase at vitamin B6 deficiency as measured in vitro [101], the in vivo flux of serine hydroxymethyltransferase is unaltered in vitamin B6 deficiency as a result of compensation by high substrate concentration. A major function of serine hydroxymethyltransferase is to balance glycine and serine concentrations. At increased glycine concentrations, more serine is formed via serine hydroxymethyltransferase, which may help maintaining remethylation during vitamin B6 deficiency.

Vitamin B6 functions as coenzyme in the transsulfuration pathway, i.e., the formation of cystathionine and cysteine from Hcy. Vitamin B6 deficiency increased plasma cystathionine concentration but did not influence plasma total Hcy concentration [101,115,117]. The fractional synthesis rate of cystathionine was unchanged, which indicated that CBS is less sensitive to vitamin B6 deficiency than cystathionine-γ-lyase [117] as seen in rat studies [118]. Also plasma cysteine concentrations and in vivo cysteine flux were unchanged after dietary vitamin B6 restriction [117] as a result of the cystathionine-γ-lyase reaction being maintained by the increase in cystathionine concentration to sustain cysteine production in all but very severe vitamin B6 deficiency. The effects of other relevant micronutrients on the in vivo function of one-carbon metabolic processes have not been examined.

VI. CONCLUSIONS

As discussed in this chapter, studies of in vivo kinetics provide a wealth of information pertaining to the metabolism of folate and its role in one-carbon metabolism. Kinetic analyses range from in vivo studies of folate and one-carbon metabolism to hypothesis generation through mathematical modeling. Such modeling can be based on fitting to experimental data or construction of a model using kinetic parameters of the biochemical processes involved. All these approaches have contributed extensively to our understanding of folate kinetics and constitute important research tools. The development of kinetically based diagnostic procedures also is likely to occur.

REFERENCES

1. O'Keefe CA, Bailey LB, Thomas EA, Hofler SA, Davis BA, Cerda JJ, Gregory JF. Controlled dietary folate affects folate status in nonpregnant women. *J Nutr* 1995; 125:2717–25.
2. Caudill MA, Cruz AC, Gregory JF, Hutson AD, Bailey LB. Folate status response to controlled folate intake in pregnant women. *J Nutr* 1997; 127:2363–70.
3. Kauwell GP, Lippert BL, Wilsky CE, Herrlinger-Garcia K, Hutson AD, Theriaque DW, Rampersaud GC, Cerda JJ, Bailey LB. Folate status of elderly women following moderate folate depletion responds only to a higher folate intake. *J Nutr* 2000; 130:1584–90.
4. Shelnutt KP, Kauwell GP, Chapman CM, Gregory JF 3rd, Maneval DR, Browdy AA, Theriaque DW, Bailey LB. Folate status response to controlled folate intake is affected by the methylenetetrahydrofolate reductase 677C-->T polymorphism in young women. *J Nutr* 2003; 133:4107–11.
5. Perry CA, Renna SA, Khitun E, Ortiz M, Moriarty DJ, Caudill MA. Ethnicity and race influence the folate status response to controlled folate intakes in young women. *J Nutr* 2004; 134:1786–92.

6. Gregory JF, Williamson J, Liao JF, Bailey LB, Toth JP. Kinetic model of folate metabolism in nonpregnant women consuming [²H₂]folic acid: Isotopic labeling of urinary folate and the catabolite para-acetamidobenzoylglutamate indicates slow, intake-dependent, turnover of folate pools. *J Nutr* 1998; 128:1896–906.

7. Gregory JF, Quinlivan EP. In vivo kinetics of folate metabolism. *Annu Rev Nutr* 2002; 22:199–220.

8. Anderson JH, Kerr DJ, Setanoians A, Cooke TG, McArdle CS. A pharmacokinetic comparison of intravenous versus intra-arterial folinic acid. *Br J Cancer* 1992; 65:133–35.

9. Bunni MA, Rembiesa BM, Priest DG, Sahovic E, Stuart R. Accumulation of tetrahydrofolates in human plasma after leucovorin administration. *Cancer Chemother Pharmacol* 1989; 23:353–57.

10. DeVito JM, Kozloski GD, Tonelli AP, Johnson JB. Bioequivalence of oral and injectable levoleucovorin and leucovorin. *Clin Pharm* 1993; 12:293–99.

11. Priest DG, Schmitz JC, Bunni MA, Stuart RK. Pharmacokinetics of leucovorin metabolites in human plasma as a function of dose administered orally and intravenously. *J Natl Cancer Inst* 1991; 83:1806–12.

12. Chanarin I, Mollin DL, Anderson BB. The clearance from the plasma of folic acid injected intravenously in normal subjects and patients with megaloblastic anaemia. *Br J Haematol* 1958; 4:435–46.

13. Metz J, Stevens K, Krawitz S, Brandt V. The plasma clearance of injected doses of folic acid as an index of folic acid deficiency. *J Clin Pathol* 1961; 14:622–25.

14. Gregory JF, Williamson J, Bailey LB, Toth JP. Urinary excretion of [²H₄]folate by nonpregnant women following a single oral dose of [²H₄]folic acid is a functional index of folate nutritional status. *J Nutr* 1998; 128:1907–12.

15. Schalhorn A, Kuhl M, Stupp-Poutot G, Nussler V. Pharmacokinetics of reduced folates after short-term infusion of d, 1-folinic acid. *Cancer Chemother Pharmacol* 1990; 25:440–44.

16. Quinlivan EP, Gregory JF 3rd. Reassessing folic acid consumption patterns in the United States (1999–2004): Potential effect on neural tube defects and overexposure to folate. *Am J Clin Nutr* 2007; 86:1773–79.

17. Quinlivan EP, Gregory JF 3rd. Effect of food fortification on folic acid intake in the United States. *Am J Clin Nutr* 2003; 77:221–25.

18. Wald DS, Bishop L, Wald NJ, Law M, Hennessy E, Weir D, McPartlin J, Scott J. Randomized trial of folic acid supplementation and serum homocysteine levels. *Arch Intern Med* 2001; 161:695–700.

19. van Oort FV, Melse-Boonstra A, Brouwer IA, Clarke R, West CE, Katan MB, Verhoef P. Folic acid and reduction of plasma homocysteine concentrations in older adults: A dose-response study. *Am J Clin Nutr* 2003; 77:1318–23.

20. Daly S, Mills JL, Molloy AM, Conley M, Lee YJ, Kirke PN, Weir DG, Scott JM. Minimum effective dose of folic acid for food fortification to prevent neural-tube defects. *Lancet* 1997; 350:1666–69.

21. Carrero JJ, Lopez-Huertas E, Salmeron LM, Baro L, Ros E. Daily supplementation with (n-3) PUFAs, oleic acid, folic acid, and vitamins B-6 and E increases pain-free walking distance and improves risk factors in men with peripheral vascular disease. *J Nutr* 2005; 135:1393–99.

22. Lamers Y, Prinz-Langenohl R, Bramswig S, Pietrzik K. Red blood cell folate concentrations increase more after supplementation with [6S]-5-methyltetrahydrofolate than with folic acid in women of childbearing age. *Am J Clin Nutr* 2006; 84:156–61.

23. Venn BJ, Green TJ, Moser R, McKenzie JE, Skeaff CM, Mann J. Increases in blood folate indices are similar in women of childbearing age supplemented with [6S]-5-methyltetrahydrofolate and folic acid. *J Nutr* 2002; 132:3353–55.

24. Hao L, Yang QH, Li Z, Bailey LB, Zhu JH, Hu DJ, Zhang BL, et al. Folate status and homocysteine response to folic acid doses and withdrawal among young Chinese women in a large-scale randomized double-blind trial. *Am J Clin Nutr* 2008; 88:448–57.

25. Shane B. Folate chemistry and metabolism. In: Bailey LB, ed., *Folate in Health and Disease*. New York: Marcel Dekker, 1995:1–22.

26. Pietrzik K, Lamers Y, Bramswig S, Prinz-Langenohl R. Calculation of red blood cell folate steady state conditions and elimination kinetics after daily supplementation with various folate forms and doses in women of childbearing age. *Am J Clin Nutr* 2007; 86:1414–19.

27. Ward M, McNulty H, McPartlin JM, Strum WB, Weir DG, Scott JM. Plasma homocysteine, a risk factor for cardiovascular disease, is lowered by physiological doses of folic acid. *Q J Med* 1997; 90:519–24.

28. Yang TL, Hung J, Caudill MA, Urrutia TF, Alamilla A, Perry CA, Li R, Hata H, Cogger EA. A long-term controlled folate feeding study in young women supports the validity of the 1.7 multiplier in the dietary folate equivalency equation. *J Nutr* 2005; 135:1139–45.

29. Homocysteine Lowering Trialist's Collaboration. Dose-dependent effects of folic acid on blood homocysteine concentrations: A meta-analysis of the randomized trials. *Am J Clin Nutr* 2005; 82:806–12.

30. Neal B, MacMahon S, Ohkubo T, Tonkin A, Wilcken D. Dose-dependent effects of folic acid on plasma homocysteine in a randomized trial conducted among 723 individuals with coronary heart disease. *Eur Heart J* 2002; 23:1509–15.

31. Jacques PF, Bostom AG, Wilson PW, Rich S, Rosenberg IH, Selhub J. Determinants of plasma total homocysteine concentration in the Framingham Offspring cohort. *Am J Clin Nutr* 2001; 73:613–21.

32. Nygard O, Refsum H, Ueland PM, Vollset SE. Major lifestyle determinants of plasma total homocysteine distribution: The Hordaland Homocysteine Study. *Am J Clin Nutr* 1998; 67:263–70.

33. Fohr IP, Prinz-Langenohl R, Brönstrup A, Bohlmann AM, Nau H, Berthold HK, Pietrzik K. 5,10-Methylenetetrahydrofolate reductase genotype determines the plasma homocysteine-lowering effect of supplementation with 5-methyltetrahydrofolate or folic acid in healthy young women. *Am J Clin Nutr* 2002; 75:275–82.

34. Lamers Y, Prinz-Langenohl R, Moser R, Pietrzik K. Supplementation with [6S]-5-meth-yltetrahydrofolate or folic acid equally reduces plasma total homocysteine concentrations in healthy women. *Am J Clin Nutr* 2004; 79:473–78.

35. Norsworthy B, Skeaff CM, Adank C, Green TJ. Effects of once-a-week or daily folic acid supplementation on red blood cell folate concentrations in women. *Eur J Clin Nutr* 2004; 58:548–54.

36. Melikian V, Paton A, Leeming RJ, Portman-Graham H. Site of reduction and methylation of folic acid in man. *Lancet* 1971; 2:955–57.

37. Whitehead VM, Cooper BA. Absorption of unaltered folic acid from the gastro-intestinal tract in man. *Br J Haematol* 1967; 13:679–86.

38. Wright AJA, Finglas PM, Dainty JR, Wolfe CA, Hart DJ, Wright DM, Gregory JF. Differential kinetic behavior and distribution for pteroylglutamic acid and reduced folates: A revised hypothesis of the primary site of PteGlu metabolism in humans. *J Nutr* 2005; 135:619–23.

39. Kelly P, McPartlin J, Goggins M, Weir DG, Scott JM. Unmetabolized folic acid in serum: Acute studies in subjects consuming fortified food and supplements. *Am J Clin Nutr* 1997; 65:1790–95.

40. Leeming RJ, Portman-Graham H, Blair JA. The occurrence of folic acid (pteroyl-L-monoglutamic acid) in human blood serum after small oral doses. *J Clin Pathol* 1972; 25:491–93.

41. Pfeiffer CM, Fazili Z, McCoy L, Zhang M, Gunter EW. Determination of folate vitamers in human serum by stable-isotope-dilution tandem mass spectrometry and comparison with radioassay and microbiologic assay. *Clin Chem* 2004; 50:423–32.
42. Kalmbach RD, Choumenkovitch SF, Troen AM, D'Agostino R, Jacques PF, Selhub J. Circulating folic acid in plasma: Relation to folic acid fortification. *Am J Clin Nutr* 2008; 88:763–68.
43. Smith AD, Kim YI, Refsum H. Is folic acid good for everyone? *Am J Clin Nutr* 2008; 87:517–33.
44. Pentieva K, McNulty H, Reichert R, Ward M, Strain JJ, McKillop DJ, McPartlin JM, et al. The short-term bioavailabilities of [6S]-5-methyltetrahydrofolate and folic acid are equivalent in men. *J Nutr* 2004; 134:580–85.
45. Prinz-Langenohl R, Fohr I, Tobolski O, Finglas P, Pietrzik K. Bioavailability of (6S)-5-methyltetrahydrofolate relative to folic acid. *Bioavailability 2001*, Interlaken, Switzerland. Berlin/Heidelberg: Springer, 2001.
46. Houghton LA, Sherwood KL, Pawlosky R, Ito S, O'Connor DL. [6S]-5-Methyltetrahydrofolate is at least as effective as folic acid in preventing a decline in blood folate concentrations during lactation. *Am J Clin Nutr* 2006; 83:842–50.
47. Venn BJ, Green TJ, Moser R, Mann JI. Comparison of the effect of low-dose supplementation with L-5-methyltetrahydrofolate or folic acid on plasma homocysteine: A randomized placebo-controlled study. *Am J Clin Nutr* 2003; 77:658–62.
48. Bostom AG, Shemin D, Bagley P, Massy ZA, Zanabli A, Christopher K, Spiegel P, Jacques PF, Dworkin L, Selhub J. Controlled comparison of L-5-methyltetrahydrofolate versus folic acid for the treatment of hyperhomocysteinemia in hemodialysis patients. *Circulation* 2000; 101:2829–32.
49. Mader RM, Steger GG, Rizovski B, Djavanmard MP, Scheithauer W, Jakesz R, Rainer H. Stereospecific pharmacokinetics of rac-5-methyltetrahydrofolic acid in patients with advanced colorectal cancer. *Br J Clin Pharmacol* 1995; 40:209–15.
50. Willems FF, Boers GH, Blom HJ, Aengevaeren WR, Verheugt FW. Pharmacokinetic study on the utilisation of 5-methyltetrahydrofolate and folic acid in patients with coronary artery disease. *Br J Pharmacol* 2004; 141:825–30.
51. Russell RM, Rosenberg IH, Wilson PD, Iber FL, Oaks EB, Giovetti AC, Otradovec CL, Karwoski PA, Press AW. Increased urinary excretion and prolonged turnover time of folic acid during ethanol ingestion. *Am J Clin Nutr* 1983; 38:64–70.
52. Krumdieck CL, Fukushima K, Fukushima T, Shiota T, Butterworth CE. Long-term study of excretion of folate and pterins in a human subject after ingestion of C-14 folic acid, with observations on effect of diphenylhydantoin administration. *Am J Clin Nutr* 1978; 31:88–93.
53. Buchholz BA, Arjomand A, Dueker SR, Schneider PD, Clifford AJ, Vogel JS. Intrinsic erythrocyte labeling and attomole pharmacokinetic tracing of C-14-labeled folic acid with accelerator mass spectrometry. *Anal Biochem* 1999; 269:348–52.
54. Lin YM, Dueker SR, Follett JR, Fadel JG, Arjomand A, Schneider PD, Miller JW, et al. Quantitation of in vivo human folate metabolism. *Am J Clin Nutr* 2004; 80:680–91.
55. Pfeiffer CM, Gregory JF. Preparation of stable isotopically labeled folates for in vivo investigation of folate absorption and metabolism. *Methods Enzymol* 1997; 281:106–16.
56. Gregory JF. Stable isotopic tracers for studies of folate bioavailability and metabolism: Development, principles and applications. In: G. Jansen, ed., *Symposia Proceedings—Chemistry and Biology of Pteridines and Folates*. Heilbronn, Germany: SPS Publications, 2007:566–83.
57. Gregory JF, Toth JP. Chemical synthesis of deuterated folate monoglutamate and in vivo assessment of urinary excretion of deuterated folates in man. *Anal Biochem* 1988; 170:94–104.

58. Gregory JF, Caudill MA, Opalko FJ, Bailey LB. Kinetics of folate turnover in pregnant women (second trimester) and nonpregnant controls during folic acid supplementation: Stable-isotopic labeling of plasma folate, urinary folate and folate catabolites shows subtle effects of pregnancy on turnover of folate pools. *J Nutr* 2001; 131:1928–37.

59. Gregory JF, Swendseid ME, Jacob RA. Urinary excretion of folate catabolites responds to changes in folate intake more slowly than plasma folate and homocysteine concentrations and lymphocyte DNA methylation in postmenopausal women. *J Nutr* 2000; 130:2949–52.

60. Kownacki-Brown PA, Wang CZ, Bailey LB, Toth JP, Gregory JF. Urinary excretion of deuterium-labeled folate and the metabolite p-aminobenzoylglutamate in humans. *J Nutr* 1993; 123:1101–08.

61. Stites TE, Bailey LB, Scott KC, Toth JP, Fisher WP, Gregory JF. Kinetic modeling of folate metabolism through use of chronic administration of deuterium-labeled folic acid in men. *Am J Clin Nutr* 1997; 65:53–60.

62. von der Porten AE, Gregory JF, Toth JP, Cerda JJ, Curry SH, Bailey LB. In vivo folate kinetics during chronic supplementation of human subjects with deuterium-labeled folic acid. *J Nutr* 1992; 122:1293–99.

63. Wright AJA, Finglas PM, Dainty JR, Hart DJ, Wolfe CA, Southon S, Gregory JF. Single oral doses of C-13 forms of pteroylmonoglutamic acid and 5-formyltetrahydrofolic acid elicit differences in short-term kinetics of labelled and unlabelled folates in plasma: Potential problems in interpretation of folate bioavailability studies. *Br J Nutr* 2003; 90:363–71.

64. Caudill MA, Gregory JF, Hutson AD, Bailey LB. Folate catabolism in pregnant and nonpregnant women with controlled folate intakes. *J Nutr* 1998; 128:204–08.

65. Bhandari SD, Gregory JF. Folic acid, 5-methyltetrahydrofolate and 5-formyltetrahydrofolate exhibit equivalent intestinal absorption, metabolism and in vivo kinetics in rats. *J Nutr* 1992; 122:1847–54.

66. Lakshmaiah N, Bamji MS. Half-life and metabolism of H-3-folic acid in oral contraceptive treated rats. *Horm Metab Res* 1981; 13:404–07.

67. Murphy M, Scott JM. Turnover catabolism and excretion of folate administered at physiological concentrations in the rat. *Biochim Biophys Acta* 1979; 583:535–39.

68. Pheasant AE, Connor MJ, Blair JA. The metabolism and physiological disposition of radioactively labeled folate derivatives in the rat. *Biochem Med* 1981; 26:435–50.

69. Butterworth CE, Baugh CM, Krumdieck C. A study of folate absorption and metabolism in man utilizing carbon-14-labeled polyglutamates synthesized by solid phase method. *J Clin Invest* 1969; 48:1131–42.

70. Clifford AJ, Heid MK, Muller HG, Bills ND. Tissue distribution and prediction of total-body folate of rats. *J Nutr* 1990; 120:1633–39.

71. Anguera MC, Stover PJ. Identification of an enzymatic folate degradation pathway. *FASEB J* 2001;15:A955.

72. Suh JR, Herbig AK, Stover PJ. New perspectives on folate catabolism. *Annu Rev Nutr* 2001; 21:255–82.

73. Anguera MC, Stover PJ. Methenyltetrahydrofolate synthetase is a high-affinity catecholamine-binding protein. *Arch Biochem Biophys* 2006; 455:175–87.

74. McPartlin J, Courtney G, McNulty H, Weir D, Scott J. The quantitative analysis of endogenous folate catabolites in human urine. *Anal Biochem* 1992; 206:256–61.

75. McPartlin JM, Weir DG, Courtney G, McNulty H, Scott JM. The level of folate catabolism in normal human populations. In: Cooper B, Whitehead V, eds., *Pteridines and Folic Acid Derivatives*. New York: de Gruyer, 1986: 513–16.

76. Pratt RF, Cooper BA. Folates in plasma and bile of man after feeding folic acid—H3 and 5-formyltetrahydrofolate (folinic acid). *J Clin Invest* 1971; 50:455–62.

77. Herbert V, Zalusky R. Interrelations of vitamin B12 and folic acid metabolism—Folic acid clearance studies. *J Clin Invest* 1962; 41:1263–76.

78. Gregory JF, Bailey LB, Thomas EA, Toth JP, Cerda JJ, Fisher WR. Stable-isotope study of long-term folate metabolism in a human subject. *FASEB J* 1994; 8:A920.
79. McPartlin J, Halligan A, Scott JM, Darling M, Weir DG. Accelerated folate breakdown in pregnancy. *Lancet* 1993; 341:148–49.
80. Higgins JR, Quinlivan EP, McPartlin J, Scott JM, Weir DG, Darling MRN. The relationship between increased folate catabolism and the increased requirement for folate in pregnancy. *BJOG* 2000; 107:1149–54.
81. Bailey LB, Gregory JF, Caudill M, Cruz A. The relationship between increased folate stetabolism and the increased requirement for folate in pregnancy. *BJOG* 2001; 108:772–73.
82. Herbert V. Recommended dietary intakes (RDI) of folate in humans. *Am J Clin Nutr* 1987; 45:661–70.
83. Gregory JF, Bhandari SD, Bailey LB, Toth JP, Baumgartner TG, Cerda JJ. Relative bioavailability of deuterium-labeled monoglutamyl tetrahydrofolates and folic acid in human subjects. *Am J Clin Nutr* 1992; 55:1147–53.
84. Lucock M. Folic acid: Nutritional biochemistry, molecular biology, and role in disease processes. *Mol Genet Metab* 2000; 71:121–38.
85. Jackson RC, Harrap KR. Studies with a mathematical-model of folate metabolism. *Arch Biochem Biophys* 1973; 158:827–41.
86. Jackson RC. Kinetic simulation of anti-cancer drug-interactions. *Int J Biomed Comput* 1980; 11:197–224.
87. Jackson RC. Toxicity prediction from metabolic pathway modeling. *Toxicology* 1995; 102:197–205.
88. Jackson RC, Harrap KR. Computer models of anti-cancer drug interaction. *Pharmacol Ther* 1979; 4:245–80.
89. Seither RL, Trent DF, Mikulecky DC, Rape TJ, Goldman ID. Folate pool interconversions and inhibition of biosynthetic processes after exposure of L1210 leukemia-cells to antifolates—Experimental and network thermodynamic analyses of the role of dihdydrofolate polyglutamylates in antifolate action in cell. *J Biol Chem* 1989; 264:17016–23.
90. White JC. Reversal of methotrexate binding to dihydrofolate reductase by dihydrofolate—Studies with pure enzyme and computer modeling using network thermodynamics. *J Biol Chem* 1979; 254:889–95.
91. Martinov MV, Vitvitsky VM, Mosharov EV, Banerjee R, Ataullakhanov FI. A substrate switch: A new mode of regulation in the methionine metabolic pathway. *J Theor Biol* 2000; 204:521–32.
92. Prudova A, Martinov MV, Vitvitsky VM, Ataullakhanov FI, Banerjee R. Analysis of pathological defects in methionine metabolism using a simple mathematical model. *Biochim Biophys Acta* 2005; 1741:331–38.
93. Nijhout HF, Reed MC, Budu P, Ulrich CM. A mathematical model of the folate cycle: New insights into folate homeostasis. *J Biol Chem* 2004; 279:55008–16.
94. Reed MC, Nijhout HF, Sparks R, Ulrich CM. A mathematical model of the methionine cycle. *J Theor Biol* 2004; 226:33–43.
95. Reed MC, Nijhout HF, Neuhouser ML, Gregory JE, Shane B, James SJ, Boynton A, Ulrich CM. A mathematical model gives insights into nutritional and genetic aspects of folate-mediated one-carbon metabolism. *J Nutr* 2006; 136:2653–61.
96. Nijhout HF, Reed MC, Lam S-L, Shane B, Gregory JF 3rd, Ulrich CM. In silico experimentation with a model of hepatic mitochondrial folate metabolism. *Theor Biol Med Model* 2006; 3:40.
97. Ulrich CM, Neuhouser M, Liu AY, Boynton A, Gregory JF III, Shane B, James SJ, Reed MC, Nijhout HF. Mathematical modeling of folate metabolism: Predicted effects of genetic polymorphisms on mechanisms and biomarkers relevant to carcinogenesis. *Cancer Epidemiol Biomarkers Prev* 2008; 17:1822–31.

98. Storch KJ, Wagner DA, Burke JF, Young VR. Quantitative study in vivo of methionine cycle in humans using [methyl-^{2}H$_3$]- and [1-^{13}C]methionine. *Am J Physiol* 1988; 255:E322–31.

99. Storch KJ, Wagner DA, Burke JF, Young VR. [1-^{13}C; methyl-^{2}H$_3$]Methionine kinetics in humans: Methionine conservation and cystine sparing. *Am J Physiol* 1990; 258:E790–98.

100. Millward DJ. Vernon Young and the development of current knowledge in protein and amino acid nutrition. Vernon Young 1937–2004. *Br J Nutr* 2004; 92:189–97.

101. Davis SR, Scheer JB, Quinlivan EP, Coats BS, Stacpoole PW, Gregory JF 3rd. Dietary vitamin B-6 restriction does not alter rates of homocysteine remethylation or synthesis in healthy young women and men. *Am J Clin Nutr* 2005; 81:648–55.

102. Davis SR, Stacpoole PW, Williamson J, Kick LS, Quinlivan EP, Coats BS, Shane B, Bailey LB, Gregory JF 3rd. Tracer-derived total and folate-dependent homocysteine remethylation and synthesis rates in humans indicate that serine is the main one-carbon donor. *Am J Physiol Endocrinol Metab* 2004; 286:E272–79; Erratum 2004; 286:E674.

103. Fukagawa NK, Yu YM, Young VR. Methionine and cysteine kinetics at different intakes of methionine and cysteine in elderly men and women. *Am J Clin Nutr* 1998; 68:380–88.

104. Raguso CA, Pereira P, Young VR. A tracer investigation of obligatory oxidative amino acid losses in healthy, young adults. *Am J Clin Nutr* 1999; 70:474–83.

105. Young VR, Wagner DA, Burini R, Storch KJ. Methionine kinetics and balance at the 1985 FAO/WHO/UNU intake requirement in adult men studied with L-[^{2}H$_3$-methyl-1-^{13}C]methionine as a tracer. *Am J Clin Nutr* 1991; 54:377–85.

106. Raguso CA, Regan MM, Young VR. Cysteine kinetics and oxidation at different intakes of methionine and cystine in young adults. *Am J Clin Nutr* 2000; 71:491–99.

107. van Guldener C, Kulik W, Berger R, Dijkstra DA, Jakobs C, Reijngoud DJ, Donker AJ, Stehouwer CD, De Meer K. Homocysteine and methionine metabolism in ESRD: A stable isotope study. *Kidney Int* 1999; 56:1064–71.

108. Storch KJ, Wagner DA, Young VR. Methionine kinetics in adult men: Effects of dietary betaine on L-[^{2}H$_3$-methyl-1-^{13}C]methionine. *Am J Clin Nutr* 1991; 54:386–94.

109. MacCoss MJ, Fukagawa NK, Matthews DE. Measurement of intracellular sulfur amino acid metabolism in humans. *Am J Physiol Endocrinol Metab* 2001; 280:E947–55.

110. Cuskelly GJ, Stacpoole PW, Williamson J, Baumgartner TG, Gregory JF 3rd. Deficiencies of folate and vitamin B(6) exert distinct effects on homocysteine, serine, and methionine kinetics. *Am J Physiol Endocrinol Metab* 2001; 281:E1182–90.

111. Gregory JF 3rd, Cuskelly GJ, Shane B, Toth JP, Baumgartner TG, Stacpoole PW. Primed, constant infusion with [^{2}H$_3$]serine allows in vivo kinetic measurement of serine turnover, homocysteine remethylation, and transsulfuration processes in human one-carbon metabolism. *Am J Clin Nutr* 2000; 72:1535–41.

112. Davis SR, Quinlivan EP, Shelnutt KP, Ghandour H, Capdevila A, Coats BS, Wagner C, et al. Homocysteine synthesis is elevated but total remethylation is unchanged by the methylenetetrahydrofolate reductase 677C->T polymorphism and by dietary folate restriction in young women. *J Nutr* 2005; 135:1045–50.

113. Lamers Y, Williamson J, Gilbert LR, Stacpoole PW, Gregory JF 3rd. Glycine turnover and decarboxylation rate quantified in healthy men and women using primed, constant infusions of [1,2-^{13}C$_2$]glycine and [^{2}H$_3$]leucine. *J Nutr* 2007; 137:2647–52.

114. Quinlivan EP, Davis SR, Shelnutt KP, Henderson GN, Ghandour H, Shane B, Selhub J, Bailey LB, Stacpoole PW, Gregory JF 3rd. Methylenetetrahydrofolate reductase 677C->T polymorphism and folate status affect one-carbon incorporation into human DNA deoxynucleosides. *J Nutr* 2005; 135:389–96.

115. Lamers Y, Williamson J, Ralat M, Quinlivan EP, Gilbert LR, Keeling C, Ueland PM, et al. Moderate dietary vitamin B-6 restriction raises plasma glycine and cystathionine

concentrations, increases in vivo serine production from glycine, while minimally affecting the rates of glycine turnover, glycine cleavage and related aspects of 1-carbon metabolism in healthy men and women. *J Nutr* 2009; 139:452–60.

116. Scheer JB, Mackey AD, Gregory JF 3rd. Activities of hepatic cytosolic and mitochondrial forms of serine hydroxymethyltransferase and hepatic glycine concentration are affected by vitamin B-6 intake in rats. *J Nutr* 2005; 135:233–38.

117. Davis SR, Quinlivan EP, Stacpoole PW, Gregory JF 3rd. Plasma glutathione and cystathionine concentrations are elevated but cysteine flux is unchanged by dietary vitamin B-6 restriction in young men and women. *J Nutr* 2006; 136:373–78.

118. Lima CP, Davis SR, Mackey AD, Scheer JB, Williamson J, Gregory JF 3rd. Vitamin B-6 deficiency suppresses the hepatic transsulfuration pathway but increases glutathione concentration in rats fed AIN-76A or AIN-93G diets. *J Nutr* 2006; 136:2141–47.

21 Folate Analytical Methodology

Christine M. Pfeiffer, Zia Fazili, and Mindy Zhang

CONTENTS

I. INTRODUCTION

Approaches to the analysis of folates in biological samples have developed and improved during the past 50 years. Initially, the microbiological assay was introduced; it exploits the fact that a specific microorganism cannot grow in a folate-free medium and therefore responds proportionally to folate present in the sample. Next, protein-binding assays were developed; these assays use the highly specific folate-binding protein to "extract" folate from the sample. Many of these assays have been automated for high-throughput clinical analysis. Finally, chromatographic methods were added to the repertoire; the distinguishing feature of these methods is that they can separate and measure individual folate forms, either in their monoglutamate state or as polyglutamates.

Many different folate vitamers can be found in biological samples, with variations in the oxidation state of the pteridine moiety, in the one-carbon substituent group at the N-5 and/or N-10 positions, and in the glutamate chain length. Furthermore, reduced folates exhibit instability at extreme pH values or when exposed to elevated temperature, oxygen, or light. These are just some issues that complicate the analysis of folates in biological samples and that lead to large method differences. Initial steps to standardize folate methods began with the development of higher-order reference methods that use isotope-dilution/liquid chromatography/tandem mass spectrometry (ID/LC/MS/MS). The development of matrix-based reference materials was also an important part of this effort. However, much more needs to be done to achieve better comparability between methods. In this chapter, we present and discuss various methods to measure folates in such biological samples as serum, blood, tissues, and foods. Rather than following the typical outline of presenting methods in the order of their historical appearance, we have opted to begin with chromatographic methods. We have done so for two reasons: (1) these methods represent the area with the greatest amount of new development, and (2) these methods require relatively extensive extraction and cleanup compared with the microbiological assay or protein-binding assays. These characteristics provide the rationale for presenting these techniques at the beginning of the chapter.

II. CHROMATOGRAPHIC ASSAYS

Chromatography-based assays were developed much later than the microbiological assay or protein-binding assays. However, in recent years the applicability of these relatively new methods has been evaluated for the measurement of folates in physiological fluids or foods. Contrary to the microbiological and protein-binding assays, where only total folate is determined, chromatographic assays provide information on individual folate species. This technology was widely explored in the 1970s and 1980s, and review articles by Gregory et al. provide comprehensive information on early chromatographic methods for folate determination in biological samples [1–3]. During the past several decades, advances have been made in the extraction and cleanup of folates, mainly owing to the introduction of commercially available solid-phase extraction (SPE) materials. Bench-top mass spectrometers became more available to specialized reference laboratories during the past 10 years, creating a surge of new method developments by liquid chromatography coupled to single (LC/MS) or tandem mass spectrometry (LC/MS/MS) [4]. Advances in automation of previously laborious manual methods have also been made. Higher-order reference methods by ID/LC/MS/MS are now available that measure folate species in biological samples.

A. FOLATE STANDARD COMPOUNDS

1. Chemical Properties and Sources for Folate Standard Compounds

Chromatographic methods use a variety of folate standards because a wide range of folate forms is present in physiological and food samples. Folates are made up of three main components: a fully aromatic pteridine that is coupled via a carbon-nitrogen (C9-N10) bond to *p*-aminobenzoic acid, which in turn is coupled via an amide bond through its carboxyl moiety to the amino group of L-glutamic acid. Different folate vitamers result from variations in the oxidation state of the pteridine moiety, in the one-carbon substituent group at the N-5 and/or N-10 positions, and in the glutamate chain length. In nature, folates exist primarily as reduced and usually as one-carbon substituted forms of pteroylglutamates. Pteroylglutamic acid (PGA), also called folic acid, is the most oxidized and stable form of folate. It is used as a vitamin supplement and in food fortification. A detailed review of chemical properties of folates is provided elsewhere [2].

Commonly used folate monoglutamates (tetrahydrofolic acid [THF], 5-methyl-THF, 5-formyl-THF, 5,10-methenyl-THF, 5,10-methylene-THF, dihydrofolic acid [DHF], PGA, 10-formyl-PGA) are commercially available (Sigma-Aldrich, St. Louis, MO; Merck Eprova AG, Schaffhausen, Switzerland; and Schircks Laboratories, Jona, Switzerland). Polyglutamyl folates of PGA, 5-methyl-THF (racemic), and 5-formyl-THF (racemic) are available (Schircks Laboratories), but other reduced polyglutamyl folates have to be custom synthesized [5,6]. Initially stable isotope-labeled folates were also custom synthesized either to be used in bioavailability studies [7] or as internal standards (IS) in stable isotope-dilution assays [8]. The compounds were either deuterium labeled ($^2H_4$) on the *p*-aminobenzoic acid ring or ^{13}C labeled on the glutamic acid moiety. More recently, commonly used stable isotope-labeled (glutamate-$^{13}C_5$) monoglutamyl folates ($^{13}C_5$-[6S]THF, $^{13}C_5$-[6S]5-methyl-THF, $^{13}C_5$-[6S]5-formyl-THF, $^{13}C_5$-[6R]5,10-methenyl, and $^{13}C_5$-PGA) can be acquired commercially (Merck Eprova AG) and have been used as IS in MS-based assays.

2. Preparation and Storage of Calibrators

The proper preparation and storage of folate standards are critical to obtaining accurate results. Because of the labile nature of reduced folates, it is prudent to avoid exposure of them to elevated temperature, light, or oxygen. The following are some general recommendations; more detailed procedures can be found elsewhere [9]:

1. It is important to keep all solid standard materials and calibration solutions frozen, ideally at approximately −70°C.
2. All handling of standards or samples should be done under subdued light (gold fluorescent) and expediently.

3. Stock solutions should be prepared with buffers degassed with inert gas (usually nitrogen or helium) to minimize oxidative breakdown.
4. The concentration of the first stock solution should be determined by ultraviolet (UV) spectrophotometry. To avoid oxidative breakdown during this step, L-cysteine (1 g/L) can be added.
5. The presence of antioxidants (typically 10 g/L ascorbic acid [AA] or a combination of AA and β-mercaptoethanol [β-MCE]) in folate stock solutions is necessary to protect reduced folates.
6. Aliquots of high-concentration stock solutions (approximately 100 μg/mL) of commonly used folates can be stored at −70°C for up to 2 years without loss of activity. Fresh aliquots of lower-concentration stock solutions (approximately 10 μg/mL) should be prepared every other month and stored at −70°C. Daily calibrators are prepared by diluting the lower-concentration stock solutions.
7. Once thawed, stock solutions should be discarded after use.

3. Folate Interconversions

Quinlivan et al. [3] provide a good overview of potential folate interconversions caused by pH or heat. In short, there is a pH-driven equilibrium between 10-formyl-THF (at neutral and alkaline pH), 5-formyl-THF (at slightly acidic pH), and 5,10-methenyl-THF (at acidic pH) [3]. Furthermore, at slightly acidic pH, heat accelerates the conversion of 10-formyl-THF to 5-formyl-THF, a process that has been exploited by some methods to yield complete conversion of 10-formyl-THF to 5-formyl-THF [10]. At physiological pH values, 5,10-methylene-THF dissociates to formaldehyde and THF. However, this conversion can be prevented at pH 10, a fact that has been exploited by methods using a high pH borate extraction buffer [11]. Folate interconversions have to be considered when one is applying different extraction or chromatographic conditions. Such interconversions are also the reason that some investigators have resorted to categorizing red blood cell (RBC) folates as methyl versus formyl folate or methyl versus nonmethyl folate [12–17].

B. Sample Preparation for Methods Measuring Intact Folates

Regardless of the analytical procedure, the accuracy of the analysis is highly dependent on the merits of the preparative methods used. The initial key preparative steps for folate analysis in biological samples are the extraction and, in many cases, the enzymatic deconjugation of the polyglutamyl folates. Sample preparation procedures for folate analysis vary considerably because of the complexity of the sample matrix and the composition of the folate pool in the sample (i.e., reduced vs. nonreduced folates, proportion of folate polyglutamates vs. monoglutamates). Furthermore, the analysis of folates by chromatographic methods requires at least some sample cleanup, and frequently the sample will need to be concentrated to enable detection of trace amounts.

1. Extraction and Cleanup Techniques

This section describes the various techniques to extract and clean up folates from biological samples, such as serum, whole blood, tissues, and foods. The next section provides an overview of techniques by sample matrix.

a. *Extraction of Folates*

Owing to the labile nature of most reduced folates, extraction always requires the addition of antioxidants, regardless of the matrix. AA and reduced thiols, such as β-MCE or dithiothreitol (DTT), have been used either alone or in combination [3]. Extraction is usually performed by heat, acid, or organic solvent. Matrices that contain polyglutamyl folates generally require deconjugation to monoglutamates. Regardless of the extraction technique, caution has to be used to prevent degradation of folates in the process, and the presence of an IS that corrects for potential procedural losses is highly desirable.

i. *Heat Extraction*   In this common form of extraction, the sample is mixed with buffer containing antioxidants and heated to release folate from its binding proteins. Often, extraction buffers have been chosen with pH values near the optimum of the conjugase used. Acidic buffers (pH 4–5) are used with hog kidney conjugase, whereas more neutral buffers are used for conjugases with approximately neutral pH optimum, such as chicken pancreas, rat plasma, and human plasma. In 1990, Gregory et al. [18] reported the superiority of the Wilson and Horne extraction buffer. This mixed Hepes/Ches buffer, pH 7.85, containing a combination of AA and β-MCE, was earlier shown to eliminate interconversion and degradation of folates at 100°C that were attributed to the formation of formaldehyde from buffers containing AA only [19]. The Wilson and Horne buffer effectively extracted radiolabeled folates from livers of rats previously dosed with [³H]folate [18]. The higher pH buffer was also superior, as judged by the microbiological assay of total folate, in the extraction of beef liver and peas compared with a pH 4.9 acetate buffer. A second extraction improved the completeness of the release of folate from the sample matrix.

ii. *Acid Extraction*   Various acids have been used to precipitate proteins and extract folate from the matrix: trichloroacetic acid (TCA) [20], acetic acid [21], perchloric acid [22–24], and most recently metaphosphoric acid (MPA) [25]. In comparing TCA with MPA, Nelson et al. [25] showed that although both acids caused total protein precipitation, only MPA avoided degrading 5-methyl-THF and maintained the sample at pH 3.5 or lower, ensuring complete release of protein-bound 5-methyl-THF. The pH of the sample treated with a minimal amount of TCA was less than 2.0, a fact that may explain the low stability of folates.

iii. *Organic Solvent Extraction*   To avoid folate degradation, acetone [26,27] and acetonitrile [28,29] have been used by some investigators as a mild form of extraction. Hahn et al. [27] reported that acetone precipitation of proteins caused less destruction of some folates and led to higher extraction rates of folates from biological materials, as examined by using an endogenous labeling technique. However, this technique could not be combined with subsequent hydrolysis of pteroylpolyglutamates because traces of acetone in the sample denature the enzyme.

iv. *Deconjugation of Polyglutamyl Folates*   Matrices that contain polyglutamyl folates generally require the deconjugation to monoglutamates. Although incubation of tissue or food homogenates under conditions providing autolytic deconjugation with endogenous conjugase(s) has been used earlier [30,31], these procedures can lead to undesirable interconversion and/or enzymatic degradation of folates by other enzymes [2,27]. Hence if the folate pattern is of interest, it is recommended to first inactivate the endogenous conjugase and then hydrolyze folate polyglutamates by addition of an exogenous conjugase. There are three main sources of exogenous conjugase: hog kidney, chicken pancreas, and rat plasma. Human plasma conjugase is used for autolytic deconjugation of polyglutamyl folates in RBCs. Hog kidney and human plasma conjugase are exopeptidases that remove the N-terminal glutamates one at a time until reaching monoglutamates; they have an optimum at acetic pH (approximately 4.5) [32,33]. Chicken pancreas and rat plasma have an optimum at neutral pH [34,35]. Whereas chicken pancreas is an endopeptidase that generates diglutamates, rat plasma is an exopeptidase producing monoglutamates. It has been shown that certain food components inhibit hog kidney conjugase activity [36].

v. *Trienzyme Treatment*   The use of a trienzyme treatment versus conjugase alone has become common practice for food extraction and has generally increased the measurable folate concentration [37,38]. This method involves the use of α-amylase and protease in addition to conjugase and allows a more complete extraction of folate trapped in carbohydrate- or protein-rich food matrices. Hyun and Tamura [37] reviewed the variations in trienzyme extraction used by different investigators. They concluded that (1) the pH of extraction buffers is less important because of the nearly complete folate extraction using the trienzyme method; (2) heat treatment is unnecessary for releasing folates from the binding protein as long as protease treatment is performed; and (3) the order and length of enzyme treatments should always be verified for a specific matrix. Generally, though, the protease treatment is performed first; then the enzyme is heat deactivated; and lastly the sample is treated with α-amylase and conjugase, either simultaneously or sequentially.

b. *Cleanup of Folates*

Sample cleanup is usually performed by SPE using ion-exchange or reversed-phase (RP) preparative chromatography or by solid-phase affinity extraction (SPAE) chromatography using folate-binding protein (FBP).

i. *SPE*   Initially investigators used preparative ion-exchange chromatography with diethylaminoethyl derivatives of beaded carbohydrates, such as cellulose or Sephadex [2]. When different types of prepacked SPE cartridges became commercially available, Rebello [39] tested a variety of RP (ethyl, octyl, octadecyl, and phenyl) and anion-exchange (aminopropyl, quaternary amine, and primary/secondary amine) cartridges for their potential to adsorb and elute folate monoglutamates from standard solutions. He found quantitative recoveries for aminopropyl and for all the RP cartridges. Indeed, many investigators have since used RP cartridges for high-performance liquid chromatography (HPLC) methods [24,40–45] and MS-based methods [9,17,25,46–49]. It has been shown that it is no longer necessary to remove proteins from serum before applying the sample to RP cartridges, as long as the pH of the diluted sample is low enough (pH 3.5) to hinder the rebinding of 5-methyl-THF to the native proteins in the sample [25]. Some investigators have used strong anion-exchange (SAX) cartridges, mainly for the cleanup of food extracts [31,50–55]. Because high salt concentrations are needed for the elution of folates from SAX cartridges but are not compatible with stable MS-based methods, the majority of these methods use RP cartridges.

ii. SPAE In SPAE, FBP is covalently immobilized to a solid support. The original method developed by Selhub et al. [56] used agarose (Sepharose) beads, suitable only for low-pressure flow conditions, whereas more recent methods used FBP immobilized to polymeric beads that can also be used under high-pressure flow conditions [11,57]. Because FBP has a high affinity for folates from pH 9 to pH 7 but virtually no binding below pH 3.5 [58], sample extracts are generally loaded onto the SPAE column under neutral conditions and are eluted under acidic conditions [56]. To preclude adsorption and blockage of the affinity medium by sample proteins, the proteins should be removed before passing the sample through the SPAE column [57]. Nelson et al. [25] showed further that excess high-affinity binding sites on the SPAE column are capable of capturing plasma folate that is strongly held by the trace amounts of native FBP and weakly held by the large amount of albumin when the pH of the sample is appropriately adjusted (pH 6.3) and controlled. SPAE columns can usually achieve a higher concentration of the sample (10-fold or more) compared with SPE columns, presenting an advantage for SPAE columns when one is measuring trace amounts. Because of the high specificity of FBP, SPAE generates much cleaner extracts and consequently lower background interference. SPAE columns are not commercially available; more recently, FBP has become commercially available [14,57], simplifying the column manufacture; however, its expense limits its use. Other disadvantages of SPAE columns are that (1) the binding capacity significantly decreases with increased usage, necessitating regular verification of the binding capacity; (2) there is a disparity in binding between the different folate species, with the lowest affinity for 5-formyl-THF [2], necessitating a significant excess of FBP for complete recovery of 5-formyl-THF [59]; and (3) FBP shows a significantly higher affinity toward natural vitamers compared with the racemic folates, a fact that can pose a problem if stable isotopically labeled racemic standards are used for LC/MS/MS [60].

2. Extraction and Cleanup Issues for Different Matrices

a. *Serum, Urine, and Cerebrospinal Fluid*

Although the extraction of intact folates from physiological fluids such as serum, cerebrospinal fluid (CSF), and urine requires removal of proteins and ionic compounds before cleanup and possibly sample concentration steps, no deconjugation is necessary because folates occur as monoglutamates in these materials. Analysis of intact folates in urine has generally been conducted as part of bioavailability or kinetic studies, and the sample was cleaned up by affinity chromatography with no previous extraction step [61]. Up to the late 1980s, protein precipitation in serum was mainly done by heat [62,63], acid [20], or organic solvent [26], typically without a subsequent sample cleanup step. 5-Methyl-THF in CSF was even analyzed by HPLC with electrochemical detection via direct injection [64]. When commercial

SPE materials became more widely available, the sample was typically cleaned by SPE-RP [40,42–45,65], omitting the protein precipitation step, yet still requiring the concentration of the sample after SPE through evaporation and reconstitution in a much smaller volume. Interestingly, some of the initial MS-based methods quantifying serum folates reverted to using heat [66,67], acid [25], or organic solvent extraction [29] for protein precipitation, followed by SPAE [66,67] or SPE-RP [25]. Other methods applied serum/buffer mixtures directly to SPAE [57] or SPE-RP columns [9,46,47,68,69] for sample cleanup.

b. Whole Blood

Extraction of folates from whole blood is more complex because RBCs first need to be hemolyzed to release polyglutamyl folates, which in turn need to be deconjugated to monoglutamates. RBCs have traditionally been hemolyzed osmotically by diluting in a hypotonic solution, usually 10 g/L AA [17,22,70,71], although sometimes the pH of the AA solution is adjusted from 2.7 to 4.0 [14,71] or 4.5 [71,72], raising the hemolysate pH from 4.0 to 4.7 and 5.2. Although the proportion of whole blood to AA solution varies from as little as 1:3 [73] to as much as 1:40 [50], the most common ratio is 1:10 or 1:11. The deconjugation step takes advantage of the endogenous plasma pteroylpolyglutamate hydrolase (conjugase), which has a pH optimum of 4.5 [33]. Hemolysates are incubated anywhere from 30 minutes at room temperature [17] to 4 hours at 37°C [71], with 60 to 90 minutes at 37°C as an intermediate condition [14,70,72,74]. In some methods, hemolysates (after incubation) are heat [14,50,70] or acid [22] extracted before further cleanup and/or chromatography.

Using HPLC with fluorescence detection and custom-synthesized 5-methyl-THF heptaglutamate, Pfeiffer and Gregory [74] confirmed that hemolysate pH is a critical factor in producing folate monoglutamates, and they concluded that dilution of whole blood with 10 g/L AA yielded fast hydrolysis of long-chain polyglutamates and that total conversion to 5-methyl-THF occurred after 90 minutes of incubation at 37°C. In a more recent report, Fazili et al. [71] expanded on those findings by incorporating the measurement of folate diglutamates by LC/MS/MS to monitor the progression of deconjugation. The LC/MS/MS method, more sensitive than the previously used HPLC with fluorescence detection (FD) method, showed that longer incubation times are needed (4 hours at 37°C for pH 4.0 hemolysates and 3 hours at 37°C for pH 4.7 hemolysates) to obtain complete (>97%) conversion of diglutamates to monoglutamates. In pilot studies designed to address the question of folate trapping by deoxyhemoglobin (deoxy-Hb) as it switches quaternary structure to oxyhemoglobin (oxy-Hb) when picking up oxygen, as hypothesized by Wright et al. [75], Fazili et al. [71] could not find any indication of folate trapping. The question of whether detergents, such as saponin [75,76] or Triton X-100 [12], aid hemolysis has also been considered [77]. It has been shown by several groups that RBCs of subjects with the *MTHFR* 677 TT genotype contain a mixture of methyl and nonmethyl folates [12,13,15,16,78,79]. Our group evaluated whether whole blood folates for subjects with the TT genotype were stable during extraction and found that approximately 50% of THF is lost during the 4-hour incubation of the hemolysate at 37°C. However, this loss can be corrected for, if the mixture of stable isotope-labeled IS is added to the hemolysate before incubation (Z. Fazili and C. M. Pfeiffer, unpublished observations).

Another approach to extract folates from whole blood is to denature the endogenous plasma conjugase by heat extraction of whole blood in a high pH borate buffer (pH 9.2) to preserve the pattern of folate polyglutamates, followed by in-line FBP affinity chromatography and HPLC analysis [11]. In older chromatographic methods, whole blood hemolysates are generally not cleaned up before analysis [22,70,73]. In newer methods, hemolysates are cleaned up by using SPE-SAX [50], SPE-RP [17,78], or SPAE columns [14].

c. Foods and Tissues

Food and tissue samples are similar when it comes to extraction of folates because the matrix is complex, the folate pool is made up of several forms, and polyglutamyl folates are present. Hence these materials always require some form of extraction after homogenation. Up to the early 1990s, methods generally used acetate extraction buffers in conjunction with hog kidney conjugase [10,21,80], whereas later the use of a neutral pH buffer (Wilson and Horne buffer or phosphate buffer) in conjunction with rat plasma conjugase prevailed [53,55,59,81–85]. The use of a trienzyme treatment versus conjugase alone has also become very common for food extraction during the past 15 years [53,55,59,82,85]. Because of the complexity of food and tissue extracts, they require good cleanup before they are analyzed chromatographically. Most applications use either SPE-SAX [51–55] or SPAE columns [11,59,83–85]. Recently, Zhang et al. [84] used ultrafiltration as a means to clean up spinach extracts by separating compounds by molecular weight. Selhub et al. specialized in the determination of folate distribution in tissues by one-carbon substituent and glutamate chain length [5,11,86]. To maintain the original folate pattern to the extent possible, they used slightly alkaline extraction buffers, denatured the endogenous conjugase, and, at least initially, used ion-pair chromatography. To enable quantitation of trace-level amounts, they used SPAE columns that generated highly purified and concentrated extracts.

C.   Measurement of Intact Folates

Two review articles by Gregory [1,2] provide detailed insight on early chromatographic methods. The current review focuses on newer HPLC and LC/MS/(MS) methods to measure intact folates. Nelson [4] recently reviewed the expanding role of MS in folate research.

1.   High-Performance Liquid Chromatography

HPLC methods provide rapid separation of individual folate species from biological samples. During the past 20 years, separation of folates was performed almost exclusively on RP stationary materials with octadecyl (C18), octyl (C8), or phenyl-bonded silica phases. HPLC columns have become very reproducible, and column life has been improved greatly through advances in manufacturing techniques, higher carbon loads, and more effective end capping. The retention of folate monoglutamates on RP columns decreases rapidly above pH 4 to 5 [73]. Two basic principles have been used to retain negatively charged folates on a nonpolar stationary phase. In ion suppression, the pH of the mobile phase is lowered to less than 4, resulting in masking of folate charges [10]. Phosphate buffer with acetonitrile as organic modifier is typically used. In ion-pair chromatography, folate vitamers can be separated at neutral pH as ion pairs with cationic surfactants [81]. Tetrabutylammonium phosphate is typically used as ion-pair reagent, and methanol is used as organic modifier. Although ion-pair chromatography at neutral pH offers the advantage of maintaining folate patterns by avoiding interconversion of folates taking place at acidic pH values, the use of ion-pair reagents has its own complications. As a result, more investigators have resorted to the use of ion suppression [11,27,40,43,45,51,53, 59,70,73,82,83,85] compared with ion-pair chromatography [5,28,44,52]. However, the selection of the separation mode depends greatly on the mode of detection and the objectives of the analysis. Both isocratic and gradient elution have been used. Isocratic separation offers the advantage of faster throughput because it does not require column re-equilibration before the next injection. However, gradient separation offers more flexibility in resolving complicated folate patterns.

Different detection modes have been used in folate analysis. UV/diode array detector (DAD), fluorescence (FL), and electrochemical (EC) are the most common detection modes. They exhibit increasing sensitivity and specificity in this order. PGA does not exhibit native fluorescence; however, it can be analyzed fluorometrically by the introduction of a postcolumn derivatization system involving hypochlorite to cleave PGA (as well as DHF and THF) oxidatively to fluorescent pterins [2]. Whereas UV/DAD detection is compatible with both ion-suppression and ion-pair HPLC, FL detection is not suitable for ion-pair HPLC because the FL of reduced folates is maximal at pH 2, but it rapidly decreases as the pH approaches 7 [31]. EC detection is typically used in combination with ion-suppression HPLC [11,26,40,45,64].

As a result of low concentrations of 5-methyl-THF in serum, most investigators used EC detection [20,26,40,45,64] and sample volumes of 0.5 to 1.0 mL. To follow drug treatment with methotrexate (MTX) and/or folinic acid, investigators used EC [65], FL [28], a combination of UV and EC [42], or a combination of UV and FL detection [43]. Investigators performed online acidification of the mobile phase to pH 2 for a 16-fold increase in 5-methyl-THF to allow FL detection in combination with ion-pair HPLC [44].

To measure different folate forms in blood or tissues, mainly FL detection was used [27,50,70,73]. Owing to the concentration potential of affinity chromatography, the group of Selhub et al. [86] was able to determine detailed tissue folate composition by HPLC/DAD, albeit gram quantities of tissue were needed because of the limited sensitivity of DAD. Later they achieved increased sensitivity by using a four-channel coulometric EC detector and peak identification by combination of retention time and response pattern across the four channels [11]. The amount of information gained with this method is tremendous. However, reduced folate polyglutamate calibrators have to be custom synthesized; the detector responses could shift over time; a coelution is possible between some THF and 5-methyl-THF chain lengths, requiring equations to calculate resolution; and the level of data reduction is highly complex.

Individual folates in foods were generally measured by a combination of UV/DAD (mainly for PGA) and FL detection (mainly for the reduced folates) [51,82,85,87–89]. Folates in cereal grain products were also measured by UV/ DAD alone [52,59]. Ndaw et al. [83] measured total folate in various foods by FL detection after precolumn conversion of all folates to 5-methyl-THF and chromatographic separation of the different 5-methyl-THF polyglutamates. Doherty et al. [53] measured 5-methyl-THF and PGA in various foods; they used FL detection, using the native fluorescence of 5-methyl-THF and performing UV-induced photolysis of PGA to generate fluorescence.

The microbiological assay has also been used as a sensitive "detector" to either quantify various folates [81,90] or PGA in serum [23,24] in fractions collected during HPLC. Although this approach is cumbersome and lengthy, it has the advantage of bringing together the specificity of a chromatographic method with the sensitivity of the microbiological assay.

Few investigators have evaluated the addition of an IS to correct for procedural losses. Lucock et al. [40] incorporated β-hydroxyethyltheophylline, a compound with similar extraction characteristics to 5-methyl-THF, into their serum assay. However, they had to use UV detection for the IS, and they used EC detection for 5-methyl-THF. Chladek et al. [44] used p-aminoacetophenon in their serum assay, but the recovery for this IS (88%) was slightly different from the recovery of 5-methyl-THF (98%). Hahn et al. [27] used MTX and 3′,5′-dichlorofolic acid (DCFA) to monitor the extraction and chromatography of tissue samples. Although these compounds showed similar stability as other reduced folates during heat or acetone extraction, they might not be universally suited. MTX is used as an antifolate drug in cancer therapy and therefore might appear in the serum of cancer patients. DCFA showed unsatisfactory recovery from SPE (50%–60%) compared with complete recovery for 5-methyl-THF and PGA when evaluated as potential IS in a food assay [53].

2. Liquid Chromatography/(Tandem) Mass Spectrometry

Mass spectrometers coupled to LC are the newest and most expensive type of detectors for chromatographic methods. However, because of their sensitivity, selectivity, and specificity, ID/LC/MS/MS methods are considered higher-order methods. During the past decade, mass spectrometers have become smaller in footprint, less expensive, more robust and user friendly, and consequently more available in specialized reference laboratories. Although they still require operation by experienced personnel and service by highly trained and specialized technicians, they can provide high-throughput measurements in a routine environment. As a result, some large clinical laboratories have already shifted over to this promising technique.

Some basic requirements of MS-compatible mobile phases are that they contain high organic content, low salt content, and low content of compounds with poor volatility, such as ion-pair reagents. This allows the sample to easily evaporate during ionization. These requirements preclude the use of ion-pair HPLC in conjunction with MS detection. To still provide adequate retention of folates on RP columns, facilitating their separation from signal-suppressing impurities eluting at or near the void volume of the LC column, ion-suppression HPLC is the method of choice, but phosphate buffers have to be replaced with buffers that provide good volatility. Electrospray ionization (ESI) is considered a softer ionization type than atmospheric pressure chemical ionization (APCI) and therefore is preferred for folate analysis. APCI is not well suited because high desolvation temperatures are required that might negatively impact folate stability [29].

One advantage of MS detection compared with other detection modes is that it can be applied to in vitro or in vivo studies with stable isotope-labeled folates, which is not possible with EC or FL detection for obvious reasons [66,67]. Ideally, a different stable isotope-labeled compound should be used as IS in addition to the labeled compound used to test bioavailability or kinetic profiles.

Tables 21.1A and 21.1B present an overview of LC/MS/(MS) methods for physiological fluids and foods. Initial MS-based methods for folate measurement in biological samples were nonisotopic—i.e., they did not use stable isotope-labeled ISs [29,48], and/or they provided less selectivity and sensitivity because of the use of single-quadrupole [25,48,57,66] or ion-trap instruments in LC/MS mode [46,49]. These methods were used to measure 5-methyl-THF alone [25,46,57] or several folate forms [29] in serum and PGA alone [46] or several folate forms [48] in foods. Another feature of early methods was that they were performed using negative-ion ESI because positive-ion mass spectra were complicated by the appearance of sodium and potassium adducts [29,46,48,66]. However, acidic mobile phases compromise the signal in negative-ion ESI. To obtain adequate signal, Garbis et al. [29] had to use a mobile phase with neutral pH and introduce triethylamine postcolumn as an organic base. To ensure adequate retention of folates at neutral pH, the authors used a hydrophilic interaction (HILIC) stationary phase that provided normal-phase retention.

More recently, LC/MS and LC/MS/MS methods have used positive-ion ESI and acidic mobile phases composed of either formic or acetic acid in water with methanol and/or acetonitrile as organic modifier. They have also used stable isotope-labeled folates as ISs to allow highly accurate quantitation at trace levels. In any method, the use of an appropriate IS helps to correct for procedural losses. In MS, however, the use of a stable isotope-labeled IS has another important function: It corrects for the variation in ionization from sample to sample. Because quantitation is based on the relative ratio of the unlabeled analyte to the labeled IS, and the IS is expected to behave identically to the analyte, complete recovery of folate during extraction and cleanup is not essential in the use of ID techniques; however, the recovery should be high enough to provide a good signal. Conversely, not using a stable isotope-labeled IS in LC/MS/(MS) can produce questionable results.

LC/MS/MS provides three levels of selectivity: chromatographic separation, mass/charge ratio (m/z) of the ionized precursor compound, and precursor to fragment ion transition. Different precursor ions with the same m/z ratio can produce distinct fragmentation patterns. One would expect that at this level of selectivity, methods no longer require sample cleanup; however, such is not the case because ion suppression caused by the matrix has to be eliminated. The only methods not requiring sample cleanup were those used for the analysis of PGA in multivitamin tablets [91,92]. All other published ID/LC/MS/MS methods have used SPE-RP (C18 or phenyl) [9,17,47,78], SPE-SAX [54,55], or SPAE columns [14,25,66,67]. Most LC/MS/MS methods for the measurement of serum folate determined only 5-methyl-THF [25,57] or 5-methyl-THF and PGA [47,67]. Pfeiffer et al. [9] published the first method that measured 5-methyl-THF, PGA, and 5-formyl-THF in serum after SPE cleanup using phenyl cartridges, and they used respective $^{13}C_5$-labeled ISs for each compound. They also published a follow-up method that conducted automated SPE on a 96-well plate for high throughput [78]. This method has been applied to both serum and

TABLE 21.1A

LC/MS/(MS) Assays for Physiological Fluids

Reference	Matrix	Extraction	Cleanup	Chromatography	Detection	Internal Standard(s)	Folates Measured	Assay Characteristics	Comments
Garbis [29]	Plasma (1.9 mL)	Protein precipitation with acetonitrile; evaporation under vacuum; reconstitution	"Online"	Hydrophilic interaction LC; ammonium acetate in acetonitrile, pH 6.9; microbore flow rate (50 μL/min)	LC/MS/MS; negative-ion ESI	Nonisotopic; MTX	PGA, 5CH3THF, 5CHOTHF, THF	Recovery of folate species from spiked plasma >97%; intra-assay CV 3.7–6.5% (n = 5); LODs: PGA 37.5, THF 425, 5CH3THF 165, 5CHOTHF 140 pM; LOQs: FA 80, THF 1,250, 5MeTHF 400, 5FoTHF 360 pM	Sample extraction essential to avoid ionization suppression or analyte interference; positive-ion mass spectra complicated by Na+ and K+ adducts; HILIC stationary phase provides normal-phase retention proportional to polarity of solute
Pawlosky [46]	Serum (0.5 mL)	N/A	SPE phenyl	RP; formic acid and acetonitrile/methanol in water	LC/MS; positive-ion ESI	ID/MS; 13C5-5CH3THF	5CH3THF	Intra-assay CV 5.4% (n = 4); interassay CV 7.6% (n = 5 days)	Confirmation of 5CH3THF in selected samples by MS/MS
Nelson [68]	Plasma (0.5 mL)	N/A	SPE C18	RP-phenyl; gradient of ammonium formate and methanol in water, pH 3.5	LC/MS; positive-ion ESI	ID/MS; 13C5-5CH3THF	5CH3THF	LOQ for 5CH3THF 0.39 ng/mL; spiking recovery of 5CH3THF for SPE 94%	Preliminary method

	Sample	Pretreatment	Extraction	Chromatography	Detection	Analyte	ID	Validation	Comments
Hart [66]	Plasma (5 mL), urine (55 mL)	Heat	SPAE (FBP)	RP-C18; acetic acid and acetonitrile in water, pH 3.3	LC/MS; negative-ion ESI	5CH3THF	ID/MS; D2-PGA	Linear range 0–9 nM; LOD 0.2 nM; LOQ 0.55 nM; CV 7.4%	Used for kinetic studies
Nelson [57]	Plasma (1 mL)	N/A	SPAE (FBP)	RP-phenyl; gradient of ammonium formate and methanol in water, pH 3.5	LC/MS; positive-ion ESI	5CH3THF	ID/MS; 13C5-5CH3THF	Linear range 0.04–40 ng/mL; LOD 0.04 ng/mL; LOQ 0.4 ng/mL; spiking recovery 98%	
Nelson [25]	Plasma, serum (0.5 mL)	Protein precipitation with MPA	SPE C18; effluent evaporated to 1/4 of volume; 4 h for 6 samples	RP-phenyl; gradient of ammonium formate and methanol in water, pH 3.5	LC/MS; positive-ion ESI	5CH3THF	ID/MS; 13C5-5CH3THF	Linear range 0.4–97 ng/mL; LOD 0.4 ng/mL; LOQ 1.2 ng/mL; CV ~3%; spiking recovery 94%	No significant difference between 5MeTHF levels whether extracts were prepared with or without protein precipitation
	Plasma, serum	Protein precipitation with MPA	SPAE (FBP); 2.5 h for 6 samples	RP-C18; formic acid and methanol in water, pH 2.3	LC/MS/MS; positive-ion ESI	5CH3THF	ID/MS; 13C5-5CH3THF	Linear range 0.03–101 ng/mL; LOD 0.03 ng/mL; LOQ 0.1 ng/mL; CV ~7%; spiking recovery 100%	SPAE/LC/MS/MS ~10x more sensitive than SPE/LC/MS—better sample purification and enhanced detection sensitivity with MRM mode

continued

TABLE 21.1A (continued)
LC/MS/(MS) Assays for Physiological Fluids

Reference	Matrix	Extraction	Cleanup	Chromatography	Detection	Folates Measured	Internal Standard(s)	Assay Characteristics	Comments
Pfeiffer [9]	Serum (0.275 mL)	N/A	SPE phenyl; 24 samples in 3 h	RP-C8; acetic acid and methanol/acetonitrile in water, pH 3.2	LC/MS/MS; positive-ion ESI	5CH3THF, PGA, 5CHOTHF	ID/MS; 13C5-labeled IS for each folate	Linear range 0.22–220 nM; LODs: 5CH3THF 0.13, 5CHOTHF 0.05, PGA 0.07 nM; CV <10%; SPE recoveries: 5CH3THF 75%, 5CHOTHF 72%, PGA 77%	First paper using appropriate stable isotope-labeled IS and measuring several folate forms
Fazili [78]	Serum (0.275 mL), WB lysate (1:11 diluted WB in 1% pH 2.7 AA; 4 h at 37°C)	N/A	SPE phenyl; 36 samples in 3 h	RP-C8; acetic acid and methanol/acetonitrile in water, pH 3.2	LC/MS/MS; positive-ion ESI	5CH3THF, PGA, 5CHOTHF, THF, 5,10CH=THF	ID/MS; 13C5-labeled IS for each folate	Linear range 0.22–220 nM; LODs: THF 2.5, 5,10CH=THF 0.7; CV 4%–8% 5CH3THF, 6%–20% minor forms; SPE recovery: 72%–81% for all forms; method recovery: 90%–101% for all forms	First automated 96-well plate ID/LC/MS/MS method that measures intact folate monoglutamates in WB lysates and serum

Kok [67]	Plasma (2 mL)	Heat	SPAE (FBP); concentrated by SPE (HLB Oasis) and evaporation	RP-C18; formic acid and acetonitrile in water, pH 2.3	LC/MS/MS; positive-ion ESI	5CH3THF, PGA	ID/MS; 13C5-5CH3THF, 2H4-PGA	LODs: 5CH3THF 0.012, PGA 0.5 nM; linear range: 5CH3THF 0.012–320, PGA 0.5–45 nM; imprecision: 5CH3THF ~9%; recoveries 80%–110%	Method also used for kinetic studies; Hart extraction method [66] improved to only use 2 mL plasma
Nelson [47]	Plasma, serum (0.5 mL)	N/A	SPE C18	RP-cyano; gradient of formic acid and methanol in water	LC/MS/MS; positive-ion ESI	5CH3THF, PGA, tHcy	ID/MS; 13C5-5CH3THF, 13C5-PGA, 2H8-homocysteine	Linear range: 5CH3THF 0.02–829, PGA 0.05–913 nM; LODs: 5CH3THF 0.02, PGA 0.05 nM; LOQs: 5CH3THF 0.07, PGA 0.14 nM; imprecision (n = 6): 5CH3THF ~2%, PGA 5%–10%	Combined folate/ Hcy method; SPE-RP is preferred over SPE-SAX for LC/ MS/MS because high salt concentrations, needed to elute folates, in particular FA from SAX, are not compatible with stable ESI MS
Satterfield [69]	Serum (0.5 mL)	N/A	SPE C18	RP-phenylpropyl; formic acid and methanol in water	LC/MS/MS; positive-ion ESI	5CH3THF	ID-MS; 13C5-5CH3THF		Similar to Nelson [25] SPE/LC/MS method, but LC/ MS/MS and isocratic mobile phase

continued

TABLE 21.1A (continued)
LC/MS/(MS) Assays for Physiological Fluids

Reference	Matrix	Extraction	Cleanup	Chromatography	Detection	Folates Measured	Internal Standard(s)	Assay Characteristics	Comments
			SPE C18	RP-C18; formic acid and methanol in water	LC/MS/MS; positive-ion ESI	5CH3THF, PGA	ID-MS; 13C5-5CH3THF, 13C5-PGA		Similar to Nelson [25] SPE/LC/MS method, but different instrument, isocratic mobile phase, and LC column
			SPAE (FBP	RP-C18; formic acid and methanol in water	LC/MS/MS; positive-ion ESI	5CH3THF	ID-MS; 13C5-5CH3THF, 13C5-PGA		Similar to Nelson [25] SPAE/LC/MS/MS method, but different instrument and isocratic mobile phase
Smith [14]	WB lysate (1 mL) (1:10 diluted WB in 1% pH 4 AA; 90 min at 37°C)	Heat	SPAE (FBP); concentrated by SPE (HLB Oasis) and evaporation	RP-C18; formic acid and acetonitrile in water, pH 2.3	LC/MS/MS; positive-ion ESI	5CH3THF, sum of nonmethyl-THF (THF, 5,10CH2THF, 5,10CH=THF, 5CHOTHF, 10CHOTHF)	ID-MS; 13C5-5CH3THF, 13C5-5CHOTHF, 2H4-PGA, 13C5-5,10CH=THF	LOQ 0.4 nM; intra- and interassay CV for 5CH3THF 1.2% and 2.8%; intra- and interassay CV for nonmethyl-THF 1.6% and 1.5%; recovery 97%–107%	Storage of WB samples in AA at low pH resulted in 53%–90% loss of nonmethyl-THF fraction

Ueland [93]	Serum, plasma (1 mL)	No information	No information	RP; acetic acid and organic solvent in water	LC/MS/MS; positive-ion ESI	5CH3THF, 5CHOTHF, PGA, 4-α-OH-5CH3DHF, pABG	ID-MS	Intraday CV ~5% (at 30 nM); 182 samples/24 h	In serum/plasma samples left at RT for days, the decline in 5CH3THF and folate detected by MA is recovered as 4-α-OH-5CH3DHF
Huang [17]	Plasma (0.3 mL), WB (0.5 mL lysate) (1:10 diluted with 1% pH 2.7 AA; 30 min at RT)	N/A	SPE C18; eluate evaporated under nitrogen and redissolved	RP-C18; gradient of acetic acid and methanol/acetonitrile in water	LC/MS/MS; positive-ion ESI	5CH3THF, PGA, THF, 5,10CH=THF	ID-MS; 13C5-5CH3THF, 13C5-5CHOTHF, 13C5-PGA, 13C5-THF	Linear range 4.5–900 nM; LODs: PGA 3, THF 6, 5CH3THF 2.5, 5,10CH=THF 1.2 pg on-column; imprecision better than 15%	First, analysis of THF, 5CH3THF and PGA; then, addition of 1 M HCl to vial, 4 h at RT to convert 5CHOTHF and 10CHOTHF into 5,10CH=THF and 13C5-5CHOTHF and 13C5-THF into 13C5-5,10CH=THF

TABLE 21.1B
LC/MS/(MS) Assays for Foods

Reference	Matrix	Extraction	Cleanup	Chromatography	Detection	Folates Measured	Internal Standard(s)	Method Characteristics	Comments
Stokes [48]	Multivitamin extract, breakfast cereal, beef extract, vegetable extract	Heat	SPE C18	RP-C18; acetic acid and acetonitrile in water	LC/MS: negative-ion ESI	PGA, 5CH3THF, THF, 5CHOTHF and/or 10CHOTHF	Nonisotopic; confirmation by monitoring ratios of three structurally significant ions	No recovery of 5CHOTHF from spiked samples; large peak at m/z 472 for 5CHOTHF in spiked and unspiked samples, but confirmation ion ratios did not match	Variation in retention time of standards and samples; decreasing peak areas of 5CHOTHF and PGA during run—no quantitation
Pawlosky [49]	Fortified food	Heat (phosphate buffer)	SPE C18; effluent evaporated; redissolved twice	RP-C18; gradient of formic acid and methanol in water	LC/MS: ion trap; negative-ion ESI	PGA	ID/MS; 13C5-FA	CV 5.6% (n = 4)	Confirmation of FA in selected samples by MS/ MS; results obtained in several test samples agreed well with listed values

Rychlik [54]	Spinach, broccoli	Heat; protease, rat serum deconjugase	SPE SAX	RP-C18; gradient of formic acid and acetonitrile in water	LC/MS/MS: ion trap; positive-ion ESI	5CH3THF, 5CHOTHF, THF (n.d.), FA (n.d.)	ID/MS; 2H4-labeled IS for each form	LODs: 5CH3THF 0.5, 5CHOTHF 1.2, THF 1.5, PGA 2.6 µg/100 g fresh weight; imprecision ~6%	SIDA method is a promising tool for the quantification of folates; differences to other published food folate values
Rychlik [91]	Multivitamin tablets	HEPES/CHES extraction buffer at RT; filtration	N/A	RP-C18; gradient of formic acid and acetonitrile in water	LC/MS/MS: ion trap; positive-ion ESI	PGA	ID/MS; 2H4-PGA	Recovery 99%; imprecision ~3%	
Freisleben [55]	Spinach, wheat bread, meat	Heat; protease, amylase, then rat serum deconjugase	SPE SAX	RP-C18; gradient of formic acid and acetonitrile in water	LC/MS/MS: ion trap; positive-ion ESI	THF, 5CH3THF, 5CHOTHF, 10CHOPGA, PGA	ID/MS; 2H4-labeled IS for each form	LODs: 5CH3THF 0.5, 5CHOTHF 1.2, THF 1.5, 10CHOPGA 0.6, PGA 2.6 µg/100 g fresh weight; imprecision ~6%; recoveries 80%–110%	SAX cleanup provided extracts with less interfering substances during LC/MS/MS than RP SPE

continued

TABLE 21.1B (continued)
LC/MS/(MS) Assays for Foods

Reference	Matrix	Extraction	Cleanup	Chromatography	Detection	Folates Measured	Internal Standard(s)	Method Characteristics	Comments
Freisleben [60]	Spinach, wheat bread, meat	Heat; protease, rat serum deconjugation	SPAE for wheat bread and beef extracts, SPE SAX for spinach extracts and plasma	RP-C18; gradient of formic acid and acetonitrile in water	LC/MS/MS; ion trap; positive-ion ESI	THF, 5CH3THF, 5CHOTHF, 10CHOPGA, PGA	ID/MS; 2H4-labeled IS for each form	10-fold higher sensitivity with SPAE compared with solid-phase anion-exchange cartridges	Comparison of LC/MS/MS with HPLC/FD; limitations of SPAE: decreasing binding capacity with use, discrimination between folate vitamers, and higher affinity toward the natural vitamers than racemic isotopomeric standards
Zhang [84]	Spinach	Heat w/ phosphate buffer; rat serum as deconjugase	Ultrafiltration (5 kDa molecular mass cutoff membrane filter)	RP-C18; gradient of formic acid and acetonitrile in water	LC/MS/MS; positive-ion ESI	THF, 5CH3THF, 5CHOTHF, 10CHOPGA, PGA, MTX	Nonisotopic; FA (because not detectable in spinach)	LODs: 5CH3THF 0.02, THF 0.09, 5CHOTHF 0.05, 10CHOPGA 0.03 ng/mL; optimal extraction parameters: 10 min at 100°C, incubation with rat serum at 37°C (pH 6.5) for 4 h, 1:10 ratio of sample vs buffer	Results are highly influenced by pH of extraction buffer (2.9–8.6); MTX could not be used as IS because the spinach matrix suppressed the ionization of MTX by about 50%

Phillips [94]	Fresh fruits and vegetables	Trienzyme treatment (modification of Doherty [53])	SPE SAX	RP-C18; gradient of formic acid and acetonitrile in water	LC/MS/MS: positive-ion ESI	5CH3THF, 5CHOTHF, 10CHOPGA	Nonisotopic		
Nelson [92]	Multivitamin tablets	Aqueous/org. extraction (pH 7.5)	N/A	RP-phenyl; isocratic formic acid and methanol in water	LC/MS/MS: positive-ion ESI	PGA	ID/MS; 13C5-PGA	Linear range 0.02–73 ng on-column; LOD 0.02 ng on-column; LOQ 0.06 ng on-column	Application to certify FA in NIST SRM 3280 multivitamin/multimineral tablets
		Aqueous extraction (pH 11.1)	N/A	RP-phenyl; isocratic acetic acid and methanol in water	LC/MS/MS: negative-ion ESI	PGA	ID/MS; 13C5-PGA	Linear range 0.02–293 ng on-column; LOD 0.02 ng on-column; LOQ 0.06 ng on-column	Application to certify FA in NIST SRM 3280 multivitamin/multimineral tablets

conventionally prepared whole blood hemolysates; it measured in addition to the above folate forms THF and 5,10-methenyl-THF. Two other groups have developed LC/MS/MS methods for the measurement of whole blood folate. Smith et al. [14] measured 5-methyl-THF, the sum of non–methyl-THF (5-formyl-THF and 5,10-methenyl-THF [the latter derived mainly from 10-formyl-THF and 5,10-methylene-THF and partially from THF]), and PGA in hemolysates that were heat extracted and cleaned by SPAE columns. Huang et al. [17] developed a two-step approach to capture whole blood folates. They first measured 5-methyl-THF, THF, and PGA in hemolysates after SPE-RP cleanup and concentration of the eluate. Then, they measured 5,10-methenyl-THF after acid conversion of 5-formyl-THF and 10-formyl-THF into 5,10-methenyl-THF. It is apparent from these different approaches that the analysis of whole blood folate by LC/MS/MS may not yet have reached a final procedure, and future modifications and improvements can be expected. Hannisdal et al. [95] have developed a method that measures 4-α-hydroxy-5-methyl-THF (an oxidation product of 5-methyl-THF) in addition to 5-methyl-THF, 5-formyl-THF, PGA, and two folate catabolites (p-aminobenzoyl glutamic acid [pABG] and p-acetamidobenzoyl glutamic acid [apABG]) after using acetonitrile to deproteinize serum. They found an average of 12% of 4-α-hydroxy-5-methyl-THF in 168 fresh serum samples from healthy Norwegian blood donors. The possible existence of 4-α-hydroxy-5-methyl-THF in vivo should be investigated in future studies, taking particular measures to avoid folate oxidation in vitro [95].

Pawlosky et al. developed an LC/MS method for the measurement of PGA in fortified foods [49], as well as the measurement of 5-methyl-THF and PGA in citrus juices [96] and in a series of food reference materials [97]. Rychlik et al. [54,55] have conducted extensive work using LC/MS/MS to measure various folate forms in foods (spinach, broccoli, wheat bread, and meat) after heat extraction, trienzyme treatment, and SPE-SAX cleanup. They found SAX cleanup to provide extracts with fewer interfering substances during LC/MS/MS than SPE-RP [55]. They also evaluated SPAE as an alternative cleanup technique for wheat bread and beef extracts [60]. In addition to the commonly cited disadvantages of SPAE, they noted that the useful load of the affinity columns for the unlabeled vitamers is further reduced by the added labeled ISs that occupy folate binding sites as well, and that the affinity columns revealed discrimination of racemic folate isotopomers compared with their unlabeled, natural analogues. Two additional LC/MS/MS for folates in spinach [84] and in green and red sweet peppers [94] were published recently; however, both did not use stable isotope-labeled ISs.

Most of the recent ID/LC/MS/MS methods have comparable method characteristics. The linear range of the methods is excellent, usually covering two orders of magnitude. Because these methods use ISs, the spiking recovery of folates added to various biological samples is nearly complete (100% ± 10%). Only few methods have determined the SPE efficiency (by adding the ISs after elution from the cartridge): Investigators reported good recovery (70%–80%) for most folates except for THF (50%) [9,78]. The imprecision is typically between 5% and 10%, and sometimes it is between 10% and 15% for low-concentration compounds. Although it is difficult to compare limits of detection and quantitation across methods because they were derived and expressed differently, it is sufficient to say that LC/MS/MS methods provide the necessary sensitivity to measure relevant folate forms in biological samples.

D. Measurement of Folate Breakdown Products as a Surrogate Indicator for Total Folate

Because the measurement of intact folates is very complex, some groups have aimed at assessing total folate via folate breakdown products. Methods have been developed for the measurement of whole blood total folate after acid hydrolysis to p-aminobenzoic acid (pABA) by GC/MS or LC/MS/MS. Serum total folate can be determined by LC/MS/MS after mild acid hydrolysis to pABG.

1. Gas Chromatography/Mass Spectrometry

One approach to extract folates from whole blood is the acid hydrolysis of native folates at 110°C to pABA for analysis of total folate by GC/MS [98–101]. The original method by Santhosh-Kumar et al. [98] is specific for folate, as FBP is used to bind all folates and remove any free pABA or pABG with one or multiple glutamate residues before acid hydrolysis, whereas all subsequent methods eliminated the need for specific binder proteins or enzymatic deconjugation steps and relied on pABA not being normally found in blood [99–101]. Individuals who use pABA as a drug would have to discontinue it for a few days before blood collection [102]. The sample preparation steps for these GC/MS methods were simplified over time to reach a sample throughput of 40 samples/3 days [100]. Yet, all of them still require a lengthy multistep preparation, including acid hydrolysis, several SPE and liquid/liquid extraction steps, and a final derivatization step to make the pABA GC viable. Stable isotope-labeled pABA ($^{13}C_6$) is used as IS; the methods display great sensitivity and excellent imprecision (≤5%), and they are appropriate for blood from patients using MTX and antibiotics.

2. Liquid Chromatography/Tandem Mass Spectrometry

Another approach to extract folates from whole blood is the acid hydrolysis of native folates at 110°C to pABA for analysis of total folate by LC/MS/MS [102,103]. Compared with the GC/MS methods, the sample preparation steps for the LC/MS/ MS method are much simpler and require only acid hydrolysis, SPE-RP cleanup, and methylesterification [102]. The method has also been adapted to a 96-well plate procedure to increase sample throughput [103]. However, it is still more complex and time-consuming than current LC/MS/MS methods that measure intact folates. It uses $^{13}C_6$-pABA as IS, recovers six different folates between 84% and 105%, and has an imprecision of 11%.

Hannisdal et al. [104] have developed an LC/MS/MS method for the measurement of serum folate species and their degradation products via controlled oxidation and limited acid hydrolysis to pABG. This method is mainly of interest in archived serum samples that have already undergone some folate degradation. The authors initially explored the possibility of measuring pABA following strong acid hydrolysis. However, compared with microbiological analysis, many serum samples seemed to contain pABA precursors that were not microbiologically active folate species. The authors concluded that measurement of serum folate as pABA equivalents after strong acid hydrolysis was not feasible. They found no native pABG in serum, except for a few samples with very high folate concentrations and if the serum was treated with 0.12 M HCl as a result of partial conversion of folate to pABG at low pH. The method cannot be used to assess folate status in patients receiving MTX because it is partially (40%) recovered as pABG. The method displays excellent imprecision (≤5%) and recovers 84% to 106% of various folates, except for 5-formyl-THF (~50% recovery).

E. SUMMARY

HPLC methods offer the possibility of measuring individual folate forms, and they can be conducted by using relatively inexpensive instrumentation. However, compared with the microbiological assay and protein-binding assays, they require a high degree of sample cleanup and concentration to compensate for suboptimal sensitivity and to some degree specificity. Such complex sample manipulation in the face of problematic folate stability begs for the use of ISs that can compensate for procedural losses. However, thus far no suitable compounds have been identified that cover the wide spectrum of folate characteristics.

The advantages of MS methods are that they offer the highest degree of accuracy (when stable isotope-labeled ISs are used) and selectivity (for MS/MS). Moreover, their sensitivity surpasses most other detectors (with the possible exception of EC). However, the instrumentation is expensive, and an experienced staff is needed to operate and maintain it.

There is general consensus that folate standards and biological samples have to be treated with great care to ensure folate integrity during storage, sample handling, and measurement. The fact that more standard compounds (polyglutamates of reduced folates, stable isotope-labeled folates) are now commercially available than 10 years ago shows that there is great interest in folate research. Advances in the area of SPE materials and instrumentation for automated SPE have facilitated sample preparation and thereby increased sample throughput. HPLC columns have been greatly improved to provide more robustness. Last, the availability of ID/LC/MS/MS has removed the "black box" and moved folate methods one step closer to knowledge of what the true value in a sample is.

III. PROTEIN-BINDING ASSAYS

Protein-binding assays were developed during the 1970s and 1980s as a simpler and faster alternative to the microbiological assay. Initially only manual methods were available, and the detection was through radiolabeled folates. A review by Gregory [1] discusses these early radioassays. Later, fully automated nonradioassays were developed for clinical analyzers. Because many of the early methods have changed or have been discontinued, this review will mainly focus on more recent assays.

A. FACTORS INFLUENCING PROTEIN-BINDING ASSAYS

Protein-binding assays have been developed for the clinical laboratory to provide high throughput measurements. Although some of the older assays were true immunoassays using folate-specific antibodies as the folate binder [105,106], most modern assays use FBP (mainly from milk or milk fractions, sometimes from porcine plasma or kidney) to specifically bind folate from the sample, and therefore are protein-binding assays [107]. The higher degree of specificity than is obtainable in the microbiological assay is a plus, but protein-binding assays are subject to all limitations pertaining to FBP. Wilson et al. [107] provide a good overview of various issues to be considered in the standardization of folate-binding assays.

1. Response to Different Folate Monoglutamates and Polyglutamyl Chain Lengths

Shane et al. [108] reported that folate monoglutamates exhibited different responses in radioassay procedures, depending on the one-carbon constituent, the oxidation state, and the stereoisomer used. Folate polyglutamates generally exhibited an increased response compared with monoglutamates, and that response varied, depending on the folate concentration. The authors concluded that this makes protein-binding assays unsuitable for the determination of mixtures of folate derivatives that are normally encountered in biological extracts, such as tissues or foods. Indeed, protein-binding assays have mainly been applied to folate measurement in serum and whole blood. Little is known about how the relative affinities of FBP for PGA and 5-methyl-THF are affected by the method of FBP incorporation into assay reagents [107].

2. Influence of pH and Protein Content of the Sample

Most protein-binding assays are conducted at pH 9.3 because PGA and 5-methyl-THF show equivalent binding affinity to FBP at that pH [109]. However, it was shown that slight deviations in pH can lead to variations in binding affinity and to erroneous measurements [110]. Blackmore et al. reported that most protein-binding assays under-recover 5-methyl-THF and over-recover PGA [111]. Effects of the pH might be one of the reasons for these inaccurate recoveries. The protein content of the sample is another important factor. Shane et al. [108] showed that differences in binding occurred depending on whether the folate standards were in serum, human serum albumin, or buffer. Therefore, protocols of modern assays always stipulate that samples should be diluted with a protein solution rather than a buffer.

3. Other Problems Encountered with Protein-Binding Assays

Protein-binding assays suffer from a limited dynamic range that typically extends only to approximately 20 ng/mL serum folate [112]. Therefore, increased blood folate concentrations in the US population as a result of folic acid fortification have necessitated dilution and reanalysis of a high proportion of samples. However, in addition to the limited dynamic range, binding assays may suffer from inaccurate dilution linearity [107,112]. These linearity problems are sometimes the result of differing dose-response characteristics between the standards and patient samples. Because the factors that cause "disharmony" between gravimetrically correct calibrators and the patient dose response may not be linear across the assay range, the linearity problems can sometimes be only resolved if gravimetrically correct standards are adjusted mathematically to fit a patient dose-response curve [107].

Binding assays are not sensitive to antibiotics in biological samples, and the FBPs used generally have little affinity for folate analogs and oxidation products [110]. However, the antifolate drug MTX has been reported to interfere with radioassays at levels attained in plasma following high-dose chemotherapy [113,114].

B. Sample Preparation

Sample preparation procedures vary depending on the type of the protein-binding assay. In competitive assays, the sample and the labeled folate conjugate are mixed before the introduction of a limited amount of FBP, ensuring competition for the binding sites. Conversely, in noncompetitive assays, an excess capacity of FBP is incubated with the sample before the addition of the labeled folate conjugate. Protein-binding assays can be either heterogeneous or homogeneous. In heterogeneous assays, excess unbound analyte or excess reaction components have to be removed, requiring that either the FBP or the folate conjugate be immobilized to a solid support [3]. In homogeneous assays, no separation step is required.

1. Radioassays

Most radiometric assay procedures are competitive binding assays in which radiolabeled tracer folate (^{125}I-PGA) and unlabeled folate from the sample compete at pH 9.3 for limited binding sites on the FBP. Endogenous proteins are either denatured through heat (boil assays) or through treatment with an alkaline reagent (no-boil assays). Although the Bio-Rad (Hercules, CA) assay was discontinued in 2007, it is still included in this review because it was used extensively for almost 20 years in large population-based surveys, and data from this assay are still used to compare with other methods and studies. Radioassays require a manual multistep procedure that takes several hours before radioactivity counting is performed on a β-counter. Typically, 0.2 mL of serum or whole blood hemolysate is required per determination, and each sample is analyzed in duplicate. Most radioassays measure both serum folate and vitamin B12.

2. Automated (Nonradioassay) Protein-Binding Assays

Different commercial kits are available for automated folate measurement in serum or whole blood hemolysates on clinical analyzers (Table 21.2). The preparation of whole blood hemolysates is always performed off line, and the conditions for this step vary across assays. Most binding assays are competitive and heterogeneous, and they use milk protein as the source for the FBP. Generally, an on-board pretreatment step with alkaline reagent and antioxidant ensures the release of folate from endogenous FBP and its stabilization to prevent oxidation. Next, folate conjugate and FBP immobilized to a solid support are sequentially added (sequence of addition is opposite for noncompetitive binding assays). Finally, a trigger solution generates chemiluminescence. The FBP can be immobilized directly on a microbead (Ortho-Clinical Diagnostics Vitros, Rochester, NY; Roche Elecsys, Indianapolis, IN; and cobas e analyzer, Roche) or paramagnetic particle (Abbott Architect, Abbott Park, IL) through a secondary anti-FBP antibody that is immobilized onto a microbead

TABLE 21.2

Protein-Binding Assays

Company	Instrument	Matrix[a]	Type[b]	Immobilization	Folate Conjugate	Detection[c]	Calibrator	Assay Characteristics	Comments
Abbott Folate assay	Architect	SE, HEP-P, WB (1:11 diluted with 0.4% AA, and guanidine HCl; 1:2 dilution w/ citric acid and guanidine HCl)	NC, HET, No-boil	FBP immobilized to paramagnetic particles	Pteroic acid acridinium-labeled	CL	PGA in HSA	LOD 0.8 ng/mL; dynamic range 0.8–30 ng/mL; throughput 200 tests/h	Standardized to NIBSC IS 03/178; extended dynamic range; not available in US; tentative launch time is 2009 or 2010; available abroad
	AxSYM	SE, EDTA-P, WB (1:11 diluted with folate lysis reagent, then 1:2 diluted with protein diluent)	NC, HET, No-boil	FBP immobilized through ion capture	Pteroic acid and alkaline phosphatase	CL	PGA in HSA	LOD 0.9 ng/mL; dynamic range 0.9–20 ng/mL; throughput 47 tests/h; sample volume 105 µL	Nonlinearity and narrow dynamic range are a problem; available in US since 2006; available abroad
Beckman Coulter Folate assay	Access 2, UniCel DxI	SE, HEP-P, WB (1:21 diluted with 0.15% AA)	C, HET, No-boil	Secondary anti-FBP antibody coupled to paramagnetic microparticles	Folic acid alkaline phosphatase	CL	PGA in buffered matrix	LOD 0.5 ng/mL; dynamic range 0–20 ng/mL; throughput 100 tests/h; sample volume 55 µL	Access instrument no longer supported; same kit used for Access2 (bench-top) and UniCel DxI (floor-model); assay available on both instruments in US and abroad
Ortho Clinical Diagnostics (OCD) Folate assay	VITROS	SE, P, WB (1:41 diluted with red cell folate reagent)	C, HET, No-boil	Biotinylated FBP coupled to streptavidin-coated well	Horseradish peroxidase-labeled folate	CL	PGA in buffer	LOD 0.2 ng/mL; dynamic range 0–20 ng/mL; sample volume 53 µL	

continued

TABLE 21.2 (continued)
Protein-Binding Assays

Company	Instrument	Matrix^a	Type^b	Immobilization	Folate Conjugate	Detection^c	Calibrator	Assay Characteristics	Comments
Roche Folate II	Elecsys 2010, E170, cobas e411, e601	SE, WB (1:31 diluted with 0.2% AA)	C, HET, No-boil	Ruthenium-labeled FBP-folate biotin complex coupled to streptavidin-coated microparticles	Biotin-labeled folate	Electro-CL		LOD 0.6 ng/mL; dynamic range 0.6–20 ng/mL	
Siemens (formerly Dade Behring) FOL Flex LOCI Folate assay	Dimension Vista 1500 Intelligent Lab System	SE, HEP-P	C, HOM, No-boil	Biotinylated FBP/streptavidin complex containing photosensitive dye; not immobilized	Folic acid derivative containing chemiluminescent dye	CL through oxygen channeling	PGA	LOD 0.5 ng/mL; dynamic range 0.5–20 ng/mL; throughput 180 tests/h; sample volume 10 μL	Low sample volume because of higher sensitivity; not for WB; available in the US since 2008
Siemens (formerly Bayer Diagnostics) Folate assay	ACS:180	SE, WB (1:21 diluted with 1% AA)	C, HET, No-boil	Biotinylated FBP/avidin complex coupled to paramagnetic particles	Acridinium ester–labeled folate	CL	5CH3THF in buffer with HSA	LOD 0.25 ng/mL; dynamic range 0–24 ng/mL; throughput 180 tests/h; sample volume 130 μL	Became obsolete at end of 2008
	ADVIA Centaur	SE, WB (1:21 diluted with 1% AA)	C, HET, No-boil	Biotinylated FBP/avidin complex coupled to paramagnetic particles	Acridinium ester–labeled folate	CL	5CH3THF in buffer with HSA	LOD 0.35 ng/mL; dynamic range 0.35–24 ng/mL; throughput 240 tests/h; sample volume 150 μL	Available in the US and abroad; XP is floor-model, CP is bench-top model; same kits can be used

Siemens (formerly DPC) Folic acid assay	Immulite 1000	SE, HEP-P, WB (1:21 diluted with 1% AA)	C, HET, Boil	Secondary anti-FBP antibody coupled to microbead	Ligand-labeled folate	CL	Traceable to an IS	LOD 0.8 ng/mL; dynamic range 1–24 ng/mL; sample volume 200 µL	Partially manual (boil step); 1000 (bench-top) available in the US and abroad; different kits than for 2000
	Immulite 2000 (or 2500)	SE, HEP-P, WB (1:26 diluted with 0.5% AA)	C, HET, No-boil	Microbead with anti-FBP antibody	Ligand-labeled folate and alkaline phosphatase labeled antiligand	CL	Traceable to an IS	LOD 0.8 ng/mL; dynamic range 1–24 ng/mL; sample volume 50 µL	Relatively low sample volume; 2000 (floor-model) available in the US and abroad; different kits than for 1000; 2500 (floor-model) may be phased out
Tosoh	AIA-Pack	SE	C, HET, No-boil	Polyclonal antibody		EIA		LOD 0.8 ng/mL; dynamic range 0–20 ng/mL; sample volume 100 µL	
Boehringer Mannheim CEDIA	Cobas-Mira, Roche		C			CEDIA		LOD 3.6 nM	

^a SE, serum; HEP-P, heparin plasma; EDTA-P, EDTA plasma; WB, whole blood; AA, ascorbic acid.

^b NC, noncompetitive; C, competitive; HET, heterogeneous; HOM, homogeneous.

^c CL, chemiluminescence; EIA, enzyme immunoassay; CEDIA, cloned enzyme donor immunoassay.

(Siemens Immulite, Deerfield, IL) or paramagnetic particle (Siemens Advia Centaur and ACS:180; Beckman Coulter Access, Fullerton, CA), or through ion capture (Abbott IMx and AxSYM). Recently, the first homogeneous chemiluminescent immunoassay was released (Siemens Dimension Vista). The luminescent oxygen channeling technology (LOCI) eliminates the need for trigger reagents or separate washing steps. It is claimed to provide greater sensitivity, precision, and accuracy. The sample preparation for enzymatic folate assays (Tosoh AIA-Pack, South San Francisco, CA; Boehringer Mannheim Cedia, Pleasanton, CA) uses the same principles as are applicable for FBP-based assays.

C. Measurement

1. Radioassays

Radiometric binding assays use radiolabeled folate conjugate (typically ^{125}I-PGA or ^{75}Se-PGA), and the folate concentration in the sample is calculated by comparing the radioactivity in the pellet with a standard curve. The folate concentration of the sample is inversely proportional to the radioactivity in the pellet, resulting in a high sensitivity of radioassays at low folate concentrations.

2. Automated (Nonradioassay) Protein-Binding Assays

Automated protein-binding assays typically use chemiluminescence as detection. The amount of folate conjugate bound to the FBP is proportional to the resulting light signal and the relationship between the folate concentration in the sample, and the resulting light signal is inversely proportional. Enzyme immunoassays typically use fluorescence detection, but everything else applies.

D. Summary

Protein-binding assays can provide reasonable assay precision and very high sample throughput with minimum operator involvement. Their lack of sensitivity to antibiotics is an advantage compared with the microbiological assay. However, they are subject to all limitations that apply to FBP, resulting in questionable accuracy when mixtures of folates (or certain antifolates such as MTX) are present in biological samples. A new challenge for protein-binding assays is to extend their reportable range to higher folate concentrations, in response to changing population values.

IV. MICROBIOLOGICAL ASSAYS

The microbiological assay has been used for total folate measurement for more than 50 years. Several important improvements were introduced between 1966 and 1986: (1) the aseptic addition of serum to autoclaved solutions, alleviating the need to autoclave serum [115]; (2) the development of a chloramphenicol-resistant strain of *Lactobacillus casei*, eliminating the need for sterilization or aseptic addition [116] and enabling the use of disposable labware [117]; (3) the ability to cryopreserve the inoculum, providing standardized growth curves for hundreds of assays [118]; and (4) the introduction of automated microtiter plate technology, miniaturizing the assay and providing dramatically improved efficiency in absorbance readings [119]. From this point, two "types" of microbiological assays were put into practice. Horne and Patterson [120,121] adopted the 96-well plate technology and cryopreservation, but they maintained the traditional organism (ATCC 7469), necessitating sterilization of reagents by filtration and stringent aseptic precautions. O'Broin and Kelleher [122] incorporated the use of a chloramphenicol-resistant organism (ATCC 27773 or NCIB 10463) in addition to the above advantages. In 1997, Molloy and Scott [123] published a protocol of this new and improved microbiological assay adapted from the O'Broin method.

Ironically, by the time all these improvements were put into place to make the microbiological assay more robust and efficient, most investigators had lost interest and had switched to automated protein-binding assays or to chromatographic methods. During the past few years, however, the microbiological assay has experienced renewed interest, mainly because of the need for an inexpensive, low-technology, yet accurate, folate method that could be used by low-resource countries interested in assessing population folate status in nutrition surveys. The small amount of biological sample needed, a result of the high sensitivity of the assay, is also an appealing aspect for nutrition surveys, particularly if the survey personnel are able to collect only limited amounts of blood through finger-stick sampling. Finally, preparation of dried blood spots (DBS) is often the only possibility to produce a valid biological sample if the population is located remotely and survey personnel are without access to reliable electricity, transportation, and other infrastructure. Total folate can be measured in DBS with the microbiological assay [124,125].

A. FACTORS INFLUENCING THE MICROBIOLOGICAL ASSAY

The principle of the turbidimetric microbiological assay is that the microorganism is dependent on folate and cannot grow in a folate-free medium. Therefore, the growth response is proportional to the amount of folate in the sample. The majority of determinations of total folate in foods and other biological samples during the early days has been performed by use of *Lactobacillus rhamnosus* (ATCC 7469), formerly known as *L. casei* [126,127]. *L. rhamnosus* has been shown to be specific to biologically active folate without responding to inactive folate stereoisomers [108,119], to folate precursors such as pteroic acid [128], or to breakdown products such as pABG [103]. The main feature of the organism is that it shows similar response to a wide variety of naturally occurring folate derivatives.

1. Response to Different Polyglutamyl Chain Lengths

L. rhamnosus responds fully to mono-, di-, and triglutamates, but its response decreases with increasing polyglutamyl chain length: On a molar basis, only 66%, 20%, 4%, and 2% of the response obtained with PGA monoglutamate is obtained with tetra-, penta-, hexa-, and heptaglutamates of PGA, respectively [129]. These response patterns mean that folate activity before conjugase treatment cannot be considered a measure of the natural "free folate" unless pteroylpolyglutamates are absent from the sample [129].

2. Response to Different Folate Monoglutamates

L. rhamnosus is generally reported to exhibit similar growth response to various monoglutamyl folates [108,120,122], albeit the growth curves shown by Horne and Patterson [120] demonstrate some variability in folate response. Phillips and Wright [130–132] showed a concentration-dependent reduced response of 5-methyl-THF compared with PGA at pH 6.8, which disappeared at pH 6.2. Using the chloramphenicol-resistant version of *L. rhamnosus* (ATCC 27773) and an adaptation of the O'Broin et al. method [122], we observed that, on a molar basis, 5-methyl-THF produced a slightly higher response curve than PGA, resulting in lower calculated results if 5-methyl-THF was used as a calibrator compared with PGA [9]. We repeated our experiments using multiple stock solutions and analyzed the results over multiple days to better account for assay variability. On average, we found a difference of 15% in calculated results between using 5-methyl-THF or PGA as calibrator (Figure 21.1; M. Zhang and C. M. Pfeiffer, unpublished observations).

3. Problems Encountered with the Microbiological Assay

The presence of antibiotics or antifolates can interfere with the growth of the microorganism and thereby result in an underestimation of folate concentrations [114,133]. Evidence of such interference is either a complete inhibition of organism growth or a partial inhibition that creates a discrepancy in the results of two dilutions [122]. Serum

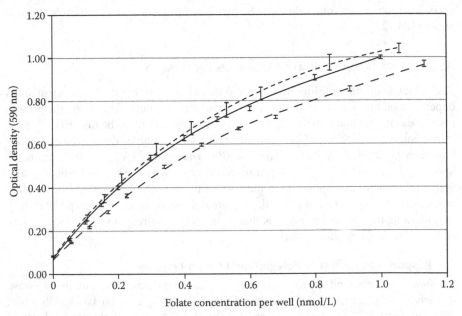

FIGURE 21.1 Average growth response of *L. rhamnosus* to different folate calibrator forms. .... 5-Formyl-THF; two independent calibrator preparations (Merck Eprova and Sigma-Aldrich) were analyzed on 1 day. _____ 5-Methyl-THF; one calibrator preparation (Merck Eprova) was analyzed over 10 independent days. _ _ _ _ _ _ PGA; four independent calibrator preparations (Merck Eprova and Sigma-Aldrich) were analyzed on 1 day. Error bars represent standard error.

preincubation with a β-lactamase preparation has shown some success in eliminating interference caused by certain antibiotics [122]. *L. rhamnosus* strains resistant to rifampicin [134] or MTX [135] have also been developed. During the past year or so, our laboratory has analyzed more than 7,000 serum and whole blood samples from the US population. Thus far, we found marked inhibition of the microorganism growth in only a few samples (far less than 1%), for which we suspected interference from either antibiotics or antifolates as a result of discrepant results of the two dilutions (M. Zhang and C. M. Pfeiffer, unpublished observations). This is consistent with other reports [122]. Because of the high folate status of the US population, we were able to use higher dilutions on reanalysis and obtained a reportable result in most cases.

Although stimulation of the growth of the organism by nonfolate factors of food extracts has been of some concern, little research has been conducted to examine the specificity of *L. rhamnosus* as used in the analysis of foods and other biological materials [131]. It is interesting to note that among the few studies that compared food folate results obtained by chromatographic methods with those obtained by microbiological assay, most found lower results by HPLC or LC/MS [53,55,82]. Pfeiffer et al. [59] used SPAE-purified cereal grain extracts as a sample for the microbiological assay and found comparable results between the two assays. It is possible that nonfolate factors that could stimulate the growth of the organism were removed.

Because of its high sensitivity, the microbiological assay is susceptible to extraneous folate and microbial contamination. Therefore, it has been recommended to carry out all operations by using PGA or other folate calibrators well away from the microbiological workstation [123] and to start over with new materials and organisms when problems are encountered, rather than wasting time trying to determine the cause of the trouble [117,127]. In our experience, contamination issues are not a frequent problem (<1 of 100 runs) if these suggestions are followed.

B. SAMPLE PREPARATION

1. Serum

No special sample preparation other than a dilution of serum, typically with freshly made 5 g/L sodium ascorbate solution, is necessary. In populations with low folate status, serum is usually diluted 1:20 [122,123], whereas in populations with normal folate status, serum may be diluted 1:40 [123]. Because of the high folate status of the US population after the initiation of folic acid fortification, we routinely dilute serum samples 1:100.

2. Whole Blood

Hemolyzed EDTA-whole blood is generally used to determine blood folate status. In the calculation of an accurate RBC folate concentration, the contribution of serum folate and the hematocrit have to be taken into consideration [136]. Alternatively, washed RBCs can be used with plasma replacement [137]. It is important to carefully mix the whole blood before removing an aliquot. Usually 100 μL of whole blood is added to 900 μL of 10-g/L freshly prepared AA solution [122,123]. This not only achieves an efficient hemolysis of RBCs [77], but it also lowers the pH of the sample to slightly acidic, so that long-chain polyglutamates are rapidly cleaved to short-chain polyglutamates and monoglutamates through the endogenous conjugase [74]. Hemolysates are usually left at room temperature [123] or at 37°C [122] for

30 minutes. Our group has shown that when freshly prepared hemolysates are frozen before analysis, there is no need to incubate the thawed sample before processing [71]. Hemolysates are usually diluted 1:40 (populations with low folate status) or 1:80 (populations with normal folate) [123]. As with serum, our group uses a greater dilution for hemolysates as well (1:140).

3. Dried Blood Spots and Serum Spots

DBS samples are useful in situations where only minute quantities of blood are available and/or the infrastructure does not allow sophisticated sample handling and storage. The samples are prepared by pipetting EDTA-whole blood (approximately 50 μL) onto filter paper cards placed horizontally on a rack and allowed to air-dry overnight at room temperature [124]. Folate and hemoglobin are coeluted from DBS center punches (1/4 inch or 6.35 mm in diameter) into an ascorbate-detergent solution (5 g/L AA, 1 mL/L Triton, or 0.5 or 1 mL/L Tween 80) by sonicating for 60 minutes [124,125]. Hydrolysis of folate polyglutamates by endogenous plasma conjugase proceeds during elution. DBS eluate folate (by microbiological assay) and Hb concentrations (by spectrophotometry) are then assayed by use of an assumed common dilution factor of 1:20. Whole blood folate results are expressed as Hb-folate after division by the Hb result as follows: Hb-folate (nmol/g) = whole blood folate (nM)/Hb (g/L). Because of this calculation, analytic precision is independent of the DBS area-volume relation, and accurate folate analysis of blood specimens of unknown volume or dilution is possible [125].

O'Broin and Gunter [138] also developed a dried serum spot (DSS) assay for folate. To maintain folate stability and avoid bias resulting from nonuniform serum distribution in the paper, serum spots had to be prepared on ascorbate-treated paper, and the entire spot, rather than a fixed-size punch, had to be used for analysis. However, the stability of DSS folate for up to 1 week at 20°C and for 2 weeks at 4°C indicated a potential for short-term storage in conventional refrigerators or for shipping by mail from collection sites.

4. Foods

The analysis of food folates by microbiological assay follows the same extraction steps as described under chromatographic methods, but no sample cleanup is performed. Because of its commercial availability and low cost compared with other conjugase enzymes, chicken pancreas has been used predominantly to generate folate diglutamates for the microbiological assay. As with chromatographic methods, trienzyme extraction is also used with the microbiological assay [37] and is part of the American Association of Cereal Chemists (AACC) Official Method 86-47 for total folates in cereal products [139].

C. Measurement

1. Total Folate by Conventional *L. rhamnosus* Assay

Historically, either PGA [122,123] or 5-formyl-THF (racemic form) [120,127] has been used as a calibrator because they are easier to handle due to their greater stability compared with other folate forms. Our group uses 5-methyl-THF because this compound is the predominant folate form in serum and whole blood, and, as noted earlier, we found slight differences in response between PGA and 5-methyl-THF.

A detailed assay procedure using the chloramphenicol-resistant organism (ATCC 27773) has been described previously [123]. Briefly, 200 μL of growth medium and 50 or 100 μL of diluted sample (made up to 100 μL with 5 g/L sodium ascorbate) are pipetted into 96-well plates; for each sample, two independent dilutions, two volumes (50 μL and 100 μL) per dilution, and two replicates per volume are used, for a total of eight wells/sample. The plates are tightly sealed and incubated at 37°C in the dark for 40 to 45 hours. After plates have cooled down to room temperature, they are thoroughly mixed by slow inversion, and the optical density is measured at 590 nm on a microplate reader. A polynomial equation (third degree), generated from a 10-point calibration curve spanning a concentration range of 0 to 50 pg/well, is used to calculate the average folate concentration (from the four replicates) in each sample.

We implemented the following modifications in our laboratory. They provide higher throughput without compromising the quality of the assay (M. Zhang and C. M. Pfeiffer, unpublished observations):

1. Because of the high dilution for hemolysates (1:140), we found it unnecessary to include a color blank for each whole blood sample as suggested by O'Broin [122]. In our assay, the color blank gives typically the same optical density as the calibration curve zero-point. However, if samples are diluted 1:40, a color blank should be used.
2. Instead of having a separate quality control (QC) plate, we prefer to distribute the QC samples across all plates to monitor the quality of each plate.
3. Furthermore, including a blank (medium and sodium ascorbate only) on each plate (four replicates) is helpful to test for contamination.
4. We have automated the sample pipetting steps using a four-probe robotic sample handler. This allows us to prepare seven plates with a total of 132 patient samples (including a standard plate) within 2 hours, whereas it would take more than twice the time to manually dilute and dispense the samples. The precision of the automated and manual assay is comparable (9%–11% CV for three levels of serum or whole-blood QC pools analyzed over several months). The automated pipetting has one drawback: Approximately 200 μL of serum or hemolysate is needed for the probe to pick up the sample.

Another important change our laboratory has introduced is the use of 5-methyl-THF as a calibrator instead of PGA [122,123] or 5-formyl-THF [120,127]. We made this choice because we observed a slightly higher response of the microorganism with this folate form, and the majority of folate in biological samples is 5-methyl-THF.

2. Differential Folate Microbiological Assay

By conducting multiple microbiological assays with different organisms, sometimes called the "differential folate microbiological assay," investigators have determined the folate composition of biological samples before chemical methods were available [127]. They would assess total folate by using *L. rhamnosus*, 5-methyl-THF by calculating the difference between the *L. rhamnosus* and *Streptococcus faecium* response, and they would assess nonmethyl folate by calculating the difference between *L. rhamnosus* and *Pediococcus cerevisiae* response. To our knowledge, these methods are no longer used.

D. Summary

The microbiological assay distinguishes itself by exceptional sensitivity, low cost, and simple instrumentation. The introduction of 96-well plate technology has dramatically improved assay efficiency. Cryopreservation of the organism and the availability of a chloramphenicol-resistant strain have made the assay more robust and precise. The disadvantages of the microbiological assay are that it measures only total folate, its imprecision is slightly higher than for other methods, antibiotics or antifolates can cause interference with the growth of the organism, and the assay can suffer from contamination issues if not performed carefully. Although the automation of the pipetting steps significantly decreased the manual labor involved with the assay, it still takes 2 days before results are available; therefore, assays can be set up only during the early part of the week.

V. PREANALYTICAL FACTORS RELEVANT FOR PHYSIOLOGICAL FLUIDS

Blood folate concentrations are influenced by numerous preanalytical factors that relate to the physiological or health status of the individual or to the handling of the sample before analysis. Although the laboratory typically has little influence on the former, it can avoid potential problems during sample handling to maintain its integrity. Clinical textbooks contain useful information on physiological factors that affect blood folate concentrations [140–142]; however, only scant information is available on proper sample handling. With more countries conducting nutrition surveys—often in low-resource settings—the demand for reliable sample handling information is continually increasing. Even the best analytical method is bound to produce poor results if the quality of the sample is inadequate.

A. Sample Collection

1. Venous versus Capillary Blood Collection

Using the microbiological assay, O'Broin et al. [124] compared Hb-folate concentrations (ratio between folate and Hb determined in the same sample) of volumetrically prepared finger-stick and venous EDTA whole blood samples from 28 healthy volunteers. They found good correlation and no significant difference ($r^2 = 0.98$; $P > .87$). This was also true for nonvolumetrically prepared samples from 45 blood bank donors, with the finger-stick sample taken secondary to a primary sampling from the identical site for Hb screening to simulate field conditions ($r^2 = 0.9$; $P > .39$). To simplify sample collection even further, they instructed 56 blood bank donors to add a drop of blood directly from the finger-stick site into an EDTA-cryovial containing 1 mL of sterile AA (5 g/L)/Triton X-100 (1 g/L) solution, to cap the vial, and to mix the solution immediately and thoroughly by inversion six times. The Hb-folate concentration in these samples also compared well with venous controls ($r^2 = 0.85$; $P > .3$). Estimation of Hb-folate overcomes the problem of accurately pipetting and diluting small sample volumes. However, it requires an additional analysis (determination of Hb in the hemolysate) and adequate mixing of the blood with the EDTA (mixing and inverting the cryovial at least six times) to avoid formation of clots in small finger-stick samples [124].

2. Influence of Various Anticoagulants

Laboratories typically prefer analyzing serum samples because plasma might contain fibrinogen clots—particularly after longer storage or multiple freeze/thaw cycles—and the clotting makes pipetting more difficult. The suitability of different sample types has to be verified for each assay. O'Broin et al. [143] found no significant difference between folate results from serum, heparinized (HEP), or EDTA plasma samples with the microbiological assay; whole blood folates collected in both HEP and EDTA did not show a difference in concentrations either. Using LC/MS/MS, Fazili et al. [78] compared serum to plasma with various anticoagulants from 26 volunteer blood donors. They found that dipotassium EDTA and acid citrate dextrose (ACD) plasma samples produced significantly lower results compared with serum (−3.8% [95% CI, −7.4% to −0.2%], $P = .009$, and −15.7% [−19.6% to −11.8%], $P < .0001$, respectively). The lower results found with ACD plasma were mostly attributable to the volume of the ACD solution in the tube (12% dilution). HEP plasma gave slightly but not significantly lower concentrations (−2.5% [−4.6% to 0.5%], $P = .11$). Our group also applied the microbiological assay to the same samples and found similar anticoagulant effects: EDTA (−12.4% [−9.5% to −15.3%], $P < .0001$), ACD (−15.0% [−12.4% to −17.6%], $P < .0001$), and HEP (2.6% [−0.8% to 6.0%], $P = .097$) (M. Zhang and C. M. Pfeiffer, unpublished observations). However, the magnitude of the difference between EDTA plasma and serum was larger with the microbiological assay. EDTA was previously reported to interact with divalent cations in the medium and to inhibit growth of the organism [144]. The addition of manganese or iron supposedly chelates excess EDTA [123,144]. Our growth medium contains manganese sulfate (15 mg/100 mL) but possibly not enough to completely remove the inhibition. As part of the same study, we investigated the effect of anticoagulants on whole blood folate measured by both assays in hemolysates from 10 blood donors. Compared with EDTA, HEP produced similar results (±5%), but ACD produced significantly lower results, even after dilution correction (10%–20% lower) (Z. Fazili, M. Zhang, and C. M. Pfeiffer, unpublished observations).

B. Sample Processing

1. Influence of Delayed Sample Processing

Because reduced folates are susceptible to oxidation and breakdown, it is recommended to process blood samples as soon as possible after collection and to keep the tubes protected from light and elevated temperatures in the interim. O'Broin et al. [124,143] tested the short-term stability of whole blood total folate under different storage conditions. They found greater than 90% recovery of folates when intact blood was stored up to 4 days at 4°C [124] and greater than 80% recovery at 22°C ($n = 14$) [124,143]; the latter was also confirmed by van Eijsden [145]. Using LC/MS/MS, we are currently conducting a long-term storage experiment (−70°C) of intact blood from subjects with *MTHFR* CC and TT genotype ($n = 13$). During the past 2 years, we obtained whole blood total folate concentrations generally comparable to hemolysates generated at the time of blood collection. However, the folate pattern for TT subjects has changed slightly over time, with a reduction of THF in favor of 5,10-methenyl-THF (Z. Fazili and C. M. Pfeiffer, unpublished observation).

Storage of unprocessed EDTA whole blood at elevated temperature is unacceptable, even for short periods: after only 1 day at 37°C, nearly 20% loss of whole blood total folate was observed [121], and 30% loss of serum total folate [146].

2. Generation of Whole Blood Hemolysate

As discussed in Section II, Chromatographic Assays, it is important to use appropriate conditions for hemolysis and deconjugation of folate polyglutamates. This step is best performed in the controlled environment of a laboratory. If possible, it is preferred to generate hemolysates at the time of blood collection. However, if accurate pipetting and prompt freezing of the hemolysate cannot be achieved in the field, it might be better to maintain the intact whole blood refrigerated for less than 1 week or to freeze an aliquot of whole blood and perform the hemolysis at a later time at the laboratory that conducts the folate assay. However, it is important to note that significant folate losses can occur when frozen whole blood is thawed inappropriately. In samples with TT genotype ($n = 2$), our group observed on average 2%, 21%, and 51% folate losses when we kept the thawed whole blood samples at ambient temperature for 1, 2, and 3 hours, respectively. We observed smaller losses in samples with CC genotype (1%, 7%, and 24%, respectively; Z. Fazili and C. M. Pfeiffer, unpublished observations). A similar rapid loss of folate activity (50%) was found by O'Broin et al. [124] when they left frozen whole blood at ambient temperature for 24 hours; they consequently recommended that blood samples that thaw during transportation should not be analyzed.

3. Dried Blood Spots

It is important to ensure complete drying of DBS cards before storage and to store the cards in resealable plastic bags with desiccant sachets. Short-term, DBS cards can be kept refrigerated for up to 1 week or at ambient temperature for a few days with more than 90% recovery of folates [125]. For long-term storage, DBS cards should be placed into frozen storage (−20°C or lower) as soon as possible, but at least within 1 week of preparation to avoid folate losses greater than 10% [125]. Once the DBS cards are frozen, unnecessary freezing/thawing should be avoided, and the exposure of the sample to room temperature should be minimized. Because of the high surface/volume ratio of DBS samples, the samples thaw very quickly once removed from the freezer.

C. Sample Storage

1. Storage Stability

Short-term storage stability of folates in refrigerated serum samples is generally good (<10% decrease) for less than 1 week [143,146–148]. Plasma samples have been reported to be less stable than serum samples, with or without the addition of

AA [143], which can help protect folates during storage [123,143]. The UK National External Quality Assessment Service (NEQAS) Haematinics scheme showed that serum samples preserved with AA (5 g/L) and stored up to 1 week at ambient temperature showed full recovery of spiked 5-methyl-THF and PGA (<5% loss) [111]. Serum stored in a frost-free freezer at −20°C for even a short period (<1 month) may be relatively unstable and sensitive to minor temperature fluctuations associated with the freeze/thaw cycles [149].

The short-term stability of whole blood total folate in unfrozen hemolysates is worse than that of intact whole blood [124,143]. The stability is acceptable if hemolysates are stored at 4°C (>90% recovery for up to 4 days) [124] but unacceptable if hemolysates are stored at 22°C (only 80% and 50% recovery after 1 and 2 days, respectively) [124,143].

Only sparse information is available on long-term storage stability of folates. Good stability of folates in serum or plasma (containing 5 g/L AA) stored at −20°C for years [143] and of hemolysates stored at −20°C for 26 months [150] was reported. Conversely, a 20% decrease in folate concentrations in serum without ascorbate after 1 year of storage at −20°C with no further decrease thereafter for up to 4 years [151] was found. Recent data from our laboratory on both serum (without ascorbate) and whole blood hemolysate QC samples seem to indicate that as long as samples are stored at −70°C they are stable for at least 4 years. Even hemolysates containing folate forms other than 5-methyl-THF (i.e., THF, 5,10-methenyl-THF, and 5-formyl-THF) showed good stability (Z. Fazili and C. M. Pfeiffer, unpublished observations).

2. Freeze/Thaw Stability

Folates are susceptible to losses as a result of repeated freezing/thawing. Pfeiffer et al. [9] observed no loss of folates when serum was subjected to three freeze/thaw cycles with only brief exposure to ambient temperature (1 hour) but up to 10% loss with extended exposure to ambient temperature (5 hours). Similarly, Drammeh et al. [146] found less than 5% loss of folates when serum was subjected to three freeze/thaw cycles with 3 hours each at ambient temperature. Our laboratory found good stability of whole blood folates not containing THF for up to three freeze/thaw cycles but approximately 20% loss in a whole blood sample containing THF after two freeze/thaw cycles (Z. Fazili and C. M. Pfeiffer, unpublished observation).

VI. METHOD COMPARISONS

A. Physiological Fluids

Many reports have shown that folate methods for serum and whole blood generally agree poorly, and this has not changed much during the past 20 years [152–157]. As a result of continuous reformulations of most commercial assays, we are limiting the presentation and discussion of such data to recent reports.

1. Results from Individual Research Studies

The three European FLAIR (Food-Linked Agro-Industrial Research) intercomparison studies [154], the two Centers for Disease Control and Prevention (CDC) international round-robin studies [155,158], and the assay comparison study conducted by the ARUP Institute for Clinical and Experimental Pathology [156] have presented a comprehensive picture of the large interassay variations of commercial kit assays and the microbiological assay for serum and particularly whole blood samples. They stressed the importance of improved standardization of diagnostic kits, the development of reference methods and suitable reference materials, and the need to use method-specific reference ranges. Laboratories performing the same commercial assay generally produced comparable results; however, results obtained with the microbiological assay by various laboratories did not necessarily agree well [154,155]. Most commercial assays demonstrated acceptable imprecision ($\leq$10%), generally good linearity, and good correlation when compared with the microbiological assay or with the Bio-Rad Quantaphase II assay [156,158]. However, they revealed poor agreement with two- to ninefold differences in concentrations between methods [155], large interlaboratory variations (approximately 20% for serum samples and 47% for whole blood samples) [158], and substantial calibration differences with different effects in serum and whole blood [156]. The lack of assay comparability for whole blood folate has also been shown by Clifford et al. [159], when they compared their GC/MS assay measuring pABA as a surrogate indicator of total folate with the microbiological, radio-, and chemiluminescence assay and received rather poor correlations (r between 0.47 and 0.83).

2. Results from External Quality Assurance Programs

Earlier reports from quality assurance programs showed that interlaboratory variation for serum and whole blood folate assays was unsatisfactory [152,153]. Some of the problems were thought to be inherent to radioassays (measuring a mixture of folate compounds), whereas other factors such as variation in dilution, diluent, and incubation of whole blood samples, calculation errors, release of bound folate, and stability of folates during the procedure could be influenced. Bock et al. [157] recently compared, as part of the College of American Pathologists (CAP) Ligand survey, serum folate results obtained by participants using two types of survey material: conventional proficiency testing material (PTM) and fresh-frozen human serum (FFS). They found no correlation of method biases between PTM and FFS samples, indicating that PTM and FFS exhibit different method biases and the biases reflect analyte heterogeneity and/or matrix effects in addition to calibration biases.

To provide up-to-date information on comparability of commercial assays for serum and whole blood folate, we have obtained permission from the CAP Ligand survey and the UK NEQAS Haematinics program to show a subset of their data from 2007 (Table 21.3 and Figure 21.2). We selected three representative serum and whole blood samples from each program at low, medium, and high folate concentration. The CAP data (Table 21.3) show that (1) the intra-assay variability for whole blood samples is approximately twofold higher compared with serum samples; (2) the interassay variability for whole blood samples is almost threefold higher compared with serum samples; and (3) the interassay range of results is two- to threefold for serum samples and 5- to 20-fold for whole blood samples. The UK NEQAS data (Figure 21.2) show slightly better inter-assay ranges of results for serum (twofold) and whole blood samples (two- to threefold), possibly because fewer methods are shown

TABLE 21.3
Method Comparisons CAP 2007

Serum Folate (ng/mL) Instrument	Serum Sample K-13 from 2007					Serum Sample K-11 from 2007					Serum Sample K-06 from 2007				
	No. Labs	Mean	CV (%)	Median	Range	No. Labs	Mean	CV (%)	Median	Range	No. Labs	Mean	CV (%)	Median	Range
Abbott Architect i	8	—	—	3.8	3.1–4.8	8	—	—	11.6	7.4–14.7	—	—	—	—	—
Abbott AxSYM	76	4.35	11.5	4.4	3.1–5.4	77	14.36	6.1	14.5	12.4–16.6	68	18.8	11.1	19.0	13.8–26.2
Bayer ACS:180	8	—	—	3.7	1.7–4.0	6	—	—	11.8	10.1–13.9	8	—	—	20.5	15.0–22.5
Bayer Advia Centaur	463	3.39	12.4	3.4	2.1–4.7	459	10.95	10.1	10.9	8.0–14.3	480	18.4	10.1	18.2	12.5–24.0
Bayer Advia Centaur CP	20	3.74	14.2	3.7	2.6–5.0	20	13.67	13.4	13.6	11.0–16.9	9	—	—	28.0	24.0–33.4
Beckman Access/2	349	3.00	7.0	3.0	2.4–3.6	355	11.04	5.9	11.0	9.2–12.9	350	18.6	6.8	18.7	14.1–24.2
Beckman Unicel Dxl	223	2.91	8.7	2.9	2.2–3.4	223	10.92	6.3	11.0	9.3–13.0	198	18.3	5.5	18.3	15.9–20.0
DPC Immulite 2000	132	4.15	10.1	4.2	3.1–5.4	132	12.71	9.1	12.6	10.4–16.1	131	20.6	9.9	20.5	15.2–28.9
DPC Immulite 1000	8	—	—	4.2	3.3–5.0	8	—	—	12.4	9.6–14.2	10	20.4	11.7	19.9	15.9–24.0
Roche COBAS e411/ Elecsys	76	4.84	10.2	4.8	3.7–6.0	76	11.41	6.8	11.4	8.7–13.5	44	23.2	18.6	22.1	14.4–37.0
Roche COBAS e601/ E170	121	4.12	8.6	4.1	3.2–5.1	121	10.16	6.4	10.1	8.5–11.8	105	18.0	7.0	18.0	14.3–20.3
Tosoh AIA-Pack	18	4.47	10.9	4.4	3.8–5.4	18	10.44	14.8	9.9	8.4–13.3	14	15.7	14.6	14.8	12.4–19.2
Vitros ECi, ECiQ	204	3.21	13.2	3.2	1.9–4.2	205	11.58	12.7	11.6	7.2–15.1	109	19.0	7.5	19.4	14.5–23.3
All results	1,730	3.47	19.0	3.3	1.7–6.0	1,733	11.34	12.0	11.2	7.2–16.9	1,554	18.9	11.5	18.7	12.4–37.0

continued

TABLE 21.3 (continued)
Method Comparisons CAP 2007

Red Blood Cell Folate (ng/mL)

Instrument	Whole Blood Sample FOL-02 from 2007					Whole Blood Sample FOL-05 from 2007					Whole Blood Sample FOL-01 from 2007				
	No. Labs	Mean	CV (%)	Median	Range	No. Labs	Mean	CV (%)	Median	Range	No. Labs	Mean	CV (%)	Median	Range
Abbott AxSYM	6	—	—	110	78–122	6	—	—	223	156–279	6	—	—	487	420–586
Bayer Advia Centaur	114	119	17.9	117	75–186	104	335	16.7	327	210–485	116	646	12.8	651	409–821
Beckman Access/2	29	101	15.9	104	32–131	24	289	16.0	285	165–420	29	544	13.6	565	356–719
Beckman Unicel DxI	25	108	14.7	106	84–146	26	265	12.5	274	172–298	25	573	8.9	560	488–711
DPC Immulite 2000	17	82	27.9	79	32–126	18	223	7.5	215	198–253	20	430	24.0	442	154–640
Roche COBAS e411/Elecsys	10	414	22.7	420	276–602	—	—	—	—	—	9	—	—	1211	606–1,804
Roche COBAS e601/E170	20	210	11.5	207	168–261	24	410	9.5	421	344–455	19	774	7.7	777	635–870
Vitros ECi, ECiQ	13	77	28.4	78	35–111	11	167	10.6	157	143–193	12	321	12.7	328	247–411
All results	239	130	55.9	112	32–602	223	312	26.1	304	123–546	242	613	29.6	605	154–1,804

CAP, College of American Pathologists.

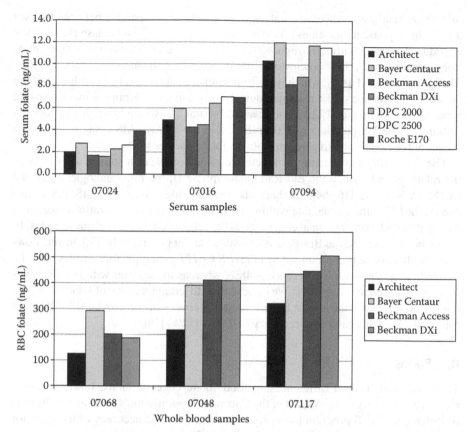

FIGURE 21.2 Serum and RBC folate results from scheme participants of the UK NEQAS 2007 Haematinics surveys using various commercial assays. The number of participants per method group was over 10, except for the Beckman DXi method for RBC folate, where the number fluctuated around 10. The method mean was not trimmed if the number of participants was 9 or fewer.

and those methods also compared more favorably in the CAP survey. Nonetheless, data from both programs indicate that there is still significant disagreement in serum and whole blood folate results generated by commercial assays.

3. Issues Related to Comparability of Data from Population Studies

Because the Bio-Rad Quantaphase II assay was used from 1991 to 2006 to generate serum and whole blood folate data for a representative part of the US population as part of National Health and Nutrition Examination Survey (NHANES), there is a lot of interest in comparing data from other studies and populations obtained with different methods with this assay [160]. Before that, an early version of the microbiological assay was used during NHANES II (1971–1975) [161], and the Bio-Rad Quantaphase I radioassay was used during the first phase of NHANES III (1988–1991) [162]. The Quantaphase I assay was initially calibrated against the microbiological assay; therefore, values were generally comparable between the two assays. In response to questions raised by Levine [163], the Quantaphase II assay was introduced in 1993 with spectrophotometrically verified PGA calibrator concentrations, resulting in a 30% downward shift in measured folate concentrations [162]. The Quantaphase II assay, which was discontinued in 2007, has been replaced by the 96-well plate version of the microbiological assay using a chloramphenicol-resistant strain of *L. rhamnosus* [122,123] to measure serum and whole blood folate concentrations for the US population (NHANES), and the LC/MS/MS assay is used on a subset of the population to generate data on folate species [9,78].

Our laboratory has recently conducted method comparison studies to determine the relationship between the Bio-Rad Quantaphase II, the microbiological, and the LC/MS/MS assays [16,164]. In short, the microbiological and LC/MS/MS assays used at the CDC are comparable within ±10%; however, the concentrations measured by the Bio-Rad assay are on average approximately 30% lower in serum samples. In whole blood samples, the Bio-Rad assay values are approximately 45% lower; however, the difference is confounded by *MTHFR* C677T genotype: for samples with the CC and CT genotype, the difference is 48%, whereas for samples with the TT genotype, the difference is only 31%. We believe that different recovery of folate forms by the Bio-Rad assay is the reason for this: under-recovery of 5-methyl-THF (51%) and 5-formyl-THF (18%) and over-recovery of THF (152%) [16].

B. Foods

There are also method differences in food folate concentrations; however, fewer reports address this issue. As part of the European Commission's Community Bureau of Reference (BCR) program to improve the reliability and accuracy of methods for the determination of vitamins in food, a first BCR intercomparison study was conducted in 1990 [165], and five subsequent intercomparison studies were completed between 1990 and 1997 [166]. The first BCR study compared folate results for lyophilized Brussels sprout material by various methods (microbiological assay, HPLC procedures, enzyme protein-binding assays, and radio-protein-binding assays) [165]. Most laboratories used the microbiological assay and obtained intralaboratory variabilities generally less than 10%; however, the interlaboratory variability was approximately 20%. The few laboratories that used HPLC had problems with resolution of folate compounds, peak identification, and calibration.

The next five BCR intercomparison studies focused on standardization of HPLC techniques [166]. Five candidate reference materials (lyophilized Brussels sprouts powder, certified reference material [CRM] 431; wholemeal flour, CRM 121; milk powder, CRM 421; lyophilized mixed vegetables, CRM 485; and lyophilized pig's liver, CRM 487) were studied, aiming to optimize the deconjugation step, the sample cleanup before HPLC analysis, and the peak identification and calibration. Recommendations were to use AA and nitrogen flushing during extraction, strong anion exchange columns for sample cleanup, and fluorescence detection for more specificity, and to determine the concentration of calibrators spectrophotometrically. The average intra- and interlaboratory variations were 6% and 15% for the determination of 5-methyl-THF by HPLC and 9% and 18% for the determination of total folate by microbiological assay.

The authors concluded that further work was needed for HPLC analysis of folate forms other than 5-methyl-THF to improve stability during extraction and sample cleanup and address interconversions between forms during deconjugation.

A recent international interlaboratory analysis of food folate evaluated three test materials (soybean flour, fish powder, and breakfast cereal) analyzed by 26 laboratories, most of which were using the microbiological assay [167]. Even though trienzyme extraction was recommended for folate extraction, only about half of the laboratories used this technique instead of single-enzyme treatment using folate conjugase. The interlaboratory variability among the 17 laboratories performing the *L. casei* microbiological assay was between 24% and 35% for the three test materials. The authors concluded that it is important to standardize the methods of folate extraction and to use reliable reference materials to obtain more comparable results for food folate analysis.

A standardized microbiological assay using trienzyme extraction is available for the determination of total folate in cereal products (AACC Method 86–47) and has been evaluated in an AACC collaborative study by 13 laboratories [136]. The interlaboratory variability ranged from 2% to 22% for 16 fortified samples and from 28% to 53% for four unfortified cereal grain samples.

C. SUMMARY

An assessment of the data from these method comparisons indicates that most progress has been made when investigators systematically study each aspect of a method. Because users of commercial assays have little to no room to evaluate potential changes, they have to rely on the manufacturers to do so. Although the comparability of assays requires improvement for measurement of both serum and whole blood folate, much more work needs to be done to standardize whole blood folate assays.

VII. STANDARDIZATION AND INTERNATIONAL REFERENCE MATERIALS

A. PHYSIOLOGICAL FLUIDS

There is no official standardization program available for folate measurements in physiological fluids. In fact, what we call "standardization" (calibrator value assignments are made based on the absolute known quantities) is often a "harmonization" of methods (calibration value assignments are made based on the values obtained by a higher-order reference method or a candidate reference method) [107]. For example, manufacturers calibrating their assays to the microbiological assay or the Bio-Rad Quantaphase II assay are examples of harmonization, a practical approach to improving comparability of results between laboratories, whereas manufacturers calibrating their assays with well-characterized primary folate standards are standardization attempts. Wilson et al. [107] nicely describe the complex difficulties in trying to standardize folate assays. Only recently have higher-order reference methods and matrix-based reference materials been developed to facilitate the establishment of a systematic standardization program.

1. Higher-Order Reference Methods

The Joint Committee for the Traceability in Laboratory Medicine (JCTLM) reviews and tracks higher-order reference methods and reference materials in the field of clinical chemistry. The JCTLM has approved CDC LC/MS/MS reference methods for the measurement of 5-methyl-THF, 5-formyl-THF, and PGA, and National Institute of Standards and Technology (NIST). LC/MS/MS reference methods for the measurement of 5-methyl-THF and PGA. A complete list of approved reference materials and reference measurement procedures is available at http://www.bimp.fr/en/committees/jc/jctlm/jctlm-db/.

2. National Institute of Standards and Technology Reference Materials

In 2005, the NIST released the first US standard reference material for serum folate, SRM 1955, "Folate and Homocysteine in Human Serum" (https://srmors.nist.gov/view_detail.cfm?srm=1955). It is a three-level material and has certified concentrations for 5-methyl-THF by LC/MS/MS, reference concentrations for PGA by LC/MS/MS, and information values for 5-formyl-THF by LC/MS/MS, as well as for total folate by LC/MS/MS microbiological assay and Bio-Rad Quantaphase II assay [69]. The commutability of this material for various assays has not yet been determined.

3. National Institute for Biological Standards and Controls Reference Materials

Also in 2006, the National Institute for Biological Standards and Controls (NIBSC) released "03/178—1st International Standard for Vitamin B12 and Serum Folate." The reference material was characterized for serum folate by LC/MS/MS for a total folate target value of 12.1 nmol/L (consisting of 9.75 nmol/L 5-methyl-THF, 1.59 nmol/L 5-formyl-THF, and 0.74 nmol/L PGA) (http://www.nibsc.ac.uk/products/cataloguefull.asp?id=03/178). Thorpe et al. [168] showed that the use of IS 03/178 to standardize serum folate assays reduced interlaboratory variability from approximately 20% to less than 10%.

An NIBSC whole blood reference material with an assigned content of 13 ng/ampoule is available (95/528—Whole Blood Folate 1st International Standard 1996). The value assignment for this reference material has been carried out by 13 laboratories using microbiological assays and radioassays against in-house standards (http://www.nibsc.ac.uk/products/cataloguefull.asp?id=95/528) [169].

B. FOODS

1. National Institute of Standards and Technology Reference Materials

There are several food reference materials available from NIST: SRM 1846 infant formula with a reference concentration for PGA of 1.29 ± 0.28 mg/kg, as well as SRM 2383 baby food composite and SRM 1546 meat homogenate, both with only an information concentration for PGA.

2. European Institute for Reference Materials and Measurement Reference Materials

The European Institute for Reference Materials and Measurements (IRMM) has several CRMs for nutrients in foods available. Three of them contain certified values for total folate: BCR-121 wholemeal flour (0.50 ± 0.07 mg/kg), BCR-485 mixed vegetables (3.15 ± 0.28 mg/kg), and BCR-487 pig's liver (13.3 ± 1.3 mg/kg) (http://irmm.jrc.ec.europa.eu/html/reference_materials_catalogue/catalogue/index.htm).

VIII. OVERALL SUMMARY

The microbiological assay is the oldest method to determine folate in biological samples, and for a period it was not used as frequently, surpassed by more user-friendly protein-binding assays and more specific and selective chromatographic assays. Usually when new methods become established and accepted, they tend to make older methods obsolete. Interestingly, for the microbiological assay this does not seem to be the case. The emergence of ID/LC/MS/MS methods has provided the folate area for the first time with higher-order reference methods. The fact that these methods show relatively good agreement with the microbiological assay reinforces the validity of the latter. The microbiological assay will not be the method of choice for highly specialized laboratories that are interested in more than total folate. However, this assay can and possibly will be the method of choice for low-resource settings.

Most clinical laboratories use protein-binding assays because these are currently the only methods that provide the high throughput coupled with a relatively low cost, and they do not require extensive technical expertise. This is not likely to change in the near future. It is hoped that manufacturers will become more engaged in standardizing their assays to reference materials that have been characterized by ID/LC/MS/MS and that more of these reference materials will become available.

HPLC-based methods can provide great detail when one is determining folate patterns in biological samples. However, because of the lack of suitable ISs, they have to be conducted with utmost care. The greatest developmental changes in recent years have been associated with MS-based methods that have contributed significantly to anchoring folate measurements, facilitating a better understanding of method differences. With increases in automation and decreases in cost, their role will continually grow.

Each method type has its own justification for specific situations. When one is monitoring trends in folate concentrations in a population over time, either the microbiological assay (low-resource settings) or ID/LC/MS/MS (specialized laboratories) is a suitable tool, whereas commercial assays are less suited because they will likely change over time. Conversely, in the clinical setting, where assay accuracy and continuity are trumped by the need for throughput and low cost, commercial assays may be the answer. Finally, in the research setting, the various types of chromatographic assays might be best suited.

ACKNOWLEDGMENTS

We thank Mary L. Paton, Surveys Technical Director, College of American Pathologists, for giving us the opportunity to present representative folate data from the 2007 Ligand survey. We also thank Sheena Blackmore, Scheme Manager, UK NEQAS, for providing us with representative folate data from their 2007 Haematinics survey. We thank Dr. Susan J. Duthie, Principal Research Scientist, Rowett Research Institute, for thoughtful discussions on the topic of folate methods and their utility.

REFERENCES

1. Gregory JF. Folacin—Chromatographic and radiometric assays. In: Augustin J, Klein BP, Becker D, Venugopal PB, eds., *Methods of Vitamin Assays*, 4th ed. New York: John Wiley & Sons, 1985:473–96.
2. Gregory JF. Chemical and nutritional aspects of folate research: Analytical procedures, methods of folate synthesis, stability, and bioavailability of dietary folates. *Adv Food Nutr Res* 1989; 33;1–101.
3. Quinlivan EP, Hanson AD, Gregory JF. The analysis of folate and its metabolic precursors in biological samples. *Anal Biochem* 2006; 348:163–84.
4. Nelson BC. The expanding role of mass spectrometry in folate research. *Curr Anal Chem* 2007; 3:219–31.
5. Selhub J. Determination of tissue folate composition by affinity chromatography followed by high-pressure ion pair liquid chromatography. *Anal Biochem* 1989; 182:84–93.
6. Bagley PJ, Selhub J. Analysis of folates using combined affinity and ion-pair chromatography. *Methods Enzymol* 1997; 281:16–25.
7. Pfeiffer CM, Gregory JF. Preparation of stable-isotopically labeled folates for in vivo investigation of folate absorption and metabolism. *Methods Enzymol* 1997; 281:106–16.
8. Freisleben A, Schieberle P, Rychlik M. Synthesis of labeled vitamers of folic acid to be used as internal standards in stable isotope dilution assays. *J Agric Food Chem* 2002; 50:4760–68.
9. Pfeiffer CM, Fazili Z, McCoy L, Zhang M, Gunter EW. Determination of folate vitamers in human serum by stable-isotope-dilution tandem mass spectrometry and comparison with radioassay and microbiologic assay. *Clin Chem* 2004; 50:423–32.
10. Gregory JF, Sartain DB, Bay BPF. Fluorometric determination of folacin in biological materials using high performance liquid chromatography. *J Nutr* 1984; 114;341–53.
11. Bagley PJ, Selhub J. Analysis of folate form distribution by affinity followed by reversed-phase chromatography with electrochemical detection. *Clin Chem* 2000; 46:404–11.
12. Bagley PJ, Selhub J. A common mutation in the methylenetetrahydrofolate reductase gene is associated with an accumulation of formylated tetrahydrofolates in red blood cells. *Proc Natl Acad Sci USA* 1998; 95:13217–20.
13. Friso S, Choi S-W, Girelli D, Mason JB, Dolnikowski GG, Bagley PJ, Olivieri O, et al. A common mutation in the 5,10-methylene-tetrahydrofolate reductase gene affects genomic DNA methylation through an interaction with folate status. *Proc Natl Acad Sci USA* 2002; 99:5606–11.
14. Smith DE, Kok RM, Teerlink T, Jakobs C, Smulders YM. Quantitative determination of erythrocyte folate vitamer distribution by liquid chromatography-tandem mass spectrometry. *Clin Chem Lab Med* 2006; 44:450–59.
15. Smulders YM, Smith DEC, Kok RK, Teerlink T, Gellekink H, Vaes WHJ, Stehouwer CD, Jakobs C. Red blood cell folate vitamer distribution in healthy subjects is determined by the methylenetetrahydrofolate reductase C677T polymorphism and by the total folate status. *J Nutr Biochem* 2007; 18:693–99.
16. Fazili Z, Pfeiffer CM, Zhang M, Jain RB, Koontz D. Influence of 5,10-methylene-tetrahydrofolate reductase polymorphism on whole-blood folate concentrations measured by LC-MS/MS, microbiologic assay, and Bio-Rad radioassay. *Clin Chem* 2008; 54:197–201.
17. Huang Y, Khartulyari S, Morales ME, Stanislawska-Sachadyn A, Von Feldt JM, Whitehead AS, Blair IA. Quantification of key red blood cell folates from subjects with defined MTHFR 677C>T genotypes using stable isotope dilution liquid chromatography/mass spectrometry. *Rapid Comm Mass Spectrom* 2008; 22:2403–12.

18. Gregory JF, Engelhardt R, Bhandari SN, Sartain DB, Gustafson SK. Adequacy of extraction techniques for determination of folate in foods and other biological materials. *J Food Comp Anal* 1990; 3:134–44.
19. Wilson SD, Horne DW. High-performance liquid chromatographic determination of the distribution of naturally occurring folic acid derivatives. In: Chytil F, McCormick DB, eds., *Methods in Enzymology*. San Diego, CA: Academic Press, 1986:269–73.
20. Lankelma J, Van der Kleijn E. Determination of 6-methyltetrahydrofolic acid in plasma and spinal fluid by high-performance liquid chromatography, using on-column concentration and electrochemical detection. *J Chromatogr* 1980; 182:35–45.
21. Holt DL, Wehling RL, Zeece MG. Determination of native folates in milk and other dairy products by high-performance liquid chromatography. *J Chromatogr* 1988; 49:271–79.
22. Leeming RJ, Pollock A, Barley C. A critical assessment of methods for measuring folate in human serum and red blood cells. In: Cortios H-C, Ghisla S, Blau U, eds., *Chemistry and Biology of Pteridines*. Berlin: Walter de Gruyter & Co., 1990:188–91.
23. Kelly P, McPartlin J, Scott J. A combined high-performance liquid chromatographic-microbiological assay for serum folic acid. *Anal Biochem* 1996; 238:179–83.
24. Sweeney MR, McPartlin J, Weir DG, Scott JM. Measurements of sub-nanomolar concentrations of unmetabolized folic acid in serum. *J Chromatogr B* 2003; 788:187–91.
25. Nelson BC, Pfeiffer CM, Margolis SA, Nelson CP. Solid-phase extraction-electrospray ionization mass spectrometry for quantification of folate in human plasma or serum. *Anal Biochem* 2004; 325:41–51.
26. Kohashi M, Inoue K. Microdetermination of folate monoglutamates in serum by liquid chromatography with electrochemical detection. *J Chromatogr* 1986; 382:303–07.
27. Hahn A, Flaig KH, Rehner G. Optimized high-performance liquid chromatographic procedure for the separation and determination of the main folacins and some derivatives. *J Chromatogr* 1991; 545:91–100.
28. Schleyer E, Reinhardt J, Unterhalt M, Hiddemann W. Highly sensitive coupled-column high-performance liquid chromatographic method for the separation and quantitation of the diastereomers of leucovorin and 5-methyltetrahydrofolate in serum and urine. *J Chromatogr B* 1995; 669:319–30.
29. Garbis SD, Melse-Boonstra A, West CE, van Breemen RB. Determination of folates in human plasma using hydrophilic interaction chromatography-tandem mass spectrometry. *Anal Chem* 2001; 73:5358–64.
30. Day BP, Gregory JF. Determination of folacin derivatives in selected foods by high performance liquid chromatography. *J Agric Food Chem* 1981; 29:374–77.
31. Gounelle J-C, Ladjimi H, Prognon P. A rapid and specific extraction procedure for folates determination in rat liver and analysis by high-performance liquid chromatography with fluorometric detection. *Anal Biochem* 1989; 176:406–11.
32. Bird OD, Robbins M, Vandenbelt JM, Pfiffner JJ. Observations on vitamin Bc conjugase from hog kidney. *J Biol Chem* 1946; 163:649–59.
33. Lakshmaiah N, Ramasastri BV. Folic acid conjugase from plasma. I. Partial purification and properties. *Int J Vitam Nutr Res* 1975; 45:183–93.
34. Mims V, Laskowski M. Studies on vitamin Bc conjugase from chicken pancreas. *J Biol Chem* 1945; 160:493–503.
35. Horne DW, Krumdieck CL, Wagner C. Properties of folic acid γ-glutamyl hydrolase (conjugase) in rat bile and plasma. *J Nutr* 1981; 111:442–49.
36. Engelhardt R, Gregory JF. Adequacy of enzymatic deconjugation in quantification of folate in foods. *J Agric Food Chem* 1990; 38:154–58.
37. Hyun TH, Tamura T. Trienzyme extraction in combination with microbiologic assay in food folate analysis: An updated review. *Exp Biol Med* 2005; 230:444–54.

38. Tamura T. Determination of food folate. *Nutr Biochem* 1998; 9:285–93.
39. Rebello T. Trace enrichment of biological folates on solid-phase adsorption cartridges and analysis by high-pressure liquid chromatography. *Anal Biochem* 1987; 166:55–64.
40. Lucock MD, Hartley R, Smithells RW. A rapid and specific HPLC-electrochemical method for the determination of endogenous 5-methyltetrahydrofolic acid in plasma using solid phase sample preparation with internal standardization. *Biomed Chromatogr* 1989; 3:58–63.
41. Priest DG, Bunni MA. A comparison of HPLC and ternary complex-based assays of tissue reduced folates. *Anal Lett* 1992; 25:219–30.
42. Etienne MC, Speziale N, Milano G. HPLC of folinic acid diastereomers and 5-methyltetrahydro-folate in plasma. *Clin Chem* 1993; 39:82–86.
43. Belz S, Frickel C, Wolfrom C, Nau H, Henze G. High-performance liquid chromatographic determination of methotrexate, 7-hydroxymethotrexate, 5-methyl-tetrahydrofolic acid and folinic acid in serum and cerebrospinal fluid. *J Chromatogr B* 1994; 661:109–18.
44. Chladek J, Sispera L, Martinkova J. High-performance liquid chromatographic assay for the determination of 5-methyltetrahydrofolate in human plasma. *J Chromatogr B* 2000; 744:307–13.
45. Opladen T, Ramaekers VT, Heimann G, Blau N. Analysis of 5-methyltetrahydrofolate in serum of healthy children. *Mol Gen Metab* 2006; 87:61–65.
46. Pawlosky RJ, Flanagan VP, Pfeiffer CM. Determination of 5-methyltetrahydrofolic acid in human serum by stable-isotope dilution high-performance liquid chromatography-mass spectrometry. *Anal Biochem* 2001; 298:299–305.
47. Nelson BC, Satterfield MB, Sniegoski LT, Welch MJ. Simultaneous quantification of homocysteine and folate in human serum or plasma using liquid chromatography/tandem mass spectrometry. *Anal Chem* 2005; 77:3586–93.
48. Stokes P, Webb K. Analysis of some folate monoglutamates by high-performance liquid chromatography-mass spectrometry. *J Chromatogr A* 1999; 864:59–67.
49. Pawlosky RJ, Flanagan VP. A quantitative stable-isotope LC-MS method for the determination of folic acid in fortified foods. *J Agric Food Chem* 2001; 49:1282–86.
50. Wigertz K, Jagerstad M. Comparison of a HPLC and radioprotein-binding assay for the determination of folates in milk and blood samples. *Food Chem* 1995; 54:429–36.
51. Vahteristo LT, Ollilainen V, Koivistoinen PE, Varo P. Improvements in the analysis of reduced folate monoglutamates and folic acid in food by high-performance liquid chromatography. *J Agric Food Chem* 1996; 44:477–82.
52. Osseyi ES, Wehling RL, Albrecht JA. Liquid chromatographic method for determining added folic acid in fortified cereal products. *J Chromatogr A* 1998; 826:235–240.
53. Doherty RB, Beecher GR. A method for the analysis of natural and synthetic folate in foods. *J Agric Food Chem* 2003; 51:354–61.
54. Rychlik M, Freisleben A. Quantification of pantothenic acid and folates by stable isotope dilution assays. *J Food Comp Anal* 2002; 15:399–409.
55. Freisleben A, Schieberle P, Rychlik M. Specific and sensitive quantification of folate vitamers in foods by stable isotope dilution assays using high-performance liquid chromatography-tandem mass spectrometry. *Anal Biochem* 2003; 376:149–56.
56. Selhub J, Ahmad O, Rosenberg IH. Preparation and use of affinity columns with bovine milk folate-binding protein (FBP) covalently linked to Sepharose 4B. *Methods Enzymol* 1980; 66:686–90.
57. Nelson BC, Pfeiffer CM, Margolis SA, Nelson CP. Affinity extraction combined with stable isotope dilution LC/MS for the determination of 5-methyltetrahydrofolate in human plasma. *Anal Biochem* 2003; 313:117–27.
58. Lyngbye J, Hansen SI, Holm J. Kinetics of folate protein binding. *Methods Enymol* 1980; 66:694–709.

59. Pfeiffer CM, Rogers LM, Gregory JF. Determination of folate in cereal-grain food products using trienzyme extraction and combined affinity and reversed-phase liquid chromatography. *J Agric Food Chem* 1997; 45:407–13.
60. Freisleben A, Schieberle P, Rychlik M. Comparison of folate quantification in foods by high-performance liquid chromatography-fluorescence detection to that by stable isotope dilution assays using high-performance liquid chromatography-tandem mass spectrometry. *Anal Biochem* 2003; 315:247–55.
61. Gregory JF, Toth JP. Chemical synthesis of deuterated folate monoglutamates and in vivo assessment of urinary excretion of deuterated folates in man. *Anal Biochem* 1988; 170:94–104.
62. Chapman SK, Greene BC, Streiff RR. A study of serum folate by high-performance ion-exchange and ion-pair partition chromatography. *J Chromatogr* 1978; 145:302–06.
63. Giulidori P, Galli-Kienle M, Stramentinoli G. Liquid-chromatographic monitoring of 5-methyltetrahydrofolate in plasma. *Clin Chem* 1981; 27:2041–43.
64. Hyland K, Surtees R. Measurement of 5-methyltetrahydrofolate in cerebrospinal fluid using HPLC with coulometric electrochemical detection. *Pteridines* 1992; 3:149–50.
65. Birmingham BK, Greene DS. Analysis of folinic acid in human serum using high-performance liquid chromatography with amperometric detection. *J Pharm Sci* 1983; 72:1306–09.
66. Hart DJ, Finglas PM, Wolfe CA, Mellon F, Wright AJ, Southon S. Determination of 5-methyltetrahydrofolate (^{13}C-labeled and unlabeled) in human plasma and urine by combined liquid chromatography mass spectrometry. *Anal Biochem* 2002; 305:206–13.
67. Kok RM, Smith DE, Dainty JR, van den Akker JT, Finglas PM, Smulders YM, Jakobs C, de Meer K. 5-Methyltetrahydrofolic acid and folic acid measured in plasma with liquid chromatography tandem mass spectrometery: Applications to folate absorption and metabolism. *Anal Biochem* 2004; 326:129–38.
68. Nelson BC, Dalluge JJ, Margolis SA. Preliminary application of liquid chromatography-electrospray-ionization mass spectrometry to the detection of 5-methyltetrahydrofolic acid monoglutamate in human plasma. *J Chromatogr B* 2001; 765:141–50.
69. Satterfield MB, Sniegoski LT, Sharpless KE, Welch MJ, Hornikova A, Zhang N-F, Pfeiffer CM, Fazili Z, Zhang M, Nelson BC. Development of a new standard reference material: SRM 1955 (homocysteine and folate in human serum). *Anal Bioanal Chem* 2006; 385:612–22.
70. Luo W, Li H, Zhang Y, Ang CY. Rapid method for the determination of total 5-methyl-tetrahydrofolate in blood by liquid chromatography with fluorescence detection. *J Chromatogr B* 2002; 766:331–37.
71. Fazili Z, Pfeiffer CM, Zhang M, Jain R. Erythrocyte folate extraction and quantitative determination by liquid chromatography-tandem mass spectrometry: Comparison of results with microbiologic assay. *Clin Chem* 2005; 51:2318–25.
72. Hoppner K, Lampi B. Reversed phase high pressure liquid chromatography of folates in human whole blood. *Nutr Rep Int* 1983; 27:911–19.
73. Lucock MD, Daskalakis I, Schorah CJ, Levene MI, Hartley R. Analysis and biochemistry of blood folate. *Biochem Mol Med* 1996; 58:93–112.
74. Pfeiffer CM, Gregory JF III. Enzymatic deconjugation of erythrocyte polyglutamyl folates during preparation for folate assay: Investigation with reversed-phase liquid chromatography. *Clin Chem* 1996; 42:1847–54.
75. Wright AJA, Finglas PM, Southon S. Erythrocyte folate analysis: A cause for concern? *Clin Chem* 1998; 44:1886–91.
76. Wright AJA, Finglas PM, Southon S. Erythrocyte folate analysis: Saponin added during lysis of whole blood can increase apparent folate concentrations depending on hemolysate pH. *Clin Chem* 2000; 46:1978–86.

77. O'Broin S, Kelleher B. Optimization of erythrocyte folate extraction. *Clin Chem* 2001; 47:2181–82.
78. Fazili Z, Pfeiffer CM. Measurement of folates in serum and conventionally prepared whole blood lysates: Application of an automated 96-well plate isotope-dilution tandem mass spectrometry method. *Clin Chem* 2004; 50:2378–81.
79. Davis SR, Quinlivan EP, Shelnutt KP, Maneval DR, Ghandour H, Capdevila A, Coats BS, et al. The methylene-tetrahydrofolate reductase 677C>T polymorphism and dietary folate restriction affect plasma one-carbon metabolites and red blood cell folate concentrations and distribution in women. *J Nutr* 2005; 135:1040–44.
80. White DR, Lee HS, Krüger RE. Reversed-phase HPLC/EC determination of folate in citrus juice by direct injection with column switching. *J Agric Food Chem* 1991; 39:714–17.
81. Wilson SD, Horne DW. High-performance liquid chromatographic determination of the distribution of naturally occurring folic acid derivatives in rat liver. *Anal Biochem* 1984; 142:529–35.
82. Konings EJM. A validated liquid chromatographic method for determining folates in vegetables, milk powder, liver, and flour. *J AOAC Int* 1999; 82:119–27.
83. Ndaw S, Bergaentzle M, Aoude-Werner D, Lahely S, Hasselmann C. Determination of folates in foods by high-performance liquid chromatography with fluorescence detection after precolumn conversion to 5-methyltetrahydrofolates. *J Chromatogr A* 2001; 928:77–90.
84. Zhang G-F, Storozhenko S, Van Der Straeten D, Lambert WE. Investigation of the extraction behavior of the main monoglutamate folates from spinach by liquid chromatography-electrospray ionization tandem mass spectrometry. *J Chromatogr A* 2005; 1078:59–66.
85. Poo-Prieto R, Haytowitz DB, Holden JM, Rogers G, Choumenkovitch SF. Use of the affinity/HPLC method for quantitative estimation of folic acid in enriched cereal-grain products. *J Nutr* 2006; 136:3079–83.
86. Varela-Moreiras G, Seyoum E, Selhub J. Combined affinity and ion pair liquid chromatographies for the analysis of folate distribution in tissues. *J Nutr Biochem* 1991; 2:44–53.
87. Vahteristo L, Ollilainen V, Varo P. HPLC determination of folate in liver and liver products. *J Food Sci* 1996; 61:524–26.
88. Vahteristo LT, Ollilainen V, Varo P. Liquid chromatographic determination of folate monoglutamates in fish, meat, eggs, and dairy products consumed in Finland. *J AOAC Intl* 1997; 80:373–78.
89. Ruggeri S, Vahteristo LT, Aguzzi A, Finglas P, Carnovale E. Determination of folate vitamers in food and in Italian reference diet by high-performance liquid chromatography. *J Chromatogr A* 1999; 855:237–45.
90. Belz S, Nau H. Determination of folate patterns in mouse plasma, erythrocytes, and embryos by HPLC coupled with a microbiological assay. *Anal Biochem* 1998; 265:157–66.
91. Rychlik M. Simultaneous analysis of folic acid and pantothenic acid in foods enriched with vitamins by stable isotope dilution assays. *Anal Chim Acta* 2003; 495:133–41.
92. Nelson BC, Sharpless KE, Sander LC. Quantitative determination of folic acid in multivitamin/multielement tablets using liquid chromatography/tandem mass spectrometry. *J Chromatogr A* 2006; 1135:203–11.
93. Ueland PM, Midttun Ø, Winderberg A, Svardal A, Skålevik R, Hustad S. Quantitative profiling of folate and one-carbon metabolism in large-scale epidemiological studies by mass spectrometry. *Clin Chem Lab Med* 2007; 45:1737–45.
94. Phillips KM, Ruggio DM, Ashraf-Khorassani M, Haytowitz DB. Difference in folate content of green and red sweet peppers (*Capsicum annuum*) determined by liquid chromatography-mass spectrometry. *J Agric Food Chem* 2006; 54:9998–10002.

95. Hannisdal R, Ueland PM, Svardal A. Liquid chromatography—tandem mass spectrometry analysis of folate and folate catabolites in human serum. *Clin Chem* 2009; 55:1147–54.

96. Thomas PM, Flanagan VP, Pawlosky RJ. Determination of 5-methyltetrahydrofolic acid and folic acid in citrus juices using stable isotope dilution-mass spectrometry. *J Agric Food Chem* 2003; 51:1293–96.

97. Pawlosky RJ, Flanagan VP, Doherty RF. A mass spectrometric validated high-performance liquid chromatography procedure for the determination of folates in foods. *J Agric Food Chem* 2003; 51:3726–30.

98. Santosh-Kumar CR, Deutsch JC, Hassell KL, Kolhouse NM, Kolhouse JF. Quantitation of red blood cell folates by stable isotope dilution gas chromatography-mass spectrometry utilizing a folate internal standard. *Anal Biochem* 1995; 225:1–9.

99. Dueker SR, Lin Y, Jones AD, Mercer R, Fabbro E, Miller JW, Green R, Clifford AJ. Determination of blood folate using acid extraction and internally standardized gas chromatography-mass spectrometry detection. *Anal Biochem* 2000; 283:266–75.

100. Lin Y, Dueker SR, Jones AD, Clifford AJ. A parallel processing solid phase extraction protocol for the determination of whole blood folate. *Anal Biochem* 2002; 301:14–20.

101. Lin Y, Dueker SR, Clifford AJ. Human whole blood folate analysis using a selected ion monitoring gas chromatography with mass selective detection protocol. *Anal Biochem* 2003; 312:255–57.

102. Owens JE, Holstege DM, Clifford AJ. Quantitation of total folate in whole blood using LC-MS/MS. *J Agric Food Chem* 2005; 53:7390–94.

103. Owens JE, Holstege DM, Clifford AJ. High-throughput method for the quantitation of total folate in whole blood using LC-MS/MS. *J Agric Food Chem* 2007; 55:3292–97.

104. Hannisdal R, Svardal A, Ueland PM. Measurement of folate in fresh and archival serum samples as *p*-aminobenzoylglutamate equivalents. *Clin Chem* 2008; 54:665–72.

105. DaCosta M, Rothenberg SP. Identification of an immunoreactive folate in serum extracts by radioimmunoassay. *Br J Haematol* 1971; 21:121.

106. Hendel J. Radioimmunoassay for pteroylglutamic acid. *Clin Chem* 1981; 27:701.

107. Wilson DH, Williams G, Herrmann R, Wiesner D, Brookhart P. Issues in immunoassay standardization: The ARCHITECT folate model for intermethod harmonization. *Clin Chem* 2005; 51:684–87.

108. Shane B, Tamura T, Stokstad ELR. Folate assay: A comparison of radioassay and micro-biological methods. *Clin Chim Acta* 1980; 100:13–19.

109. Givas JK, Gutcho S. pH dependence of the binding of folates to milk binder in radioassay of folates. *Clin Chem* 1975; 21:427.

110. Waxman S, Schreiber C. Determination of folate by use of radioactive folate and binding proteins. In: McCormick DB, Wright LD, eds., *Methods in Enzymology, vol. 66.* New York: Academic Press, 1980:468–83.

111. Blackmore S, Pfeiffer C, Hamilton MS, Lee A. Recoveries of folate species from serum pools sent to participants of the UK NEQAS Haematinics Scheme in February and March 2004. *Clin Chim Acta* 2005; 355:S459.

112. Billen J. Zaman Z, Claeys G, Blanckaert N. Limited dynamic range of a new assay for serum folate. *Clin Chem* 1999; 45:581–82.

113. Lindemans J, Van Kapel J, Abels J. Evaluation of a radioassay for serum folate and the effects of ascorbate and methotrexate. *Clin Chim Acta* 1975; 65:15–20.

114. Carmel R. Effects of antineoplastic drugs on *Lactobacillus casei* and radioisotopic assays from serum folate. *Am J Clin Pathol* 1978; 69:137–39.

115. Herbert V. Aseptic addition method for *Lactobacillus casei* assay of folate activity in human serum. *J Clin Pathol* 1966; 19:12–16.

116. Davis RE, Nicol DJ, Kelly A. An automated method for the measurement of folate activity. *J Clin Pathol* 1970; 23:47–53.
117. Scott JM, Ghanta V, Herbert V. Trouble-free microbiologic serum and red cell folate assays. *Am J Med Technol* 1974; 40:125–34.
118. Grossowicz N, Waxman S, Schreiber C. Cryoprotected *Lactobacillus casei*: An approach to standardization of microbiological assay of folic acid in serum. *Clin Chem* 1981; 27:745–47.
119. Newman EM, Tsai JF. Microbiological analysis of 5-formyletrahydrofolic acid and other folates using an automatic 96-well plate reader. *Anal Biochem* 1986; 154:509–15.
120. Horne DW, Patterson D. *Lactobacillus casei* microbiological assay of folic acid derivatives in 96-well microtiter plates. *Clin Chem* 1988; 34:2357–59.
121. Horne DW. Microbiological assay of folates in 96-well microtitre plates. *Methods Enzymol* 1997; 281:38–43.
122. O'Broin S, Kelleher B. Microbiological assay on microtitre plates of folate in serum and red cells. *J Clin Pathol* 1992; 45:344–47.
123. Molloy AM, Scott JM. Microbiological assay for serum, plasma, and red cell folate using cryopreserved, microtitre plate method. *Methods Enzymol* 1997; 281:43–53.
124. O'Broin SD, Kelleher BP, Davoren A, Gunter EW. Field-study screening of blood folate concentrations: Specimen stability and finger-stick sampling. *Am J Clin Nutr* 1997; 66:1398–405.
125. O'Broin SD, Gunter EW. Screening of folate status with use of dried blood spots on filter paper. *Am J Clin Nutr* 1999; 70:359–67.
126. Keagy PM. Microbiological and animal assays. In: Augustin J, Klein BP, Becker D, Venugopal PB, eds., *Methods of Vitamin Assays*, 4th ed. New York: John Wiley & Sons, 1985:445–71.
127. Tamura T. Microbiological assay of folates. In: Picciano MF, Stokstad ELR, Gregory JF III, eds., *Folic Acid Metabolism in Health and Disease*. New York: Wiley-Liss, 1990:121–37.
128. Bogner AL, Shane B. Bacterial folylpoly(γ-glutamate) synthase-dihydrofolate synthase. *Methods Enzymol* 1986; 122:349–59.
129. Tamura T, Shin YS, Williams MA, Stokstad ELR. *Lactobacillus casei* response to pteroylpolyglutamates. *Anal Biochem* 1972; 49:517–21.
130. Phillips DR, Wright AJA. Studies on the response of *Lactobacillus casei* to different folate monoglutamates. *Br J Nutr* 1982; 47:183–89.
131. Phillips DR, Wright AJA. Studies on the response of *Lactobacillus casei* to folate vitamin in foods. *Br J Nutr* 1983; 49:181–86.
132. Wright AJA, Phillips DR. The threshold growth response of *Lactobacillus casei* to 5-methyl-tetrahydrofolic acid: Implications for folate assays. *Br J Nutr* 1985; 53:569–73.
133. Beard MEJ, Allen DM. Effect of antimicrobial agents on the *Lactobacillus casei* folate assay. *Am J Clin Pathol* 1967; 48:401–04.
134. Cole AJL, Bate J, Gyde OHB. Rifampicin and folate and vitamin B12 assays. *BMJ* 1973; 2:53.
135. Mehta BM, Hutchison DJ. A microbiologic disc assay for 5-methyltetrahydrofolate in the presence of methotrexate. *Cancer Chemother Rep* 1977; 61:1657–63.
136. Kelleher BP, O'Broin SD. High serum folate and the calculation of red cell folate. *Clin Lab Haematol* 1995;17:204–5.
137. Philpott N, Kelleher BP, Smith OP, O'Broin SD. High serum folates and the simplification of red cell folate analysis. *Clin Lab Haematol* 2001; 23:15–20.
138. O'Broin S, Gunter E. Dried-serum spot assay for folate. *Clin Chem* 2002; 48:1128–30.
139. DeVries JW, Keagy PM, Hudson CA, Rader JI. AACC collaborative study of a method for determining total folate in cereal products—Microbiological assay using trienzyme extraction (AACC method 86-47). *Cereal Foods World* 2001; 46:216–19.

140. Tietz NW, ed. *Clinical Guide to Laboratory Tests*, 3rd ed. Philadelphia: WB Saunders, 1995.
141. Young DS. *Effects of Drugs on Clinical Laboratory Tests*, 4th ed. Washington, DC: AACC Press, 1995.
142. Young DS. *Effects of Preanalytical Variables on Clinical Laboratory Tests*, 2nd ed. Washington, DC: AACC Press, 1997.
143. O'Broin JD, Temperly IJ, Scott JM. Erythrocyte, plasma, and serum folate: Specimen stability before microbiological assay. *Clin Chem* 1980; 26:522–24.
144. Tamura T, Freebert LE, Cornwell PE. Inhibition of EDTA of growth of *Lactobacillus casei* in the folate microbiological assay and its reversal by added manganese or iron. *Clin Chem* 1990; 36:1993.
145. van Eijsden M, van der Wal MF, Hornstra G, Bonsel GJ. Can whole blood samples be stored over 24 hours without compromising stability of c-reactive protein, retinol, ferritin, folic acid, and fatty acids in epidemiologic research? *Clin Chem* 2005; 51:230–32.
146. Drammeh BS, Schleicher RL, Pfeiffer CM, Jain RB, Zhang M, Nguyen PH. Effects of delayed sample processing and freezing on serum concentrations of selected nutritional indicators. *Clin Chem* 2008; 54:1883–91.
147. Kubasik NP, Graham M, Sine HE. Storage and stability of folate and vitamin B-12 in plasma and blood samples. *Clin Chim Acta* 1979; 95:147–49.
148. Komaromy-Hiller G, Nuttall KL, Ashwood ER. Effect of storage on serum vitamin B12 and folate stability. *Ann Clin Lab Sci* 1997; 27:249–53.
149. Lawrence JM, Umekubo MA, Chiu V, Petitti DB. Split sample analysis of serum folate levels after 18 days in frozen storage. *Clin Lab* 2000; 46:483–86.
150. Kelleher B, O'Broin S. Choice of materials for long-term quality control of blood folate assays. *Clin Chem* 1996; 42:652–54.
151. Ocké MC, Schrijver J, Obermann-de Boer GL, Ploemberg BPM, Haenen GR, Dromhout D. Stability of blood (pro)vitamins during four years of storage at -20°C: Consequences for epidemiologic research. *J Clin Epidemiol* 1995; 48:1077–85.
152. Dawson DW, Fish DI, Frew IDO, Roome T, Tilston I. Laboratory diagnosis of megaloblastic anaemia: Current methods assessed by external quality assurance trials. *J Clin Pathol* 1987; 40:393–97.
153. Brown RD, Jun R, Hughes W, Watman R, Arnold B, Kronenberg H. Red cell folate assays: Some answers to current problems with radioassay variability. *Pathology* 1990; 22:82–87.
154. van den Berg H, Finglas PM, Bates C. FLAIR intercomparisons on serum and red cell foalte. *Int J Vit Nutr Res* 1994; 64:288–93.
155. Gunter EW, Bowman BA, Caudill SP, Twite DB, Adams MJ, Sampson EJ. Results of an international round robin for serum and whole-blood folate. *Clin Chem* 1996; 42:1689–94.
156. Owen WE, Roberts WL. Comparison of five automated serum and whole blood folate assays. *Am J Clin Pathol* 2003; 120:121–26.
157. Bock JL, Endres DB, Elin RJ, Wang E, Rosenzweig B, Klee GG. Comparison of fresh frozen serum to traditional proficiency testing material in a College of American Pathologists Survey for ferritin, folate, and vitamin B12. *Arch Pathol Lab Med* 2005; 129:323–27.
158. Pfeiffer CM, Gunter EW, Caudill SP. Comparison of serum and whole blood folate measurements in 12 laboratories: An international study. *Clin Chem* 2001; 47:A62 (abstract 203).
159. Clifford AJ, Noceti EM, Block-Joy A, Block T, Block G. Erythrocyte folate and its response to folic acid supplementation is assay dependent in women. *J Nutr* 2005; 135:137–43.

160. Pfeiffer CM, Johnson CL, Jain RB, Yetley EA, Picciano MF, Rader JI, Fisher KD, Mulinare J, Osterloh JD. Trends in blood folate and vitamin B12 concentrations in the United States, 1988–2004. *Am J Clin Nutr* 2007; 86:718–27.
161. Senti FR, Pilch SM. Analysis of folate data from the Second National Health and Nutrition Examination Survey (NHANES II). *J Nutr* 1985; 115:1398–402.
162. Life Sciences Research Office. *Assessment of Folate Methodology Used in the Third National Health and Nutrition Examination Survey (NHANES 1988–1994)*. Prepared for the Center for Food Safety and Applied Nutrition, Food and Drug Administration, Department of Health and Human Services. Washington, DC: US Government Printing Office, 1994.
163. Levine S. Analytical inaccuracy for folic acid with a popular commercial vitamin B12/folate kit [Letter]. *Clin Chem* 1993; 39:2209–10.
164. Fazili Z, Pfeiffer CM, Zhang M. Comparison of serum folate species analyzed by LC-MS/MS with total folate measured by microbiologic assay and Bio-Rad radioassay. *Clin Chem* 2007; 53:781–84.
165. Finglas PM, Faure U, Southgate DAT. First BCR-intercomparison on the determination of folates in food. *Food Chem* 1993; 46:199–213.
166. Finglas PM, Wigertz K, Vahteristo L, Witthoft C, Southon S, De Froidmont-Gortz I. Standardisation of HPLC techniques for the determination of naturally-occurring folates in food. *Food Chem* 1999; 64:245–55.
167. Puwastien P, Pinprapai N, Judprasong K, Tamura T. International inter-laboratory analyses of food folate. *J Food Comp Anal* 2005; 18:387–97.
168. Thorpe SJ, Sands D, Heath A, Blackmore S, Lee A, Hamilton M, O'Broin S, Nelson BC, Pfeiffer C. International standard for serum vitamin B12 and serum folate: International collaborative study to evaluate a batch of lyophilized serum for B12 and folate content. *Clin Chem Lab Med* 2007; 45:380–86.
169. Thorpe SJ, Sands D, Heath AB, Hamilton MS, Blackmore S, Barrowcliffe T. An international standard for whole blood folate: Evaluation of a lyophilized haemolysate in an international collaborative study. *Clin Chem Lab Med* 2004; 42:533–39.

Index

Page numbers followed by t indicate table; those followed by f indicate figure.

Printed in the United States
by Baker & Taylor Publisher Services

Printed in the United States
by Baker & Taylor Publisher Services